THE COMPLETE
MEDICAL
ASSISTANT

THE COMPLETE
MEDICAL ASSISTANT

Janet R. Sesser, MS, BS, RMA (AMT)
Faculty Medical Assisting on Campus and Medical Billing and Coding Online
The Allen School of Health Sciences
Phoenix, Arizona

Deborah L. Westervelt, AS, RMA (AMT)
Registered Medical Asssitant III/Clinical Supervisor
Washington University Orthopedics
St. Louis, Missouri

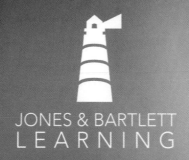

JONES & BARTLETT
LEARNING

World Headquarters
Jones & Bartlett Learning
5 Wall Street
Burlington, MA 01803
978-443-5000
info@jblearning.com
www.jblearning.com

Jones & Bartlett Learning books and products are available through most bookstores and online booksellers. To contact Jones & Bartlett Learning directly, call 800-832-0034, fax 978-443-8000, or visit our website, www.jblearning.com.

21990-6

Production Credits
VP, Product Management: Amanda Martin
Product Manager: Cathy Esperti
Product Specialist: Ashley Malone
Product Coordinator: Elena Sorrentino
Digital Project Specialist: Angela Dooley
Director of Marketing: Andrea DeFronzo
Marketing Manager: Suzy Balk
Production Services Manager: Colleen Lamy

VP, Manufacturing and Inventory Control: Therese Connell
Composition: S4Carlisle Publishing Services
Project Management: S4Carlisle Publishing Services
Cover Design: Briana Yates
Senior Media Development Editor: Faith Brosnan
Rights Specialist: Becky Damon
Printing and Binding: LSC Communications

Library of Congress Cataloging-in-Publication Data
Library of Congress Cataloging-in-Publication Data unavailable at time of printing.

LCCN: 2020936183

6048

Printed in the United States of America
24 23 22 21 20   10 9 8 7 6 5 4 3 2 1

Dedication

The authors wish to dedicate this book to the medical assistant students who decided to devote their future career to providing compassionate patient care in the delivery of health care and to the health care educators who encourage and mentor their students throughout the medical assistant program.

Reviewers

Ramona Atiles
Medical Assisting
Career Institute of Health and Technology
Brooklyn, New York

Delena Kay Austin, BTIS, CMA (AAMA)
Faculty, Medical Assistant Program
Health Science Technology, Medical Assistant
Macomb Community College
Warren, Michigan

Julie Benson, AS, RMA, RPhbt, EKG
Medical Assistant Program Coordinator
Platt College
Los Angeles, California

Suzanne Bitters-Woods
Director of Education
Harris School of Business
Cherry Hill, New Jersey

Felicia Burns
Instructor
Remington College
Garland, Texas

Ursula Backner Cole
Medical Assisting
Platt College
Los Angeles, California

Beverly Connor, AAS, CMAS, CPC
JC Medical Assistant
Metro Business College
Cape Girardeau, Missouri

Deneen Dotson, CCMA, MA
Program Director, Medical Assisting
Brookline College Tucson
Tucson, Arizona

Anna Fritz
Department Chair, Medical Assisting
South College
Knoxville, Tennessee

Todd Gervais
Clinical and Administrative Medical Assisting
San Joaquin Valley College
Visalia, California

Henry Gomez
Medical Assistant
Division of Health Disciplines
Asa College
Miami, Florida

Angela Guyott
Medical Assisting/Specialist
Metro Business College
Cape Girardeau, Missouri

Sharyn Ketcham
Medical Assisting
Phoenix College
Phoenix, Arizona

Seth Lang
Medical Assisting/Patient Care Technician
Anamarc College
El Paso, Texas

Alice Macomber
Medical Assisting Instructor
Keiser University—Port Saint Lucie Campus
Port Saint Lucie, Florida

Shannon McCoy
Academic Coordinator for the Medical Assisting Program
Virginia College
Birmingham, Alabama

Elizabeth Olson, AAMA
Certified Medical Assistant
Rasmussen College
Maitland, Florida

Valerie A. Reed
Lead Instructor, Medical Assisting
Heritage Institute of Technology
Fort Myers, Florida

Christopher Riser
Program Director, Health Sciences
Remington College
Garland, Texas

Raiza Rodriguez, PA-C
Medical Assistant
Keiser University
Fort Lauderdale, Florida

Donna Rowan
Medical Assisting/Allied Health Coordinator
Harford Community College
Bel Air, Maryland

Clifford Schmidt
Medical Assistant Program
Cerritos College
Norwalk, California

Jewel Scott, RN, RMA
Medical Assisting
Keiser University
Fort Lauderdale, Florida

Angela Senger
Medical Assisting
St. Louis College of Health Careers
Fenton, Missouri

Vivek Sharma
North-West College
Los Angeles, California

Richard St. Clare, RMA, CAHI, BSHHS, MBA
Medical Assistant/Medical Administrative Specialist/
    Phlebotomy
Seattle Vocational Institute
Seattle, Washington

Deanna Stephens, RMA
Director of Allied Health
Virginia College—Baton Rouge
Baton Rouge, Louisiana

Helen Weeks
Medical Office Assistant Program
Henry Ford Community College
Dearborn, Michigan

Marybeth Wilson, BS
Medical Specialties
College America, Denver Campus
Denver, Colorado

Saydee Wilson, AAS, BA, MBA
Medical Assisting Program Director
Associate Director of Education
Pioneer Pacific College
Portland, Oregon

Petra York
Program Director, Medical Clinical Assistant with X-Ray
    Technology
Western Tech
El Paso, Texas

About the Authors

Janet R. Sesser, a Registered Medical Assistant, holds a Master of Science in Health Education, Bachelor of Science in Health Care Management, and an Associate Degree in Medical Assisting. She is currently teaching in a Medical Assisting program as well as online instruction in Medical Billing and Coding program for a private postsecondary school in Phoenix, Arizona. Her background includes many years working as a practicing medical assistant for various types of practices and as a cardiopulmonary technician. For the past 25 years, she has worked in postsecondary education teaching and writing allied health curricula. Sesser is actively involved with American Medical Technologists, serving as an appointed member on the AMT Examinations, Qualifications, and Standards Committee. She is a recipient of the Medallion of Merit Award, the highest honor bestowed by AMT to a medical assistant, and a frequent presenter at national and state medical conferences.

Deborah L. Westervelt, a Registered Medical Assistant, holds an Associate Degree in Science. She is currently a Clinical Supervisor for an Orthopedic Physiatry practice in Chesterfield, Missouri. Her background includes many years working as a practicing medical assistant and office manager for various types of practice. Deborah worked for 20 years in postsecondary education teaching, supervising, and writing allied health curricula. Westervelt is also actively involved with American Medical Technologists, serving as a board member and co-chair of the AMT RMA Examinations, Qualifications and Standards Committee. She is a recipient of the Medallion of Merit Award and serves on the Missouri State Society as the state treasurer.

Preface

Health care is constantly evolving and expanding, developing improved, more efficient ways to deliver patient care. Science and research are finding new ways to prevent and treat disease and improve a person's well-being. The health care system depends on knowledgeable health care professionals to provide this health care. Physicians, hospitals, and other health care providers rely on versatile, multiskilled medical assistants to assist with the management of their patients.

Medical assistants need to be educated in the entry-level knowledge necessary to meet the expectation of the health care providers and to ensure patient safety during the delivery of procedures and treatments. Just as the medical field has expanded knowledge and technology, the medical assistant needs to adopt an attitude of life-long learning in order to keep pace with the anticipated changes to the future medical field landscape.

The Complete Medical Assistant textbook serves as a comprehensive collection of entry-level knowledge and skills necessary for the medical assistant to be confident to practice medical assisting under the supervision of a licensed health care provider. This first edition textbook includes the 2015 curriculum requirements set forth by the Commission on Accreditation of Allied Health Education Programs (CAAHEP). It also includes the content and skills required by the Accrediting Bureau of Health Education Schools (ABHES).

The textbook was designed with the student in mind as the primary reader and user. The level of presentation takes into account the typical entry-level medical assistant student, using a writing style that will make it easy to read and comprehend for long-term retention of information. As medical assistant students use this textbook to learn and understand the theory and concepts of the health care environment, we hope that they will appreciate and fully understand their responsibility as a health care professional to provide quality service to their health care practitioners and patients. As students progress from the classroom, to the externship experience, and then to their employment, we encourage them to adopt an attitude of lifelong learning and continuing education in health care. In their future experiences, they will encounter diversity in the workplace, with their employers, coworkers as well as their patients. With the higher incidence of global travel and relocation, it is more likely for medical assistants to participate in the treatment of conditions such as the Zika virus and victims of natural disasters. Medical assistants serve to protect us by educating, immunizing, practicing sound aseptic technique throughout the medical office, keeping up with standards, supporting certification and other indicators of competency, and remaining vigilant to the health risks of our populations.

We believe that this textbook will challenge the student but at the same time introduce the student to the essentials of becoming a complete medical assistant.

ORGANIZATION OF THE TEXT

The textbook design is a sequential progression of information divided into five sections. The chapters are intended to stand alone in content so the medical assistant program can implement them in the sequence desired. This textbook will fulfill the requirements of a certificate or diploma program and satisfy the clinical and administrative components of the associate level program. The main areas presented in each chapter are as follows.

Section I General Skills for the Medical Assistant

Chapter 1 introduces essential communication techniques the medical assistant need for effective and appropriate interaction with patients, staff, and supervisors in the workplace. Chapter 2 provides information regarding the basic legal and ethical principles for the safe and lawful practice of medical assisting. Chapter 3 information includes the medical office operations involving the computer operation of the office and the function of the intranet and Internet to support the business practice.

Section II Anatomy and Physiology

This section includes six (6) chapters that introduce the medical assistant to the anatomy of the human body and the functions of the major body systems. The information includes an overview of the organization of the body, the integumentary, skeletal, muscular, nervous, endocrine, digestive, cardiac, respiratory, urinary, and reproductive systems.

● Section III Administrative Medical Assistant Skills

Chapter 10 presents the concepts of scheduling appointments in the health care facility used to maximize the provider's effectiveness in meeting the needs of the patients. Chapter 11 provides information about the appropriate methods to document the patient's medical record and maintain HIPAA requirements. Chapters 12, 13, and 14 introduce the concepts of medical insurance coding, medical office finances, and health insurance claims processing. These chapters explore the practice methods used in medical facilities to support financial activities in the medical business and comply with policies set forth by insurance reimbursement requirements.

● Section IV Clinical Medical Assistant Skills

Chapter 15 provides critical information on practicing quality medical asepsis in the medical office. Infection control is a primary focus throughout this chapter. Chapter 16 examines the techniques of obtaining a medical history and the basic elements involved in patient assessment procedures. Chapter 17 provides essential information for the medical assistant to prepare the patient and assist the physician with a physical examination. Chapter 18 includes concepts of maintaining a surgical environment, setting up sterile trays, and assisting the physician throughout minor office surgical procedures. Chapter 19 introduces basic pharmacology math required to determine accurate dosages ordered by the physician. Injection techniques presented include intradermal, subcutaneous, and intramuscular methods of administration. Chapter 20 discusses various diagnostic tests the medical assistant will encounter in the ambulatory medical setting. Chapter 21 gives information about developing patient education materials based on the patient needs. Chapter 22 presents the key elements for recognizing and managing medical office emergencies. First aid procedures are included in the chapter as well as how to prepare for catastrophic emergencies in the community.

● Section V Clinical Laboratory

Chapter 23 describes the role of the medical assistant in the clinical laboratory. Information includes CLIA and OSHA requirements to work legally and safely within the clinical laboratory. Chapter 24 explores the components and function of the blood. The elements of the complete blood count and normal values are included. Also discussed are various types of anemia and their causes. Chapter 25 presents the practice of phlebotomy including the equipment used, patient techniques, and safety measures required. Capillary puncture techniques are introduced. Chapter 26 examines the different types of immunity and immunological testing. The antigen–antibody reaction is examined focusing on the major blood types and the importance of blood type testing.

Chapter 27 presents the purpose of the urinalysis, performance of the test including the methods of proper specimen collection. Urine drug testing and specimen chain of command are discussed. Chapter 28 discusses the purpose of performing clinical chemistry tests and the common chemistry panels ordered by the physician. The information includes how the chemicals in the body affect the function of the various systems and how the physician uses the test results to diagnose metabolic problems. Chapter 29 presents information including the use of microbiological cultures and the different types of bacteria, fungus, and viruses found in the human body. Various specimen collection methods are discussed.

FEATURES

The textbook design is user friendly and student centered. Essential elements of medical assisting presented are easy to implement into a medical assisting program. The key chapter features, where applicable, are designed to stimulate the student's learning and retention and include the following:

- Chapter objectives
- CAAHEP and ABHES competencies
- Chapter terms
- Medical abbreviations
- Icons to indicate content that is part of the cognitive, psychomotor, and affective learning domains
- Case scenarios emphasizing critical thinking
- Cultural connections to introduce students to different customs and beliefs
- Study skills for students
- Patient education
- Detailed procedures
- Externship preparation
- National certification examination preparation questions
- Electronic medical records exercises

User's Guide

This User's Guide introduces the helpful features of *The Complete Medical Assistant* that enable you to master new concepts and put your new skills into practice.

CHAPTER OPENING ELEMENTS

Each chapter begins with the following elements, to help orient you to the material:

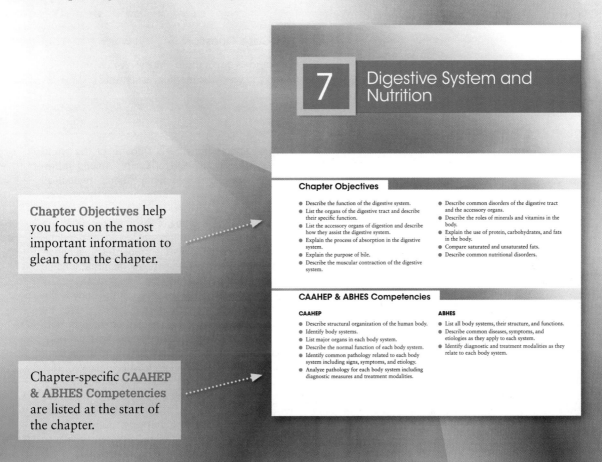

Chapter Objectives help you focus on the most important information to glean from the chapter.

Chapter-specific **CAAHEP & ABHES Competencies** are listed at the start of the chapter.

Chapter Terms and Abbreviations that are defined in the chapter are listed for quick reference.

7 Digestive System and Nutrition

Chapter Objectives

- Describe the function of the digestive system.
- List the organs of the digestive tract and describe their specific function.
- List the accessory organs of digestion and describe how they assist the digestive system.
- Explain the process of absorption in the digestive system.
- Explain the purpose of bile.
- Describe the muscular contraction of the digestive system.
- Describe common disorders of the digestive tract and the accessory organs.
- Describe the roles of minerals and vitamins in the body.
- Explain the use of protein, carbohydrates, and fats in the body.
- Compare saturated and unsaturated fats.
- Describe common nutritional disorders.

CAAHEP & ABHES Competencies

CAAHEP

- Describe structural organization of the human body.
- Identify body systems.
- List major organs in each body system.
- Describe the normal function of each body system.
- Identify common pathology related to each body system including signs, symptoms, and etiology.
- Analyze pathology for each body system including diagnostic measures and treatment modalities.

ABHES

- List all body systems, their structure, and functions.
- Describe common diseases, symptoms, and etiologies as they apply to each system.
- Identify diagnostic and treatment modalities as they relate to each body system.

134   Section II Anatomy and Physiology

Chapter Terms

Anorexia	Cirrhosis	Hepatitis	Parotitis
Appendicitis	Defecation	Ingestion	Peristalsis
Chyme	Diverticulosis	Mastication	Ulcerative colitis
Cholecystectomy	Endoscopy	Nausea	Villi
Cholelithiasis	Gastritis	Oral thrush	Vomiting

Abbreviations

BMR	HBV	IBD	LES
GERD	HCL	IBS	LDL
GI			

SPECIAL FEATURES

Unique chapter features will aid your comprehension and retention of information:

Case Study

Mary Ann Gibson is a 14-year-old and a new patient of the clinic. She recently relocated to this area with her family. When the family moved, she had to leave behind her friends that she has gone to school with since first grade. She is entering the new high school as a freshman this year. She is accompanied by her mother who is concerned that

Mary Ann is losing weight although she seems to have a good appetite and eats regularly. Mary Ann is reluctant to step on the scale to obtain her height and weight. Rosa, the medical assistant, continues to escort her to the examination room. Mary Ann asks Rosa quietly if she can see the doctor without her mother in the room.

Case Studies challenge you to think through real-world situations and are tied to Case Questions emphasizing critical thinking throughout the chapter.

Case Question

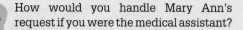 How would you handle Mary Ann's request if you were the medical assistant?

Cultural Connections introduce you to different customs and beliefs.

Cultural Connection

Asthma affects individuals throughout the world in various cultures and ethnicity. Among different cultures, there are many "home remedies" that have been passed down through generations and are still being used to alleviate symptoms of respiratory illness. Some of these preparations are herbal products that have mucolytic, anti-inflammatory, and bronchodilation properties. It is important that patients are questioned about any home treatments that they may be using as these may interact or exaggerate the effect in the body when combined with prescription medications. This information will help the physician provide the safe and appropriate medication for asthma patients. Examples of these herbs include Puerto Rican families that use chamomile and eucalyptus tea, East Indian use of Indian gooseberry and frankincense, the Chinese use of ginkgo biloba and Ma-huang (ephedra), and the European communities that use mustard, horseradish, elderberry, primrose, rose hips, and thyme. The medical assistant needs to make sure to include these home remedies in the

Study Skill

To study the digestive system build a roadmap. Use a large the mouth, and draw a highw of the digestive tract. For ea road, build a city that lists th or structure, how the struct digestion of food, and what functions. This exercise will to study from. Make it colorfu

Study Skills offer helpful tips for studying.

Ethics boxes help you learn how to respond to ethical dilemmas that might be encountered on the job.

Ethics

There are numerous cases in which physicians have lost their practice, and their freedom, due to Medicare and/or Medicaid fraud. Know what services were provided and code accordingly. If you have questions, ask. Never submit claims for procedures or services that were not provided. Protect your professional reputation. Always ask questions if you have any doubts before submitting a claim. If you witness fraud, be sure to report it to CMS, or OIG.

Patient Education boxes contain information on topics you need to know in order to help educate patients.

Patient Education

When a physician orders certain tests or procedures, they may require preauthorization the insurance company. Sometimes, this can be difficult to explain to the patient. It is important that the patient understands that even though the physician ordered the test or procedure we must follow the insurance companies guidelines. Be sure they understand that failure to obtain a preauthorization can result in the insurance company not paying for the test or procedure. MRI is one example of a test that must be preauthorized. The patient is responsible to pay for the cost of the test if the insurance company does not cover it.

Domain Icons indicate content that is part of the cognitive, psychomotor, and affective learning domains.

Detailed, step-by-step Procedures show you how to perform essential medical assisting tasks properly.

Procedure 10-1 Making Appointments for New Patients

Follow these steps when making an appointment for a new patient:

1. Obtain the patient's full name, address, day and evening phone numbers, reason for the visit, and name of who referred the patient. This information helps you determine how soon and for how long the patient will need to be seen.

2. Explain the office's payment policy. Ask the patient to bring insurance information to the office. Patients cannot be expected to make any required payments unless they are aware of the policy. You should also verify insurance to determine whether your office participates in their plan.

3. Make sure the patient knows where the office is located. Give directions if needed. This helps patients arrive on time.

4. Ask the patient if it's acceptable to call them at home or work. Some patients don't want medically related messages left on voicemail or with a coworker.

5. Double-check your appointment book or computer screen to make sure you have recorded the appointment for the correct date and time. Mistakes can cause overbooking, angry patients, and irritated physicians and staff.

6. Before hanging up, confirm the day, date, and time of the appointment with the patient. Repeating this information ensures that no mistakes or misunderstandings have occurred.

7. If another physician referred the patient, make a note to contact the referring physician's office for copies of the patient's records. This will give the physician information about the patient that he needs. It also may eliminate the need to repeat some tests.

Procedure 10-2 Making Appointments for Established Patients

Follow these steps to schedule a return appointment.

1. Find out the reason for the return visit. If a specific test is to be done, check the schedule to see when the equipment is available. This will help you offer a good date and time.

2. Offer the patient a specific date and time. If the patient doesn't agree, offer one or two other dates and times. Just asking the patient, "When would you like to return?" can create indecision in the patient.

3. Enter the patient's name and telephone contact number in the appointment book or the computer. Also, confirm their current insurance to verify that they are still with a participating plan. Having this information with the appointment makes it easier to call the patient if you have to cancel or reschedule it.

4. Place the information on an appointment card and give it to the patient. Repeat aloud to the patient the day, date, and time of the appointment as you hand over the card. This step helps the patient remember the appointment.

5. Double-check your record of the appointment to be sure you have not made an error. Appointment errors waste time for everyone, including the patient, staff, and physician.

6. End your conversation with a pleasant word and smile. Your friendliness will feel good to a patient who may be anxious about having to return to the physician.

Preparing for Externship sections offer helpful information and tips to help you prepare for your externship experience.

Chapter Recap reinforces learning by reviewing key points from the chapter.

At the end of each chapter, an **Online Resources for Students** section lists available ancillary resources on the text's online site.

Certification Preparation Questions at the end of each chapter allow for exam practice.

Electronic medical records exercises, **CareTracker Connection,** help you master content as you learn to use the Harris CareTracker software for patient scheduling, charting, coding, and billing.

Preparing for Externship

You should treat your externship as a job, but remember that you are still a student. The externship does not pay students for hours worked at the site. Some students adopt the attitude that if they are not paid they do not need to apply 100% of their effort each day. This is a negative approach to the externship. You should always strive to give your best in all you do. Think of the patients that you work with and the coworkers that rely on you. You need to be assertive asking what you can do to help everyone. Be prepared to be on your feet most of the time. Students who do not appear to be alert and busy give the perception of being lazy or uninterested. Ask a lot of good questions and be involved observing as much as you can. There is always something to do in the medical office.

Chapter Recap

- The digestive system includes the structures of the mouth, esophagus, stomach, small and large intestine, rectum, and anus.
- Accessory organs that support the digestive process include the liver, gallbladder, and pancreas.
- The digestive process requires substances to help breakdown the food into usable nutrients that can be absorbed into the bloodstream. These include saliva, hydrochloric acid, bile, and pancreatic enzymes.
- Minerals and vitamins are essential to the function of the body. Vitamins are primarily responsible for assisting in metabolism and the manufacture of red blood cells.
- Disorders and diseases of the digestive organs can affect the overall health of the body due to the inability of nutrients to get into the body cells. These include infections, organ malfunction and defects, and lack of enzyme secretion for the breakdown of nutrients for absorption.
- Protein, carbohydrates, and fats are necessary in the daily diet in order to provide the proper nutrition for healthy body cells. These nutrients are required for cell production and repair and energy for adequate functioning of the cells.

Online Resources for Students

Student Resources available on the text's online site include:
- Audio Glossaries
- Animations
- Competency Evaluation Forms
- Videos
- Anatomy & Physiology Module with Heart and Lung Sounds
- Weblinks
- Worksheets

Exercises and Activities

Certification Preparation Questions

1. Which of these is the substance produced in the stomach that breaks down protein and destroys foreign organisms?
   a. Vitamin K
   b. Chyme
   c. Hydrochloric acid
   d. Bile
   e. Pepsin

2. Which of these are the three sections of the small intestine in the order they are located?
   a. Duodenum, ileum, jejunum
   b. Ileum, sigmoid, jejunum
   c. Jejunum, duodenum, ileum
   d. Sigmoid, ileum, duodenum
   e. Duodenum, jejunum, ileum

CareTracker Connection

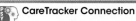 **HARRIS** CareTracker   Entering Prescriptions and Documenting Patient Medications

CareTracker Activities Related to This Chapter
- Case Study 12: Create and Print Prescriptions

NOTE: *Case Study 12 has prerequisite cases (in addition to Cases 1 to 11), which must be completed first.*
Many patients today are on multiple prescription medications. Accurately documenting a patient's

---

ADDITIONAL LEARNING RESOURCES

Valuable ancillary resources for both students and instructors are available on the text's online site. See the inside front cover for details on how to access these resources.

- Students Resources include worksheets, competency evaluation forms, audio glossaries, videos, animations, and more!
- Instructor Resources include lesson plans, image bank, slides in PowerPoint format, answer keys, CAAHEP and ABHES competencies mapping spreadsheets, and more.

Available for purchase separately:

- *Study Guide for The Complete Medical Assistant* comes with procedure skill sheets and a variety of question types to meet the needs of different learning styles and to reinforce content and knowledge.

STUDY GUIDE for
THE COMPLETE
MEDICAL
ASSISTANT

Janet R. Sesser
Deborah L. Westervelt

Acknowledgments

This adventure would not have been possible without the initial encouragement from Michael Nobel, Acquisitions Editor. He supported the concept of this textbook to provide the need to know information in a format that is easy to read, comprehend, and retain format. From start to finish of this project, Amy Millholen, Senior Product Development Editor, was there for support, encouragement, and expert advice. Her positive attitude and constant oversight kept the momentum going. Without her ability to manage and direct the production, the end resulting product would not be possible. A huge thank you to both Michael and Amy.

Also, thank you to C. Lynn Phillips Karvanek, RN, DC, for her contribution writing the test bank that accompanies this book. Her experience and knowledge teaching medical assistants and understanding of the practice of medical assisting allows her to relate to the entry-level expectations of the new graduate medical assistant.

Contents

Section V

CLINICAL LABORATORY

Section I

General Skills for the Medical Assistant

Communication Skills for Medical Assistants

Chapter Objectives

- Recognize and respond to verbal communications.
- Identify and describe six interviewing skills.
- Recognize and respond to nonverbal communications.
- Describe the skill of active listening.
- List special techniques to use when talking to children and patients who are impaired or emotionally upset.
- Summarize how to act professionally in your communications with patients and with other health care providers.
- Identify community resources.
- Explain why having a professional image in the office is important.
- List the duties of a medical office receptionist.
- Explain general office policies.

- Demonstrate telephone techniques.
- Identify the common types of incoming calls and explain how to handle each type.
- Describe how to triage incoming calls.
- Explain how to identify and handle calls that involve medical emergencies.
- Respond to and initiate written communications.
- List six key guidelines for medical writing.
- Summarize how to write a business letter.
- Name the ways written materials can be sent and explain how each method is used.
- Describe the process for handling incoming mail.
- Demonstrate proper patient education technique.
- Summarize the theories of Maslow, Erikson, and Kubler-Ross.

CAAHEP & ABHES Competencies

CAAHEP

- Identify styles and types of verbal communication.
- Identify types of nonverbal communication.
- Recognize barriers to communication.
- Identify techniques for overcoming communication barriers.
- Recognize the elements of oral communication using a sender–receiver process.

- Define coaching a patient as it relates to health maintenance, disease prevention, compliance with treatment plan, community resources, and adaptations relevant to individual patient needs.
- Recognize elements of fundamental writing skills.
- Discuss applications of electronic technology in professional communication.
- Define the principles of self-boundaries.
- Define patient navigator.

- Describe the role of the medical assistant as a patient navigator.
- Relate the following behaviors to professional communication: assertive, aggressive, and passive.
- Differentiate between adaptive and nonadaptive coping mechanisms.
- Differentiate between subjective and objective information.
- Discuss the theories of Maslow, Erikson, and Kubler-Ross.
- Discuss examples of diversity (cultural, social, and ethnic).
- Use feedback techniques to obtain patient information.
- Respond to nonverbal communication.
- Use medical terminology correctly and pronounced accurately to communicate information to providers and patients.
- Coach patients regarding office policies, health maintenance, disease prevention, and treatment plans.
- Explain cultural diversity, developmental life stage, and communication barriers.
- Demonstrate professional telephone techniques.
- Document telephone messages accurately.

- Respond to nonverbal communication.
- Compose professional correspondence utilizing electronic technology.
- Develop a current list of community resources related to patients' health care needs.
- Facilitate referrals to community resources in the role of a patient navigator.
- Report relevant information concisely and accurately.

ABHES

- Display professionalism through written and verbal communications.
- Effectively screen patients' needs by utilizing effective communication.
- Assist in accurate patient education.
- Demonstrate the ability to teach patients self-examination, disease management, and health promotion.
- Perform the essential requirements for employment such as resume writing, effective interviewing, dressing professionally, time management, and following up appropriately.
- Demonstrate professional behavior.

Chapter Terms

Adaptive mechanism	Discrimination	Nonadaptive mechanism	Referral
Aggressive	Established patient	Objective	Stat
Assertive	Feedback	Passive	Stereotyping
Bias	Grief	Patient navigator	Subjective
Clarification	Kinesics	Prejudice	Terminal disease
Communication	New patient	Proxemics	

Abbreviations

ADA	HIPAA	PMH	SH
FH			

Case Study

Susan McNeil called the office today to request an appointment and to report no improvement from her visit last week. She states that she has been getting progressively worse all week and now it hurts to breathe. Upon review of her file, you notice she was to call if not improved within 24 hours or follow up in a week if improving. Susan states she struggled to make it a week to call as directed.

Communication is the sending and receiving of information. As a medical assistant, you will need good communication skills. You'll have to share information accurately with patients, physicians, and other health care workers. As in the case with Ms. McNeil, effective communication is key to quality patient care. In this chapter, you'll learn about the various factors that can affect the accurate exchange of messages. You'll also learn techniques for communicating effectively in writing, over the telephone, and face-to-face in the medical office.

 COMMUNICATION BASICS

Most information is communicated in messages. When we hear the word *message*, we probably think of voice mail or e-mail. These are just two kinds of messages. Messages may be spoken or written or they may take some other form. When dealing with patients, physicians, and coworkers, you must be able to receive and understand the messages they are sending. You also must be able to respond to those messages appropriately. You have to know what information to share as well as when and how to provide it.

Most likely, you'll be the first person a patient meets in the office. Your attitude and communication skills will set the tone for the rest of the patient's experience.

Communication Flow

Communication requires three things:

- A message
- A person to send the message
- A person to receive the message

Figure 1-1 is a diagram showing the flow of communication between a patient and the medical assistant.

In a conversation, people swing back and forth between the roles of sender and receiver. The receiver seeks **clarification** (understanding) of the message by sending a response called **feedback.**

As a medical assistant, one of your duties will be to communicate with patients. Good communication requires the following skills:

- Clarifying—State your message in a clear and direct way. For example, you can say, "I'm going to draw

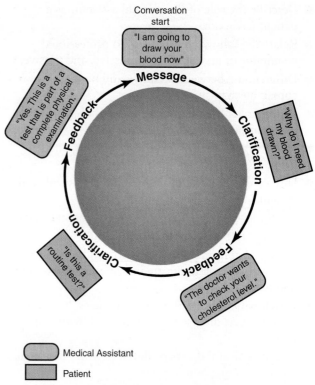

Figure 1-1   Flow of communication. (Reprinted from Kronenberger J, Ledbetter J. *Jones & Bartlett Learning's Comprehensive Medical Assisting.* 5th ed. Burlington, MA: Jones & Bartlett Learning, LLC; 2016.)

some blood now because the doctor would like to check your cholesterol level."
- Validating—Make sure your message answers the patient's questions or concerns. What if the patient asks if it is going to hurt? You might say, "You will feel a pinch when I insert the needle. I'll let you know when I'm going to do that."
- Adapting—Keep the patient's level of understanding in mind when stating a message. What if the patient asks if this is a routine test? You can answer, "Yes. This blood test is just part of a routine physical exam."
- Questioning—Ask the patient for feedback to be sure the message he received is the message you intended to send. For example, after you have drawn the blood, check in with the patient to be sure he doesn't have any questions. "We will contact you with the results of your cholesterol level. Do you have any further questions that I can answer?"

Types of Communication

The most common way of sending messages is by verbal communication. This form of communication uses language—words that are spoken or written. But not all messages involve the use of words. For example, you can often tell how a person feels about something by the expression on her face. Nonverbal communication

---

Case Questions

 Why do you think a patient would wait so long to call for an appointment if they were that ill?

Is there something the medical assistant should have done prior to the time the patient called for a follow-up appointment?

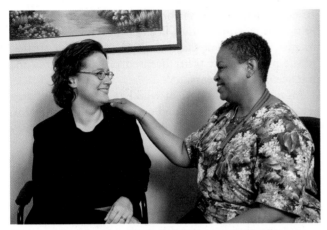

Figure 1-2 Therapeutic touch sends a message to the patient that you are caring and concerned. (Reprinted from Kronenberger J, Ledbetter J. *Jones & Bartlett Learning's Comprehensive Medical Assisting.* 5th ed. Burlington, MA: Jones & Bartlett Learning, LLC; 2016.)

is the sending and receiving of messages without using words. Much of your communication will be conversations with patients about office policies, procedures, and patient care. Figure 1-2 is a photo of a medical assistant with a patient. It demonstrates the value of therapeutic touch when talking with a patient.

Verbal Communication

Most of your communications as a medical assistant will be verbal communication. Much of that will involve oral communication—verbal communication that uses spoken words.

You'll need good oral communication skills to carry out many of your duties. You'll need to make appointments and referrals. You'll also educate patients about their conditions. And, of course, you'll be sharing information with the physician. These communication guidelines will help:

- Speak in a polite manner. A pleasant way of speaking is one sign of a professional.
- Use proper English. Bad grammar and slang expressions will give an unprofessional image.
- Don't talk down to patients.
- Avoid using medical terms a patient might not know.

For example, the medical assistant may ask the patient "Have you ever had a myocardial infarction?" and then the patient answers "No, but I've had two heart attacks."

Other kinds of oral communication can change the meaning of spoken messages. Two examples of nonverbal "speech" are paralanguage and nonlanguage sounds.

- Paralanguage includes a voice's tone, volume, and pitch. For example, someone who shouts, "I'm not angry!" at the top of his voice is sending a different

message than a person who says the same thing in a quiet tone.
- Nonlanguage sounds include sighs, sobs, laughs, grunts, and so on. Such sounds can give spoken words very different meanings. For example, someone who says, "Everything is fine!" while sobbing is sending a message that he may not feel fine at all.

Knowing how to interpret paralanguage and nonlanguage sounds can help you plan your responses to the patient.

Using language to send written messages is another type of verbal communication. The ability to write clearly and accurately is another communication skill that is important in health care work.

After treatment, a patient usually receives oral instructions first. You or the physician will explain key areas of concern. Then, the patient is generally given written instructions to take home. It's important that instructions are detailed and clear.

Nonverbal Communication

Nonverbal communication—sending messages without using words—is sometimes called body language. Body language includes several types of behavior, such as kinesics, proxemics, and touch. Nonverbal communication can show more accurately a person's true feelings and attitude than verbal communication can. You must read people's nonverbal clues in addition to what they tell you.

Kinesics is the study of body movements. These include facial expressions, gestures, and eye movements. A patient's face can show inner feelings—such as anger or fear—that conversation may not reveal. The eyes can hint at what a person may be thinking or feeling. For example, a patient whose eyes wander while you are talking may be impatient or disinterested. Or he may not understand what you're saying.

Proxemics refers to a person's "comfort zone" and how she reacts to others in the space around her. People think of the area immediately around them as "personal space." Many people prefer that this space not be invaded by strangers. For most Americans, personal space extends out about 3 feet from their bodies.

To provide care to patients, you must enter their personal space. Some people get very uncomfortable when their space is invaded. Therefore, it is important that you approach patients in a professional manner. You should explain clearly what you plan to do. Your explanation will make patients less anxious about what is going to happen. Figure 1-3 demonstrates how a medical assistant would talk with a child at their eye level.

For some patients, a kind, gentle touch can provide emotional support. But for other people, being touched by a stranger is a negative experience. It can make them very uncomfortable. Take time to explain what you will

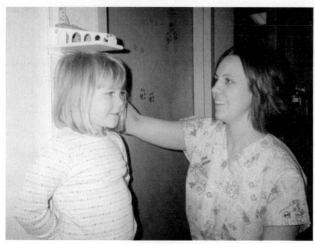

Figure 1-3   The medical assistant communicates at eye level with a child. (Reprinted from Kronenberger J, Ledbetter J. *Jones & Bartlett Learning's Comprehensive Medical Assisting*, 5th ed. Burlington, MA: Jones & Bartlett Learning, LLC; 2016.)

be doing prior to performing any task on the patient. Be in tune with your patients' feelings by observing their expressions and behaviors. Keep in mind that to some patients, a simple touch can be extremely unpleasant. Utilize your observation and communication skills to determine if a gentle, supportive touch is appropriate for your patient at that moment.

Active Listening

Active listening helps you understand the messages the patient is sending. If you do not receive and interpret a patient's messages correctly, you will not be able to provide the best care.

Active listening is a skill that must be developed. You become an active listener by following these practices:

- Give your full attention to the person who is speaking.
- Keep interruptions to a minimum.
- Pay attention to the speaker's paralanguage, body language, and other clues, in addition to what she is saying.

Interviewing Patients

As a medical assistant, it's likely that one of your duties will be taking information from patients. You'll perform this duty by interviewing the patient. You'll need to ask certain questions and interpret the patient's responses. Some information will be **subjective**, information only the patient can provide (such as description of location and degree of pain), and some will be **objective**, information gained by observation or examination.

New patient interviews cover several topics. They include the patient's past medical (**PMH**) and family history (**FH**), a brief review of body systems, and the patient's social history (**SH**) and medications. A new

patient is defined as someone who has never been seen by the physician or other licensed provider within the practice or a patient that has not been seen or treated by the physician or other licensed provider within the practice in over 3 years.

An interview of a patient who has seen the physician before—called an **established patient**—is quite different. You should take these steps when interviewing an established patient.

1. Review the patient's chart for information about health problems.
2. Make a list of questions to ask the patient to update health information about current medical problems and any changes in health.
3. Confirm with the patient that medications and treatments listed on the chart are current and accurate. Be sure to verify dosage and use of medications.
4. Ask about any allergies.

Effective interviews with new and established patients require good communication skills. Show professionalism during the interview. Begin by introducing yourself. Listen actively. Ask the appropriate questions and carefully record answers. Finally, always conduct the interview in a private area. Table 1-1 provides a list of subject areas that will be asked of a new patient in the initial interview.

Ethical Dilemma

Oftentimes, patients will bring family members or friends with them to the physician office. Sometimes, their main function is transportation, while others are there for support. Regardless, you need to consult with the patient in private prior to allowing family, friends, or guests in the room. Keep in mind information discussed in room is confidential.

Patient Education

As a medical assistant, you'll need good communication skills to teach patients about their medical conditions. Teaching can involve something as simple as explaining how often a patient should take a medication.

The communication skills involved in patient teaching include skills for active listening and interviewing. Follow these guidelines to provide effective patient education:

- Find a quiet room away from the main office flow, if possible.
- Have useful handouts or information sheets available.
- Allow enough teaching time so you're not rushed.
- Give information in a clear, organized, and to-the-point manner.
- Follow the oral teaching with written instructions.
- Allow the patient time to review the written instructions.
- Encourage the patient to ask questions.

Table 1-1	Key Subjects in a New Patient Interview
Key Subjects	**What You Need to Know**
Medical history	Any hospitalizations and dates Any surgeries and dates Any chronic problems
Female patients	Any pregnancies and complications Any miscarriages, stillbirths, or abortions (spontaneous and/or therapeutic)
Family history	Age and health of parents (if deceased, cause and age at death) Age and health of brothers and sisters Any genetic problems in family
Body system review	General questions about all body systems: cardiovascular, pulmonary, integumentary, musculo-skeletal, sensory, neurological, gastrointestinal, immune, endocrine, urological, and reproductive
Social history	Alcohol use Tobacco use Any drug use Hobbies Education Employment
Medications	Any prescription medicines (when taken and how much) Any over-the-counter medicines (when taken and how much)

- Ask the patient questions in a way that will help you determine understanding.
- Invite the patient to call the office if any other questions come to mind. Be sure to record your name and the office number on correspondence given to the patient.

Stay aware of current medical issues, discoveries, and trends, as well as useful community services that are available in your area. This knowledge will make you an even better patient educator.

Patient Education

The physician informs you that Susan McNeil will need education on the proper use of a MDI (metered-dose inhaler) and peak flow meter. You provide Susan with a sample of the MDI prescribed along with her personal peak flow meter to take home. You review all of the steps with Susan first and then watch as she attempts to execute the procedure. During her practice, you notice that she is not making a tight seal on the peak flow meter, which of course is affecting her results; you correct the issue and have her repeat the procedure. You feel confident in Susan's understanding of the procedure so you have her sign the patient education completion form. You give Susan a written copy of the procedural steps to follow for home use.

Practice instructing a fellow student on the proper use of an inhaler and peak flow meter.

Challenges to Good Communication

Sometimes, no matter how hard you try, people may not receive your message accurately. This is especially true if you use slang and clichés. A cliché is an expression that has lost its original meaning and therefore can result in misunderstanding. You should avoid the use of slang terms for the same reason.

There are some other common reasons why patients may misunderstand your message. These include:

- *You used medical terms.* Keep in mind that most patients will not understand many medical terms and abbreviations. If you use such terms in speaking to patients, be sure they understand what the terms mean.
- *The patient was distracted.* A common cause of distraction is pain. For example, teaching a patient how to use crutches is much more difficult if his ankle or knee still hurts. He will be concentrating on the pain, not on what you are saying. The same is true of patients who have just received good news. Their focus will be on calling family members and not on your conversation.
- *Environmental factors interfered.* Noise or interruptions can distort messages. For example, staff lounges or break rooms can be noisy. Keep the doors to these areas closed. Also, workers should not be vacuuming or emptying trash while patients are present.

Cultural Differences

In your medical assisting career, you'll come into contact with people from many backgrounds and cultures. Each person's culture shapes his values and beliefs. A person's background often influences the way that person views other people and situations. Understanding these differences can help you give each patient the best care.

Patients from some cultures may be offended by the personal questions asked when their medical history is taken. They may view such questions as an invasion of their privacy. In such cases, the physician may need to get involved to lessen the patient's concerns.

It might seem harmless to casually touch a patient on the arm when talking to him. Many people, however, don't like to be touched—especially by someone they don't know. There are also cultural differences that you must consider.

Cultural Connection

In Asian cultures, it is not appropriate to touch a person's head. The head is considered sacred in certain countries and should not be touched. If, this comes up during a medical procedure, you should explain yourself and make sure the patient is comfortable. Personal space can also be an issue. Most Americans feel comfortable with about 3 feet of personal space; however, this varies in different cultures. Look for nonverbal clues that show a patient's comfort level before you move in for an exam. Be sensitive to these cultural differences when you interact with patients. This reduces misunderstandings and helps avoid offending patients.

Study Skill

Practice various discussions you might have with a patient with different classmates. At first, practicing phone calls or other interactions with a classmate might seem silly or funny; however, there is much to be gained through practice. The more you practice, the more at ease you should feel with addressing different topics. Start out by practicing phone calls for appointments, then progress all the way to emergency situations. This practice will aid in understanding of how communication works and help you to develop good listening skills.

Bias and Stereotyping

As a medical assistant, you'll meet people of differing ages, races, and sexual orientations. Your values may sometimes differ greatly from a patient's values. But you should never let your values or your **bias**, opinions about something, affect your dealings with patients; to treat them differently because of their backgrounds, cultures, or personal values is **discrimination**.

Stereotyping is holding an opinion about all members of a group based on oversimplified views about some of its members. Stereotyping is a form of **prejudice**.

Bias, discrimination, stereotyping, and prejudice have no place in health care. These damaging views don't allow for patients' individual differences. They also prevent equality in the receiving of quality medical care.

As a health care professional, you have a duty to treat all people fairly and equally. The following practices will help you do this:

- Avoid letting stereotypes shape your opinions.
- Don't make value judgments about people.
- Have a professional attitude and manner.
- Guard against discrimination in your practices.

By doing these things, you send patients the message that you accept human differences. This will give them confidence that you provide quality care to all who seek it.

Language Barriers

The best communication takes place when language is used. But some people cannot speak or understand enough English for effective communication. You may need to use an interpreter in such cases. Someone on the office staff might also be able to help. In either case, be sure the interpreter accurately understands what you are saying.

It may seem logical to use an English-speaking member of the patient's family as an interpreter. However, this should only be a last resort. Family members might feel uncomfortable sharing bad news or information of a sensitive nature. Additionally, there may be information that needs to be shared with the patient that they wouldn't want the family member to know.

When choosing an interpreter, try to find someone of the same gender as the patient. Some cultures ban members of the opposite gender—even family members—from discussing personal issues about the body.

Other Communication Challenges

Many situations present special challenges for communication. Some patients may have sight or hearing problems. Patients may be young children or they may be too ill or medicated to understand. Other patients may have limited understanding due to mental or emotional conditions. Patients who are frightened or anxious may require even more special attention.

In each case, you need to evaluate the situation and the patient's ability to understand. Many times, a family member will be present who can help you. Make sure to obtain all needed information, whether that involves the patient or the family member. But never completely ignore the patient. Patients should feel they are part of the exchange, even when it requires the help of others.

For example, sharing information with a parent of a young child is appropriate. However, if you have an adult patient who has not consented (in writing) to the sharing of medical information with another person (regardless if they are related, unless it is a legal guardian, guardian ad litem, or durable medical power of attorney), you must refrain from sharing information. Information may be obtained from these sources (document as such); however, no information can be given to them.

Hearing Impaired

Patients with hearing impairments can range from partial hearing loss to complete hearing loss. Patients with complete hearing loss are usually able to communicate with sign language, interpreters, or other tools. Those with partial hearing loss can be a bigger challenge.

Communicating with all hearing-impaired patients requires sensitivity and patience. These suggestions may help:

- Touch the patient gently to gain his/her attention.
- Talk directly in front of the patient, face to face. Don't place yourself at an angle to the patient or talk with your back turned.
- Make sure you are near a bright light, so that your face is illuminated.
- Do not shout. Raising your voice will not increase the patient's understanding.
- Use pictures and other communication aids if necessary.
- Use short sentences with short words. Speak clearly. Don't exaggerate your facial movements.
- Lower the pitch of your voice. People with some kinds of partial hearing loss cannot hear high-pitched sounds.
- Use notepads and demonstrations as needed. Pictograms—flash cards that show basic medical terms—can be helpful.
- Eliminate all distractions. Nearby noises can make communication more difficult for those with partial hearing loss.

Sight Impaired

Sight impairments range from complete blindness to blurred vision. Patients who can't see lose information others gain from nonverbal communication.

Here are some ideas for communicating with sight-impaired patients:

- Identify yourself by name each time the patient comes into the office.
- Speak in a normal tone without raising your voice.
- At all times, let the patient know exactly what you'll be doing. Alert the patient before touching him or her.
- Offer the patient your arm and escort him to the examining or interview room.

- Have the patient touch the examining table, counter, chair, etc., to help him gain a mental image of the room.
- Explain the sounds of any machines to be used in the examination or procedure and what each machine does.
- Tell the patient when you are leaving the room and knock before entering.

Speech Impairments

Speech impairments can come from a number of medical conditions. One common condition is stroke. Oral surgery and cancer of the tongue or voice box also can affect a patient's ability to communicate, as can stuttering.

These suggestions will help you communicate with a patient who has impaired speech:

- Allow such patients time to gather their thoughts.
- Allow plenty of time for them to communicate.
- Don't rush conversations.
- Be aware of your own facial expressions.
- Offer a notepad to write questions.

Mental Health Conditions

Many mental disorders can damage a patient's ability to communicate. These disorders present a wide range of challenges. Some illnesses can cause the patient to have uncontrolled outbursts. Others cause the patient to be **passive**, without resistance or response, keeping the patient from communicating at all.

Communicating with patients who have moderate to severe mental disorders requires special training and practice. But many patients with mental illnesses will not offer such challenges. Most mental illnesses can be controlled with medication and other treatments.

Use these methods when communicating with patients who have mental illnesses:

- Tell the patient what to expect and when things will happen.
- Keep conversations professional and focused.
- Don't force or demand answers from patients who will not speak.
- Don't agree with a patient who asks if you are hearing voices or seeing objects that are not there.

If you feel unsafe with the patient, speak to your supervisor or the physician about your concerns.

Substance Abuse

It also can be difficult to communicate with patients who have histories of substance abuse, alcoholism, or other addictions. If they are withdrawing from addiction, they may be very upset and aggressive. When dealing with such patients, keep the following points in mind:

- Identify the reason for their visit and follow your regular assessment duties.
- Keep your communication professional.

- Avoid making any judgments about them.
- Speak in a calm voice.

Angry or Distressed Patients

Illness, long waiting times, and financial issues are among the things that can make some patients angry or upset. The key to communicating with such patients is to keep the problem from getting worse. Tell patients about waiting times, billing and insurance practices, and office policies as early as possible.

It's common for patients to get upset when they hear bad news about their health. Most patients take such news in a calm manner. But it's important to offer assistance as needed.

Provide written instructions for the patient to read later. They should include information of the diagnosis, causes of the illness, treatment choices, and phone numbers to call for more information.

Most importantly, you don't want to get defensive. Here are some suggestions to help you communicate with an angry or distressed patient:

- Be supportive.
- Be open and honest.
- Don't give the patient false reassurances.
- Don't make light of the patient's problem or concern.
- Avoid using humor and sarcasm.
- Ensure your own safety if the patient becomes aggressive or threatening.
- Speak in a low, calm voice.

Children

The levels of understanding in children vary greatly. Communication must be adjusted to each child's needs. The following general suggestions will help you.

- Children respond to eye contact on their level. Raise them to your height, or, better yet, lower yourself to theirs.
- Keep your voice low pitched and gentle.
- If you think the child doesn't understand a question, ask it in a different way.
- Keep your movements slow and visible. Tell children when you need to touch them.
- Allow a child to express fear, to cry, and so on.
- Be prepared for the child to return to an earlier stage of development during an illness. For example, a child may go back to thumb-sucking for comfort during times of stress.
- If a child doesn't want to talk, use play to ask your question and get the child's cooperation.

There are also hints for communicating effectively with adolescents. Here are some tips.

- Many adolescents resent authority. Some teenagers may not want a parent in the room during the interview. Assess the situation before including the parent.

- Never show shock or judgment when dealing with adolescents. Doing so will immediately close communication.

Grieving Patients

At times, you'll encounter patients or family members who are dealing with **grief**, or great sadness. Grieving starts when a person suffers an important loss. This might be the death of a loved one, the end of a relationship, the loss of a job, or the loss of good health or a body part.

Grieving is a complex process that usually takes place in the following stages.

1. Denial
2. Anger
3. Bargaining
4. Depression
5. Acceptance

The stages don't have to occur in this order. Some people might experience the stages in a different order. Others might skip stages in the process. Every person is different.

Each stage in the process can produce certain emotions and behaviors. In the anger stage, a patient may blame the physician or the care he received at the medical office. The depression stage can lead to unusual quietness, isolation, and increased crying. Acceptance is the last stage. The patient may say, "I am going to die." A **terminal disease** is a fatal illness that is in its final stages.

The stages of grieving can spread over many months. Each person grieves at his own pace and in his own way. There's no set time period and no right way to grieve. Some grieving patients may want to talk about their feelings. Patients with a terminal disease might want to discuss their fears of dying. They may express concern for loved ones they will leave behind.

Support grieving patients in the following ways:

- Give grieving patients the time to express themselves. Practice active listening.
- Use touch to show your understanding if the situation is appropriate.
- Provide education for patients if some of their concerns are because of a lack of understanding about their condition.
- Be familiar with local resources such as grief or other counseling services and hospice care. Your awareness allows you to suggest such services when they are ordered by the physician.

Dr. Kubler-Ross identified the stages of grief an individual experiences when dealing with death and dying of a loved one. Figure 1-4 shows the five stages of grief identified by Dr. Kubler-Ross.

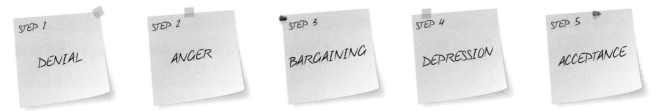

Figure 1-4 Dr. Kubler-Ross five stages of grief. (Image from Shutterstock.com.)

Professional Distance

How people act toward each other is determined by their relationships. For instance, you treat a friend differently than you would a stranger. Your dealings with patients must be at a level that allows you to carry out your duties effectively. You must not let personal relationships affect how you do that.

It's easy to get attached to patients, especially elderly patients who may be lonely. But getting personally involved with patients is not a good idea. It can damage your ability to make objective decisions about these patients and their needs. For example, don't offer to drive patients to appointments, pick up prescriptions, or do their grocery shopping. Keep your professional distance. This helps you stay objective. It also makes the care you deliver more professional and effective.

PROFESSIONAL COMMUNICATIONS

Good communication with your coworkers and employer is just as important as good communication with your patients.

Communicating with Coworkers

Conversations with coworkers must be appropriate and professional throughout the work day. Discussions that aren't related to work should be limited to break times. It's not appropriate to discuss TV shows, family problems, and so on in front of patients. Loud talking, whispering, and a lot of laughing also create an unprofessional environment.

Communicating with Physicians

Physicians depend on medical assistants for information they need to provide quality patient care. This communication always must be professional. Follow these guidelines when talking with a physician:

- Always call the physician *doctor* unless she tells you otherwise.
- Never call the physician by his or her first name in front of a patient.

- Speak confidently to earn the physician's trust and respect.
- Be honest if you don't know something. It's better to say, "I'm not sure what to do with this specimen," than to do something and make a mistake.

Addressing Patients

How you address patients sends them clues about your attitude and how you will provide care.

- A proper form of address, such as *Mrs. Smith* or *Mr. Jones*, shows respect and sets a professional tone.
- Nicknames, such as *sweetie*, *honey*, and *kiddo*, aren't appropriate in a medical setting. They can offend patients' dignity. Using nicknames also puts communication on a personal level instead of a professional one.
- Avoid identifying patients by their medical condition, such as "the broken arm in the waiting room." Patients who come to a medical office often feel anxious. This can make them very sensitive to things they see and hear. Using medical conditions instead of names can be insulting to many patients. It sends the message that staff members see them as nothing more than an illness.
- Avoid using slang in place of proper medical terms. For example, say *urine* instead of *pee*. If you're unsure of the correct term, explain the condition instead. That's better than using a term that might be incorrect.

Psychological Considerations

As a medical assistant, it is important to understand the emotional and mental needs of your patients. A basic understanding of human needs and the stages of psychosocial development will aid in your ability to effectively relate to your patients. Some patients will demonstrate **adaptive mechanisms**, the ability to learn to adjust to changes and thrive, even in the most stressful of times. Others will demonstrate **nonadaptive mechanisms**, inability to cope with changes such as increased stress, causing changes in physical and/or mental health.

Maslow's theory (Hierarchy of Needs) was developed by Abraham Maslow in 1943. Based on his research and observations, Dr. Maslow determined that psychological

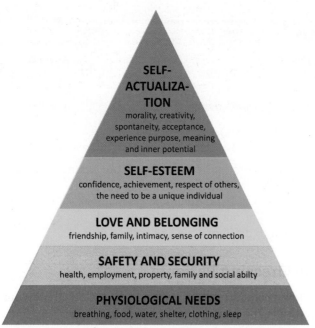

Figure 1-5   Maslow's Hierarchy of Needs. (Image from Shutterstock.com.)

development was determined by the Hierarchy of Needs. There are five levels in the Hierarchy of Needs:

1. Self-actualization
2. Esteem
3. Love/Belonging
4. Safety
5. Physiological

Figure 1-5 is a pyramid demonstrating the five levels of Maslow's Hierarchy of Needs.

Eric Erikson researched the psychosocial stages of development. Through his research, he identified the eight steps healthy individuals pass through. Based on Erikson's theory, or Erikson's Stages of Development, failure in any of the steps or stages results in confusion or conflict. Figure 1-6 shows details on ages at which different stages occur.

Communicating with Other Offices

Physicians sometimes send patients to other offices for special treatments, tests, or services. This action is called a **referral**. Physicians often depend on their medical assistants to make the arrangements. Keep these key points in mind when you make a referral:

- The patient's privacy always comes first. Make sure that you give no more medical information about the patient than the other office needs.
- Follow all legal requirements for giving the information to the new office.
- Be careful when using fax machines, e-mail, and other electronic devices. Make sure the intended receiver is the one who gets the information and use a fax sheet that identifies the information as confidential.

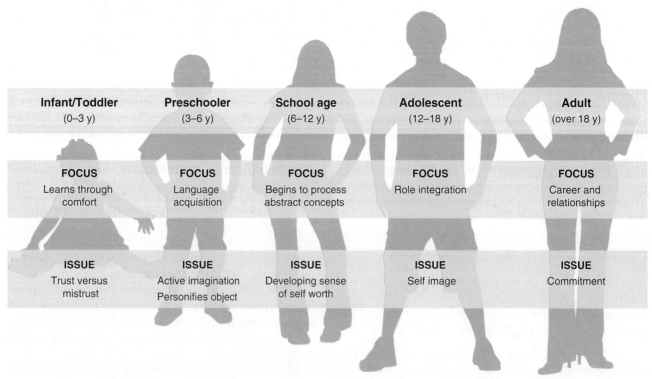

Figure 1-6   Erikson's Stages of Development. (Reprinted from Houser H, Sesser J. *JBL's Medical Assisting Exam Review for CMA, RMA & CMAS Certification*. 4th ed. Burlington, MA: Jones & Bartlett Learning, LLC; 2016.)

- Provide only facts and don't relay suspicions or assumptions about the patient.
- Don't make judgments about the information or the patient when communicating with the other office.
- Make sure the other office received the information and that it can do the referral.

Protecting Patients' Privacy

Information about patients is confidential. This means it must be kept private. To help keep patient information from being revealed accidentally, practice these behaviors in the office each and every day:

- Be careful not to speak too loudly.
- When calling coworkers over an intercom, do not reveal the patient's name or other information. For example, don't say, "Bob Smith is on the phone. He wants to know if his blood test results are back." Instead, just say, "There's a patient on line 1."
- Don't discuss patients in cafeterias, elevators, parking lots, or other public places. A patient's friends or relatives might overhear you.
- Before going home, destroy any slips of paper in your pockets that have notes about patients on them.
- If there is a window between the reception desk and the waiting area, keep it closed when not speaking to visitors.

ATTITUDE, APPEARANCE, AND IMPRESSION

As a medical assistant, you'll be the patient's main contact with the physician. In some cases, a patient may spend more time with you than with the physician. You're also likely to be the first office professional the patient meets. If your duties include working at the reception desk or answering the phone, this will always be true.

Your attitude and appearance send messages to patients as much as your verbal and nonverbal communications do. First impressions are lasting ones. The way you look and the way you interact with the patient will set the tone for the visit. It will influence how the patient views the office and the quality of care it provides.

The importance of presenting yourself to patients as a qualified and caring professional cannot be overemphasized.

- A positive view of the office helps create a good physician–patient relationship.
- Patients who feel positive about their experience are more likely to follow their treatment plan.
- Patients with a negative view of the office may choose to find another physician.
- Loss of patients will cause a loss of income for the office. A medical office is like any other business. It will not keep operating if it does not make money.

Courtesy and Diplomacy

Success as a medical assistant requires courtesy and diplomacy. Courtesy is politeness and good manners. Diplomacy is the art of dealing with people in difficult situations without offending them. Both skills are basic to good human relations.

Here are just a few ways to show courtesy and respect to coworkers.

- Before borrowing supplies, ask permission; do not use someone else's desk without permission.
- Always knock before entering a room, even if the door is open.
- Refer to physicians by their title and last name, unless they tell you otherwise.

Every day, you will deal with many different people in different circumstances. You have to remain positive and professional, even at difficult times.

Use diplomacy in touchy situations. For example, patients may want to know what's wrong with other patients. Family members may want to know what the physician told the patient. You must politely refuse to give out such information. It is confidential.

Pain, worry, and waiting can make a patient angry or unreasonable. You must use self-control and continue to act professionally. Never argue with a patient. Try to calm the patient and show your desire to help. Finally, any situation that you can't handle should be referred to the physician or office manager.

The Importance of Attitude

Your attitude is the way you feel about something. It can be either positive or negative. How you feel influences how you act. You transfer your attitude to others through your behavior. You have the power to influence a patient's attitude and behavior.

As a medical assistant, you must be able to transfer a positive attitude to patients. This requires that you view every person as someone who is worthy of care and respect. Ask yourself: "If I were in this patient's situation, how would I want to be treated?" Your positive attitude toward a patient will influence her own attitude and behavior. In this way, your actions can lead to a more positive response from the patient. Remember, you are the **patient navigator**—as such, you navigate or guide the patient through the health care system. Your main goal is to insure patients receive timely, quality care.

Case Question

 How can the medical assistant become a better patient navigator for the patient in the case study, Susan McNeil?

The Importance of Appearance

Your appearance is another factor that will influence how a patient views the medical office. Good health and good grooming present a positive image to the patient.

One way you can affect your appearance is by taking good care of yourself. Taking "good care" of yourself means:

- Eating the "right" foods (having a balanced diet)
- Exercising regularly (even walking will help)
- Getting enough sleep (but not at work, of course)

These tips will help not only your appearance but also your performance. If you are tired or sluggish, you cannot provide good patient care.

Personal Hygiene

Pay special attention to personal hygiene. People who are ill are often very sensitive to odors. Even smells that are normally pleasant can be distressing to them. A daily shower or bath is important, followed by an unscented deodorant. Do not wear perfume, cologne, or scented lotions or hair spray. Good oral hygiene is also important. During the day, avoid foods that may produce an offensive odor, such as garlic or onions.

Grooming

Keep your hair clean and styled. Fingernails must be clean and trimmed. If you wear nail polish, use only clear or neutral polish. Vivid colors are not appropriate for a medical office. Long nails also are not appropriate. If you wear makeup, keep it natural and apply it lightly.

Dress

Most offices have a dress code. Here are some general guidelines.

- Whether you wear a uniform or not, your clothes should be clean and pressed. Wrinkles, stains, missing buttons, and tears do not create a professional image.
- Your shoes should always be clean and polished.
- Women's stockings should be neutral in color and free of runs and holes.
- Women's jewelry should be plain and simple. Large rings, long chains, dangling earrings, and showy bracelets are not appropriate for the medical office. Multiple bracelets also are not appropriate jewelry for a medical setting.
- If you have pierced ears, many offices require that you wear only small stud earrings. In some offices, you can only wear one pair of earrings and you must remove any facial piercings.

- Fingernails should be less than a quarter-inch long and unpolished. The CDC strongly discourages health care workers form wearing artificial nails due to the increased chance passing infection between the provider and a patient.
- If you have any tattoos, don't be surprised if you're asked to cover them up while at work. This is standard practice for many offices.

 ## THE MEDICAL ASSISTANT AS RECEPTIONIST

Medical offices often hire a nonmedical person to serve as receptionist. The receptionist is the employee who greets patients and alerts the appropriate staff members when patients arrive. In many offices, the receptionist also answers the telephone. If you work in this kind of office, your duties may include filling in for the receptionist while he is at lunch or on break.

In some offices, you may work as a receptionist all or most of the time. These offices prefer to have a medically trained person in this role. But whichever type of office you are in, you need to know and be able to perform the duties of a receptionist.

Before the Office Opens

A receptionist's duties start before the first patient arrives. Her first duties might include:

- Unlocking the door and turning on the lights
- Turning off an alarm, if necessary
- Turning on computers, printers, copiers, and other electronic equipment
- Checking that the examination rooms have been cleaned and are stocked with needed supplies
- Checking that the reception room, bathrooms, and other public spaces are clean
- Checking for any messages on the answering machine or voice mail, on the fax machine, in e-mail, or left with the answering service overnight
- Checking that the thermostat is set to a comfortable temperature

Preparing for Patients

One of your most important duties is to gather supplies and equipment for all procedures performed during the day.

Paperwork that is manually completed and scanned into the medical record should be printed and readily available for use. For example, periodically, your office may have patients complete a new health history form to insure that all information is current. Additionally, your office may have HIPAA-based forms, which is completed periodically.

When the Office Is Open

During the medical office's business day, your main responsibilities as receptionist will include:

- Welcoming patients and visitors
- Registering and orienting patients
- Managing the reception area

Welcoming Patients and Visitors

Try to greet all patients in person and by name, if possible. A smile and cheerful greeting make the patient feel welcome. This helps create a positive image of the office for the patient. Try to recall something personal about the patient. Ask about a hobby or pet.

Sometimes, a patient will arrive while you are away from your desk. Check the reception area for new arrivals when you return. Many offices have a bell or chime on the door. Some have a sign asking patients to check in with the receptionist.

Registering and Orienting Patients

Patients who are new to the office will have to fill out a registration form, or a patient information sheet. They also must sign a privacy notice that's required by federal law.

The registration form asks the patient to provide some basic information:

- Patient's name, address, phone number, and social security number
- Name, address, and phone number of the patient's insurance company or whoever is responsible for paying the bill
- Name and address of the patient's employer
- Patient's marital status and spouse's name, if appropriate
- Name of the person who referred the patient

Many information sheets also ask about the patient's health history. Sometimes, you will complete this part of the form while interviewing the patient. Most offices have the patient fill in this information. He can ask for your help if he has any questions.

The Health Insurance Portability and Accountability Act (**HIPAA**) requires medical offices to inform patients how they handle patients' personal and health information. The patient is given this notice at the patient's first visit and is reviewed at least annually. By signing it, the patient agrees that he understands and accepts the office's privacy policies.

After the patient has completed this paperwork, briefly explain the office's general policies. When it's the patient's turn to be seen, you may also be responsible for escorting the patient to the examination room.

Reception Area Management

Another important receptionist duty is managing the reception area. This area should provide safety and comfort for patients waiting to be seen by medical staff. It should be clean and uncluttered with plenty of room for walking. Check the reception area several times a day to make sure it is clean and tidy.

Managing Waiting Time

Patients expect to be seen at their appointment time. They've taken time from their schedules to see the physician. They don't want to be kept waiting.

Be sure to tell patients if the physician is behind schedule. If you expect the wait will be more than 30 minutes from their appointment time, offer patients some choices.

- Ask the patient if he wants to reschedule her appointment for another day.
- Suggest that the patient leave the office and come back, if she wishes, at a later time that day.

The Reception Area and Contagious Diseases

It's important that patients in the reception area not exposed to others with contagious diseases. This is a greater concern in some offices than in others. Family practice physicians and pediatricians (children's physicians) often treat highly contagious diseases. If you work for a pediatrician, you'll need to learn how to look at rashes and tell if they are contagious.

Managing patients with contagious diseases requires good communication with the clinical staff. They may know if one of the day's patients has a contagious disease. If so, they should alert you.

Many infectious diseases cannot be passed by routine contact, such as shaking hands, talking, or touching. Examples of such diseases are HIV and hepatitis. Some diseases, however, are highly contagious, and patients who have those should not be left to wait in the reception area.

If a patient has one of these conditions, she should not wait in the reception area with other patients. Patients with the following conditions should be taken to an examination room at once:

- Chickenpox
- Conjunctivitis
- Influenza
- Measles and rubella
- Meningitis (and suspected cases)
- Mumps
- Pertussis
- Pneumonia (if patient is coughing)
- Smallpox
- Tuberculosis
- Wounds (if open and draining)

Other patients may have impaired immune systems. For instance, medications they are taking may lower their resistance to infection. "Germs" that would be harmless to other people can be dangerous to such patients. To reduce their risk of exposure, they also should wait in an examination room. Every office should have guidelines for handling these patients.

Case Question

How do you think this information about contagious patients in the waiting area applies to the patient in the case study, Susan McNeil?

Patients with Disabilities

Federal law requires that all public places be available to people with disabilities. A medical reception area is a place that is open to the public. The "public" in this case includes patients and their families.

The Americans with Disabilities Act (**ADA**) sets requirements for buildings so that people with disabilities can use them. Table 1-2 is a list of requirements that must be provided in public buildings to accommodate persons with disabilities. As a receptionist, you have no control over the structure of the office. But there are some things you can do to help make its public areas friendly to people with disabilities.

- Ask that all deliveries are left in a safe place. They shouldn't be left in the reception area or where they block doorways.

- Keep toys clear of pathways into and through the waiting room.
- Check that chairs aren't placed where they might block the movement of a wheelchair.
- Make sure doors are not blocked or propped open with objects.
- Check the restroom occasionally to make sure the entrance is open and not blocked.
- Limit stacks of papers on counters that might limit patients' access to you.

TELEPHONE TECHNIQUES

The telephone is the main communication tool of the medical office. You must be able to create a positive image of the office when you answer the phone. This can be more difficult than in a face-to-face conversation.

In a phone conversation, nonverbal aids such as appearance and body language cannot help. For this reason, excellent verbal skills are needed to project a caring and professional attitude over the phone. It also helps to smile when you answer the phone. This may sound silly, but you will come across sounding cheerful and professional.

Phone Courtesy

The tone and quality of your voice and speech shape the impression you send over the phone. Here are some guidelines for answering the phone in a way that is courteous and professional.

Table 1-2	Summary of ADA Requirements for Public Buildings
Area	**Requirements**
Access	Route must be at least 36 inches wide. Route must be stable, firm, and have a no-slip surface.
Ramps	Ramps must be 36 inches wide. Railings must be 34–38 inches high. Ramps longer than 6 feet must have two railings. All public levels must have ramps and elevators.
Doors	Doors must be 32 inches wide. Door handles must be no higher than 48 inches. Handles must allow doors to be opened with a closed fist. Inside doors must open without using great force.
Restrooms	Restrooms must be identified by signs that can be read by touch. Doorway must be at least 32 inches wide. Doors (including stall doors), soap dispensers, hand dryers, and faucets must be able to be operated by a closed fist. A wheelchair stall is required; it must be at least 5 × 5 feet in size.
Other	Carpeting must be no more than a half-inch high. Emergency exit system must have flashing lights and sound signals. Tables and counters must be 28–34 inches high. Space for wheelchair seating must be available.

- Answer incoming calls promptly—by the second ring, if possible. Answering calls promptly lets patients know they're important.
- Identify the office and yourself to the caller and offer assistance. This lets the caller know he has reached the correct number. For example, answer by saying, "Dr. Smith's office, Ms. Jones speaking. Can I help you?"
- Always speak politely, even if the call has interrupted your work. Do not allow your voice to show impatience or irritation.
- Never answer the phone and immediately put the caller on hold. Ask if the caller would mind holding. Courtesy requires that you wait for an answer. Also, you must find out if the call is an emergency before putting it on hold.

Handling Calls on Hold

If you cannot take a call off hold after 90 seconds, check back and ask the caller whether he wants to continue holding. Again, wait for an answer before putting the call back on hold. If the hold lasts longer than 3 minutes, apologize to the caller for the delay. Offer to call the caller back as soon as you can.

Often, you'll be on the phone and have to answer another line. Ask the person you're talking with if she would mind holding. Wait for a reply before answering the second call. Explain to the second caller that you're on another line. Tell him that you need to finish that call. Don't handle the second call while the first caller waits *unless* the second call is:

- An emergency
- A long distance call that cannot be given to another worker
- A physician calling to speak with your physician

You'll often find yourself juggling phone calls and patients in the office. Use your judgment. If the call is going to be a long one, ask the caller to wait for a moment. Take care of the office patient first. Then return to the phone call.

Incoming Calls

Several types of routine calls will come into the office each day. Patients typically call the office to:

- Make appointments
- Report health emergencies
- Seek medical advice
- Request prescription refills
- Obtain test results
- Question a bill

Be careful when talking on the phone in front of patients. Remember, all conversations with or about a patient are confidential. Labs, health insurance providers, and other physicians also will commonly call the office throughout the day.

Medical Emergencies

You must be able to tell the difference between panicked callers and true medical emergencies. First, try to calm the caller. You may need to be **assertive**, confident, and forceful, to help calm the caller. Then ask specific questions about the patient's condition. The following conditions are true phone emergencies:

- Chest pain
- Severe pain of any kind
- Difficulty breathing
- Heavy bleeding
- Loss of consciousness
- Severe vomiting
- Severe diarrhea
- Fever above 102°F

Patients with such urgent needs should be directed to the emergency room. Be sure to follow your office protocol for such occurrences. You should know how to handle such situations prior to them occurring. If a situation arises that you are uncertain how to handle, be sure to ask for assistance.

Billing Inquiries

Your duties may include handling calls with questions about fees, bills, and insurance. At times, callers will be upset with the amount of their balance and may become **aggressive**, hostile, or pushy; remain calm and professional. Other callers may want to know what the physician charges for a certain service or treatment. Don't quote prices. Instead, tell the caller that charges depend on the type of examination needed and the tests that are performed.

Additional calls may be from a patient's health insurance provider. The caller may want information about the patient. Be careful about giving out confidential patient information over the phone until you're sure of the caller's identity. Always follow HIPAA guidelines and office policy when releasing information regarding a patient's care.

Test Results

Many test results are called into the physician's office before the written report is sent. Enter the information into the EHR. Oftentimes, you are able to populate the form directly into the patient's file and then enter the results. Once results are entered, a task (electronic notice) should be sent to the physician alerting her to look at the results.

If the test was ordered **stat**, this means the results are needed right away. Record the results immediately into the EHR and send a stat task to the provider to review the results. It is also helpful to verbally inform the physician of the results so that action can be taken as soon as possible. Patients often call the office for their test results. Many physicians allow their medical assistants to give favorable test results to patients. Your office will have a policy for handling these kinds of calls. Remember, however, that you may not give test results to anyone but the patient without the patient's permission. And never take it upon yourself to give a patient test results without the physician's permission.

If a patient's test results are seriously unsatisfactory, the physician will want to discuss them with the patient.

Progress Reports

Patients may be told to call the office in a few days to report how they're feeling. If the patient says she's better, record all information in her medical record, and task the physician for review.

Hospital, home health workers, and other health care providers also may call with progress reports on a patient. For example, a home care nurse may call to say that the patient's blood pressure is now within normal limits. A physical therapist may call to report that a patient's ability to use his arm is improving. Again, record the information in the record and send a task for the physician to review. You should always bring calls that report new symptoms or seriously worsening conditions to the physician's attention immediately.

Prescription Refills

As a medical assistant, you can handle requests for refills of prescribed medicines if the chart shows that refills are permitted. If there's any doubt, tell the patient or pharmacist that you'll check with the physician and call back. There are specific categories of drugs that are not permitted by law to be refilled over the phone.

Other Routine Calls

Other kinds of calls you'll receive are:

- Requests for referrals to other physicians
- Questions from patients about the physician's instructions
- Business calls related to running the office

Ask the physician which types of calls he wants to handle immediately, which he prefers to return later, and which should be transferred to other office staff.

Calls from other physicians are generally put through at once, unless your office's policy is to handle them differently. Physicians also get personal calls. Your supervisor will tell you what kinds of calls to put through and when you should take a message.

Unidentified Callers

Sometimes, a caller who asks to speak to the physician will not give you her name. Others may not wish to tell you the reason they are calling.

You should politely tell unidentified callers that the physician is busy and that you will be happy to take a message. If the caller persists, ask him to call again at a specific time the physician is available. Then alert the physician about the time of the expected call. Most physicians will not take calls from unidentified callers as they are often times salespeople.

Angry Callers

When a caller is angry, you must be careful to not lose your own temper. Try to calm the caller and assure her that you want to help. Listen carefully and take notes. If the caller is a patient and you cannot take care of the situation, tell her that you must talk to the physician or office manager. Offer to call her back. The physician or office manager may want to speak with the patient personally. Always tell the physician about complaints regarding fees or care.

Taking Phone Messages

Taking phone messages will be a large part of your daily duties. If a message pertains to a patient, you should enter the information received and given in the EHR.

At minimum, the telephone messages should include the following information:

- The phone number where the caller can be reached
- a short description of the caller's concern

After you take a phone message, tell the caller when to expect a return call. Some physicians wait to return calls until the end of the day (except for emergencies, of course). Others return calls as they can throughout the day. Know your office's policy.

Outgoing Calls

You will be making, as well as answering, calls as a medical assistant. You should prepare carefully for your calls. Have all the information you will need in front of you before you call the number. Plan ahead of time what you are going to say.

For example, suppose the physician has an emergency and you must call a patient to reschedule his appointment. Have the scheduling program open before you make the call so that a new appointment can be offered. Be ready to explain why the physician is canceling.

Conference Calls

Your employer may ask you to set up a conference call. This is a call that puts three or more people on the line at the same time. Contact all the parties to the call in advance. This will ensure that they'll all be available at the planned time of the call. The exact procedure for making the call will depend on the kind of phone equipment your office has.

Outgoing Emergency Calls

When emergencies happen in the office, clinical staff may be busy trying to save a patient's life. They will direct you to call the local emergency medical service (EMS) to take the patient to a hospital.

Dial the EMS number. This number should be posted on every phone. Also, in most parts of the United States, you can reach EMS by dialing 911. Stay calm and speak clearly and slowly to the person who answers. Be prepared to provide:

- The patient's name, age, and gender. Age is especially important if the patient is an infant or a child. It allows the dispatcher to send the most appropriate responders.
- A brief description of the problem—for example, chest pain, the patient has stopped breathing, severe bleeding, etc.
- The level of service the physician is requesting—basic life support (BLS) or advanced life support (ALS). This also lets the dispatcher know how to respond.
- The street address of the office. Include any specific instructions for locating it. For example, "We're the Medical Office Group. Our office is on the fourth floor, third door on the left from the elevator."
- Any added information, instructions, or requests the physician asks you to provide.

After you give the information, if the dispatcher has additional questions, answer them. Ask the dispatcher when the ambulance is expected to arrive. Don't end the call until the dispatcher tells you to do so.

When you get off the phone, tell staff of EMS's estimated arrival time. Next, make sure the path through the office is clear for EMS to reach the patient. Then, reassure other patients in the reception area. If the patient has family members present, offer them reassurance and support. If an extra staff person is available, have him wait outside to flag down the EMS unit.

WRITTEN COMMUNICATIONS

Good writing skills are important to medical assisting work. You'll be responsible for either writing or producing many types of documents. These might include:

- Letters
- Memos
- Consultation reports
- Agendas for meetings
- Minutes from meetings
- Instructions to patients

Poorly written letters and other documents will reflect badly on the office and on you. They also may affect a patient's quality of care.

Writing a Business Letter

You may be asked to write various kinds of letters. These may be sent to patients, insurance companies, drug companies, various other businesses, and other health care providers. Some examples include:

- Letters welcoming new patients to the practice
- Letters to patients about their test results
- Consultation reports to other health care professionals
- Explanations of treatments to insurance companies
- Cover letters for transferring patients' records to other physicians
- Explanations to patients about charges or other billing concerns
- Thank-you letters to salespeople
- Announcements of changes in office policies or services

Follow these three steps to create a professional business letter preparing, composing, and editing. Figure 1-7 shows a computer-generated letter that has errors in it. The computer helps to identify spelling and grammar problems with documents.

Preparation

Good preparation is key when writing professional business letters. Preparation includes planning the letter's content and mechanics, as well as what the letter will look like.

Planning Content

Before you begin to write, plan your message. It may help to imagine yourself talking to the person who will receive the letter. Answering these questions also will help you prepare your message.

1. Who is my reader? Think about the reader's level of understanding. For example, letters to patients should be less technical and use fewer medical terms than letters to physicians.
2. What do I want to say, and how shall I organize my message? Briefly outline the information you want to include in the letter. Asking yourself *who, what, when, where, why*, and *how* may help you with this task.
3. What do I want the reader to do? If the reason for the letter is to ask for some action, you must tell the reader what to do. Be specific. If there's a deadline, state it. Enclosing an addressed and stamped reply envelope also may encourage the reader to act.

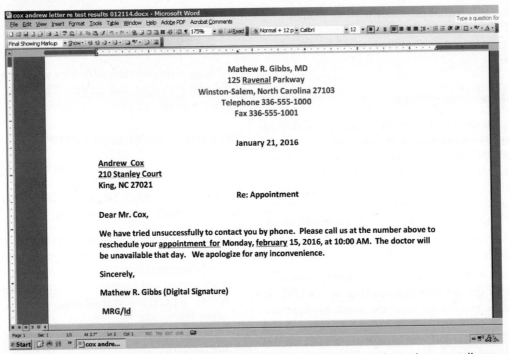

Figure 1-7 A document generated in Microsoft Word automatically underlines words or phrases noting spelling and grammar errors. A digital signature is available using the software license. (Reprinted from Kronenberger J, Ledbetter J. *Jones & Bartlett Learning's Comprehensive Medical Assisting.* 5th ed. Burlington, MA: Jones & Bartlett Learning, LLC; 2016.)

Planning Letter Mechanics

You should also plan what the letter will look like before you begin to type. This means deciding on the letter's margins, font, and template. The margin is the blank space between the type and the edge of the paper. A business letter might have margins of 1 to 1.5 inches on the left and right sides of the page. Whatever margin you choose, it should be the same on each side.

Organization of Information

There are three basic ways to organize information—or the message—in written verbal communication:

- Chronological—Discuss items in sequence; begin with the earliest date related to the information. Then go the next date, and the next, up to the most recent date. For example, this organization style could be used in writing about the physician's background for the office's brochure for new patients.
- Problem oriented—Identify the problem, explain it, and provide instructions for correcting it. A letter to a patient reporting abnormal blood test results would first state the problem—a low potassium level, for example. Then it would explain the possible causes for this problem. Finally, it would suggest treatments and follow-up procedures.
- Comparison—Evaluate two or more items of information. For instance, if asked to evaluate two computer software packages the office was considering for purchase, you would use this approach.

Composition

When you compose your letter, state your message clearly and accurately. The message should be short and to the point. Avoid wordy phrases and long sentences.

A clear message ensures that your reader knows exactly what is expected. An unclear message leaves room for doubt.

Editing

After you've typed the letter, edit it. Review your writing for errors in the information and grammar. Editing is a key step in making your letter a success.

Check the following areas:

- Accuracy of all information
- Clarity in language used
- Grammar
- Spelling
- Punctuation
- Capitalization
- Paragraphs appropriate in length
- Logical organization and flow

Make any changes that result from this review.

If possible, print out a hard copy of the letter and have a coworker edit it. He may spot errors that you missed. He also can tell you if language that seemed clear to you may not be clear to someone else. Use proofreading notations when reviewing to show areas in need of change.

The Parts of a Business Letter

A typical business letter has 11 parts. Figure 1-8 is a sample of a letter identified with these various parts of a professional business letter.

The 11 parts include:

1. Letterhead—contains the name of the physician or practice, the address, and the telephone number. It also might contain the office fax number and e-mail address. It's often in color, and it can be made part of the template itself.
2. Date—placed two to four spaces below the letter-head. Don't use abbreviations.
3. Inside Address—the name and address of the person who will be receiving the letter. Place the inside address four spaces below the date, unless a window envelope is being used. If that's the case, you may need to use different spacing to make the address visible through the window. If the letter is going to a business, insert the receiver's title as the second line, between the name and street address. The business name becomes the third line.
4. Subject line—this is an optional line. If it's used, it appears on the third line below the inside address. It begins with *Re:* (the abbreviation for "regarding") followed by the subject.
5. Salutation—the greeting that starts the letter. Place the greeting two spaces below the inside address or the subject line. Make sure it contains the title and last name of the person receiving the letter—for example, *Dear Mr. Smith* or *Dear Ms. Jones.* If the letter is to a physician, write out *Doctor—Dear Doctor Smith*, not *Dear Dr. Smith.*
6. Body—the part of the letter that contains the message. Single-space the body using a double space between paragraphs. Use letterhead only on the first page, if the body goes onto a second page.
7. Closing—concludes or closes the letter. Place the closing two spaces below the body. Capitalize only the first word. Insert a comma after the closing.
8. Signature and name—type the name and title of the person signing the letter four spaces below the closing. If you're told to sign the letter, write the physician's name, followed by a slash mark and your name.
9. Identification line—the uppercase initials tell who composed the letter. The lowercase letters tell who prepared it. Like the subject line, this element is optional.
10. Enclosure—if something is included with the letter, use the initials Enc. to indicate that. If more than one document is included, show the total number in parentheses.
11. Copy—use the letter "*c*" to show that a duplicate of the letter was sent somewhere else.

Writing a Memorandum

A memorandum, or memo, is a form of written communication used within the office. Often, memos are used for brief announcements. Memos are never sent to patients. They are less formal than letters. See Figure 1-9, which is a sample memo with the necessary formatted information.

In some ways, memos are like letters in style. But in many other ways, their style is different.

- Heading—Type the word memorandum across the top of the page.
- To—List the names of everyone who's going to receive the memo. If it's to an entire group, the group name can be typed instead of the individual names.
- From—Type the name and title of the person sending the memo.
- Date—Use the same rules as you do for letters when typing memo dates.

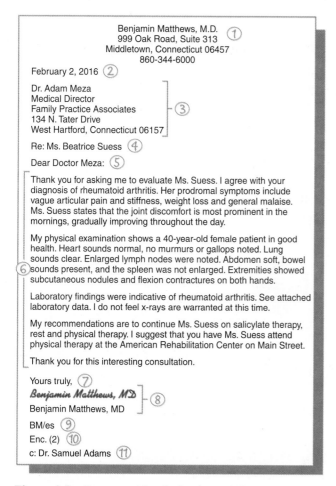

Figure 1-8 Components of a business letter in full block format contains the following elements: (1) letterhead, (2) date, (3) inside address, (4) subject line, (5) salutation, (6) body, (7) closing, (8) signature and typed name, (9) identification line, (10) enclosure, and (11) copy. (Reprinted from Kronenberger J, Ledbetter J. *Jones & Bartlett Learning's Comprehensive Medical Assisting.* 5th ed. Burlington, MA: Jones & Bartlett Learning, LLC; 2016.)

```
                              Franklin Dermatology Center
                                        123 Main Street
                                      Rockfall, Kansas
                                       913-755-2600
  Memorandum
  To:     All Medical Assistants
  From:   Patty Stricker, Office Manager
  Date:   12/03/16
  Re:     Holiday time
  ────────────────────────────────────────────────
  Please notify me by December 10 of any requests you have for
  taking time off during Christmas or New Year's. Remember that
  holiday requests will be based on seniority. The office will be
  closed at noon on December 24. The office will be closed on
  the 25th and reopen on the 26th. The office will also close on
  December 31st at noon. The office will be closed on January 1,
  reopening on the 2nd.

  If you have any questions, please e-mail me.
```

Figure 1-9 Sample memorandum (memo). (Reprinted from Kronenberger J, Ledbetter J. *Jones & Bartlett Learning's Comprehensive Medical Assisting.* 5th ed. Burlington, MA: Jones & Bartlett Learning, LLC; 2016.)

- Subject—Type a brief phase describing the purpose of the memo.
- The abbreviation Re:—Is sometimes used in place of Subject.
- Body—Insert the message of the memo.
- Copy—Use the same rules as you do for letters.

Memos don't use salutations and closings. Writing a memo requires the same preparation, composition, and editing steps that letters do. Your computer software should have a memos template as well.

Guidelines for Medical Writing

Writing letters to medical professionals is similar to writing business letters. Some additional guidelines apply including appropriate medical terms, symbols, and numbers.

Accuracy

Medical writing requires even more accuracy and clarity than writing business letters does. Pay careful attention to detail when you write medical letters and documents. Some of your letters are filed in patients' permanent medical records. Mistakes here could cause injury or death, lawsuits, and harm to the physician's practice.

When the physician asks you to draft a letter about a patient, he/she may or may not give you notes to follow. Either way, your duty in typing the letter is to be as accurate as possible. You should question anything you're not sure about.

Spelling

The spell-check feature in word processing programs can be a great help. But it has limitations. For instance, it will not find mistakes in which words are spelled correctly but are misused. Here's an example:

- "The patient's mucus was yellow."
- "The patient's mucous was yellow."

Mucus is a sticky secretion. Mucous is a membrane that secretes mucus. Both words are spelled correctly. The spell check will not flag either as an error but the second sentence is wrong.

Also, be careful about plural forms of words. Making many medical terms plural can be tricky. For example, the plural of *bulla* (a blister) is not *bullas*. It is *bullae*.

Capitalization

Pay special attention to how words and abbreviations are capitalized. Never change how a word is capitalized unless you are told to do so. If you question a capitalization, mark a hard copy of the typed document with a question mark for the physician to answer.

Some common medical terms with unusual capitalizations are pH, RhoGam, rPA, ReoPro, and aVR.

Abbreviations and Symbols

Using abbreviations and symbols saves time in writing notes by hand. When typing medical information, however, spell out all abbreviations that are not part of everyday English. For example, PM is commonly understood as an indicator of time. But NPO (meaning *nothing by mouth*) is not. Be familiar with the abbreviations and symbols that are used where you work. Most offices have a list of their approved ones.

Box 1-1 lists many medical terms that are either misspelled or misused.

Box 1-1 | **Commonly Misspelled or Misused Medical Terms**

Here are some common medical words than can be misspelled and misused easily:

- Anoxia and anorexia
- Aphagia and aphasia
- Bowl and bowel
- Emphysema and empyema
- Fundus and fungus
- Lactose and lactase
- Metatarsals and metacarpals
- Mucus and mucous
- Parental and parenteral
- Postnatal and postnasal
- Pubic and pubis
- Rubella and rubeola
- Serum and sebum
- Uvula and vulva

Be careful when interpreting what abbreviations and symbols mean. Here are some examples of what can go wrong:

- The physician wrote "The patient had good BS." You assumed that BS meant bowel sounds. So you typed, "The patient had good bowel sounds." But what the physician meant by BS was *breath sounds*.
- Do not change < or > signs to *less than* or *greater than* unless you are sure what the symbol means. If the statement means, "Her hemoglobin is less than 13," and you mistakenly type, "Her hemoglobin is greater than 13," a treatment error could occur.
- The symbols for male (♂) and female (♀) are commonly used and understood. But you should replace them with words when writing a medical or business letter.

Numbers

Numbers 1 to 10 should usually be spelled out in medical and business writing. There are exceptions, however.

- Units of measurement are always written as numbers, no matter how small—for example, 5 mg.
- Numbers referring to an obstetrical patient's condition are not spelled out. "The patient is gravida 3, para 2." Don't convert these numbers to words.

Be careful about placement of decimal points. There's a huge difference in dose between 1.25 and 12.5 mg of medication. Also, make sure you don't switch the order of numbers when you type them. Double-check for this very important kind of error.

SENDING WRITTEN COMMUNICATIONS

Once a document has been typed, edited, and signed (a letter), the next step is sending it. Most routine business letters are delivered by the United States Postal Service (USPS) through regular US mail. Other means of sending documents are also available.

- Overnight delivery by express mail—USPS offers this option as well as private delivery services such as FedEx and UPS.
- Immediate delivery by electronic mail (e-mail) or fax— These methods have drawbacks, however, despite their ease and speed. These limitations are discussed later.

There are two key things to remember when sending any written communication:

- Make every attempt to ensure that confidential material is kept confidential. Mark the outside of such envelopes "confidential." This applies to all correspondence that contains information about a patient.

- Send letters only to known addresses. Include a return address on all mail, so that it can be returned if the person is no longer at that address.

Using US Mail

When written communications are sent by regular mail, USPS guidelines should be followed to prevent errors or delays in delivery.

Addressing Envelopes

Number 10 business envelopes are used to mail most letters. Medical records, multipage test results, and some other reports and documents may be sent in larger, 9- × 12-inch mailing envelopes. Figure 1-10 is an example of an appropriately addressed No. 10 envelope with return address and recipient address.

The USPS expects the delivery address to be placed in the center portion of the envelope. The equipment USPS uses to scan the envelope for address information does not recognize writing at its edges. Addresses on large envelopes can be printed on labels and then attached to the envelope. Addresses on business envelopes will usually be printed on the envelope itself.

On a No. 10 business envelope, type the address 12 spaces down from the top, centered on the face of the envelope. Single-space the address. Provide a line each for the addressee's name, name of the business (if any), street address, and the city and state. If you abbreviate the state name, use only the official USPS abbreviation.

The five-digit zip code must appear at the end of the line for city and state. You should include the four-digit expanded zip code whenever possible. Your computer software also may let you include a USPS PostNet bar code. This is generally inserted two or three lines below the address. This bar code will speed USPS handling of the envelope.

Place the return address in the upper left corner of the envelope. It should not exceed five lines, and it is also single-spaced. Many medical offices will have their return address preprinted on their envelopes. Place

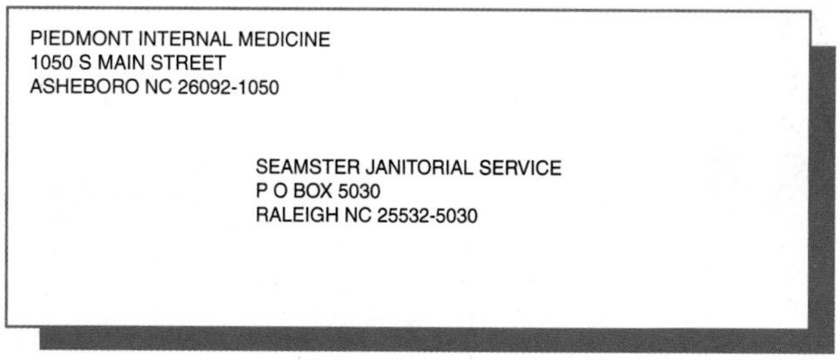

PIEDMONT INTERNAL MEDICINE
1050 S MAIN STREET
ASHEBORO NC 26092-1050

SEAMSTER JANITORIAL SERVICE
P O BOX 5030
RALEIGH NC 25532-5030

Figure 1-10 Sample No. 10 Envelope demonstrates position of mailing address and return address. (Reprinted from Kronenberger J, Ledbetter J. *Jones & Bartlett Learning's Comprehensive Medical Assisting.* 5th ed. Burlington, MA: Jones & Bartlett Learning, LLC; 2016.)

special notations such as "personal" or "confidential" two lines below the return address.

Special Services

Sometimes, it's necessary for the office to have proof that a letter was sent. For example, the physician might decide to end his/her relationship with a patient. This requires that the patient be notified and proof of delivery should be scanned into the patient's record. Proof of delivery is available from USPS by sending the letter by certified mail. This type of mailing requires an extra fee. Private express-delivery companies such as FedEx and UPS also offer tracking services that prove a letter was delivered. Figure 1-11 is a sample of a delivery notice used to identify the sender and recipient. Many companies use an electronic tablet and can e-mail verification to the sender. The device is also used as a tracking mechanism.

Faxing Documents

Facsimile machines (commonly called *fax machines*) allow you to send and receive printed materials over a phone or Internet line. They're an easy and cheap way of sending records, physician's orders, test results, and other documents that must be received quickly.

When you send documents through a fax machine, include a cover sheet with them. The cover sheet is always the first page to be faxed. Most offices have a supply of printed cover sheets that you fill in for each fax. The cover sheet should contain the following information:

- Name, address, telephone, and fax number of the office
- Name of the person the fax is intended for
- Telephone number of the receiver's fax machine

- Date and time of the fax
- Number of pages being sent (count the cover sheet too)
- Confidentiality statement

Figure 1-12 is a sample of a fax cover sheet used as the first sheet sent through the fax machine. It includes the information required to identify the fax message.

The confidentiality statement located at the bottom of the fax cover sheet is necessary because the faxed information may be private. Patient test results, for example, are confidential and often are sent by fax. For legal purposes, a statement such as this one must appear on the cover sheet:

This sheet and any documents accompanying it are confidential. They are intended only for use by the person or entity named above. If you are not the intended recipient of these documents, you are hereby notified that any disclosure, copying, or distribution of this information is strictly prohibited. Notify the sender immediately by telephone.

Lack of confidentiality is one drawback of sending written communications by fax machine. You can't

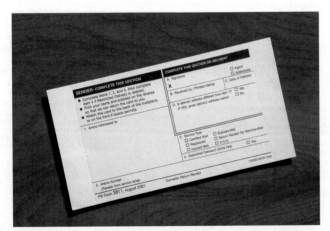

Figure 1-11 Return receipt proving recipient received the delivered document. (Reprinted from Kronenberger J, Ledbetter J. *Jones & Bartlett Learning's Comprehensive Medical Assisting*. 5th ed. Burlington, MA: Jones & Bartlett Learning, LLC; 2016.)

Cardiology Associates
Maria Sefferin, MD
897 Bayou Drive
Philadelphia, PA
215-112-9999

facsimile transmittal

To:	Fax:
From:	Date:
Re:	Pages:
CC:	

☐ Urgent ☐ For Review ☐ Please Comment ☐ Please Reply ☐ Please Recycle

Comments:

CONFIDENTIAL INFORMATION

The information in the facsimile message and any accompanying documents is confidential. This information is intended only for use by the individual or entity name above. If you are not the intended recipient of this information you are hereby notified that any disclosure, copying or distribution of this information is strictly prohibited. Please notify the sender immediately by telephone.

Figure 1-12 Sample fax cover sheet. (Reprinted from Kronenberger J, Ledbetter J. *Jones & Bartlett Learning's Comprehensive Medical Assisting*. 5th ed. Burlington, MA: Jones & Bartlett Learning, LLC; 2016.)

know for sure that it's the addressee who will actually pick up the fax at the other end.

Sometimes, when you fax documents to another fax machine, that machine may be busy sending or receiving other faxes. If this happens, your fax machine will keep redialing the number until it can send the fax. Don't use this feature, however, if unauthorized persons might have access to the documents while they are waiting to be faxed. Also, never leave unattended documents in a fax machine.

Electronic Mail

Electronic mail, or e-mail, allows you to send files from your computer to another computer anywhere in the world. When communicating by e-mail, follow the same rules that you use when writing letters.

There are two ways of sending e-mails:

- You can send the document—a letter, for example—as an e-mail.
- You can send the document as an attachment to an e-mail.

Sending the document as an e-mail requires that you type it at the time you send it. If the document already exists in your computer somewhere, you can select it and attach it to a short e-mail letter that explains what is attached. Confidentiality still cannot be guaranteed. Be sure you know your office policies on e-mail prior to sending any information or include a confidentiality statement in e-mails that contain confidential information. This is similar to the statement included on a fax cover sheet. You can easily adapt that sample cover sheet statement for use with e-mails. If you're attaching documents to an e-mail, open and look at them before you hit send to be sure you attached the correct documents.

HANDLING INCOMING MAIL

Part of your duties may be handling the incoming mail. Many types of mail will come into the office each day. They may include:

- Advertisements
- Bills from suppliers of goods and services
- Consultation letters
- Hospital communications and newsletters
- Laboratory and radiology reports
- Waiting room magazines
- Professional journals
- Literature from professional organizations
- Samples of drugs and lab test kits
- Payments from insurance companies and patients
- Other patient correspondence

Opening and Sorting Mail

Some physicians may want you to sort, open, respond to, and file mail without their review. In other offices, all mail is handled only by the physician or office manager.

Most physicians will open and handle their own personal mail. Mail about patients, however, should be opened and dealt with as soon as possible.

Any mail marked "urgent" should be processed first, whether you're permitted to open it or not. Records, test results, and other patient-related materials are next in order. Ads, announcements, and other promotional materials are handled last.

Your office may have established policies and procedures for processing the daily mail. Some additional general procedures to follow that will help you do the job efficiently include the following:

1. Gather the needed equipment: a letter opener, paper clips, and a date stamp.
2. Open all letters and check for enclosures. Attach these with a paper clip to the letter. If the letter states there were enclosures and none were sent, contact the sender. Write on the letter that enclosures were missing and the name of the person you contacted.
3. Stamp all mail with the date it was received.
4. Sort the mail into categories and handle each according to office policy. In general, this will mean:
5. Test results—Scan into EHR as soon as possible.
6. Payments—Record all checks and insurance payments and process them according to office policy.
7. Advertisements—Dispose of all advertisements unless you are told differently.
8. Employee mail—Distribute to the proper staff member.
9. Magazines—Place in the waiting room. Do not put medical journals in the waiting room.

CAREER COMMUNICATION

Another form of professional communication that you will need to work on is your resume and letter of application. Your resume will serve to represent you and the skills you possess. As such, you should take time to inventory what you have to offer a potential employer. When applying to a position, it is important that you follow the directions from the potential employer. The employer will list what items are required and those that are optional. If a letter of application is optional, you could elect not to submit one; however, it would not count against you if it were included. Imagine the impact of the submitting something that is not required but is optional. The impact is not measurable, but you would know that you took the extra step.

Letter of Application

Your letter of application, or cover letter, should serve to introduce you to the employer. This is your opportunity to explain why you are interested in the position being offered and what makes you the ideal candidate for the job. Selling yourself is never easy, so it's extremely important that you know your value. Type your letter as you would any business letter. Pay close attention to the details; such as spelling, format, content.

Resume

Your resume is a snapshot of your professional career. It should highlight your education, special training, employment, professional associations, and awards or special honors received. There are many different formats for your resume, research styles specific to the type of position you seek. Your resume should be organized in chronological order ascending from the most recent to the past. Confine your resume to one page, this allows the employer to see all your information at a glance. Be sure to include the following information:

1. Personal Information: Name, address, phone number, and e-mail
2. Educational Background: College name, dates attended, degree or program completed
3. Special Training: Name of training, dates of training
4. Professional Association: Organization name, title held such as RMA, CMA, etc., and any positions held within the organization
5. Awards or Special Honors: Perfect attendance throughout your education, Academic Honors, awards from professional organizations such as Student of the Year or RMA of the Year

Many companies have job applicants complete on-line applications and will not accept paper copies. Usually, there is an opportunity to attach a cover letter or introductory letter of intent explaining why you are applying for the position.

Remember the purpose of your letter of application is to introduce yourself, highlight why you are the best candidate for the job, and ask for an interview. Your resume should demonstrate your training and experience and secure the interview for you.

Procedure 1-1   Documenting Patient Education

The purpose is to document the instruction and education given to patients. Equipment includes a computer with an EHR program that is used to document the procedure.

1. Obtain an electronic copy of printed materials that the patient will receive.

2. In the patient's EHR, record the date, time, subject of education provided, and the names of those present during the education. It is important to include the names of those present including the educator, patient, and any family member or guest that is present.

3. Document, in detail, the manner information was presented. For example, "The patient and his mother were educated on the proper use of crutches. We reviewed written instructions, watched the Mayo Clinic Orthopedic video "How to properly use crutches," and practiced proper use.

4. Evaluate the effectiveness of your teaching and record the results of the instruction. For example, "The patient practiced ambulating through the hall. Corrections were made in crutch placement and patient continued practiced. The patient expressed understanding of materials given and demonstrated proper use of crutches."

5. Document information regarding future appointments, evaluations, or follow-up reports. For example, "The patient's mother will report to the office, via phone, on the patient's progress in 7 days. She verbally expressed understanding and will notify the physician immediately if there are any changes in symptoms."

Procedure 1-2 | Explaining General Office Procedures and Policies to the Patient

The purpose is to provide the patient with information on office practices in an effect to insure the best possible care. Equipment and supplies include the General Office Procedure and Policies brochure, highlighter, business card, and pen.

1. Welcome the patient to the practice. Introduce yourself to the patient and explain your role in the office.

2. Review the office brochure with the patient. Highlight areas of importance such as office hours, appointment scheduling, prescription refills, and after hours contact.

3. Answer any questions the patient may have. Encourage the patient to contact you if they have questions after they leave.

4. Give the brochure to the patient along with a business card. Write your name and contact information on the back.

5. Document the review of policies in the patient's record.

Procedure 1-3 | Writing a Professional Business Letter

The purpose is to create a clear and concise business letter that is professional in appearance and content. Equipment need is a computer with word processing program, 8½ × 11 paper, and a No. 10 envelope. The medical assistant was asked by Dr. Georgia Parks to compose a letter to patient, Dwayne Waterman, 12105 Quality Lane, Chesterfield, MO 63017, terminating the physician–patient relationship. She is terminating Mr. Waterman's care due to his noncompliance and failure to adhere to the narcotic use agreement he signed. Dr. Parks has advised you she will terminate the patient's care 15 days after the receipt of the letter. She will provide urgent and emergency care until that time. Dr. Parks also wants the patient informed that she will no longer prescribe any narcotic pain medications. She will release his medical records to the physician taking over his care upon receipt of a signed release of medical information. This letter will be sent certified with return receipt. Use block format, all line with start flush with the left margin.

1. Compose a rough draft of the body of the letter. Take time to insure all the information needed is covered. Have others review the letter for content and accuracy.

2. Create a "header" to serve as letterhead for Dr. Georgia Parks, include a mailing address and phone number.

3. Return down two lines and insert the date or dateline of your letter.

4. Double-space and enter the inside address. This will include Mr. Waterman's full name address.

5. Double-space and type the salutation.

6. Double-space and enter the subject line. Such as: RE: Termination of care

7. Double-space and type the body of your letter.

8. Double-space and type the complimentary close. There are numerous complimentary closures. Select one that is professional in nature.

9. Enter or return four to six times then type the physician name. This will leave space for the physician to sign. Typically, four lines are enough space for a signature.

10. Double-space, type the initials of the sender in capital letters followed by a backslash or colon, then, your initials in lower case.

Preparing for Externship

Your externship is the opportunity for you to experience the "real world" while you are still a student. Most medical assistant programs require an externship assignment in a medical facility, typically a minimum of 160 clock hours. During your time at the externship facility, you will perform the duties taught throughout the program. This chapter discusses communication essentials, which you will need to use to communicate with your school and the medical facility. Your school assigns an instructor or externship coordinator who will guide you throughout the externship experience. The medical facility will assign a supervisor, sometimes called a preceptor, who will oversee your performance of duties. It is essential that you communicate well with your supervisor and frequently ask for constructive criticism. Constructive criticism is a way of providing you feedback about how you can improve your performance. The externship course is the time to refine your skills and prepare you for your first position as a professional medical assistant.

Chapter Recap

- Effective communication includes delivery of a message, clarification that the message was received, feedback, further clarification, and final feedback.
- Dr. Kubler-Ross discovered the five steps to grieving. These steps can occur in any order and are important in dealing with loss.
- There are five levels in the Hierarchy of Needs: self-actualization, esteem, love/belonging, safety, and physiological.
- Patients and visitors should be welcomed in a professional and friendly way.
- A professional appearance includes clean, wrinkle-free clothing and well-groomed hair and nails.
- Medical letters and documents need to be well organized, concise, and free of spelling and grammar errors.
- When faxing or e-mailing documents from the medical office, a confidentiality statement must be on the document or cover page.
- USPS guidelines are used to format envelopes to prevent delays in delivery.
- Certain correspondence may require special mailing such as certified, used when a return receipt is needed to prove delivery of the item.
- A letter of application allows you to outline your qualifications and explain to a potential employer why you are the best candidate for the position.
- Your resume represents you to potential employers; therefore, it should be flawless and professional in appearance.

Online Resources for Students

Student Resources available on the text's online site include:
- Audio Glossaries
- Animations
- Competency Evaluation Forms
- Videos
- Anatomy & Physiology Module with Heart and Lung Sounds
- Weblinks
- Worksheets

Exercises and Activities

Certification Preparation Questions

1. When creating a business letter, the salutation is the:
   a. subject line.
   b. greeting.
   c. closing.
   d. body.

2. Paralanguage is:
   a. body language.
   b. sobs, sighs, or grunts.
   c. tone, volume, and pitch.
   d. facial expressions.

3. Proxemics deals with:
   a. personal space.
   b. the study of body movements.
   c. paralanguage.
   d. nonverbal communication.

4. A patient's social history includes:
   a. information on the health of the patient's brothers and sisters.
   b. past surgeries or procedures the patient has had.
   c. smoking, exercise, and alcohol habits of the patient.
   d. allergies to medications.

5. A patient schedules an appointment with the doctor through a friend as the patient does not speak English. Which of the following represent the best way to handle this situation?
   a. Ask the friend that is scheduling the appointment to come along to help with communication.
   b. Have the patient come alone and give her the information in writing to take with her for someone else to explain.
   c. Schedule a professional interpreter for the visit.
   d. Just speak to the patient in English and hope they understand.

6. When dealing with patients, it is important to establish/maintain a professional relationship by:
   a. picking up their prescriptions and delivering to the patient.
   b. offer to drive patients to appointments on your day off.
   c. being friendly while maintaining a professional distance.
   d. helping them by picking up groceries.

7. In business letters, the closing would include the words:
   a. Sincerely
   b. Dear
   c. Enclosure
   d. Re

8. Your resume should include your:
   a. hobbies and titles of recently read books.
   b. marital status and number of children you have.
   c. past medical history.
   d. education and employment history.

9. In Maslow's Hierarchy of Needs, the end result of all needs being met is:
   a. self-actualization.
   b. esteem.
   c. safety.
   d. basic needs.

10. If multiple lines require answering, the proper procedure for answering would be to answer the line, identify the office and yourself, and then:
    a. state, "please hold" and place them immediately on hold.
    b. complete one call at a time, allowing the other lines to ring because they will either wait or call back.
    c. ask the caller if they can hold, wait for answer, then place on hold if they say "yes."
    d. forward the calls to the night service and wait for things to calm down.

 Internet Activity

Using the Internet, locate five (5) positions that you would be interested in applying for. Research the qualifications for each of the positions and then create an action plan for success. In your plan, explain in detail the steps you will follow to insure that you are qualified for the positions you plan to hold in the future.

2 Law and Ethics

Chapter Objectives

- Explain why a knowledge of law and ethics is important when working in a medical facility.
- Describe the difference between law, ethics, etiquette, morals, and values.
- Distinguish how law and ethics are related.
- Compare the consequences of unlawful and unethical behavior.
- Define the three main sources of law.
- Describe the three different types of law.
- Compare and contrast criminal and civil law.
- Define *respondeat superior* and explain how it relates in a health care setting.
- Identify the three parts of a valid contract.
- Differentiate between expressed and implied contracts.
- List the steps a physician must follow when terminating a contract.
- Describe the medical assistant's scope of practice and explain resources available to answer medical assistant questions.
- Explain standard of care as it relates to physicians and medical assistants.
- Explain the difference between intentional and unintentional torts.
- Define and explain the difference between malfeasance, misfeasance, and nonfeasance.
- Identify the four Ds of negligence.

CAAHEP & ABHES Competencies

CAAHEP

- Identify and respond to issues of confidentiality.
- Perform within legal and ethical boundaries.
- Demonstrate knowledge of federal and state health care legislation and regulations.

ABHES

- Comply with federal, state, and local health laws and regulations as they relate to health care settings.
- Define scope of practice for the medical assistant within the state that the medical assistant is employed.

- Describe what procedures can and cannot be delegated to the medical assistant and by whom within various employment settings.
- Perform risk management procedures.
- Understand the importance of maintaining liability coverage once employed in the industry.
- Display compliance with Code of Ethics of the profession.
- Follow established policy in initiating or terminating medical treatment.

Chapter Terms

Abandonment
Arbitration
Assault
Battery
Beneficence
Breach
Contract
Defendant
Dilemma

Embezzlement
Ethics
Etiquette
Felonies
Fidelity
Fraud
Integrity
Libel
Malfeasance

Malpractice
Misdemeanor
Misfeasance
Negligence
Nonfeasance
Plaintiff
Precedents
Res ipsa loquitur
Respondeat superior

Slander
Stare decisis
Statutes
Subpoena
Tort
Tortfeasor
Veracity
Verdict

Abbreviations

AAMA
ADAAA
AMT

CAAHEP
CMA
DEA

HHS
HIPAA
NPP

PHI
PSDA
RMA

Case Study

Elizabeth is a medical assistant employed in a busy internal medicine practice that performs x-rays on site. Although the state where the practice is located does not allow medical assistants to do any x-ray procedures, Elizabeth recently relocated from a state where the scope of practice for medical assistants includes performing chest and extremity x-rays. One day, when the x-ray tech was out of the office on vacation, the physician asked Elizabeth to do a chest x-ray since she was trained to do x-rays. This way, the patient would not have to come back the next day when the x-ray tech returned from vacation. Not wanting to lose her new job, Elizabeth agreed to do the x-rays.

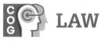 **LAW**

Everyone knows that it's important to obey the law. That's fairly easy to understand. But other forces affect our actions, too, and some of them have little to do with the law. Morals, values, ethics, and etiquette also shape our behavior. Also, there are consequences if our behavior falls short in these areas.

The law is usually straightforward. However, sometimes, it can be harder to define what's "right" when it comes to ethics and morals. In this chapter, you'll read about the connections and differences between law, ethics, and other forces that determine how we should behave.

What does any of this have to do with work in a medical office? Health care professionals are expected to demonstrate proper behavior on the job. The medical practice's success is closely linked to the actions of its employees. Most importantly, a good understanding of law and ethics can help make your career as a medical assistant pleasant, satisfying, and successful.

Laws are rules of conduct that the government creates and requires us to obey. They ensure that we receive the rights we enjoy as Americans. They also help protect us from being harmed by others. Laws protect us in two ways:

- By prohibiting possibly harmful behavior or acts
- By discouraging people from committing these acts for fear of punishment

To help you understand why we have laws, think about what life would be like without traffic laws.

Case Question

 What consequences might Elizabeth face for performing outside her legal scope of practice in that state? What are the potential issues the clinic or physician may encounter?

Suppose there were no speed limits or traffic signals requiring drivers to stop at intersections. How safe would travel be on roads and highways?

Many laws exist to protect the rights and safety of patients. Physicians must abide by certain laws. As a medical assistant, you'll need to have a basic understanding of these laws. It's your responsibility to abide by these laws and to help the physician stay within the boundaries of the law. You may not yet have heard of many of these laws but ignorance of the law is no excuse. Just one act of wrongdoing can harm a patient and cause a lawsuit. Knowledge of the laws will help you follow legal guidelines.

At some point in your career as a medical assistant, your employer may be involved in a lawsuit. You may even be involved—either as a witness or as the result of something you did or failed to do. Or, your employer may ask you to provide records to the court or to attorneys for one side or the other. In any case, a lawsuit can be a frightening thing. The good news is that knowledge of the law can help reduce that fear. This chapter will provide you with a basic knowledge of the law and the legal system, as well as describe what to expect if your office is ever sued.

 ## HOW LAWS ARE MADE

There are three branches of American government that contribute to the development, enforcement, interpretation, and application of laws (Table 2-1):

- Legislative branch—makes laws
- Executive branch—enforces laws
- Judicial branch—interprets and applies laws

Congress is the most important of the three legislative levels. No law passed by a state legislature can replace or contradict a law passed by Congress. In general, laws passed by a city or town council can't replace or contradict laws passed by that state's legislature. And they can never replace or contradict laws passed by Congress. This makes the laws that Congress passes, which are called federal laws, the most powerful laws in the land.

At each level of government, the executive branch consists of agencies or departments that enforce certain laws. One example is a city's police department, which enforces traffic laws and many other statutes (laws). Another example of an executive agency is a state's medical licensing board. The board's responsibility is to enforce the state's medical practice act. Still another example is the U.S. Drug Enforcement Administration (DEA), which helps to enforce the nation's drug laws.

 ## THREE TYPES OF LAW

Each branch of government produces a different kind of law.

- Statutory law comes from the legislative branch.
- The executive branch creates administrative law.
- Case law results from the actions of the judicial branch.

Statutory Law

The laws passed by Congress or by state legislatures are called **statutes**. Laws passed at the local level—for example, by a city council—are called ordinances. Statutes and ordinances form a body of law known as statutory law.

Table 2-1	Provides an Understanding of the Three Sources of Law	
	Understanding the Three Sources of Law	
Branch of Government	**What They Do**	**Types of Law Produced**
Legislative Branch	The legislative branches make the laws for the country, state, and cities or towns. Congress is the most important law-making body in the legislative branch. Congress passes federal laws that are the most powerful in the country.	The legislative branch creates statutory law.
Executive Branch	The executive branch enforces the laws passed by the legislative branch. Each level of government has a chief executive who is responsible for seeing that the laws are properly followed. These chief executives include the president of the United States, state governors, and mayors.	Government agencies in the executive branch create administrative law.
Judicial Branch	The judicial branch is made up of the courts that interpret and apply the law. There are federal, state, and local courts.	The courts in the judicial branch are responsible for case law.

Statutes are the main type of statutory law that will affect your work as a medical assistant.

Statutes begin as bills that are introduced into Congress or your state's legislature by one of its members. If the legislature passes the bill, it becomes a law—unless the President or state governor vetoes, or rejects, it. However, if a bill is vetoed, the legislature can sometimes pass the bill again and make it law anyway.

Once it has been passed, a law can be changed or replaced by another law. It can also be repealed, which means it is officially withdrawn as a law. Individuals also may challenge the law in court as being a violation of the state or U.S. Constitution.

Medical Assistants can be affected on the job by statutes including the Controlled Substances Act, governed by the **DEA** and the Health Insurance Portability and Accountability Act (**HIPAA**). The Controlled Substances Act regulates how your office handles and prescribes certain drugs. HIPAA sets standards for the privacy of patients' medical records and for the filing of claims to patients' health insurance providers.

Administrative Law

A government agency creates administrative law. Because administrative laws are not passed by legislatures, they are not statutes. Instead, they are called administrative rules or regulations. Violation of these laws can be considered as serious an offense as breaking a statutory law.

The main purpose of administrative law is to provide details that make statutes more clear. For example, a state's medical practices statute may require a physician to be a graduate of an accredited medical school. What exactly does that mean? Accredited by whom? Many groups rate and approve medical schools. In this case, the state medical board would create an administrative rule, or regulation, specifying the accreditation needed for a medical school's graduates to be licensed in that state.

Another example is HIPAA. The statute requires that a patient's privacy be protected, but Congress authorized a U.S. government agency, the U.S. Department of Health and Human Services (HHS), to create regulations about how that can be done. The procedures you follow when you handle patients' records in the office are probably based on HHS regulations, which are part of administrative law. Breaking one of these regulations is also a violation of HIPAA, the statutory authority behind the regulations.

Case Law

The courts of the judicial branch are the third source of law. When judges decide cases, they first look at previous cases tried under the same law to determine how the law was applied. Those earlier decisions become

Box 2-1 History of Common Law

The first common law came from decisions made by judges in English courts about 800 years ago. The English colonists brought this body of law to America in the 1600s. But life on the American frontier was very different than in England. Some of the old common law precedents didn't fit the conditions in the colonies. So, colonial courts made decisions that set new precedents. This caused the body of common law to grow in America.

Common law continues to grow and change as new conditions require new precedents. Every state except Louisiana follows English common law. In Louisiana, which was first colonized by France, common law is based on early French law.

A good example of common law is a physician's duty to provide good care to a patient. This requirement is hardly ever stated in a statute or in administrative law. But decisions in court cases have established that it's a physician's professional responsibility to provide good care. This makes it a legal requirement for physicians under common law.

precedents, or guides, that the judge applies in deciding the current case.

The legal principle is called **stare decisis**, which is Latin for "let the decision stand." It means that decisions in current court cases are based on decisions in similar past cases. Because this type of law comes from past court cases rather than from legislatures or government agencies, it's known as case law. It's also called common law, because it applies in all situations for which the facts are the same (see Box 2-1).

CRIMINAL LAW AND CIVIL LAW

You just read that there are three types of law—statutory law, administrative law, and case law—depending on who makes the law. There is also another way of looking at the law: by whom or what it applies to, rather than its origin. Looking at the law this way identifies two broad divisions of law.

- Criminal law, the most common type of public law, affects everyone. Although crimes are committed against individuals, criminal law exists to protect all of society.
- Civil law involves relationships between individuals, or between a person and the government. For this reason, civil law is also sometimes called private law.

Criminal Law

Crimes are violations of criminal law. These violations can occur in either of two ways:

- When someone takes an action that's been banned, such as driving while drunk
- When someone fails to take an action that's required, such as failing to stop for a red light at an intersection

There are two types of crimes.

- **Felonies** are serious crimes that are punishable by long prison sentences or even by death. Some of the more notorious felonies include murder, rape, kidnapping, robbery, and arson.
- **Misdemeanors** are less serious crimes that are punishable by fines or short jail sentences. Examples include traffic offenses, stealing something worth a small amount of money, and disturbing the peace.

Crime Encountered in the Medical Office

Although it's unlikely that you'll be involved with any crimes in your work as a medical assistant, they can and do sometimes occur. This section includes examples of crimes that you might encounter in a medical office.

Abuse

Child abuse is a felony and one of the leading causes of death in children under the age of 5 years. According to federal law, child abuse is any act or failure to act by a parent or caregiver resulting in the death or serious emotional or physical harm of a child, including sexual abuse and exploitation. Those actions that put a child at risk of death or harm are also considered abuse. The federal Child Abuse Prevention and Treatment Act mandates that threats to a child's physical and mental welfare be reported. State laws vary regarding the procedure for reporting abuse. However, as a medical assistant, you're professionally and ethically responsible for reporting any suspected abuse to the physician. The physician will know how to proceed. This applies not only to child abuse but also to spousal abuse and elder abuse.

Embezzlement

Embezzlement is the wrongful taking of money or property that you're responsible for and using it for your own personal needs. An employee who steals money from his employer is committing embezzlement, which is a felony.

Fraud

Fraud is any deceitful act with the intention of concealing the truth. Submitting a claim that you know to be false to a patient's health insurance plan is one example of fraud. Falsifying medical records can also be considered fraud in some cases. Fraud is a felony, too.

Battery

Battery is the actual physical touching of a person without her consent. This can range from acts such as striking an employee or a patient to various kinds of sexual contact. All acts are felonies.

Accessory to Crime

If you're aware of a crime and do nothing about it, your lack of action is also a criminal act. An accessory is someone who does not actually commit the crime, but who directly or indirectly contributes to it. Here are some behaviors that could cause someone to be charged as an accessory to a crime:

- Encouraging another person to commit a crime
- Witnessing a crime and doing nothing
- Helping cover up a crime after it has been committed

Criminal Court Cases

A person is accused of a crime when charges are brought by the local, state, or federal government. The level of government bringing the charges depends on whether the person is accused of breaking a local, state, or federal law.

Defendants and Plaintiffs

The person accused of breaking the law is called the **defendant**. The party that charges the wrongdoing is called the **plaintiff**. Because in criminal cases the government is the plaintiff, the plaintiff is also called the prosecution.

The Attorneys

An attorney (lawyer) usually represents each side in a court case. In a criminal proceeding, the prosecution's case against the defendant is presented by a city attorney, district attorney, or state's attorney, who is called the prosecutor. The defense attorney is a private attorney hired by the defendant. If the defendant can't afford an attorney, the judge will appoint an attorney to handle the defendant's case.

The Judge and the Jury

The judge conducts the trial and decides controversies over points of law and the introduction of evidence. The jury is a group of citizens from the community chosen to listen to the evidence presented and to decide the defendant's guilt or innocence. In a criminal case, this decision is called the **verdict**. If there is no jury, the judge decides the verdict. Whether there's a jury or not, if the verdict is "guilty," the judge then decides the defendant's punishment. A jury's verdict must be unanimous. If the jurors can't all agree, the defendant must be released or tried again.

Civil Law

Civil law covers wrongful acts that are not crimes. Under civil law, such charges arise when one party (the plaintiff) claims to have been injured by the actions of another party (the defendant) and sues the accused party. The plaintiff and defendant in a lawsuit are usually either a person or a business. But the government also can be a party in a suit under some circumstances.

Most civil suits fall into one of three categories.

- Family issues—These often involve matters such as divorce, child support, or disputes over child custody.
- Contract disputes—These often involve charges that someone has broken a contractual agreement. You'll read more about contracts later in this chapter.
- Torts—Wrongs committed against a person or property that don't involve violation of a contract. Torts can be intentional or unintentional. Because some intentional torts can also be crimes, we're going to discuss them briefly now.

Intentional Torts

Intentional torts involve deliberate misconduct. Two common intentional torts are slander and libel.

- **Slander** is speaking lies about another person that harms the person's reputation or employment.
- **Libel** is damaging a person's reputation in writing.

For example, if you tell your coworkers that you've heard one of the medical assistants is an alcoholic—even though you don't know for sure that it's true—then you've slandered her. If you include this information in an e-mail to one of your coworkers, then you're guilty of libel. In either case, the medical assistant can sue you for your actions.

Here are some other intentional torts that might occur in a medical office. These torts can result in criminal charges in addition to a lawsuit:

- Assault
- Battery
- Fraud

Assault

Assault is threatening a person or acting in a way that causes the person to fear harm. For example, suppose you're trying to examine a squirming child. If you threaten to strike the child if he doesn't remain still, you've just committed assault.

Battery

Battery is unlawful touching, whether or not the touching causes bodily harm. To avoid the tort of battery, you should never touch a patient without his consent. This doesn't necessarily mean that you have to ask permission, however. For example, if you're preparing to give a patient a flu shot and he rolls up his sleeve, he has indirectly given his consent. Or if you tell a patient that you're about to take her blood pressure and she doesn't object, this is also considered a form of consent.

Fraud

Fraud is any dishonest practice that's intended to deceive another person. In a medical setting, convincing a patient to accept treatment by promising her a cure, when the treatment has no reasonable chance of curing her, would be one example of fraud.

Civil Trials

Most of the actions you just read about are crimes as well as torts. This means a person accused of doing them could be tried in criminal court in addition to being sued in civil court.

Civil cases are like criminal cases in many ways. But some important differences do exist.

- In a civil case, both parties are likely to be persons or businesses—for example, *Smith v. Jones* or *Taylor v. Acme Medical Clinic*. As you've already read, in a criminal case, one party (the plaintiff) is *always* the government or "The People."
- The jury's decision does not have to be unanimous in a civil trial. If more than one-half of the jurors agree, a verdict has been reached. Also, the judge or jury in a civil case does not reach a "guilty" or "not guilty" verdict. Instead, the verdict is a finding in favor of the plaintiff or the defendant.

If a case is decided in the plaintiff's favor, the jury (or judge, if there's no jury) also decides how much money the defendant must pay. Civil cases don't involve jail sentences; instead, the defendant must compensate the plaintiff for the harm he caused. This sum of money is called compensatory damages.

In some cases, a judge or jury may award the plaintiff money beyond the value of the harm done. This additional award is called punitive damages. Its purpose is to punish the defendant for especially bad behavior.

Defenses Against Torts

Of course, one response to charges of wrongdoing is to deny that it ever took place. In such situations, the best defense may be the patient's chart or medical record. That's one reason why it's important that all contact with a patient be accurately recorded in her chart. Other defenses in civil suits include the following.

- Statute of limitations—the legal time limit that exists for filing a lawsuit
- Respondeat superior—a common law principle that employers are responsible for the actions of their employees

Statute of Limitations

Every state limits the length of time a patient has to file a suit against a health care provider. This time limit is called the statute of limitations. After that time, the person loses the right to file a law suit.

Generally, the statute of limitations expires 1 to 3 years after the alleged tort took place. However, statutes of limitations vary from state to state. For example, in some states, the statute of limitations might be as long as 8 years. Other variations occur because several states measure the time from the date that the patient discovers or should have discovered that wrongdoing may have occurred.

State laws also vary when the victim of an alleged tort is a minor. In such cases, the statute of limitations might not even begin until the patient becomes an adult. Then it might extend 2 or 3 years from that point. Some states also allow for longer statutes of limitations if the wrongdoing may have caused a patient's death.

To find the statute of limitations for your own state, contact the state board of medical examiners. The board's legal department should be able to provide you with information about the statute of limitations for your state and answer any questions you may have. The statute of limitations applies to most crimes, as well as to charges of civil wrongdoing. This means that a person can't be charged with a crime after a set length of time has passed. Some crimes, such as murder, have no statute of limitations, however. Even if it takes 30 years to find a murder suspect, that person can still be charged with the crime.

Respondeat Superior

Respondeat superior is a legal principle also known as the law of agency. It's a Latin term that means "let the master answer." This legal principle makes employers responsible for the actions of their employees. It's not a defense for your employer, but it can be an important protection for you if you're ever accused of a tort.

For example, imagine the physician you work for has asked you to administer an injection. You gather all your equipment, ensure that the rights of administering an injection have been followed, and maintain aseptic technique. However, when you inject the needle into the patient, you inadvertently hit a nerve. The patient suffers nerve damage and sues. Under *respondeat superior*, even though the physician was not the person who administered the injection, she is ultimately responsible for your actions.

Respondeat superior applies only to civil law. If an employee commits a crime, he can be arrested, brought to trial, and punished. The employer shares no responsibility for the crime unless the employer ordered, encouraged, or knowingly allowed the employee to commit it.

Keep in mind that *respondeat superior* is not always applicable. In a medical setting, your employer is responsible for your actions only when those actions are within your scope of practice. Your scope of practice is the range of tasks you're trained to perform. You should always be on guard against acting outside your scope of practice. If you do, your employer generally won't be legally responsible for your actions. If the result is a tort, you could be personally sued, and *respondeat superior* wouldn't protect you.

Case Question

How does the respondeat superior principle apply to Elizabeth, the medical assistant in the case study regarding performing x-rays?

TORTS

Torts are wrongful acts committed against a person or property. Intentional torts are deliberate acts that cause harm. For this reason, many intentional torts are also crimes. Unintentional torts are accidental rather than deliberate. In these cases, the **tortfeasor** (the person who commits the tort) does not mean to harm the person or property.

In either case, a tort always involves some sort of harm, whether it's mental, emotional, or physical.

If you hit someone with your car because you aren't paying attention to your driving, you're negligent because a reasonable person would be paying attention. Your inattentive behavior does not meet the reasonable person standard and makes you guilty of the tort of negligence.

Tort cases are tried in civil courts, and the injured person may recover money damages from the tortfeasor. Intentional torts can also be tried as crimes in criminal courts. The tortfeasor becomes the defendant and can be jailed or fined if found guilty. Since a criminal court can't award damages to the injured party, in order to collect damages, the injured party must sue the tortfeasor in a separate action in civil court.

Negligence and Malpractice

As you just learned, **negligence** results from failing to act with reasonable care, causing harm to another person. Negligence can occur in either of two ways:

- By doing something that a reasonable person would *not* do
- By *not* doing something that a reasonable person *would* do

When a professional person is negligent in his or her duties, it's known as **malpractice**. Negligence by a medical professional is called medical malpractice. This separate category for negligence by professionals is based on the principle that their level of knowledge gives them a greater duty of care than the reasonable person standard requires.

Like ordinary negligence, harm or injury must result for malpractice to occur. Accusations of malpractice are the most common reason for lawsuits against health care professionals. There are three types of malpractice claims:

- **Malfeasance**—taking an improper action
- **Misfeasance**—taking a proper action but in an improper way
- **Nonfeasance**—not taking a necessary action

Malfeasance

Malfeasance is the performance of a wrong and unlawful act. For example, a medical assistant who tells a patient to treat her symptoms by taking an aspirin is committing an act of malfeasance because only a physician can prescribe treatments.

Misfeasance

Misfeasance is the performance of a lawful act in an improper manner. For example, a medical assistant fails to use a sterile bandage when dressing a patient's wound, resulting in an infection for the patient.

Nonfeasance

Nonfeasance is the failure to perform a necessary act. For example, a patient stops breathing in the waiting room, and the medical assistant, who is trained in CPR, does not perform CPR on the patient.

The Four Ds of Negligence

For a health care provider to be sued for malpractice successfully, the plaintiff (the accuser) usually must prove four things occurred. They are sometimes called the "four Ds of negligence":

- *Duty*—the responsibility to provide a reasonable standard of care to the patient
- *Dereliction of duty*—not providing a reasonable standard of care to the patient
- *Direct or proximate cause*—the direct or indirect cause of a patient's injury
- *Damages*—the harm suffered by a patient

Direct Cause

To prove *direct cause*, there must be an unbroken chain of events that connect the improper action to the harm done. For example:

1. A child comes in sick.
2. The medical assistant administers an adult dosage of medication to the child.
3. The child dies as a result of the overmedication.

In this example, the medical assistant's failure to provide the proper dosage to the child was the direct cause of the patient's death.

However, it isn't always possible to prove direct cause. Suppose emergency services (EMS) had come to the clinic, revived the patient, and taken her to the hospital, where she later died. Proving malpractice would require proving that the medical assistant's failure to administer the correct dosage was the *proximate cause* of the patient's death. That is, it must be proven that some intervening act—such as a medication error in the hospital—didn't cause the death instead.

Damages

Many kinds of damages can cause patients to seek financial compensation from the accused in a malpractice case. Compensation is something good that is given to reduce the bad effect of some damage, loss, or injury. Some of the more common reasons for financial compensation in malpractice cases are as follows:

- Personal injury
- Pain and suffering
- Mental anguish
- Loss of enjoyment of life
- Permanent physical or mental disability
- Loss of past and future income
- Hospital and medical expenses

When malpractice causes a patient's death, a family member will often be the plaintiff in the lawsuit against the health care provider. This is called a wrongful death suit. In that case, the compensation the defendant must pay can be based on harm done to the plaintiff as well as to the patient. For example, the patient's spouse or parent (if the patient was a child) will likely have suffered mental anguish from the death. If the patient was employed, the spouse will have suffered loss of income, too. In fact, "loss of service" of spouse or child is a common cause for damage awards if the act of malpractice kills a patient.

Res Ipsa Loquitur

Sometimes, a patient does not have to prove the four Ds to win a malpractice suit. In some cases, the common law doctrine of *res ipsa loquitur* applies. (A doctrine is a principle of law.) **Res ipsa loquitur** is a Latin term that means "the thing speaks for itself." Operating on the wrong leg to fix a broken leg is a perfect example of when a patient would claim *res ipsa loquitur* in court. In an instance such as this, the surgeon's mistake would be so obvious that no more evidence is needed. For this reason, surgeons now verify the leg that needs the operation with the patient along with two or three other witnesses well before the surgery takes place. They then mark the correct leg to make sure no mistakes are made during surgery.

These precautions help keep patients safer and also protect the surgeon from committing *res ipsa loquitur*.

Three conditions must exist for the doctrine of *res ipsa loquitur* to apply:

- The defendant had direct and complete control over the cause of the injury.
- The injury would not have occurred if the defendant had exercised reasonable care.
- The plaintiff (patient) did not in any way contribute to the cause of the injury.

When a plaintiff claims *res ipsa loquitur*, the burden of proof shifts to the defendant. The defendant must prove that negligence did *not* occur.

CONTRACTS

A **contract** is a voluntary agreement between two parties from which each party benefits. If the agreement is spoken or put into writing, it's called an expressed contract. Contracts also can result from the behavior or actions of each party. This type of agreement is called an implied contract. Figure 2-1 is an example of a consent form that would be used to obtain consent to perform a procedure. It includes the name of the procedure and any risks associated with the procedure.

Whether a contract is expressed or implied, three conditions must exist to make it legally binding on each party.

- Offer and acceptance—One party makes an offer, and the other party accepts it. For example, a physician offers medical services by opening an office. Patients accept this offer by scheduling appointments.
- Consideration—Each party must exchange something of value with the other. The physician's consideration is the service she provides to the patient. The patient's consideration is payment of the physician's fee. Once each party has provided its consideration, the contract is complete.
- Competence—Each party must be able to understand the terms and conditions of the agreement. For example, a mentally incompetent person can't enter into a contract. Nor can a minor—which usually means anyone under age 18. That's why the consent of a parent or legal guardian is generally needed before treating a minor.

Expressed Contracts

Some contracts a medical office makes must be in writing in order to be enforceable. These include third-party contracts and credit agreements. Usually, such contracts involve the payment of fees.

Third-Party Contracts

Suppose a man becomes ill but can't afford to see a physician. His adult daughter makes an appointment for him to see his physician. She tells the medical assistant that she'll pay the bill for her father's care. By making this promise, the daughter has entered into an expressed contract with the office.

This is not a typical expressed contract, however. It's different because the party who's receiving the physician's consideration (the patient) is not the one providing the return consideration (the daughter). A third party, who is receiving nothing of value from the physician, is completing the exchange. This type of contract is called a third-party contract or a third-party payer contract.

Under common law, third-party contracts must be in writing to be legally binding. This means that unless the daughter signs a written contract to pay her father's bill, the office can't sue her if she later refuses to pay. The office can sue the father to collect its fees, but he may not have the means to pay.

Insurance policies are another type of third-party payer contract. Whether a third-party payer is involved or not, most offices require patients to sign written

---

I hereby authorize Dr._____ , and such assistants as may be designated, to perform:

_____
(Name of treatment/procedure)

and any other related procedures or forms of treatment, including appropriate anesthesia, transfusions that they deem necessary for the welfare of:

_____
(Name of patient)

I consent to the administration of anesthesia and/or such drugs as may be necessary. I understand that all anesthetics involve risks of complications, serious injury, or rarely death from both known and unknown causes.

I consent to the examination and retention for educational, scientific and research purposes by the Medical Staff of

_____

of all body fluids, tissues and organs removed during the course of the above treatment/procedure with privilege of ultimate use and disposal resting with said medical staff.

The following has been explained to me and I understand:

A. The nature and character of the proposed treatment/procedure.
B. The anticipated results of the proposed treatment/procedure.
C. The recognized alternative forms of treatment/procedure.
D. The recognized serious possible risks and complications of the treatment/procedure and of the recognized alternative forms of treatment/procedure, including non-treatment.
E. The possible consequences of no treatment.
F. The anticipated date and time of the proposed treatment/procedure.

Additional M.D. comments: _____
_____
_____

My physician has offered to answer all inquiries concerning the proposed treatment/procedure. I understand that I am free to withhold or withdraw consent to the proposed treatment/procedure at any time.

Witness	Signature of Person Giving Consent
Date Signed	Time ☐ A.M.	Relationship to patient (if applicable)
	☐ P.M.	

☐ Please check if this is a telephone monitored consent.
No treatment will be performed until this consent has been executed. This consent will be permanently filed in the patient's medical record.

Pt. No. _____	**Gastroenterology Associates** Anytown, PA
Name _____	**Special Consent to Treatment**
D.O.B. _____	(Diagnostic & Surgical Procedures, Anesthesia, Medical Treatment & Other Procedures)

Figure 2-1 Sample consent form. (Reprinted from Kronenberger J, Ledbetter J. *Jones & Bartlett Learning's Comprehensive Medical Assisting.* 5th ed. Burlington, MA: Jones & Bartlett Learning, LLC; 2016.)

agreements to pay any charges not paid by insurance. These agreements should be signed before treatment begins.

Credit Agreements

Another financial matter that can involve a written contract is an agreement with a patient to pay his bill over time. Federal law requires written contracts for credit arrangements under the following four conditions.

1. The credit is offered to the consumer of the goods or services.
2. The business offers credit on a regular basis.
3. Interest is charged, or there are more than four installments.
4. The credit extended is for personal or family use.

The patient must be given a copy of the signed credit contract. A second copy should be placed in the patient's billing records.

Implied Contracts

Implied contracts are contracts in which agreement between the parties is not shown by words, but by action, lack of action, or silence. Implied contracts are very common in a medical office. Here's a typical example: A patient describes her symptoms to the physician. The physician examines the patient, writes her a prescription, and tells her to schedule a follow-up appointment.

A contract has been made in this example, even though it was never directly stated. Both parties must now follow through on their implied agreement. The patient is responsible for:

- Filling the prescription and taking the medication as instructed
- Making and keeping the follow-up appointment
- Paying the bill if it is not covered by insurance

The physician has obligations, too. He must:

- Be willing to see the patient again
- Continue to treat the patient if their condition persists

If either party fails to do these things, the contract has been broken. This is known as breach of contract. Breach of contract occurs when either party fails to live up to the terms of the agreement.

Termination of Patient

The contract usually ends when the patient's treatment is complete and the physician has been paid. However, sometimes issues arise that causes a contract to end before both parties have fulfilled their obligations.

The patient has the right to terminate the contract at any time. Under certain circumstances, the physician

also has a right to end a contract early. The physician may want to end the physician–patient relationship for personal reasons. More often, however, breach of contract is the reason for early termination. Figure 2-2 is an example of a letter that can be sent to a patient when the medical practice determines that it is necessary to terminate the patient–physician relationship. This letter of notice will protect the practice from being charged with abandonment of a patient.

Breach of Contract

A physician may terminate a contract with a patient in the following situations, each of which involves breach of contract.

- The patient does not keep appointments.
- The patient does not follow the physician's instructions.
- The patient fails to pay his bill.

Abandonment

If the physician wishes to terminate the contract and the patient still seeks treatment, the physician must follow specific legal procedures to end the physician–patient relationship. If the physician doesn't terminate the

Amy Fine, MD
Charlotte Family Practice
220 NW 3rd Avenue
Charlotte, NC 25673

October 11, 2016

Regina Dodson
Jones Hill Road
Charlotte, NC 25673

Dear Ms. Dodson,

Due to the fact that you have persistently failed to follow my medical advice and treatment of your diabetes, I will no longer be able to provide medical care to you. Since your condition requires ongoing medical care, you must find another physician within the next 30 days. I will be available to you until your appointment date with a new physician.

To ensure continuity of your care, I will make your records available to your new physician. As soon as you make an appointment with a new physician, please come by our office to sign an authorization form enabling us to send your records.

Sincerely,

Amy Fine, MD

Figure 2-2 Letter of intent to terminate physician-patient relationship. (Reprinted from Kronenberger J, Ledbetter J. *Jones & Bartlett Learning's Comprehensive Medical Assisting.* 5th ed. Burlington, MA: Jones & Bartlett Learning, LLC; 2016.)

contract properly, the patient can sue the physician for **abandonment.**

Abandonment occurs when the physician ends the relationship without proper notice while the patient still needs treatment. Here are some other situations that also can be considered abandonment.

The physician doesn't see the patient as often as the patient's condition requires.

- The physician incorrectly tells the patient that no more treatment is needed.
- The physician does not arrange for another physician to care for the patient when the physician must be away.

Terminating a Contract

To end the contract with a patient and avoid a charge of abandonment, the office must send the patient a letter. As a medical assistant, you may be responsible for preparing this letter. Here's what it must contain:

- A statement that the physician intends to end the relationship
- The reasons for this action
- A termination date that is at least 30 days from the date on the letter
- A statement that the patient's medical records will be transferred to another medical facility at the patient's written request
- A recommendation urging the patient to seek any additional medical care that may be required

The termination letter must be sent by certified mail with a return receipt requested. Place a copy of the letter and the returned receipt in the patient's record.

 THE LAWSUIT

Only about 1 of every 10 lawsuits brought by patients against health care providers actually ends up in court. If the patient's case is very weak, the judge may dismiss it before the trial even begins. Other suits are settled out of court by agreement between the plaintiff, the defendant, and the defendant's liability insurance company. If there's a settlement, the defendant may agree to pay the plaintiff a certain amount of money to avoid going to trial.

Settlements also may be reached at any time once the trial is under way—until the jury actually reaches a verdict. In fact, only about one in a hundred lawsuits that are filed actually reach a final decision by a judge or a jury.

But no matter how the case ends, lawsuits can cause great stress in a medical office. Health care providers can become concerned for their jobs, their reputations, and their ability to practice their profession. Staff members may have extra demands on their time as the office prepares to defend against the suit. There are specific steps in the process of settling a lawsuit from the time the suit is filed until the conclusion in court.

Arbitration

Arbitration is an alternative method to settle a dispute without going to court. An arbitrator is selected to oversee the process. This person will review the case and make a decision on the outcome. Both parties agree in advance to accept the arbitrator's decision as final. Arbitration is an efficient way to settle an argument or disagreement. It is cheaper, faster, and easier than preparing for a trial. It is also a more private way to settle a complaint.

The Complaint

If a patient suspects that something went wrong with her treatment, she may first seek information from the medical office. In many cases, she will view the physician as unapproachable and direct her questions to the medical assistant. This creates a delicate situation, which must be handled with both caution and tact. On one hand, you should not provide any information without the physician's approval. On the other hand, you must try to avoid angering the patient.

If the patient does not get satisfactory answers at the medical office, her next step probably will be to consult an attorney. The attorney will request a copy of the patient's medical records and may also have another physician examine the patient. If the attorney thinks the patient has a case, he'll probably contact the medical office, or the practice attorney, about a settlement.

If settlement negotiations fail, the attorney's next step will be to file a written charge of wrongdoing, called a complaint, with the court. The complaint will explain in detail the torts or other violations of civil law the attorney believes have occurred. The court then serves the medical office with a copy of the complaint. At this point, the patient becomes the plaintiff, and the office becomes the defendant. Office employees who were involved in the patient's care probably will be named as defendants, too.

Discovery

Discovery is a legal process to uncover facts about the situation before the trial begins. Both sides conduct discovery. It can include the following actions.

- **Subpoenas** are orders issued by the court to obtain evidence. The term subpoena is often used to refer to an order requiring you to provide spoken testimony in court as evidence in a trial. However, you may also encounter another form of subpoena in the medical office. *Subpoena duces tecum* is an order requiring you or your employer to provide evidence in the form of documents to the court.

- Interrogatories are written questions about the case that each side submits to the other. These questions must be answered truthfully and in writing.
- Depositions are oral answers that the parties to the case and witnesses provide to questions by each side's attorney before the trial begins. They are made under oath and may be used as evidence at trial.
- Motions are requests to the judge on which he must rule. One motion the defense usually makes is that the case be dismissed, or thrown out of court. The judge generally does not rule on this motion until each side is heard at the pretrial conference.

Negotiations to settle the case out of court often continue during the discovery phase and the pretrial conference.

Collecting Evidence

As a medical assistant, it may be your job to gather records subpoenaed in a lawsuit. Here are some guidelines to follow.

- Unless instructed otherwise by your employer, do not provide records unless they've been subpoenaed.
- Provide only the exact records listed on the subpoena—nothing more or less.
- Unless the subpoena asks for original records, provide only photocopies. Again, copy only what has been asked for.
- Electronic records should be printed and not sent electronically.
- If the subpoena requires original records from a paper record, make a copy of them to replace the originals in the office files.

The Pretrial Conference

The pretrial conference is the first meeting of the plaintiff and the defendant in court. Its main purpose is to determine if the case for wrongdoing is strong enough to proceed to trial. After hearing arguments from both sides, the judge may rule on the defense's motion to dismiss the case. If the motion is granted, the case ends. If the case is not dismissed, either side may present a motion for a jury trial.

The Trial

If the case is not settled or dismissed, it goes to trial. During the trial, each side produces evidence and witnesses that present the facts of the case as that side sees them. In a jury trial, 6 to 12 citizens from the community decide whose "facts" are correct and make a decision in favor of the plaintiff or the defendant. In a bench trial, the judge determines the final decision. The judge also decides any points of law that arise during the trial.

Opening Arguments

The trial begins with opening arguments. They consist of a short speech by each side's attorney and state what each attorney intends to prove during the trial.

The Plaintiff's Case

The plaintiff's attorney presents evidence and calls witnesses first. Each witness swears to tell the truth and then, under questioning by the attorney, tells what he knows about the situation that caused the suit. Then the witness can be cross-examined by the defense attorney. The defense attorney asks questions that are designed to weaken the witness's testimony and the plaintiff's case.

The Defendant's Case

After the plaintiff's case has been presented, it's the defendant's turn. Witnesses and evidence for the defendant's version of events are introduced. Like the plaintiff's witnesses, some defense witnesses may be expert witnesses. These are witnesses with special professional or technical knowledge, who can help shed light on the facts of the case.

Closing Arguments and Jury Instructions

The trial ends with the attorneys for each side summarizing the case they presented. Next, in a jury trial, the judge instructs the jury about the law as it applies to the case. Then the jury goes to another room so it can consider the evidence and come to a decision about the case.

The Medical Assistant Testifies

So what do you do if you're asked to testify as a witness in a lawsuit? Here are some points to remember:

- Require a subpoena—It's best not to volunteer to be a witness, especially if you'll be testifying against an employer or coworker. If you're subpoenaed, you have to appear whether you want to testify or not.
- Be truthful—You'll be testifying under oath. This means that if you lie, you'll be committing perjury, which is a crime. If you gave a deposition before the trial began, your answers are compared to your answers in court. Major differences can make your testimony less believable.
- Be professional—The image you present contributes to whether your statements are considered believable. Be dignified and remain calm and serious at all times.
- Answer the question—Do not give any information that was not asked for. Unless you're asked for your

opinion, give only the facts. If you don't know something, say so.

- Cooperate with your attorney—If your attorney objects to a question from the other side's attorney, don't answer the question unless the judge tells you to do so.
- Pay attention—It's important to pay attention, especially when you're being cross-examined. The opposing attorney will be trying to get you to say things that will weaken your side's case. Think before you speak. If you get tired and your mind starts to wander, ask the judge for a recess. This is a short break in the trial.

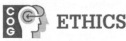 ETHICS

Ethics are guidelines for determining proper behavior. Laws do this, too, but they come from government. Ethics come from two sources.

- Personal ethics are guidelines to behavior that result from a person's morals and values.
- Professional ethics are standards of conduct that are set by professional organizations or that are generally accepted or expected by the people who work in a field.

Medical Ethics

Medical ethics are principles of conduct that govern the behavior of health care professionals. They focus on the rights, welfare, and concerns of patients. Medical ethics will affect your professional ethics as a medical assistant.

As there are more advances in the medical field, there are more ethical boundaries that must be explored. Bioethics deals with moral issues and questions that arise from advances in medicine and in the biological and health sciences. Some current bioethics issues involve:

- Questions of when life begins
- The morality of genetic engineering
- The ethics of stem cell research

When it comes to bioethical issues, religion and culture often play a significant role in what individuals believe to be right or wrong. This is especially the case with topics including stem cell research and abortion. As a medical assistant, it's important that you're aware and sensitive when dealing with such issues.

No medical professional can be successful for long if his conduct toward patients, physicians, or coworkers is unethical. Medical ethics determines medical customs, proper behavior in medical settings and situations, and professional courtesy. For example, stealing medications or prescription pads from the physician is not only illegal but unethical as well.

Values and Ethics

A person's values play an important role in how he or she acts. You may call on your own values when determining proper behavior in a professional setting.

- **Beneficence** means doing good, especially doing things that will benefit other people. Someone who possesses this value is caring and concerned with helping others.
- Humility is another value that affects personal behavior, showing modesty in your opinion of your own importance. A humble person doesn't think of himself as more important than someone else.

By having strong personal values, you'll find that it will be easier to behave correctly in a professional setting. And these personal values will not go unnoticed by your supervisors and staff. The physician will appreciate your contributions toward the success of her practice, and you'll benefit from great opportunities on the job.

Concern for Others

One sure sign of ethical behavior is that it shows respect and concern for others. The values discussed above focus more on other people than they do on the person who holds them.

But even values that don't appear to focus primarily on other people actually do. For example, look at the value of responsibility. Showing responsibility means being dependable and willing to accept the consequences of your actions. Acting responsibly means that you don't blame other people if something goes wrong. We all make mistakes, but it shows responsibility to admit when you've made a mistake and to take corrective action. Like beneficence and humility, responsibility shows that you consider other people's situations and feelings as important as your own.

Never forget that professional ethics require you to put other people's interests ahead of your own. In most professions, that means putting customers first. In health care, patients are the customers. Medical ethics require that medical professionals *always* put what's best for the patient ahead of all other concerns.

 LAWS VERSUS ETHICS

Learning and applying the principles of law and ethics can be complicated since they are closely related. At the same time, they are different in many ways.

For example, ethics often shapes behavior before laws do. Discrimination is a good example. Racial and gender discrimination were moral issues for some people long before laws made them illegal.

Legal and Ethical Limits

Another difference is that laws are more limited than ethics. That's because most legal standards are negative. Behaving lawfully often involves *not* doing something.

Think about this, unethical behavior can get you fired, and unlawful behavior can get you arrested.

Laws forbid us to harm people, but they usually don't require us to help them. It's illegal to rob someone, but no law requires you to call the police if you see someone being robbed. Ethical standards are more positive. Many people's ethics would cause them to call the police. Their morals would tell them it's the right thing to do.

Other people believe that they have no responsibility beyond obeying the law. They believe that a behavior is "wrong" only if the law forbids it. There are times when behaving lawfully is not necessarily acting ethically. Lying is one example. With the exception of slander and perjury, there's no law against lying, but most people would consider lying unethical. As a medical assistant, you'll encounter similar situations. That's just one more reason why understanding ethics is so important.

Ethical Dilemmas

This overlap of law and ethics can be confusing. As you just read, a behavior or action may be unethical, but it still may be legal. In other words, not all unethical acts are illegal. Again, lying is a good example.

On the other hand, most illegal acts are also unethical. Some illegal acts *can* be ethical, however. For example, although it's illegal to break into someone's home with the intent to rob the owners, however, it would be ethical to do so if an injured person inside needed help and breaking in was the only way to enter the home.

To make things even more complicated, as you've already read, personal ethics and professional ethics can sometimes clash. When ethics and law—or ethical standards—differ, a dilemma can result. A **dilemma** is a problem caused by a conflict between choices. In an ethical dilemma, the conflict is between rights, responsibilities, and values.

PROFESSIONAL ETHICS FOR THE MEDICAL ASSISTANT

As a medical assistant, your behavior must meet certain standards. This is important if you and your office are going to provide good customer service. But it's even more important to comply with the medical profession's ethical standards.

At the very minimum, medical ethics require that you:

- Protect the privacy of patient information
- Follow all state and federal laws
- Be honest in all your actions

You must always follow ethical standards as you perform your duties. Medical ethics require that your concern and focus always be on the rights, welfare, and concerns of patients. This means that you should show all patients the same kindness and respect.

At the same time, you must never share your personal opinions about medical issues with them. You also must ignore your personal feelings of right and wrong in dealing with patients. For example, if you believe that sexual relations between unmarried persons are immoral, you must not let your feelings affect how you treat single women seeking information about birth control.

Code of Ethics

Many professional groups write ethics codes to help their members understand how to behave ethically. The American Association of Medical Assistants (**AAMA**) is one of the national professional organizations for medical assistants. It has created five guidelines for medical assistants to follow.

1. Provide services with respect for human dignity.
2. Respect patient confidentiality, except when information is required by law.
3. Uphold the honor and high principles set forth by the AAMA.
4. Continually improve knowledge and skills for the benefit of patients and the health care team.
5. Take part in community services and activities that promote good health and welfare to the general public.

Confidentiality

Patient confidentiality is one of the most important ethical principles a medical assistant must observe. The medical assistant needs to understand and apply the laws that dictate when a patient's medical information can and can't be released. Any interactions with a patient are confidential, including your conversations and treatment. Patients will often reveal some of their innermost feelings, thoughts, and fears to their medical caregivers. Remember that this information is not for public knowledge.

So what do you do when a family member, clergy, or friend may want to know how a patient is doing? These questions are almost always asked with good intentions. However, it's both illegal and unethical to answer them or divulge any information about the patient without the patient's consent.

Being a Valued Medical Assistant

The most important value in any medical office is a commitment to putting patients first. This behavior is equally true for medical assistants. Your most important responsibility will be to place the patient's best interests first at all times. To do otherwise is highly unethical.

For example, are you familiar with the oath physicians take that states, "First do no harm"? Beneficence is the value expressed in this oath. As a medical assistant, you'll be representing the physician in many situations. Therefore, this standard of ethical behavior applies to you, too.

Empathy Not Sympathy

It's important to have empathy for patients. Empathy is imagining, understanding, and being sensitive to another person's experiences, thoughts, and feelings. Think of having empathy for others as putting yourself "in their shoes." However, empathy should not be confused with sympathy, which is feeling pity for someone. It's easy to feel sorry for patients sometimes, especially if they're suffering. But most patients will react better to someone who has empathy for them instead. It's important to show understanding for their situation, feelings, and views without feeling sorry for them. You should never say to a patient, "I know what you're going through!"

Professionalism and Personality

A medical assistant needs to exhibit personality as well as professionalism in the medical office. Acting professionally keeps you focused on ethical and legal standards of care. Being friendly makes your dealings with patients easier. It also makes patients feel like you know them, respect them, and care about them.

It's helpful to review the patient's medical record prior to his visit. This will help remind you about each particular patient and the information in the record. For example, if there's a note from the patient's last visit that said he was preparing to go on a cruise, ask how the trip was. Patients are very impressed when you show this kind of interest in them.

If you don't have specific questions, simply ask patients how they're feeling or if you can do anything else for them. They will remember that you went out of your way to help them, whether it was listening to their concerns or speaking in a kind manner. A cheerful, warm, and professional attitude will be a big help in doing your job.

Demonstrate Fidelity

Fidelity is faithfulness and loyalty to others. Professional ethics require you to perform your duties in a way that shows loyalty to your employer. But you have to be careful here. If your employer wants you do to something that is harmful to patients or is illegal or unethical in some other way, fidelity does *not* require you to do as the physician asked.

The Truth and Nothing But the Truth

Showing honesty means that you're truthful in every situation. **Veracity**, which means being truthful and honest, is an especially important value in professional ethics in the medical field. You must have the personal strength of character to admit you made an error. For example, if you give the wrong medication to a patient, you must notify your supervisor or the physician immediately.

In the medical profession, failing to admit mistakes can have very serious results, including great harm to patients and possible lawsuits.

High Standards

People with integrity are dedicated to maintaining high standards. **Integrity** is the quality of strongly sticking to your principles. For example, having integrity means that you wash your hands after all contact with every patient, even if no one is looking. Dependability and integrity go hand in hand. Integrity is demonstrated by being on time for work each day and not abusing your time at work. Once you arrive at work, you should be working. This means not tending to personal matters during the workday. You should leave personal matters such as phone calls until breaks, lunchtime, or even your day off.

 ETHICS IN ACTION

The American Association of Medical Assistants (AAMA) and the American Medical Technologists (**AMT**) have ethical codes that medical assistants need to adopt into their daily professional life.

AAMA Medical Assistant Creed

The AAMA Medical Assistant Creed focuses on integrity, fidelity, and other important values of professional ethics. Using the creed as a guide in working with patients and coworkers will help you act in an ethical manner.

- I believe in the principles and purposes of the profession of medical assisting.
- I endeavor to be more effective.
- I aspire to render greater service.
- I protect the confidence entrusted to me.
- I am dedicated to the care and well-being of all people.
- I am loyal to my employer.
- I am true to the ethics of my profession.
- I am strengthened by compassion, courage, and faith.

(Reprinted with permission from American Association of Medical Assistants.)

AMT Standards of Practice

The American Medical Technologists certifies medical assistants as Registered Medical Assistants (RMA). The organization adopted the following Standards of Practice, which define the essence of competent, honorable, and ethical behavior for an AMT-certified allied health care professional. Reported violations of these Standards are referred to the AMT Judiciary Committee and may result in revocation of the individual's certification or other disciplinary sanctions.

   I. While engaged in the Arts and Sciences that constitute the practice of their profession, AMT professionals shall be dedicated to the provision of competent and compassionate service and shall always meet or exceed the applicable standard of care.
  II. The AMT professional shall place the health and welfare of the patient above all else.
 III. When performing clinical duties and procedures, the AMT professional shall act within the lawful limits of any applicable scope of practice and when so required shall act under, and in accordance with appropriate supervision by an attending physician, dentist, or other licensed practitioner.
  IV. The AMT professional shall always respect the rights of patients and of fellow health care providers, shall comply with all applicable laws and regulations governing the privacy and confidentiality of protected health care information, and shall safeguard patient confidences unless legally authorized or compelled to divulge protected health care information to an authorized individual, law enforcement officer, or other legal or governmental entity.
   V. AMT professionals shall strive to increase their technical knowledge, shall continue to learn, and shall continue to apply and share scientific advances in their fields of professional specialization.
  VI. The AMT professional shall respect the law and pledges to avoid dishonest, unethical or illegal practices, breaches of fiduciary duty, or abuses of the position of trust into which the professional has been placed as a certified health care professional.
 VII. AMT professionals understand that they shall not make or offer a diagnosis or dispense medical advice unless they are duly licensed practitioners or unless specifically authorized to do so by an attending licensed practitioner acting in accordance with applicable law.
VIII. The AMT professional shall observe and value the judgment of the attending physician, dentist, or other attending licensed practitioner, provided that so doing does not clearly constitute a violation of law or pose an immediate threat to the welfare of the patient.
  IX. AMT professionals recognize that they are responsible for any personal wrongdoing and that they have an obligation to report to the proper authorities any knowledge of professional abuse or unlawful behavior by any party involved in the patient's diagnosis, care, and treatment.
   X. The AMT professional pledges to uphold personal honor and integrity and to cooperate in protecting and advancing, by every lawful means, the interests of the American Medical Technologists and its Members.

(Reprinted with permission from American Medical Technologists.)

Case Question

How do the AMT Standards of Practice apply to Elizabeth, the medical assistant in the case study at the beginning of this chapter?

Justice, Tolerance, and Perseverance

Justice is fairness in your actions toward all people. You behave justly when you apply the same rules to everyone. Another closely related value is tolerance, which means showing respect for people with opinions, beliefs, practices, or backgrounds that are different from your own. It's part of your ethical duty to show all patients the same kindness and respect, regardless of your personal feelings and opinions about them. These principles apply to your coworkers as well as the patients.

Health care can be a demanding field to work in. Perseverance, or continuing with an action despite obstacles, is a desirable quality for a medical assistant. It means that you're likely to get the job done, even when it's difficult.

The Responsible Employee

Responsibility is closely related to honesty and integrity. As you read earlier, it means being willing to answer for your actions, whether they were right or wrong. It also means that you can be depended on to do your job and to do it correctly. Responsibility is a sign of maturity in an employee.

Striving for Excellence

The duties of your position as a medical assistant will give you a high profile with patients. You'll be an important patient contact and provider of care. Professional ethics exist to guide you as you do this work. Professional ethics keep you focused on proper behavior and on providing outstanding customer service and care.

Behaving ethically shows dedication to your profession. Dedication to the standards of medical ethics will make you a model of excellence for patients, for your coworkers, and within the medical assisting community. Remember that your actions and words all reflect your values, ethics, and dedication to the profession of medical assisting.

THE MEDICAL ASSISTANT SCOPE OF PRACTICE

Every employee in a medical office must be careful to work within his scope of practice. A scope of practice is the range of activities that a health care worker is qualified to perform. In most cases, being "qualified" depends on the employee's level of education and training. For some medical professionals, such as physicians and nurses, scope of practice is determined by the laws governing the license they hold.

For medical assistants, scope of practice is less clear for a number of reasons.

- No state offers licensure to medical assistants.
- Training for medical assistants varies.
- Education levels vary from a few months to 2-year degree programs.

However, despite these obstacles, a general scope of practice for medical assistants does exist.

Study Skill

The study of law and ethics can be overwhelming with all the new terms and concepts. You need to make sure you are involved in your class. That means that you are there to learn, not to be taught. If you don't understand a term or something that the instructor says, YOU say something and ask questions. Confusion is definitely your worst enemy. Many students are embarrassed to ask questions publicly in class because they are concerned about what their classmates will think. Think about this— you are probably asking the very question that other students wish they would have asked. In a way you are probably doing them a favor. Take ownership of your education.

The Practice of Medical Assisting

Most states allow medical assistants to perform certain duties under the supervision of a licensed practitioner, such as a physician, nurse practitioner, or podiatrist. In fact, more than half the states allow a physician to assign basic clinical tasks to a medical assistant under the following conditions:

- The state's medical practice and nursing practice laws don't limit the task to physicians or nurses.
- The medical assistant has the training to perform the task safely.
- The medical assistant carries out the task under the physician's supervision.
- The physician takes responsibility for the medical assistant's actions.

A few states have laws that recognize the profession of medical assisting. Some of them even provide a scope of practice for medical assistants. South Dakota's law is a good example of a general guide. On the other hand, Arizona relies largely on the clinical and administrative competencies for medical assistants established by the Commission on Accreditation of Allied Health Education Programs (**CAAHEP**). These competencies are the skills you must master if you want to become a Certified Medical Assistant (**CMA**) by the American Association of Medical Assistants (AAMA) or a Registered Medical Assistant (**RMA**) by the American Medical Technologists (AMT).

What Medical Assistants Can Do

Over the years since medical assisting became a well-recognized profession, the tasks and duties have been identified based on medical assistant surveys conducted by national certification agencies. These tasks have been classified into administrative (front office) and clinical (back office) duties. Common administrative tasks include the following:

- Answering phones and scheduling appointments
- Greeting patients
- Setting up referral appointments
- Arranging for hospital admissions and lab services
- Updating and filing patient medical records
- Completing and submitting insurance claim forms
- Handling correspondence, billing, and bookkeeping

Clinical duties as a medical assistant can depend on the laws of the state where you work. They also can depend on the size and specialty of your medical office as well as the state medical practice laws. Common clinical tasks for medical assistants include:

- Obtaining patient medical histories
- Explaining treatment procedures to patients
- Preparing patients for examination
- Assisting the physician during examinations
- Collecting and preparing laboratory specimens
- Performing waived laboratory tests
- Instructing patients about medications and special diets
- Preparing and giving medications as directed by the physician
- Managing prescription refills as directed by the physician

- Performing venipuncture
- Performing electrocardiograms and setting up Holter monitors
- Removing sutures and changing dressings

Limits of the Scope of Practice

It's important for you to be aware of any limits your state puts on the activities of medical assistants—especially in the clinical area. For example, in some states, medical assistants may initiate and administer intravenous fluids. However, most states do not allow medical assistants to be involved with IV therapy.

It's the physician's responsibility to know what medical assistants can and can't do—either as set by state law or by a medical assistant's training and experience. A physician must not assign you activities that are beyond your scope of practice. Nor can the physician assign you tasks that are clearly not permitted by your state's laws. It's equally important that you don't perform them on your own. Exceeding your scope of practice, whether by the physician's order or on your own, is illegal as well as unethical. You're only covered under your physician's malpractice insurance if you're acting within your scope of practice. So, not only is exceeding your scope of practice poor customer service to patients, but it could also get both you and your employer sued.

Do Not Do List

Now we know what a medical assistant could do but remember that the scope of practice varies from state to state. Here are some tasks that have been identified in various states that medical assistants *cannot* perform:

- Independently diagnose symptoms, interpret test results, or treat patients
- Advise patients about their condition or treatment
- Independently write or refill prescriptions or give out medication samples
- Flush or discontinue IVs or inject medications into veins (vessels that carry blood from other parts of the body to the heart)
- Insert urinary catheters (tubes used to drain fluid from the body) or perform punctures of arteries (vessels that carry blood from the heart to other parts of the body)
- Perform tests that involve penetration of human tissues, except for skin tests and drawing blood from veins, where permitted by law
- Administer anesthetics (substances that make the body unable, or less able, to feel pain), except for anesthetic skin creams
- Operate laser equipment, practice physical therapy, or place splints on injured limbs

 # STANDARD OF CARE

The medical assistant must understand the importance of working within the legal and ethical scope of practice. But your legal and ethical responsibilities as a medical assistant don't end there. You must also provide an acceptable standard of care. Standard of care is the level of performance that's expected of a health care worker in carrying out assigned duties.

Like scope of practice, standard of care is closely linked to education and training. For example, physicians are held to a higher standard of care than are medical assistants. That's because physicians have more education and training than medical assistants do.

Unlike your scope of practice, standard of care as a medical assistant does not depend on your *own* skills and training. That's because the standard of care for each medical profession is set by the knowledge that's typical for workers in that profession. No matter what your own background is, the standard of care expected from you depends on what's reasonable to expect from the average medical assistant. This is called the reasonable person standard.

Both standard of care and scope of practice are important in avoiding the legal problems.

Duty of Care

Duty of care is another important part of standard of care. Duty of care is the legal obligation, or duty, a health care worker has to patients and sometimes to nonpatients as well.

For example, you must keep a patient's health information private and confidential. If you don't, you've breached your duty of care to the patient and have therefore not provided the proper standard of care. **Breach** is a failure to do what's required or what you have been expected to do under contract.

Duty of Obedience

The duty to follow orders is a duty of care that you owe both to your employer and to your patients. It includes the duty to:

- Interpret the physician's instructions and carry them out.
- Ask for clarification if the instructions are unclear or seem wrong.
- Immediately tell the physician if the orders appear to be harmful or dangerous for the patient. You must *not* follow any orders that seem inappropriate.

Duty of Truth

Telling the truth is a legal duty. It means that health care professionals must deal honestly and openly with patients at all times. Patients have a right to know their past and current medical status. Physicians have a duty to tell patients when their diagnosis changes as test results and other information are analyzed. It also involves making sure patients understand the risks of any treatments they agree to have. Medical assistants have the duty to be truthful with physicians and coworkers no matter the consequences. Not telling the truth may ultimately cost the medical assistant their job but more importantly it may cause harm or injury to a patient.

The Reasonable Person Standard

Has a health care worker provided an acceptable standard of care to a patient? Has the worker met his duty of care to the patient? Both questions are central to knowing whether a patient who feels wronged has a legal case against the health care provider. One way such questions are answered in court is by applying the reasonable person standard.

The reasonable person standard is a legal principle that every person has a duty to behave as a "reasonable person" would in the same circumstances. What's "reasonable" partly depends on the person involved. For example, a medical assistant who's assisting victims at an accident scene would be held to a higher standard of reasonable behavior than a person with no medical training. The standard for the medical assistant would be the behavior that could reasonably be expected from a medical assistant in that situation. The question that is usually asked is, "What would someone with the same level of training have done in this situation?" Failure to meet the reasonable person standard could lead to charges of negligence, the failure to act with proper or reasonable care.

PRIVACY AND CONFIDENTIALITY

One of the most important duties of care that you—and all health care professionals—owe to patients is the confidentiality of their personal information. Breaking patient confidentiality is a breach of professional ethics as well as a serious violation of federal law.

Patient Privacy and HIPAA

The Health Insurance Portability and Accountability Act of 1996 (HIPAA) protects the privacy of a patient's personal and health information. This law has brought sweeping changes to the health care industry. Its original purpose was to:

* Improve health benefits for workers who change jobs
* Reduce costs by streamlining the health care system
* Simplify the processing of health insurance claims

HIPAA changed how the health care system operates in four major areas:

1. Transactions
   * Creates a single national standard for how diagnoses and treatments are identified and coded on bills for services
   * Requires that bills to insurance companies be submitted electronically (by computer)
2. Privacy
   * Defines what patient information must be considered private
   * Regulates how patient information must be handled and used
   * Sets the conditions under which private patient information can be disclosed
3. Security
   * Sets standards for protecting patient information that is stored on computers and sent to others electronically, including lab test results and electronic medical records
   * Requires the use of passwords, firewalls, antivirus software, and encryption software on computers that contain or transmit patient information
4. Identification
   * Creates a national system of codes for identifying individual health care providers, health insurance plans, employers, and patients
   * Requires that each provider or health insurance plan include its identifying code on all electronic transmissions

HIPAA and its privacy rule are extremely important and will affect your work as a medical assistant.

Congress empowered the U.S. Department of Health and Human Services (**HHS**) to issue rules that set the standards for patient privacy. These administrative rules have the same authority as statutes. They must be obeyed.

Except where its release is required or allowable by law, all information about a patient is confidential. In general, however, here are some basic things you need to know on this subject to avoid allegations of breach of duty and malpractice.

* All of a patient's personal data are confidential, including name and address, phone number, employment information, and insurance information.
* All health information is confidential. This includes the patient's medical history, diagnosis, tests ordered, test results, treatments, medications administered in the office, and prescriptions.
* All written or oral communication between the patient and medical office employees is confidential.
* A patient's current appointment and appointment history is confidential.
* Even the information that a person is a patient of the practice is confidential.

The Privacy Rule

The HHS privacy rule is a huge document that greatly affects how a medical office must operate. Here are some of the rule's key provisions that are important for you to know.

- All records containing any items (called "patient identifiers") that could link their contents to a specific patient must be treated as protected health information (**PHI**).
- Except as required by law or allowed by the privacy rule, PHI may not be disclosed to others without the patient's written permission.
- Only the information that is needed should be supplied. For example, if an insurance company is being billed for a specific treatment, only the parts of the medical record related to that treatment should be disclosed.
- Patients have a right to view and receive copies of their own medical records, except in very limited and specific circumstances.
- Patients have a right to know to whom their PHI has been disclosed, except in very limited circumstances.
- Each health care provider must have a privacy notice—a document that states its privacy policies and practices, referred to as a Notice of Privacy Practices (**NPP**).
- Each health care provider must train its employees about the HHS privacy rule and appoint a privacy officer to be in charge of its enforcement.

Patient Identifiers

HIPAA recognizes the following items as patient identifiers. If even one of them appears in any patient materials, it makes those materials PHI. Unless all of these identifiers are removed from the information, the privacy rule applies:

- Name
- Address
- Zip code
- Phone number
- Fax number
- E-mail address
- Date of birth
- Birth certificate
- Social Security number
- Medical record number
- Health plan numbers
- Driver's license
- Vehicle identification number
- License plate number
- Web site address
- Fingerprints and voiceprints
- Photos

To truly protect a patient's identity, if any of these patient identifiers appears in a patient's medical records, the records must be treated as private information.

Cultural Connection

What's in a name? In the Hmong culture, there are 18 clans (groups) and all members of each clan have the same last name. The Hmong are an Asian ethnic group from the mountainous regions of Thailand, China, and Vietnam. Within the United States, the Hmong population is located in the upper Midwest, predominately in Wisconsin and Minnesota, and also in California. Most Hmong men have three names: (1) the clan name, (2) the name given to a newborn during a naming ceremony, and (3) an adult name given at the rite of passage into manhood. When dealing with patients of this ethnicity, it is important to correctly reflect the person's full legal name for documentation purposes.

The Privacy Notice

Patients visiting the office for the first time must receive a copy of the office's privacy notice, NPP, stating its policies and practices for protecting patient confidentiality and handling PHI. The notice must contain the following information:

- The ways the office uses PHI—for example, using the patient's phone number to call with appointment reminders—and the patient's right to object to such uses
- The circumstances in which the office may disclose a patient's PHI without obtaining the patient's consent
- The patient's legal rights concerning how his PHI is handled
- The name, address, and phone number of the office's privacy officer, should the patient have any questions or requests

Many offices ask patients to sign a second copy of the privacy notice to show that they received the notice and understand its contents. The signed copy is placed in the patient's record.

When Confidentiality Doesn't Apply

The privacy rule allows providers to release PHI without the patient's permission in the following circumstances:

- To a family member or other individual who is directly responsible for the patient's care, such as in the case of a mentally incompetent adult who is cared for by an adult sister or brother
- To other health care providers who become involved in the patient's care
- To attorneys, public health officials, and law enforcement authorities, where required by court order or state law

To Tell or Not To Tell

A patient's lab tests show that he has a sexually transmitted disease. He begs the medical assistant to say nothing to his wife about his test result. He says, "My marriage will be ruined if she finds out I've been unfaithful!" The medical assistant knows the wife needs to be tested—and treated if she's contracted the disease. Should the medical assistant say something to the wife?

Whether the patient asks that his secret be kept or not, the medical assistant must not say anything to the wife. The law may require that the positive test result be reported to the health department. But it's up to the health department to contact the patient's sexual partners. Professional ethics requires the medical assistant to respect patient confidentiality.

These exceptions are generally listed on the privacy notice that providers are required to give to patients. Though it isn't required that a patient sign a consent form for the medical office to obtain payment from a health plan for treatment every time the patient comes in, the patient is required to sign a consent form that allows the medical office to release the patient's information to their insurance company. This consent is signed during the patient's first visit and is valid for that day's visit as well as subsequent visits and treatments.

REGULATORY CONCERNS IN THE MEDICAL OFFICE

Medical practices need to be aware of the laws that affect the management of patients within the practice. Most of these exist to protect the patient and provide rights to the patients.

Patient Self-Determination Act

In1991, Congress passed the Patient Self-Determination Act (**PSDA**). The act states that a patient has the right to make decisions regarding their own medical care. The decisions include the right to accept or refuse treatment and the right to have an advance directive. Health care institutions (not individual doctors) are required by law to provide patients with a summary of the PSDA when they are admitted to the institution. Figure 2-3 is a sample of an advance directive form that a person will complete and have notarized when they are still able to make decisions regarding their health care. The advance directive states that when the person becomes terminal that they do not wish to have lifesaving measures taken. For example, if the person's heart stops beating, the caregivers would not perform CPR to resuscitate the person.

Durable Power of Attorney for Health Care

This is very similar to a financial power of attorney but only covers medical decisions. The person selects an agent who will act on behalf of the person if the person is unable to make their own decisions. A physician needs to certify that the person lacks the competence to make their own health care decisions.

Living Will

A Living Will, also known as an Advance Medical Directive, allows a person to declare their wishes for managing end of life care when diagnosed with a terminal condition or in a permanently unconscious state of mind or conscious but with irreversible brain damage. A Living Will usually indicates that the person does not want to be kept alive with the use of mechanical or support systems including hydration and supplemental nutrition.

Uniform Anatomical Gift Act

The Uniform Anatomical Gift Act (UAGA), initially passed in 1968, establishes the standards used when donating body organs for the purpose of transplant or research. It also sets the criteria for donation of the entire body (cadaver) for use in medical education and research. The Act allows for a surviving spouse or specific relative(s) to authorize the gift of donation. The UAGA also prohibits trafficking of human organs or making any profit from the donation of human body organs. Most states allow anatomical gift donation to be noted on the state driver's license.

Americans with Disabilities Act Amendments Act

The Americans with Disabilities Act, 1990, was designed to protect individuals with disabilities from discrimination. The Americans with Disabilities Amendments Act (**ADAAA**), enacted in 2008, was intended to provide a more clear and comprehensive definition regarding individuals with disabilities. The Act describes a disability as a physical or mental impairment that substantially limits one or more major life activities including, but not limited to:

- Caring for oneself
- Performing manual tasks
- Seeing, hearing, eating, sleeping, walking, standing, lifting, bending, speaking, breathing, learning, reading, concentrating, thinking, communicating, and working
- Major bodily functions of the immune system, normal cell growth, digestive, bowel, bladder, neurological, brain, respiratory, circulatory, endocrine, and reproductive systems

ADVANCE DIRECTIVE

UNIFORM ADVANCE DIRECTIVE OF [list name of declarant]

To my family, physician, attorney, and anyone else who may become responsible for my health, welfare, or affairs, I make this declaration while I am of sound mind.

If I should ever become in a terminal state and there is no reasonable expectation of my recovery, I direct that I be allowed to die a natural death and that my life not be prolonged by extraordinary measures. I do, however, ask that medication be mercifully administered to me to alleviate suffering, even though this may shorten my remaining life.

This statement is made after full reflection and is in accordance with my full desires. I want the above provisions carried out to the extent permitted by law. Insofar as they are not legally enforceable, I wish that those to whom this will is addressed will regard themselves as morally bound by this instrument.

If permissible in the jurisdiction in which I may be hospitalized I direct that in the event of a terminal diagnosis, the physicians supervising my care discontinue feeding should the continuation of feeding be judged to result in unduly prolonging a natural death.

If permissible in the jurisdiction in which I may be hospitalized I direct that in the event of a terminal diagnosis, the physicians supervising my care discontinue hydration (water) should the continuation of hydration be judged to result in unduly prolonging a natural death.

I herewith authorize my spouse, if any, or any relative who is related to me within the third degree to effectuate my transfer from any hospital or other health care facility in which I may be receiving care should that facility decline or refuse to effectuate the instructions given herein.

I herewith release any and all hospitals, physicians, and others for myself and for my estate from any liability for complying with this instrument.

Signed:

_____
[list name of declarant]

City of residence: _____
[city of residence]

County of residence: _____
[county of residence]

State of residence: _____
[state of residence]

Social Security Number: _____
[social security number]

Date: _____

_____
Witness

_____
Witness

STATE OF _____

COUNTY OF _____

This day personally appeared before me, the undersigned authority, a Notary Public in and for _____ County, _____ State,

_____   _____ (Witnesses)

who, being first duly sworn, say that they are the subscribing witnesses to the declaration of [list name of declarant], the declarant, signed, sealed, and published and declared the same as and for his declaration, in the presence of both these affiants; and that these affiants, at the request of said declarant, in the presence of each other, and in the presence of said declarant, all present at the same time, signed their names as attesting witnesses to said declaration.

Affiants further say that this affidavit is made at the request of [list name of declarant], declarant, and in his presence, and that [list name of declarant] at the time the declaration was executed, in the opinion of the affiants, of sound mind and memory, and over the age of eighteen years.

Taken, subscribed and sworn to before me by _____ (witness) and

_____ (witness) this _____ day of _____, 20_____.

My commission expires: _____

_____ Notary Public

Figure 2-3 Sample of advance directive form. (Reprinted from Kronenberger J, Ledbetter J. *Jones & Bartlett Learning's Comprehensive Medical Assisting*, 5th ed. Burlington, MA: Jones & Bartlett Learning, LLC; 2016.)

Health Information Technology for Economic and Clinical Health Act

The Health Information Technology for Economic and Clinical Health Act (HITECH) was designed to allow patients the right to inspect, amend, and restrict access to his/her medical record. Patients are allowed to have access to their Protected Health Information (PHI) and request amendments to the record if errors are found. They also can select who can receive their medical information and what specific information can be released.

Genetic Information Nondiscrimination Act

GINA, the Genetic Information Nondiscrimination Act of 2008, was designed to prohibit the use of genetic information when determining health insurance coverage or benefits and during employment decisions including hiring and deciding promotions of individuals. Individuals cannot be denied health insurance coverage nor can they be charged a higher premium because of their genetic information that might indicate that they are predisposed to develop a specific disease in the future.

Preparing for Externship

During your externship, you must perform within the medical assistant scope of practice. You should also only perform those procedures taught in class and that you feel confident to complete. Remember that one of the most important professional qualities of a professional medical assistant is confidentiality. HIPAA should be on your mind with everything you do at the externship. Although you may be tempted to discuss your externship experience with your friends and family, you cannot even share patient information with your classmates. Your school has developed an official affiliation with your externship facility. In the affiliation agreement, there are numerous requirements of the students when assigned to the site. One of these is the requirement that students maintain the Privacy Laws of HIPAA.

Chapter Recap

- Medical office employees need to have a good understanding of law and ethics in order to act appropriately, to make decisions in difficult situations, and to provide a high standard of customer service and medical care. Failure to act legally and ethically at all times can lead to lawsuits and loss of income for the office. It can also put you in conflict with the law.
- Laws are rules of conduct that government creates and requires people to obey. Ethics are guidelines for proper behavior that come from other sources than government. The main sources of ethics are personal morals, values, codes of conduct established by professional organizations, and standards that are generally expected by professionals who work in that field.
- Morals are a person's ideas about right and wrong, while values are generally accepted principles of importance and worth. Both may result from the influences of the person's family and culture. Rules for polite behavior are called **etiquette**. Like values and morals, etiquette is determined by culture.
- Law and ethics overlap but are not identical. Some behaviors that are legal may be unethical. However, nearly all behaviors that are illegal are unethical, too.

- Unethical behaviors can cause a medical professional to be fired. Illegal behaviors can lead to a medical professional's arrest. Both types of behaviors can result in lawsuits.
- Medical assistants who perform their duties in a legal and ethical manner show high levels of professionalism, provide good customer service, and reduce the possibility that lawsuits will result from their actions.
- A medical assistant's scope of practice is determined by her training and experience, as well as by any state laws that may apply.
- The American Association of Medical Assistants (AAMA) and American Medical Technologists (AMT) maintain lists of knowledge, skills, and duties common to the profession of medical assisting.
- Standard of care is determined by the education and training needed to practice a particular profession. Because physicians have more education and training, they are held to a higher standard of care than medical assistants are.
- Each health care professional is expected to follow orders, be truthful, and generally act as a reasonable member of the profession.

- A harmful act that's purposely committed is called an intentional tort. Many intentional torts are also crimes.
- An unintentional tort is a wrongful act that's committed accidentally, without intent to do harm.
- A person who commits an intentional or unintentional tort is called a tortfeasor.
- Negligence can occur in any of three ways: malfeasance is a wrong and unlawful act; misfeasance is a lawful act performed improperly; and nonfeasance is the failure to perform an act that should have been performed.
- In general, to prove negligence, the injured party must prove that: the tortfeasor owed a *duty* of care, the tortfeasor is guilty of *dereliction of duty* by not providing a proper standard of care, harm or injury was a *direct cause* of that failure of duty, and the harm was serious enough to require the tortfeasor to pay *damages* to the injured party.
- HIPAA rules establish which patient information is confidential and when a patient's information may and may not be disclosed. They also require that patients be given a printed notice of the medical office's policies and practices regarding privacy.
- Laws come from three sources: legislative, executive, and judicial branches.
- Criminal law involves felonies and misdemeanors.
- Civil law covers wrongful acts that aren't crimes, including family issues, contract disputes, and torts.

- Civil suits come about when one party (the plaintiff) claims to be injured by the actions of another party (the defendant) and sues the accused party. A judge or jury then finds in favor of the plaintiff or defendant and awards damages, if applicable.
- In the medical office, *respondeat superior* means your employer is responsible for your actions when you act within your scope of practice.
- For a contract to be valid, three things must be present: offer and acceptance, consideration, and competence.
- Contracts may be expressed in writing or implied through action or lack of action.
- When terminating a contract, the physician must notify the patient by letter, allowing the patient 30 days to choose another physician. The letter should state the reason for termination, make the patient's records available for transfer to another physician, and recommend further treatments and care, if necessary.
- The Patient Self Determination Act was designed to provide individuals with the ability to make decisions about their end of life care.
- The HITECH Act was passed to include rules that protect the patient's health information and their access to that information.
- The Genetic Information Non-Discrimination Act was designed to protect individuals from discrimination when applying for health insurance or during the employment process.

Online Resources for Students

Student Resources available on the text's online site include:
- Audio Glossaries
- Animations
- Competency Evaluation Forms

- Videos
- Anatomy & Physiology Module with Heart and Lung Sounds
- Weblinks
- Worksheets

Exercises and Activities

Certification Preparation Questions

1. The range of activities a medical professional is qualified to perform is called:
   a. scope of practice.
   b. standard of care.
   c. duty of care.
   d. reasonable person standard.
   e. standard of practice

2. Which of the following is not legally performed by a medical assistant?
   a. Taking medical histories
   b. Removing sutures and changing dressings
   c. Performing venipuncture
   d. Interpreting test results
   e. Performing electrocardiograms

3. What is a tortfeasor?

   a. A victim of a tort.
   b. A person who commits a tort.
   c. An attorney who sues a physician for a tort.
   d. A person who fails to take the proper action.
   e. The plaintiff in a lawsuit.

4. In the medical profession, negligence is known as:

   a. malpractice.
   b. duty of care.
   c. dereliction of duty.
   d. direct cause.
   e. a misdemeanor.

5. Who is always the plaintiff in a criminal case?

   a. The government
   b. The person accused of a crime
   c. The judge
   d. The person who has been harmed
   e. The physician

6. Which of the following does *not* have to be proven in a medical malpractice case?

   a. Direct or proximate cause
   b. *Res ipsa loquitur*
   c. Duty of care
   d. The reasonable person standard
   e. *Respondeat superior*

7. When is the *only* time you should provide someone with the original of a patient's medical record?

   a. If the patient has signed a release of medical records
   b. If the patient's attorney asks for it
   c. If photocopies of the records are not readable
   d. If the original record is subpoenaed
   e. If the patient's family requests it

8. An order issued by the court to obtain evidence is:

   a. a deposition.
   b. a discovery.
   c. an interrogatory.
   d. a subpoena.
   e. an implied contract.

9. Threatening a person or acting in a way that causes the person to fear harm is called:

   a. assault.
   b. battery.
   c. fraud.
   d. libel.
   e. slander.

10. The common law principle that employers are responsible for the actions of their employees is:

    a. *res ipsa loquitur.*
    b. *respondeat superior.*
    c. *stare decisis.*
    d. *subpoena duces tecum.*
    e. *tortfeasor.*

 Internet Activities

1. Access the Web site www.genome.gov to read more about GINA, the Genetic Information Non-Discrimination Act of 2008. Research-specific information regarding hiring practices and the illegal use of genetic information.

2. Access the Web site www.uslegal.com and research the age of majority in various states throughout the United States.

3 Medical Office Procedures

Chapter Objectives

- Review of functions of computers in the medical office.
- Explain the proper use and function of an organization's intranet.
- Discuss general guidelines for computerized appointment scheduling.
- Review various computer programs used within the health care environment.
- Discuss the importance of proper computer ethics.
- Create professional e-mails.
- Review guidelines for opening of e-mail attachments and potential hazards.
- Maintaining password and computer security.
- Understand basic Internet safety and usage.
- Discuss the role and goals of quality improvement.
- Summarize the guidelines for completing incident reports.
- Perform an inventory of supplies and equipment.

CAAHEP & ABHES Competencies

CAAHEP

- Perform routine maintenance of administrative and clinical equipment.
- Perform an inventory with documentation.
- Explain the purpose of routine maintenance of administrative and clinical equipment.
- List steps involved in completing an inventory.
- Explain the importance of data backup.

ABHES

- Maintain inventory of equipment and supplies.
- Perform routine maintenance of administrative equipment.

Chapter Terms

Cookies
Encryption
Firewalls

Incident reports
Intranet
Inventory

Meaningful Use
Privileged information
Risk management

Service contract
Unsecure information
Viruses

Abbreviations

CLIA	EHR/EMR	HIPAA	QI
CMS	HHS	POL	SSL

To be successful, a medical office must function efficiently and effectively. As a medical assistant, you'll have an important role in making sure the office runs smoothly. Appointment schedules must be made and followed. Patients' electronic medical records (**EMR**)/electronic health records (**EHR**) along other privileged information must be accurately and securely maintained. Systems must be in place to ensure that the office has a steady flow of income and that it provides high-quality care. This includes insuring that equipment is kept in good working order and needed supplies are on hand at all times.

 ## THE OFFICE COMPUTER SYSTEM

Computers are vital to the daily operation of a medical office. You will utilize the computer for almost every function in the office including, but not limited to:

- Electronic health records
- Preparing letters and memos
- Scheduling patient appointments
- Processing insurance claims
- Posting charges and payments to patients' accounts
- Ensuring lab results are available for the physician
- Ordering and charting physician prescribed medications

As you can see, being a medical assistant requires good computer skills. One of the most important aspects of computer use in the health care environment is security. There are steps that must be followed and maintained to ensure privileged information is protected. First, keep all computer passwords secure. Do not share your password with anyone. If you must record your password, never leave it out where others can view it.

Computer Care

Computers are key pieces of administrative equipment. Computers do require special attention, however. Here are some guidelines for taking care of your computer.

- Keep your computer in a cool, dry area out of direct sunlight. Excess heat and humidity can damage its parts.
- Keep computers away from magnets.
- Do not eat or drink while working at the computer.

- Plug your computer into a surge protector instead of directly into the electrical outlet. Without surge protection, changes in the office's power supply could damage the computer's parts.
- Your computer should have a battery backup power source. This will prevent loss of data in the effort of a power outage.
- Your office computer should be cleaned regularly. Follow these steps:
  - Remove any CDs, DVDs, or flash drives and close all programs that are running.
  - Shut down the CPU and turn off the monitor.
  - Clean the monitor screen with antistatic wipes. Do not use a regular glass cleaner.
  - Turn the keyboard face down so any loose debris can fall out. Do not shake or tap the keyboard.
  - Use a can of compressed air to blow the remaining dust and particles from under the keyboard's keypads.

Electronic Tablet

Many physicians and office staff use handheld devices such as tablets. Information can be entered with a stylus or on a small keyboard. The physician can use this device to send information to the main system and receive information from it. Figure 3-1 shows a physician using a handheld tablet device, which can be used to access the Internet or the practice software system to review patient data.

Some offices use this system to send messages to and from the physician regarding patient care. These are

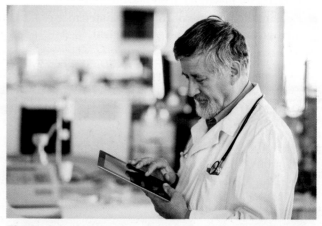

Figure 3-1 Doctor using handheld tablet. (Image from Shutterstock.com.)

often referred to as tasks. Here are some other things a physician or staff can do with their handhelds:

- Access patients' charts.
- View financial data.
- Access medical and pharmacy information.
- View procedures, x-rays, and labs.

The Intranet

An **intranet** is an internal business system that gives you quick access to company information including:

- Policy and procedure manuals
- Common office forms
- Phone lists
- Staff schedules
- Office newsletters or job postings
- Agendas for upcoming meetings
- Local hospital information
- Support for videoconferencing
- Links to other departments; like human relations and educational opportunities

Computer Scheduling

Scheduling patients by computer is more efficient than using a paper appointment book. User-friendly scheduling software helps you find open appointment times more quickly. It also lets you make changes more easily. Good scheduling software should perform the following functions:

- Offer an unlimited comment area near the patient's name; this lets you add special reminder notes for the appointment—for instance, "Patient wants a pregnancy test."
- Keep a list of patients who want to move their appointments if a more suitable one becomes available.
- Print notices to remind patients that they need to make appointments; for example, the program could be set to alert patients who regularly have an annual Pap smear that it's time to make an appointment.

Specific types of appointment software can connect to the appointment software of other offices. This is useful if a patient needs to be seen by a health care provider in another office. You can make the patient an appointment with the other provider without having to call his or her office. Some software allows patients to schedule their own appointments using the Internet. This convenience can result in fewer calls to the office and happier patients.

Patient Tracking

Software programs are designed to help the office run more efficiently by tracking the flow of patients. Here are just of few of the things this software can do:

- Show which days of the week tend to be busiest or the slowest and which have the most canceled appointments; this information can help schedule staff more efficiently.
- Track the activity of providers; for example, one physician may average 45 minutes per patient. Another may average 30 minutes. This kind of information can help you in scheduling appointments.
- Track the time patients wait in the reception area or an examination room; long waiting times can show a need for better procedures or more staff.

Insurance Submission

Software programs are used to send claims via the computer's modem or cable lines to the patient's health insurance company. Filing claims this way results in faster payment. It also allows you to track the progress of claims better and identify any problems that could cause a delay in payment.

Other insurance programs perform other functions, such as:

- Allow you to check that the patient is eligible for coverage.
- Provide preapproval of certain procedures and hospital admissions.
- Help you properly code health care services when submitting claims for insurance.

Federal law now requires that nearly all insurance claims be submitted by computer.

Financial Management

A large number of programs can help you with the office's finances. Some of them track accounts receivable (money that's owed to the office) and accounts payable (money the office owes to others). Other programs will figure what each patient owes and prepare the bills the office mails out each month. Here are some examples of even more financial software:

- Some programs alert you when a patient's account is seriously past due. They even have form letters that you can send to demand payment.
- Some software accepts and automatically deposits insurance payments directly in the office's bank account. This saves you from having to handle, record, process, and deposit these payments yourself.
- Special software will let the office take payments by credit card. Some patients will want to pay what they owe this way.

Always check a patient's account before having the computer prepare a collection letter. Collection letters should be sent only when necessary.

Other Software

A medical office needs a word processing system to run effectively. This is the software that lets you compose letters, address envelopes, and prepare other kinds of documents.

Software programs are also available that manage the office payroll and employees' personnel records.

Some programs can even document that your office is complying with **HIPAA**—the Health Insurance Portability and Accountability Act. This federal law requires health care providers to follow certain rules about patients' privacy.

Clinical Software

Medical software is not just for office administration. Some programs have valuable clinical uses. Software assists the delivery of health care, too. Here are just three examples of what clinical software can do.

- Some programs insert lab reports directly into a patient's chart. This eliminates errors that can occur when a person records the results in the chart. Most of these programs also alert the physician when a new report has been received.
- Programs help physicians write prescriptions. This eliminates errors from poor handwriting. Some programs warn the physician if the prescription is not correct for the patient's medical condition or with other drugs the patient is taking.
- With some programs, physicians can view x-rays and other tests on the computer. The physician does not have to wait for the written report. She can judge the test results herself.

In an effort to encourage physicians to utilize certified EHR technology as an avenue to increase the quality of patients' care the CMS created Meaningful Use. CMS defines **Meaningful Use** as "the use of certified EHR technology in a meaningful manner..." (cdc.gov/ehrmeaningfuluse/introduction.html).

Computer Ethics

Computers aid in the efficient operation of the office. They also make it much easier to gather and provide information. However, a computer's usefulness also has a potential for abuse. Misuse can lead to invasion of patients' privacy and other unethical behavior.

Here are some tips for using the office computers. If you follow these guidelines, your computer use will remain ethical and legal:

- Never share your password. Each employee should have his or her own password.
- Never use another person's password to get patient information. If you're authorized to see this information, ask for a password of your own.
- If you can access a lab's computer to get test results, don't obtain results on people who are not office patients. For example, suppose that your son had a test at another doctor's office that was sent to a lab to which you have access. You shouldn't look up his test results, even though he's your son.
- Never leave a patient's information displayed on the monitor and walk away from a computer. Close the file before leaving your computer.
- Don't use the office computer to surf the Internet for personal reasons. This isn't appropriate behavior at work.
- Never load any software into your office computer unless you have permission. Doing this could cause conflicts with the office software as well as other problems.

Ethical Dilemma

Your office has been working short staffed for months. A new medical assistant has joined the team. She is eager and willing to help alleviate the workload everyone has been enduring. The office manager has not received a password for her and mentions to you that if you were to share your password just for a few days so that things could run smoother, she would not report it. Passwords are linked directly to the person to whom they are assigned; therefore, anything that is entered using a specific password becomes that person's responsibility.

Case Study

Your office has a strict policy on e-mailing of patient's **privileged information**. As part of their HIPAA compliance, they maintain a policy prohibiting the e-mail of privileged information. Matthew McNeil, a well-established patient, called to report that he and his family are out of the country on vacation and he needs a copy of the x-ray report for his daughter, Sarah, who injured her arm while under that care of your office physician. He is asking for the report to be e-mailed to him. While on this family vacation, Sarah was skiing and injured her arm, and he wants to have the x-ray report to show the physician where they are vacationing. You explain your office policy to Mr. McNeil and he becomes very upset. He pleads for you to make an exception, just this once. He promises not to tell anyone.

Case Questions

How would you respond to Mr. McNeil if you were the office medical assistant? Is there anything you might do to try to assist Sarah's father with his request?

Professional E-mail

It is critical that all correspondence that leaves the medical office is professional and appropriate. This includes all e-mail messages sent. Use these tips to maintain a professional tone in your e-mail messages:

- Follow office protocol regarding what can and can't be e-mailed. As in the case study, it would only take one e-mail to breach compliance.
- Always check your spelling, grammar, and punctuation before you send any e-mails. Poor grammar or incorrect spelling can take away from your message.
- Keep messages short and to the point. Remember, you are not entertaining the reader. You are communicating information to him or her.
- Avoid colored fonts or cute figures in your e-mails. Imagine your e-mail as a typewritten business letter.
- Always fill in the subject line. Give the reader a sense of what your e-mail is about. For example, "Staff meeting tomorrow," tells your reader the essence of the message.
- Never send an e-mail to the physician about an emergency situation. Call or page the physician instead.

Here are some guidelines for using your office computer's e-mail program:

- Don't read e-mails for the physician or other staff that are sent to the office's general e-mail address. Each staff member should have his or her own office e-mail address. You should forward the e-mail to that person's address.
- It's never appropriate to receive personal mail at your office e-mail address. It's also not appropriate to access your personal e-mail while at work.

- Never send sensitive patient information by email unless it has been encrypted. **Encryption** is a process of encoding information so that only authorized individuals can view it. This usually involves entering a special password.

Computer Passwords

Many of the things you'll do on the computer will require a password. Here are some guidelines for creating and protecting the passwords you choose:

- Combine letters and numbers in each password you create.
- Avoid using your name, initials, birth date, phone number, and the word *password* as passwords.
- Do not tape your password on your computer or leave it in your desk.
- Change your password from time to time, often systems are set to require that you change your password at set intervals.

 ## INTERNET BASICS

Your office probably can connect to the Internet. Most medical offices can. The Internet can be helpful to the office in a number of ways. It provides quick access to information such as medications; you could look to ensure that you are spelling a medication correctly or verify dosage, side effects, and other valuable information. It also provides a way to locate the name and phone number to other physicians, hospitals, or physical therapy centers. Remember to limit computer use to approved use only. Do not send personal e-mails, play games, or use social media while on your work computer.

Internet Research

The Internet is a great tool for researching topics in the medical office. Table 3-1 is a list of some common sites that might have relative information required in the office.

Table 3-1	Basic Medical Sources on the Internet	
Site	**Internet Address**	**Description**
American Medical Association (AMA)	www.ama-assn.org	Contains information on many subjects related to the practice of medicine
Centers for Disease Control (CDC)	www.cdc.gov	Offers information on a variety of health care topics
CINAHL Information Systems	www.cinahl.com	Includes articles for nurses and other allied health care professionals
NLM Gateway	gateway.nlm.nih.gov	Connects users with 18 different collections of medical information
PubMed Central	pubmedcentral.nih.gov	Contains thousands of articles on many health care subjects from different journals

Occasionally, the physician will ask the medical assistant to provide patient education materials to the patients. Here is a list of Internet resources that have a vast amount of information that can be used to develop patient education training materials, or the patient may be referred to the site for additional information.

- American Dental Association: www.ada.org/public/index.asp
- American Sleep Apnea Association: www.sleepapnea.org
- Consumer health information: www.health.nih.gov
- Health information for seniors: www.nihseniorhealth.gov
- MedlinePlus: www.medlineplus.gov
- *Merck Manual*: www.merckhomeedition.com
- National Attention Deficit Disorder Association: www.add.org
- Smoking cessation: www.QuitNet.org
- Sources for children with cancer: www.cancersourcekids.com
- Travel health: www.cdc.gov/travel
- General health: mayoclinic.com

Financial Help on the Internet

Sometimes, patients who are having trouble paying for their prescriptions can find help on the Internet. If you know of such a patient, here are some ways you can assist:

- Tell the patient to visit the home page of the company that makes the drug—for example, www.Pfizer.com.
- Suggest a patient assistance site that can help the patient to find discounted drugs or coupons to help with the cost, for example, www.needymeds.com.
- Patients on Medicare can find help at www.medicare.gov/prescription/home.asp.
- Physicians can find assistance for patients at www.Rxhope.com.

COMPUTER SECURITY

The Internet connects you to computers around the world. This can expose the office computer system to a number of dangers. Here are some dangers and some guidelines to keep your computer safe and working well.

- **Cookies**—tiny files that many sites will leave in your hard drive.
  - Some cookies track what you do on the Internet and report it to the site.
  - You can block cookies by setting limits on them on your Web browser.

- **Unsecure information**—information you fill out on a site might be seen by unauthorized people.
  - Never provide private information to a site that does not have a Secure Sockets Layer (SSL).
  - The SSL scrambles information as it leaves your computer and unscrambles it when it reaches the site.
  - A tiny picture of a lock in your browser's status bar shows if a site is secure.
- **Viruses**—can invade your computer and destroy your files and software. They are a major security problem.
  - Never download information, screen savers, or other programs onto your computer from suspicious sites.
  - Only open attachments to e-mail that are sent by known sources. Attachments from unknown sources could contain viruses.
  - Make sure your computer is equipped with virus protection software. Use the updating service that most antivirus programs offer.
- **Firewalls**—computer programs or devices that prevent unauthorized users from accessing private information on your computer's network through the Internet.
  - Firewalls are used to prevent people from gaining entry to private computer networks from outside the network.
  - A firewall builds a list of acceptable Web sites based on your past use of the computer. Attempts to access sites not on the list are denied.
  - Some firewalls limit the type or content of files your computer can receive.

Figure 3-2 is a sample of what the https and lock symbol would look like when you are accessing a secured Web site.

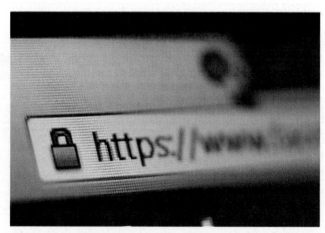

Figure 3-2   Computer security https and lock. (Image from Shutterstock.com.)

QUALITY IMPROVEMENT

Quality improvement, or **QI**, is an effort to improve every part of an organization. In health care, QI's main goal is to provide services that meet and exceed patients' needs. Many medical providers are required by law to have QI programs. QI programs encourage teamwork and raise morale in the office.

QI in Medical Offices

QI programs exist in medical offices mainly because two federal agencies require them.

- The Occupational Safety and Health Administration (OSHA) requires QI programs to protect employees and patients. You'll learn more about them in your clinical training.
- The Centers for Medicare & Medicaid Services (CMS) requires providers who treat patients covered by Medicare and Medicaid to have QI programs.

Here are some of the ways QI programs can benefit health care organizations:

- Identify delays and failures in the delivery system for care.
- Improve service to patients and their families.
- Encourage teamwork within the organization.
- Increase efficiency and productivity.
- Increase employee morale.
- Improve patient satisfaction and outcomes.

Patient Outcomes and QI

Patient outcomes are the final results of the care patients receive. Here's an example. A patient arrives in the office with a cut on her leg. The cut is sutured. Six days later the patient returns to have the sutures removed. The wound healed with no complications. This patient's outcome was acceptable. Patient outcomes are reported to various agencies that oversee health care. Currently, only hospitals are required to produce "report cards" on their patient outcomes. But pressure is building in Congress to require all health care providers to do so.

Patients can view report cards on various sites on the Internet. They can use this information to help them select a provider whose services best meet their needs.

Regulatory Agencies and QI

CMS (Centers for Medicare & Medicaid Services) is a division of the U.S. Department of Health and Human Services (**HHS**). HHS and CMS monitor two federal laws—the Clinical Laboratory Improvement Amendments (**CLIA**) and the Health Insurance Portability and Accountability Act (HIPAA). Both laws are related to QI because they set standards in many areas of health care. Some of these standards will affect what you do as a medical assistant.

CLIA

Congress passed the Clinical Laboratory Improvement Amendments in 1988. The standards they set improved accuracy in lab test results. Before CLIA, some lab tests, such as Pap smears, were notoriously inaccurate. Patients died as a result. CLIA set three levels of complexity for lab tests:

- Waived
- Moderate complexity
- High complexity

HHS approves clinical laboratories and physician office labs (**POLs**) to perform tests at one of these levels. Most POLs can perform only waived or moderate complexity tests. Here are some of the tests a POL can perform:

- Waived: urine dipsticks, fecal occult blood packets, urine pregnancy tests, ovulation kits, centrifuged microhematocrits, and certain blood glucose tests
- Moderate complexity tests: white blood cell counts, Gram staining, packaged rapid strep test, and automated cholesterol testing

All labs must have a QI program to identify and correct testing problems.

HIPAA

HIPAA, Health Information Portability and Accountability Act, was passed to:

- Set standards for the security and privacy of patients' health information; these standards are covered in detail in other chapters of this book.
- Set standards for submitting claims to patients' health insurers.

As with CLIA, medical offices need to have QI programs in place to make sure HIPAA standards are being met. For example, HIPAA requires that each medical office have a privacy officer. This person is responsible for seeing that patients' information is handled in the ways HIPAA requires.

> ### Study Skill
>
> You will discover that the health care industry has numerous abbreviations used. These are found not only in the clinical or back office but also in the administrative or front office part of the practice. Start developing a flash card system using 3 × 5 index cards with the abbreviation on one side and the meaning on the other side. As you collect these, sort them by administrative or clinical abbreviations.

RISK MANAGEMENT

Risk management is the process of identifying problems before they cause injury to patients or staff. Potential problems are directly related to risk factors. A risk factor is anything that could be a safety concern. A few typical risk factors in a medical office include:

- Poor lighting
- Frayed wires on electrical instruments or machines
- Improper disposal of needles
- Poor procedures for identifying patients

The risk factors just listed could result in these problems:

- Patients falling
- Electric shock
- Needlesticks of employees
- Treatment mistakes

Incident Reports

One way to find risk factors in your office is to look for trends in the office's **incident reports**. These are written accounts of negative events experienced by patients, visitors, or staff. Incident reports should be completed for even minor negative events.

If you're involved in or witness a negative event, you'll be expected to file an incident report. Your office probably has a standard form for incident reports that you would fill out. Here's what usually happens next:

- A supervisor reviews the report for completeness and accuracy and sends it on.
- The report will be given to the office manager or the physician. (In a hospital, it would go to the risk manager.)
- The physician may add comments to the report. This will depend on the type of event and the office's policy. If the event involved a patient, the physician will probably assess the patient and record the findings on the report.

Bad things can happen, even in the safest offices. Sometimes, they result from human errors. Other times, their causes are unknown or unavoidable. For instance, if you give a patient the wrong medication, that's a human error. You must complete an incident report. Now, suppose you gave the patient the correct medication and he had an allergic reaction to it. You still must complete an incident report, even though there was no human error. That's an example of an unavoidable event.

Here are some events that always require an incident report:

- All medication errors
- Any fall by a patient, employee, or visitor
- Drawing blood from the wrong patient

- Incorrect labeling of blood tubes or other lab specimens
- Accidental needlesticks of employees
- Workers' compensation injuries (work-related injuries)

A good rule to follow is, "When in doubt, complete an incident report."

Completing an Incident Report

Your office will have its own incident report form. The following information always should be included:

- The name, address, and phone number of the injured person
- The birth date and sex of the injured person
- The date, time, and location of the event
- Names and addresses of any witnesses
- A brief description of the event and what was done to deal with it
- Any tests or treatments that were performed
- Patient examination findings, if any
- The signature and title of the person completing the form
- Any other signatures required by office policy

Incident Reports and QI

Groups of incident reports can be studied to look for patterns. Finding patterns in negative events can help identify problem areas. These problems can then be corrected through QI programs. For example, there might be a trend like the day of the week when most events happen. If many events occur on Friday afternoons, staffing for that time period might be evaluated.

 Case Question

Do you think the case study scenario would require an incident report for the office? If so, why?

OFFICE EQUIPMENT AND SUPPLIES

The average medical office contains a lot of expensive equipment. It also uses a huge amount of supplies. Making sure equipment works correctly and that the office doesn't run out of needed supplies is an important part of quality control. Broken equipment can keep the office from running smoothly or from running at all. Computer breakdowns could keep you from scheduling appointments, for instance, or from sending out monthly bills. You also wouldn't want to turn away a patient because a piece of clinical equipment wasn't working right.

Service Contracts

A **service contract** is an arrangement with a company to care for office equipment. For a yearly fee, the company will inspect and service certain equipment, such as a photocopier or an EKG machine. One of your duties may be to keep track of these contracts and make sure that equipment is serviced regularly.

Routine Care of Equipment

Another of your duties may be to make regular checks of clinical equipment to be sure it's working correctly. Your office's QI program may have a schedule that tells how often each type of equipment should be checked. Checking the accuracy of a blood glucose meter is one example of this task. This responsibility is commonly given to a medical assistant. Medical assistants also may have to check other lab equipment to help the office meet CLIA requirements. Specifically, CLIA requires:

- A system to assure that each piece of lab equipment is producing accurate results on lab tests
- A log for each piece of equipment that shows each time its accuracy was checked and the results of the check

If federal inspectors visit your office lab, they will want to see these records.

Equipment Inventory

You may need to keep track the inventory of office machines as well as their performance and accuracy. To run smoothly, every business needs to know what pieces of equipment it has and how many. This list of the number of each item is called an **inventory**.

It's important to have an inventory of equipment in case of a theft, a fire, or some other damage to the office.

Maintaining Supplies

It's very important that the office is properly supplied. Medical supplies—bottles of sterile water, for instance—often have expiration dates. If too much is on hand, it may expire. And once the sterile water expires, it shouldn't be used. Always discard expired stock. If a patient is harmed because outdated medicines or supplies are used, the office could be sued. Also, too much inventory on hand is quite costly for the office. On the other hand, you don't want to have so little of something that you might run out of it.

Keeping good records is the key to avoiding both situations. You should make a weekly or monthly inventory of the office's supplies. Comparing these numbers over time will give you an idea of how fast the office uses its stock of each item. This will help you know how much of that item to keep on hand and when it's time to order more.

You may be responsible for the office's entire stock of supplies. Or your job may include tracking only certain types of supplies.

Inventory of Office Equipment

A well-run medical office keeps close track of its administrative and clinical equipment. Use these guidelines when preparing an inventory of the equipment in your office:

- Determine exactly what should be included in the inventory. Your supervisor or employer should provide this guidance.
  - Should all equipment be included or only equipment that costs more than a set amount of money?
  - Should office furnishings, such as examining tables and waiting room lamps and chairs, be included?
- Create an inventory sheet for each category of equipment. Categories could be defined by the type of equipment or by its location.
  - There might be a sheet for all computers and a separate sheet for all EKG machines, for example.
  - There might be a separate sheet for each room, on which all the equipment in that room is listed.
- Prepare columns on the sheet with the following titles:
  - Location (or equipment type)
  - Manufacturer
  - Serial number
  - Purchased or leased
  - First year of service
  - Service contract
  - Expiration date
- Record the information for each piece of equipment, as available, in each row on the sheet.
  - Not all items will have a serial number. For this reason, some offices assign and attach an inventory number to each piece of equipment.
  - The lease or purchase date helps in identifying old equipment that may need to be replaced.
  - Service contracts should be tracked so managers can decide when and if to renew them.
- Follow office policy in what you do with the completed inventory.
- Update the inventory at regular intervals to show the following changes:
  - Disposal of old equipment
  - Addition of new equipment
  - Relocation of equipment
  - Renewal or expiration of service contracts

Inventory of Office Supplies

It's important to keep track of supplies so your office doesn't run out of critical items, keep too much stock on hand, or use outdated medical supplies. Your office software can help you with this task. Follow these steps to use the computer to inventory supplies:

- Open the spreadsheet software on your computer and create a document called *Supply Inventory*. If you use the computer when doing inventories, it will make calculating the use rate of supplies easier and more accurate.

- Type the title of the file—for example, *Medical Supplies Inventory*—in the appropriate cell of the spreadsheet. You may want to inventory medical supplies and office supplies separately.
- Create a row for each type of supply and columns across the spreadsheet to show the following data for each month of the year:
  - The amount on hand for that month
  - The amount used since the last inventory
  - The amount that needs to be ordered
- Create formulas in the appropriate cells to automatically calculate the amount used and the number to be reordered.
- Count the number of each item in the supply stock and record the number in the correct place on the spreadsheet.

- As you count, check for supplies with expiration dates that have passed. Properly dispose of any such items. You should not use outdated supplies.
- Pull items with the oldest expiration dates to the front of each type of supply. This will help to ensure that these items will be used first.
- When the counts are complete and recorded on the spreadsheet, save your work and print out the spreadsheet.
- Use the printed spreadsheet to reorder supplies. The spreadsheet formulas will have calculated how many of each item has been used and how many more you need to order.
- When the new supplies arrive, stock them behind the existing supplies. This allows the oldest supplies to be used first.

Procedure 3-1 Conducting an Inventory of Supplies

The purpose is to maintain adequate levels of all supplies (administrative, clinical, and laboratory) needed to ensure quality patient care. Equipment includes supply inventory sheets, requisition/order forms, and a pen.

1. Create a list of supplies (administrative, clinical, and laboratory) used in your office.

2. Determine par or minimum levels for each item on the supply list. This will be on past use or estimated if a new product. Estimated supplies will need frequent monitoring to ensure a proper par is set for the future. Records par levels on the supply inventory sheet. It's best to create an electronic master that you can use either electronically or manually.

3. Document current amounts on hand and then determine the amount needed by subtracting the par from the amount on hand.

4. Complete the requisition/order form for supplies needed.

5. Submit the requisition/order form to your office manager.

6. Document actions taken to prevent duplication of work and orders.

Procedure 3-2 Performing Routine Equipment Maintenance

The purpose is to maintain proper function of equipment and to prolong equipment life. Equipment includes Office equipment, Lint-free towel, water, mild soap, other supplies as listed by manufacturer guidelines, and an equipment maintenance log.

1. Review manufacturer guidelines of your office equipment. It is important to follow these guidelines as failure to do so can damage equipment and void its warranty.

2. Clean the exterior of the equipment. Check to ensure that equipment that is not used frequently is covered and protected against dust and particles.

3. Perform maintenance step provided in the user's manual. If the manual has been misplaced, use the Internet to search for a replacement.

4. Record maintenance completed for each piece of equipment on the maintenance log. Your office should maintain a log that lists all maintenance performed on each piece of equipment in the office. Routine maintenance should be completed on a monthly basis. Any concerns discovered during these checks should be noted and corrected by appropriately skilled individuals.

Preparing for Externship

While you are completing coursework at the school, you will start preparing for your externship by completing various items that the externship site will probably request prior to your first day on site. Most medical facilities require that students provide documentation of a health exam. This may be a simple statement of good health provided by your health care provider, or it may require that you have some medical testing including proof of hepatitis B vaccination, screening for rubella or proof of MMR (measles, mumps, rubella), and recent negative tuberculosis test. Many sites want to see proof of completion of a CPR course. Medical assistant programs usually include this training as part of the requirement to complete the program. You should be prepared to present a current resume to the potential externship site when you do your interview. When you are at the externship site, you will probably be required to have your own stethoscope and a wristwatch with a second hand that is used to count pulse and respiration rates. The watch may be necessary since most facilities do not allow the use of cell phones, and there is no certainty that each exam room will have a clock with a second hand. Some sites routinely use pulse oximeter devices to measure the pulse rate, but there is no way to determine respiration rates except manually using a watch or clock.

Chapter Recap

- Computers are essential to the operation of a medical office.
- Protection of EHR is vital, never share your password.
- Computer software helps medical assistants do their jobs more efficiently.
- The Internet plays a key role in health care by providing medical information to patients and health care professionals.
- Use caution when sharing information on the Web; visit only sites trusted and approved by your employer.

- Quality improvement programs benefit medical offices by identifying potential problems and creating solutions for them.
- CLIA and HIPAA require attention to maintaining standards in both clinical and administrative areas of health care service.
- Risk management helps achieve quality improvement through the filing and review of incident reports.
- Medical assistants play key roles in maintaining equipment and supplies that are critical to a medical office.

Online Resources for Students

Student Resources available on the text's online site include:
- Audio Glossaries
- Animations
- Competency Evaluation Forms

- Videos
- Anatomy & Physiology Module with Heart and Lung Sounds
- Weblinks
- Worksheets

Exercises and Activities

Certification Preparation Questions

1. While working on the computer, you need to step away for a quick minute. What should you do?
   a. Leave the system up, as is.
   b. Turn off the screen and stay logged in.
   c. Lock the system using the window and "L" key.
   d. Lock the system using the control and "L" key.
   e. Turn off the computer.

2. Cookies are defined as:
   a. tiny files left on your hard drive by a Web site.
   b. a program that prevents unauthorized users.
   c. something that invades and destroys files and software.
   d. Secure Sockets Layers.
   e. a device used for memory storage

3. Electronic health records are protected under:
   a. CLIA.
   b. HON.
   c. HIPAA.
   d. SSL.
   e. OSHA.

4. Anytime a person is injured, a ____ must be completed as soon as possible.
   a. confidentiality statement
   b. incident report
   c. HIPAA form
   d. CLIA form
   e. release of information form

5. Which of the following invade and destroy files and software?
   a. Firewall
   b. SSL
   c. HON
   d. Viruses
   e. Cookies

6. A rapid strep test performed in a physician office laboratory would fall under which of the following CLIA categories?
   a. Low complexity
   b. Low-to-moderate complexity
   c. Moderate complexity
   d. Moderate-to-high complexity
   e. High complexity

7. Which of the following regulations set standards designed to ensure improved laboratory accuracy?
   a. CLIA
   b. HIPAA
   c. OSHA
   d. CMS
   e. AMA

8. A urine dipstick performed in a physician operated laboratory would fall under which of the following CLIA categories?
   a. Low complexity
   b. Low-to-moderate complexity
   c. Moderate complexity
   d. Moderate-to-high complexity
   e. High complexity

9. Inventory controls are designed to:
   a. ensure that the office has more than enough supplies to last 60 days.
   b. ensure that the office runs efficiently and has the supplies it needs when they are needed.
   c. allow items to run out so that you can always have the newest items on the market.
   d. limit the use of supplies to urgent needs only.
   e. limit the amount of supplies used per patient to ensure cost management.

10. Which of the following represents an important rule in password security?
    a. Post your password to your computer screen so you don't forget it.
    b. Change your password frequently to ensure that no one else knows it.
    c. Share your password with coworkers so that it looks like you do most of the work.
    d. Use your birthday as your password as it will be easy to remember.
    e. Use one password for everyone in the office to make it easy for the entire staff.

CareTracker Connection

Medical Office Management

 HARRIS CareTracker Activities Related to
CareTracker This Chapter
- Getting Started
- Case Study 1: Basic Administration and Setup

In this chapter, you learned that computers and applications are essential to the day-to-day operations of medical offices. One application widely used in medical office management is Harris CareTracker Practice Management and Physician Electronic Medical Record, or CareTracker for short.

Tasks discussed in this chapter that can be performed in CareTracker include the following:

- Creating and maintaining patient electronic health records
- Scheduling patient appointments

- Entering patient demographic and insurance information
- Entering patient medical and family history
- Entering patient clinical data
- Ordering labs and medications
- Composing letters and memos
- Posting charges and payments to patients' accounts
- Processing insurance claims
- Tracking accounts payable and receivable
- Tracking patient data

As you can see, CareTracker can be used to do a lot! Many of these tasks are discussed in CareTracker Connection features in other chapters. A task we'll consider here is building provider schedules.

To schedule patient appointments, you first must know the availability of the health care providers in the office. CareTracker allows you to create a custom schedule for each provider that consists of templates for different types of days, each with its own start and end times, and different types of weeks.

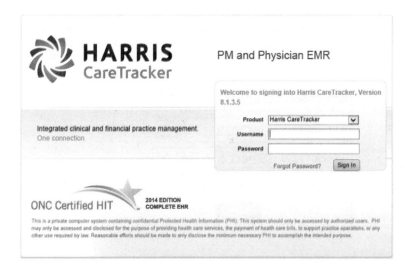

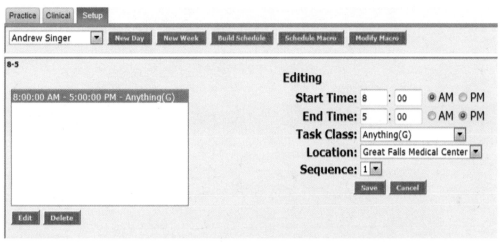

Using these building blocks, you can then set up the provider's schedule for a whole year.

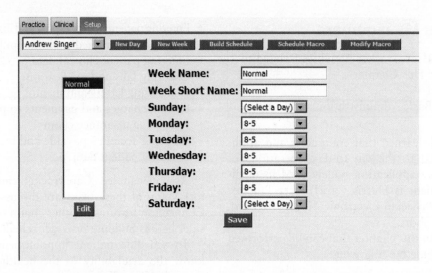

Once a provider's schedule is built, you can then schedule patients for that provider.

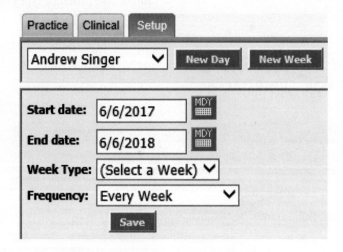

Section II

Anatomy and Physiology

4 Organization of the Body and Integumentary System

Chapter Objectives

- Define the terms anatomy, physiology, and pathology.
- Describe the organization of the body from chemicals to the whole organism.
- List 11 body systems and give the general function of each.
- Define and give examples of homeostasis.
- Using examples, discuss the components of a negative feedback loop.
- Define metabolism and name the two types of metabolic reactions.
- List and define the main directional terms for the body.
- List and define the three planes of division of the body.
- Name the subdivisions of the dorsal and ventral cavities.
- Name and locate the subdivisions of the abdomen.
- Cite some anterior and posterior body regions along with their common names.
- Show how word parts are used to build words related to the body's organization.
- Name and describe the layers of the skin.
- Provide the location and function of the accessory structures of the integumentary system.
- List the major functions of the integumentary system.
- List the main disorders of the integumentary system.
- Describe the classification and danger of burns.

CAAHEP & ABHES Competencies

CAAHEP

- Describe structural organization of the human body.
- Identify body systems.
- Describe body planes, directional terms, quadrants, and body cavities.
- List major organs in each body system.
- Describe the normal function of each body system.
- Identify common pathology related to each body system including signs, symptoms, and etiology.
- Analyze pathology for each body system including diagnostic measures and treatment modalities.

ABHES

- List all body systems, their structure, and their functions.
- Describe common diseases, symptoms, and etiologies as they apply to each system.
- Common diseases, diagnoses, and treatments.
- Identify diagnostic and treatment modalities as they relate to each body system.

Chapter Terms

Adipose	Dermatosis	Jaundice	Psoriasis
Albinism	Epidermis	Keratin	Sebum
Anabolism	Erythema	Melanin	Urticaria
Anatomy	Extracellular fluid	Melanoma	Vitiligo
Catabolism	Homeostasis	Metabolism	
Cerumen	Impetigo	Negative feedback	
Cyanosis	Intracellular fluid	Physiology	

Abbreviations

BSA   HPV   SLE

All medical sciences rely on the study of the anatomy and physiology of the human body. **Anatomy** refers to the structure of the body and **physiology** the function of those body parts. When you understand the structure and function of the body, it is easier to study and analyze the disease process.

ORGANIZATIONAL STRUCTURE OF THE HUMAN BODY

The best way to study the anatomy of the body is to begin with the organization of the body from the simple level, or smallest components, to the more complex level, the body systems. The cells of the body are the smallest components and are the basic units of life. The body's cells are specialized meaning that they all have a specific function. A nerve cell functions differently than a muscle cell. These specialized groups of cells form the tissues of the body, for example, muscle tissue or nerve tissue. The tissues work together as an organ. Organs work together to make up a body system. Now we have a whole organism, the human body.

Body Systems

The human body is composed of eleven (11) different systems, all responsible for a different function within the body.

The systems and major function include:

- Integumentary system
- Skeletal system
- Muscular system
- Nervous system
- Endocrine system
- Cardiovascular system
- Lymphatic system
- Respiratory system
- Digestive system
- Urinary system
- Reproductive system

Integumentary System

The word integument means skin. The integumentary system is composed of the skin and accessory structures including the hair, nails, sweat glands, and oil glands. The main function of the skin is to protect the body. Later in the chapter, we will cover the integumentary system.

Skeletal System

The skeletal system provides the basic framework for the body. There are 206 bones with joints between the bones allowing for movement. Ligaments are the structures that hold the bones together. The skeleton also protects internal organs from injury.

Muscular System

Muscles are attached to the bones allowing movement of body parts. Muscles help the body to maintain posture and provide protection to internal organs. Muscles produce heat in the body. In addition to skeletal muscle, which is voluntary, there are smooth muscles found in blood vessels and internal organs and cardiac muscle only found in the heart.

Nervous System

The brain, spinal cord, and nerves are the major parts of the nervous system. The body relies on the nervous system for control and coordination. The special sense organs require the nervous system to act as a relay system sending electrical signals to and from the brain.

In the chapter discussing the nervous system, the special senses are included.

Endocrine System

Endocrine glands are organs that produce hormones, which regulate the body activities. The hormones affect growth and reproduction as well as metabolism and nutrient utilization.

Cardiovascular System

The heart and blood vessels, arteries and veins, make up the cardiovascular system of the body. The heart pumps blood through the arteries to carry oxygen and nutrients to the body tissues. The veins carry blood back to heart from the body. The blood in the veins contains carbon dioxide and waste products from the tissues.

Lymphatic System

The lymphatic system assists the circulatory system. Lymph vessels return fluids from the tissues to the blood. The tonsils, thymus, and spleen are organs of the lymphatic system and support the immune system of the body. Lymphatic fluid (lymph) fills the lymphatic vessels.

Respiratory System

The lungs are the primary organs of the respiratory system. The respiratory system is responsible for conducting air to the lungs where the exchange of oxygen and carbon dioxide takes place. The blood transports oxygen to the body, and carbon dioxide, a waste product, is transported back to the lungs and expelled from the body by breathing out.

Digestive System

This system is responsible for changing our foods into nutrients that the body can use for cell metabolism. Organs of the digestive system include the mouth, esophagus, stomach, and small and large intestines. Accessory organs are the liver, gallbladder, and pancreas.

Urinary System

The primary organs of the urinary system are the kidneys. They filter the body's blood removing waste products and excess water. Other structures associated with the urinary system include the ureters, bladder, and urethra.

Reproductive System

This system includes external and internal structures concerned with reproduction of offspring. Male and female sex organs are different, but both systems provide the necessary components to reproduce.

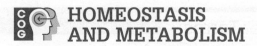

HOMEOSTASIS AND METABOLISM

Homeostasis means that there is a state of internal balance in the normal body. Literally, the term means "staying the same." Environmental conditions may change the balance; however, the body is equipped with the ability to maintain the balance or homeostasis. In order to stay healthy, conditions need to be maintained including body temperature, volume and composition of body fluids, blood gas concentrations, and blood pressure.

Body Fluids

The body fluids must remain in constant balance, volume, and composition, in order for homeostasis to be maintained. Fluids include extracellular fluid found outside the body's cells and intracellular fluid on the inside of cells. **Extracellular fluid**, outside the cell, includes blood plasma, the liquid portion of blood, and lymphatic fluid. Blood plasma carries nutrients to and from the cells. The **intracellular fluid**, inside the cells, maintains the homeostatic internal environment of the cell.

Negative Feedback

Homeostasis is primarily maintained through the process of **negative feedback**, a method that reverses any shift from normal range by upward or downward changes. Negative feedback responds to stimuli. This feedback loop requires three components:

- A sensor gathering information about a body condition
- A control center receiving input and sending corrective action if necessary
- An effector responding to the signal or action

A common example of this is a household thermostat, the sensor, set at a preferred temperature called the "set point." The thermometer responds to changes in the room temperature. When the temperature in the room drops below the set point, the control center notifies the furnace, the effector, to turn on and produce heat to warm the room. When the temperature reaches a set point, the furnace shuts off. Figure 4-1 demonstrates how a furnace responds to the thermostat either activating it or shutting it off.

Our body works in the same way regulating internal body temperature. A region of the brain is the control center sending signals to effectors such as sweat glands when the body temperature is too hot and to the muscles, to shiver, when the body is too cool. The nervous system acts to relay electrical

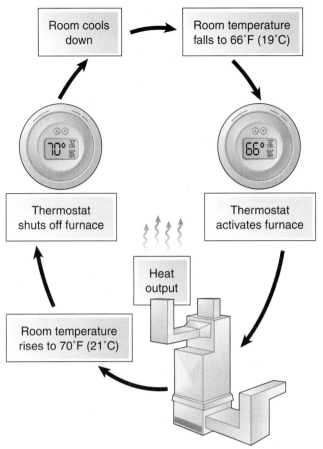

Figure 4-1 Thermostat regulation (negative feedback). (Reprinted from Cohen BJ. *Memmler's The Human Body in Health and Disease.* 13th ed. Burlington, MA: Jones & Bartlett Learning, LLC; 2014.)

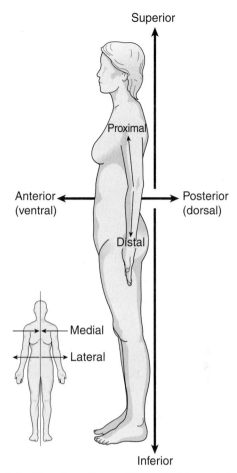

Figure 4-2 Directional terms. (Reprinted from Cohen BJ. *Memmler's The Human Body in Health and Disease.* 13th ed. Burlington, MA: Jones & Bartlett Learning, LLC; 2014.)

impulses, signals, between the components of the feedback loop.

Metabolism

Metabolism is the sum of all chemical and physical changes that occur in the body's tissues. There are two types of metabolism:

- **Catabolism**—the breakdown of complex substances into simpler compounds
- **Anabolism**—the building up of tissues through growth and repair

 BODY DIRECTIONS

Before the exploration of body directions, it is necessary to understand the anatomical position of the body. When a person is in anatomical position, they are standing upright facing forward, arms to the side of the body with the palms forward, and feet parallel

to the ground. Figure 4-2 shows each of the directional terms.

Directional Terms

The main terms used to describe the body directions are:

- Superior—above or in a higher position
- Inferior—below or lower
- Anterior or ventral—toward the belly surface or front of the body
- Posterior or dorsal—nearer the back or backside of the body
- Medial—midline of the body dividing it into left and right sides
- Lateral—away from the midline, toward the side
- Proximal—nearer to the origin or attachment point of a structure
- Distal—farther from the point of attachment

Body Planes

A plane describes a two-dimensional flat surface. Body planes are used to describe the body as it is divided

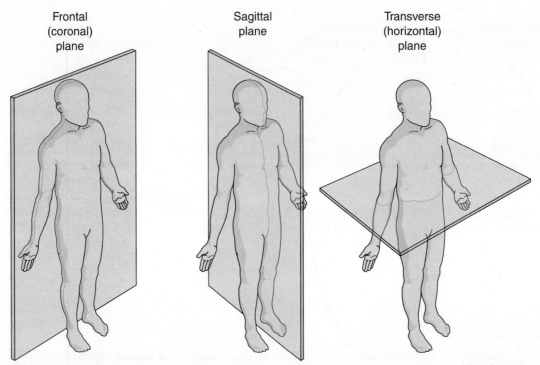

Frontal
(coronal)
plane

Sagittal
plane

Transverse
(horizontal)
plane

Figure 4-3 Body planes. (Reprinted from Cohen BJ. *Memmler's The Human Body in Health and Disease.* 13th ed. Burlington, MA: Jones & Bartlett Learning, LLC; 2014.)

into different directions. Figure 4-3 shows each of the body planes.

- Frontal plane—an imaginary line down the middle of the body dividing it into anterior and posterior sections; also called the coronal plane.
- Sagittal plane—an imaginary line down the body separating it into right and left portions. If the line is exactly down the midline of the body, dividing it into equal right and left halves, it is a midsagittal plane.

- Transverse plane—an imaginary horizontal line made across the body separating it into superior (upper) and inferior (lower) parts. Also called a horizontal plane.

Body Cavities

The internal body is divided into cavities or spaces that contain the body's organs. The two main cavities are the dorsal cavity and ventral cavity. See Figure 4-4, which demonstrates the cavities of the body.

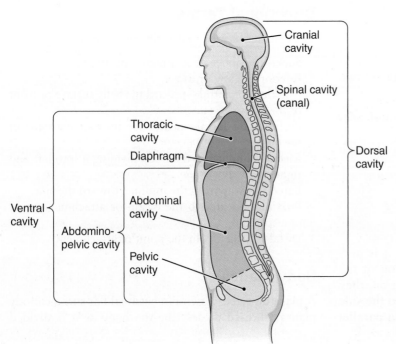

Cranial
cavity

Spinal cavity
(canal)

Thoracic
cavity

Diaphragm

Abdominal
cavity

Dorsal
cavity

Ventral
cavity

Abdomino-
pelvic cavity

Pelvic
cavity

Figure 4-4 Body cavities. (Reprinted from Cohen BJ. *Memmler's The Human Body in Health and Disease.* 13th ed. Burlington, MA: Jones & Bartlett Learning, LLC; 2014.)

Dorsal Cavity

The dorsal cavity lies on the posterior side of the body and is divided into the cranial cavity and the spinal cavity. The brain is contained within the cranial cavity and the spinal cord is found in the spinal cavity.

Ventral Cavity

The ventral cavity lies on the anterior side of the body and is divided into the thoracic cavity and the abdominopelvic cavity. These two cavities are separated by the diaphragm, the major muscle of breathing. The heart, lungs, and large blood vessels that join the heart are located in the thoracic cavity. The heart and vessels are located in the middle space of the thoracic cavity called the mediastinum.

The abdominopelvic cavity is the subdivision of the ventral cavity that lies below the diaphragm. It is further divided into two sections, the abdominal cavity and the pelvic cavity. The abdominal cavity contains the stomach, liver, gallbladder, pancreas, spleen, and most of the intestine. The pelvic cavity is below the abdominal cavity separated by an imaginary line across the top of the hip bones. This cavity contains the urinary bladder, rectum, and internal reproductive organs.

Abdominal Regions

The abdomen is divided into nine regions that assist in describing areas of examination. The regions as shown in Figure 4-5 are:

* Epigastric region—centrally located just inferior to the breastbone
* Umbilical region—centrally located around the umbilicus (navel)
* Hypogastric regions—centrally located just inferior to the umbilical region
* Hypochondriac regions, right and left—located just inferior to the ribs
* Lumbar regions, right and left—level with the lumbar region of the spine
* Iliac or inguinal regions, right and left—iliac is named for the upper rounded edge of the hip bone and inguinal for the groin region

Body Quadrants

There are four quadrants of the body, which are more general than the regions. They include the right and left upper and the right and left lower quadrants. These quadrants represent an equal division of the abdominal region into four parts. Figure 4-6 shows the four abdominal quadrants.

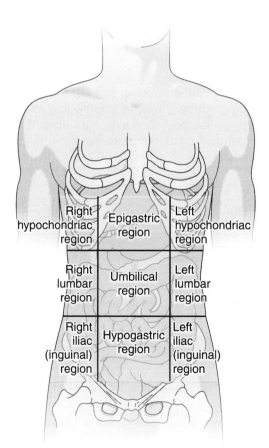

Figure 4-5   Regions of the body. (Reprinted from Cohen BJ. *Memmler's The Human Body in Health and Disease.* 13th ed. Burlington, MA: Jones & Bartlett Learning, LLC; 2014.)

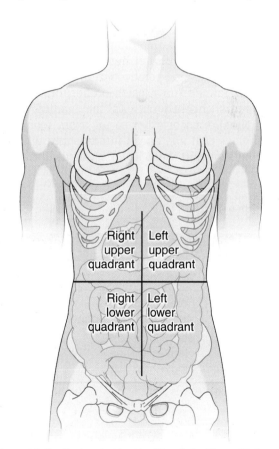

Figure 4-6   Body quadrants. (Reprinted from Cohen BJ. *Memmler's The Human Body in Health and Disease.* 13th ed. Burlington, MA: Jones & Bartlett Learning, LLC; 2014.)

MEDICAL TERMINOLOGY

Throughout the chapters of this textbook, you encounter medical terms used to describe anatomy, physiology, pathology, procedures, and treatments. Medical terminology can seem complicated and hard to understand unless you look at each term and literally break it apart into word parts, prefix, root, and suffix. The root is the main part of the word. Some terms have more than one root. The prefix starts the word and modifies the root, giving it more meaning. The suffix is at the end, following the root, and modifies the root. When the prefix, root, and suffix combine, a complete term is formed. Putting these parts together may require the addition of a vowel to the root in order for it to blend together. When a prefix is written alone, it requires a dash after the prefix, and when the suffix is written by itself, a dash is placed in front of the suffix. Table 4-1 provides an example of how the word parts are put together to make a full term.

Study Skill

As you begin to study the anatomy and physiology of the body, you will understand that although there are many systems, organs, and functions, the body is very organized. The trick to studying this information is to organize your thoughts. Mind mapping is a technique or method of building a diagram on paper to visually organize the information. The mind map resembles a spider web when finished. You start at the center of the diagram with a circle, and there are extensions coming out of various points on the circle. For example, if you want to mind map the body systems and organs in each, start the middle of the diagram with the word body systems, and draw a line away from the circle for each body system. Next, draw a line away from each body system to represent each organ in that system. You can go further and add the function of the organ. When finished, you will have a visual diagram of the body systems with each one represented as a separate extension of the circle.

Case Study

Evelyn Miller is a 56-year-old patient who frequently sees the dermatologist to evaluate new lesions she discovers on her skin. She had four skin cancer lesions removed from her face and now has found a new lesion on her forearm that she wants checked out. As the medical assistant, Natalie, escorts her to an exam room, Ms. Miller says that she doesn't understand why she is always getting these lesions. She said that she does not recall any of skin cancer in her family. She has always been a healthy woman who loves working in her garden and swimming in the community pool. She still continues to do these things and loves to wear a tank top and shorts when she does her gardening and of course she wears a swimsuit to the pool. She says that even though she is aging, she still wants to keep her beautiful bronze skin.

Table 4-1   Terminology Word Parts

Medical Term	Word Parts	Example
Homeostasis	homeo—same stat or stasis—stoppage, consistency	*Homeostasis* is the steady state (sameness) within an organism.
Pathology	path/o—disease ology—study of ology—study of	*Pathology* is the study of diseases or the disease process.
Intracellular	intra—within -ar—pertaining to	Intracellular means pertaining to inside of or within a cell.
Anatomy	ana—apart tomy—to cut, incision dissect	*Anatomy* means to cut apart to discover the structure of an organism.

Case Question

If the physician asks Natalie to provide patient education to this person, what should she tell her? If the patient asks about skin cancer and if it is fatal, what should the medical assistant explain to the patient?

THE INTEGUMENTARY SYSTEM

The integumentary system is the natural place to start introducing each of the body systems. The skin provides the first line of defense against infections and harmful agents that would damage the body. The term integumentary means "covering" and can reflect a person's health and emotional state. The accessory structures that are associated with the integumentary system are the sweat and oil glands, hair, and nails. Figure 4-7 shows a cross section of the skin with the structures contained within each layer.

Structure of the Skin

There are three layers associated with the skin:

- Epidermis
- Dermis
- Subcutaneous

Epidermis

The **epidermis** is the top layer of the skin and contains no blood vessels. It is entirely made of epithelial cells. The epidermal cells are constantly sloughed off, and replaced by new cells. The new cells are produced in the stratum basale, the deepest layer of the epidermis. These new cells are pushed toward the top layer of the epidermis. They also undergo changes replacing the cell's cytoplasm with protein called keratin. Keratin thickens

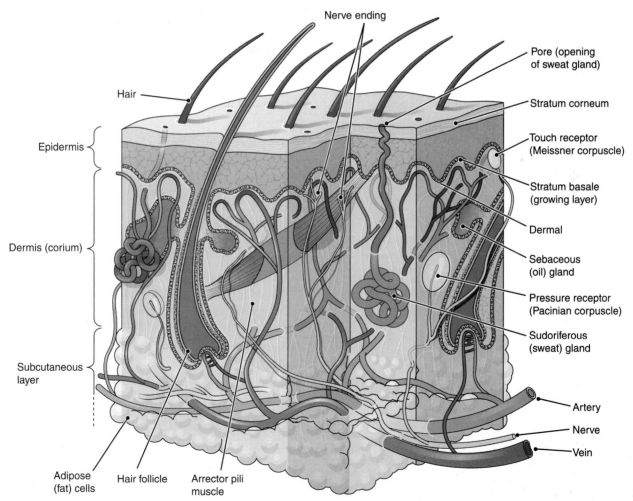

Figure 4-7   Skin structure. (Reprinted from Cohen BJ. *Memmler's The Human Body in Health and Disease*. 13th ed. Burlington, MA: Jones & Bartlett Learning, LLC; 2014.)

and protects the skin. This thickened, uppermost layer of the epidermis is the stratum corneum. This layer is more prominent in thick skin, found on the palms of hands, than in thin skin, as found on the eyelids. **Melanin** is a dark pigment that colors the skin and protects it from the harmful rays of the sun. The cells that produce melanin are call melanocytes.

Dermis

The dermis is referred to as "true skin." It is where the skin's vital functions take place. Blood vessels and nerves supply this layer of skin. Dense irregular connective tissue allows the dermis to be elastic and able to stretch. This layer of true skin also contains the sweat and oil glands and the hair follicles.

The dermal papillae are superficial projections of the dermis that forms a pattern of ridges that help prevent slipping. The pattern of the ridges is inherited and is unique to each person. Fingerprints and footprints are an example of the pattern of ridges. They are used for a personal identification since there are no two persons with the same pattern.

Subcutaneous Layer

The subcutaneous layer is a connective tissue membrane also referred to as the hypodermis since it lies beneath the dermal layer. This layer connects the skin to the deep fascia covering the muscles. The subcutaneous layer is primarily made of areolar connective tissue and varying amounts of **adipose** (fatty tissue). The adipose tissue acts as insulation and provides a reserve energy supply. The blood vessels, supplying this layer of skin, help to regulate the body temperature.

Accessory Structures of the Skin

Structures that are included with the integumentary system are:

- Sebaceous glands (oil)
- Sudoriferous glands (sweat)
- Hair
- Nails

Sebaceous Glands

The sebaceous glands are structures that secrete **sebum** (oil), which lubricates the skin and hair preventing dryness. The ducts of the glands open into the hair follicles.

Sudoriferous Glands

The sudoriferous glands are sweat glands. They are coiled, tube-like structures located in the dermis and subcutaneous tissue. Their function is to cool the body. As they release sweat (perspiration), heat is drawn from the skin as the moisture evaporates at the surface of the skin. The eccrine-type sweat glands secrete perspiration and excrete water and waste through this process. Another type of sudoriferous gland is the apocrine sweat gland located in the armpits and groin area. Secretions from these glands increase with emotional stress and sexual stimulation. Body odor is caused through the action of bacteria breaking down organic cellular materials, which are excreted from the apocrine glands.

Another type of gland is the ceruminous glands in the ear canal that produce ear wax, **cerumen**.

Hair

The body is covered with hair even though some hair is barely visible, very soft, and fine. Hairless areas of the body are the palms of the hands, soles of the feet, lips, nipples, and parts of the external genitalia. Hair develops from stem cells located in the bulb at the base of the hair follicle. Melanocytes add pigment to developing hair. The visible part of the hair seen above the skin is the shaft and the portion below the skin is the root.

Most hair follicles have an attached thin band of involuntary muscle, the arrector pili. This muscle contracts when a person is cold or frightened, raising the hair causing "goose bumps."

Nails

The fingers and toes are protected by the nails. Nails also help us grasp items too small to pick up with the hands. They are comprised of hardened **keratin** (protein). Parts of the nail are:

- Nail root—growth region located under the proximal end of the nail
- Nail plate—main portion of the visible nail
- Lunula—visible "little moon" at the proximal end of the nail
- Cuticle—an extension of the skin that seals the space between the nail plate and the skin above the root

Figure 4-8 shows a photo of a nail from the top and a cross section of a nail.

The nails can tell us a little something about a person's general health. Changes in the nail's appearance might indicate the presence of chronic diseases such as heart disease, peripheral vascular disease, malnutrition, and anemia. With these types of diseases, the nail may have an abnormal color, thickness, shape, or texture such as grooves or splitting.

Functions of the Integumentary System

The main functions of the integumentary system include:

- Protecting against infection
- Protecting against dehydration or drying
- Regulating the body temperature
- Collecting sensory information

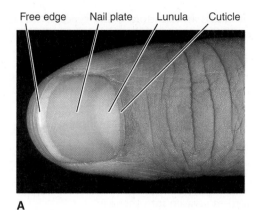

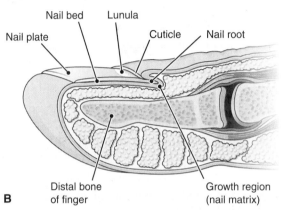

Figure 4-8   Nail structure. **A.** Healthy nail. **B.** Internal nail and finger structures. (Reprinted from Cohen BJ. *Memmler's The Human Body in Health and Disease.* 13th ed. Burlington, MA: Jones & Bartlett Learning, LLC; 2014.)

Protecting Against Infection

Pathogens are all around us just waiting to invade the body. One common route of entry is through broken skin. However, intact skin forms a primary barrier against invasion of pathogenic organisms. The skin's surface cells are constantly shed, removing the pathogens with those dead cells. There are harmful chemicals in our environment that do not enter the body due to the protective layer of the skin.

Protecting Against Dehydration

The skin is a waterproof surface protecting the body from drying out. Keratin and oil keep it moist and soft. Even though some water is lost through perspiration and evaporation, these substances prevent excessive water loss. When the skin is significantly damaged, excessive fluid is lost through the skin. An example is a person who has experienced serious burns.

Regulating Body Temperature

The skin is essential in the homeostatic management of heat and cold. Heat increases when blood flow increases to a part of the body, and when blood flow decreases, the body part becomes cooler. In a cold environment, body heat is maintained in the core of the body. This is why our feet and hands are colder. In warm climates, blood flow is increased bringing blood closer to the surface of the skin. Heat dissipates through this process. When we are warm, the skin actually becomes red. In cold temperatures, the skin can become pale or bluish in color.

Collecting of Sensory Information

The skin is one of the chief sensory organs containing many nerve endings and special receptors. The receptors detect pain, temperature changes, touch, and pressure. These skin receptors initiate reflexes that cause our body to respond to the stimulus. For example, if you touch something very hot, the immediate reaction is to pull away from the heat.

Observing the Skin

During physical examination of a patient, the physician inspects the skin for characteristics that indicate the general health of the individual. The physician will observe the color and texture of the skin as well as any damaged areas or abnormalities. Terms associated with the skin color are:

- Discoloration—distinct change in skin color.
- Melanin—skin's main pigment produced by melanocytes, darker people have a larger quantity of melanin because their melanocytes are more active.
- **Albinism**—impairs melanin production resulting in lack of pigment in the skin, hair, and eyes. See Figure 4-9, a photo of an infant with albinism.
- **Vitiligo**—blanching of the skin to near whiteness, due to the defective action of the melanocytes.
- Pallor—paleness of the skin usually caused by reduced blood flow or reduced hemoglobin (anemia).
- Flushing—redness caused by increased blood flow to the skin, usually around the face and neck.
- **Cyanosis**—bluish discoloration when there is not enough oxygen in the blood, may indicate heart or respiratory condition.
- **Jaundice**—yellowish skin discoloration, which may be caused by excessive amounts of bile pigments (bilirubin) or may be due to hepatitis or bile flow obstruction.
- **Erythema**—redness of the skin.

Disorders of the Integumentary System

Physical and chemical trauma or disease can cause various skin conditions. They can be very simple or quite intense. The general term used for any skin disease is **dermatosis**. Lesions are wounds or damage to the skin. Figure 4-10 shows various lesions of the skin.

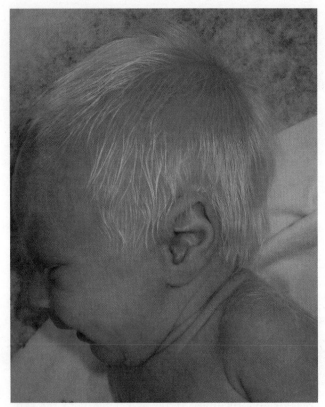

Figure 4-9   Albinism. (Reprinted from Kronenberger J, Ledbetter J. *Jones & Bartlett Learning's Comprehensive Medical Assisting.* 5th ed. Burlington, MA: Jones & Bartlett Learning, LLC; 2016.)

Lesions are classified by their type and location, above or below the surface of the skin. A rash is a type of surface skin lesion. A diaper rash is an example of a localized rash and a disease like the measles can cause a generalized rash over the entire body. A raised rash is on the skin is called an eruption. Other types of surface skin lesions are:

- Papule—a firm, raised area (pimple)
- Macule—a spot on the skin, not raised or depressed (freckles)
- Nodule—a large firm papule
- Vesicle—a blister or fluid filled sac (shingles)
- Pustule—vesicle filled with pus

Many lesions develop from trauma, sounds, or injury to the skin. These result in deeper lesions and include:

- Excoriation—a scratch into the skin
- Laceration—a rough, jagged wound caused by tearing the skin
- Ulcer—death of the tissue resulting in a deep sore
- Fissure—a crack in the skin

Burns

Burns can be minor or very serious. They can be caused from contact with hot objects and chemicals, exposure to sunlight, and electrical injuries. Burns are classified by the depth of damage and the amount of surface area affected.

- First-degree burn—superficial involving only the epidermis; skin is red, dry with minimal pain; an example is a mild sunburn.
- Second-degree burn—partial-thickness burn involves the epidermis and dermis forming blisters; an example is scalding with water or severe sunburn.
- Third-degree burn—full-thickness burn involving destruction of the entire skin, extend into subcutaneous fat, muscle, or bone; skin is broken, dry and pale, or charred; may require skin grafting or may result in loss of digits or limbs; an example is exposure to open flames.

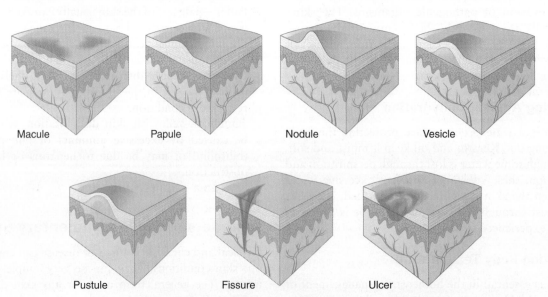

Figure 4-10   Skin lesions. (Reprinted from Kronenberger J, Ledbetter J. *Jones & Bartlett Learning's Comprehensive Medical Assisting.* 5th ed. Burlington, MA: Jones & Bartlett Learning, LLC; 2016.)

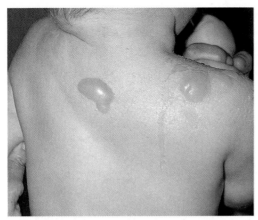

Figure 4-11 Second-degree burn. (From Fleisher GR, Ludwig S, Baskin MN. *Atlas of Pediatric Emergency Medicine.* Philadelphia, PA: Lippincott Williams & Wilkins; 2004.)

Figure 4-11 shows a second-degree burn.

In addition to the level or intensity of the burn, the **BSA**, body surface area, of the burn is evaluated to determine the percentage of the body that has been involved. The rule of nines is the formula used to estimate the burned surface area. The rule of nines applies 9% of the skin to the head; 9% for each arm, including front and back; 18% to the front of the trunk; 18% to the back of the trunk; 18% to each lower extremity; and 1% to the genital area. Figure 4-12 shows the rule of nines and percentage distribution of burns to the body.

When a person is burned, there is always concern for infection. The skin is a major defense against invading microorganisms. Damaged, burned skin becomes an avenue of entry for pathogens that cause infection. Smoke and chemical inhalation may cause respiratory complications. Burn patients need to be monitored carefully for wound care and pain control. Fluid replacement is also essential.

Skin Cancer

In the United States, skin cancer is the most common form of cancer. Sun exposure is the skin's worst enemy especially for fair skin people who live in climates where the sun is intense such as the Southwest. Early detection and treatment are crucial to managing any cancer. Basal cell and squamous cell carcinomas form in the epidermis usually on the neck, face, and hands.

Melanoma is a malignant tumor of melanocytes. This cancer can be anywhere in the body originating from a mole or birthmark called a nevus. Although it may appear as a mole, melanoma will have irregular, uneven borders, increase in size, and change color. Figure 4-13 shows two types of melanoma, superficial and nodular.

Case Question

How would you respond to the patient if she asks if she should continue going to the pool every day?

Skin Infections

Skin infections can be caused from bacteria, viruses, and fungi. The physician needs to determine the type of infection in order to properly treat each type of infection.

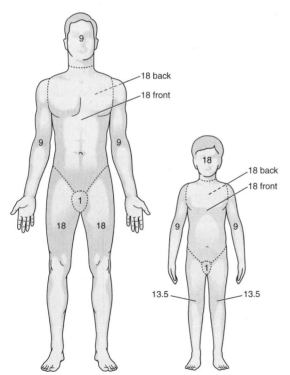

Figure 4-12 Rule of nines. (Reprinted from Kronenberger J, Ledbetter J. *Jones & Bartlett Learning's Comprehensive Medical Assisting.* 5th ed. Burlington, MA: Jones & Bartlett Learning, LLC; 2016.)

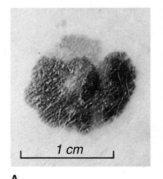 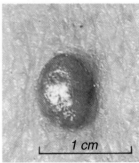

A   **B**

Figure 4-13 Malignant melanoma. **A.** Superficial melanoma. **B.** Nodular melanoma. (Reprinted from Kronenberger J, Ledbetter J. *Jones & Bartlett Learning's Comprehensive Medical Assisting.* 5th ed. Burlington, MA: Jones & Bartlett Learning, LLC; 2016.)

Bacterial Infections

Bacterial infections can be caused by simple scratches on the skin or deep lacerations. The pathogen causing the infection invades the skin tissue and, if it spreads, may lead to cellulitis, a more serious condition requiring antibiotics. Figure 4-14 shows a cellulitis infection of the toe.

Impetigo is another type of infection caused from a staphylococcal bacterial. It is acute and highly contagious. Blister-like lesions form filled with a watery fluid or pus. The blisters frequently form around the mouth and nose.

Viral Infections

Herpes is a virus that affects the skin. Type I herpes, herpes simplex virus, causes cold sores and fever blisters, watery vesicles. The most common place for these to form is around the mouth and nose and on the skin and mucous membranes. Type II herpes causes genital infections. Herpes zoster is the virus that causes shingles. It is the same virus that causes chickenpox (varicella) but is seen in adults. The viral infection follows the nerves and causes skin lesions along the course of the nerve. The most common place for shingles to form is on the trunk of the body around or near the waist. This infection is very painful and the affected area is highly sensitive to touch. There is a singles vaccine available now that is recommended for adults. See Figure 4-15.

Another viral skin infection is caused by the human papillomavirus, **HPV**, group. This virus causes warts. These small tumors can appear anywhere on the body

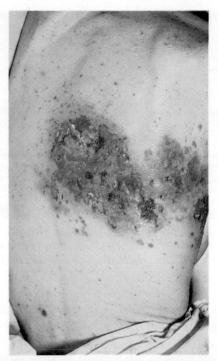

Figure 4-15 Shingles. (Reprinted from Kronenberger J, Ledbetter J. *Jones & Bartlett Learning's Comprehensive Medical Assisting.* 5th ed. Burlington, MA: Jones & Bartlett Learning, LLC; 2016.)

but are commonly found on the soles of feet (plantar wart) and on the hands. Genital warts are usually benign but may be associated with cancer of the cervix.

Fungal Infections

Mycotic (fungal) infections, commonly known as tinea, may appear on the face, body, scalp, hands, or feet. Tinea corporis is knows as ringworm because of the red, ring-shaped lesions it forms. It has nothing to do with worms. See Figure 4-16.

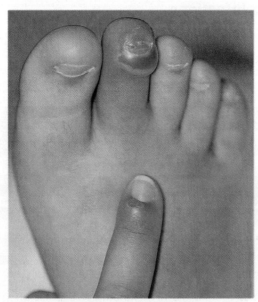

Figure 4-14 Cellulitis infection. (Reprinted from Kronenberger J, Ledbetter J. *Jones & Bartlett Learning's Comprehensive Medical Assisting.* 5th ed. Burlington, MA: Jones & Bartlett Learning, LLC; 2016.)

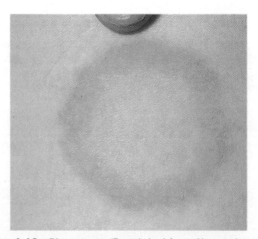

Figure 4-16 Ringworm. (Reprinted from Kronenberger J, Ledbetter J. *Jones & Bartlett Learning's Comprehensive Medical Assisting.* 5th ed. Burlington, MA: Jones & Bartlett Learning, LLC; 2016.)

Athlete's foot is a fungal growth on the feet promoted by dampness and perspiration. Fungal infections can be caused from wearing acrylic nails. The moisture forms under the nail and the fungus has an ideal environment for growth. Antifungal agents are available in topical and oral preparations.

Inflammatory Skin Disorders

Dermatitis refers to any inflammation of the skin and may be acute or chronic. The cause of the inflammation may not be realized and the skin may clear on its own. Chronic inflammation may be more serious and problematic.

Acute Inflammatory Disorders

Urticaria, or hives, is caused from an allergic reaction. The allergen may be a known substance such as certain foods or medications, or it might be in response to a toxin such as venom or contact with animal dander. Hypersensitivity to these agents causes elevated red patches called wheals. Eczema is a skin inflammation that causes intense itching. The affected area appears red with blisters or pimple-like lesions. Scaling and crusting of the skin also is present. Eczema may be the result from contact with irritants such as poison ivy, detergents, and other chemicals. See Figure 4-17.

With the intense itching, the affected person will want to scratch the skin, which may lead to a secondary bacterial infection due to the broken skin. Patients with inflammatory skin disorders benefit from the effects of corticosteroids or antihistamines to reduce the inflammation.

Chronic Inflammatory Disorders

Systemic lupus erythematosus, **SLE,** is a chronic inflammatory disease, which is an autoimmune disease of connective tissue. An autoimmune disease results from an immune reaction to one's own tissues. SLE may affect

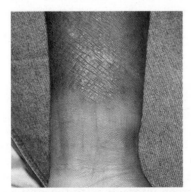

Figure 4-17   Eczema. (Reprinted from Kronenberger J, Ledbetter J. *Jones & Bartlett Learning's Comprehensive Medical Assisting.* 5th ed. Burlington, MA: Jones & Bartlett Learning, LLC; 2016.)

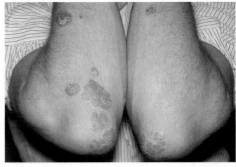

Figure 4-18   Psoriasis. (Reprinted from Kronenberger J, Ledbetter J. *Jones & Bartlett Learning's Comprehensive Medical Assisting.* 5th ed. Burlington, MA: Jones & Bartlett Learning, LLC; 2016.)

the skin and other body organs. On the skin, there may be light purple papules on the face and scalp. One specific sign associated with this disease is a butterfly-shaped rash that appears on the nose and cheeks. SLE lesions are worsened by exposure to sunlight. This disease is more common in women than men. Scleroderma is another autoimmune disease with unknown cause. There is an overproduction of collagen causing thickening and tightening of the skin. Severe scleroderma causes hardening of the skin making movements impossible especially on the face, around the mouth, and the forearms.

Psoriasis is caused from an overgrowth of keratinocytes in the epidermis. Large areas of red flat areas appear covered with silvery scales. Psoriasis is treated with topical corticosteroids and exposure to ultraviolet light. See Figure 4-18.

Accessory Organ Disorders

Acne is a common disorder caused by oversecretion of oil from the sebaceous glands. Acne vulgaris is a form of acne typically found in people between the ages of 14 and 25 years. The hormones that control sebaceous secretions become particularly active during this time period. Acne is characterized by the formation of blackheads and pimples. Excessive oil, sebum, combines with keratinocytes and form a plug within the hair follicle. The plug darkens resulting in a blackhead. When the oil forms a plug within the hair follicle and becomes blocked, it bulges, forming a whitehead, or pimple. Antibiotics, topical and oral, may be used to treat acne.

Alopecia is baldness and most commonly occurs in men as a condition known as male pattern baldness. It usually is linked to heredity and aging. Baldness may also be caused by systemic conditions such as uncontrolled diabetes and thyroid disease. Topical medications are somewhat effective in producing hair growth. Chemotherapeutic drugs, used in treating cancer, are also linked to baldness, but when the drugs are discontinued, the hair growth resumes.

WOUND HEALING AND CARE

When the skin is damaged or injured, repair of the damage starts to take place. After the area heals, a scar, called a **cicatrix**, may remain on the skin's surface. A scar is formed from connective tissue and is strong when healed but is not as flexible as the surrounding tissue. When a wound is sutured together, the scarring is minimized since there is not as much connective tissue needed for repair.

Wound Care

The medical assistant will provide wound care for patients who present with new injuries and for those who need follow up care. For initial care, water or saline solution is used to cleanse the wound. It is important to wear disposable gloves when providing wound care. The physician will examine the wound and decide if sutures are indicated for the wound. The key to healing any wound is infection control. Antibacterial ointments may be used if needed. Sterile dressings are the most effective way to protect the wound from infection. Patients should be instructed to keep the wound dry and clean. The medical assistant may need to demonstrate to the patient how to change the dressing without contaminating the wound.

The Healing Process

The goal with wound care is to promote proper and efficient healing of the wound. There are factors that may affect the healing process.

- Proper nutrition—patients should maintain a balanced diet with the nutrients needed for cell repair and regrowth. Vitamins and minerals are important especially vitamins A and C needed for the production of collagen.
- Rich blood supply—blood supplies tissues with oxygen and nutrients and carries away the waste products that could increase during the healing process. White blood cells are necessary to attack the bacteria at the site of the wound. Diseases such as diabetes

may delay the healing process due to poor circulation of some patients.
- Prevent infection—when a wound is contaminated, the healing process is prolonged due to inflammation of the tissues. Infection also interferes with the formation of materials needed to heal the wound.
- Age—as we age, the healing process also slows due to the slower replacement of cells. Older persons may also have a lowered immune response to infection causing the healing to take longer.

DERMATOLOGY

Dermatology is the study of the skin and a dermatologist is a physician specialist who treats patients with various conditions of the skin and accessory organs. Diagnostic procedures, performed by the physician, include the initial physical examination of the skin. The medical assistant will be asked to assist in the collection of wound cultures and bandaging wounds. Dermatologists rely on a skin biopsy to exam lesions for malignant growth. Medical assistant need to provide patient education to ensure compliance with wound care.

Cultural Connection

Working in any medical practice, the medical assistant may observe patients with marks or bruises on their skin. Although some of these may be caused from trauma, falls, and abuse, there are other reasons for specific discolorations of the skin. Among the Asian culture, specifically Chinese, there is a practice called cupping. It is a method or treatment that involves creating a vacuum, or suction, by heating and applying hot glass cups to the body. Circular areas of bruising are left on the skin once the cups are removed. This strange practice is thought to help blood disorders, skin problems (eczema and acne), as well as other health conditions.

Preparing for Externship

It is never too early to start thinking about your externship course and preparing as much as you can ahead of time. One of the things that most sites require is an interview so they can initially meet the student and determine if it will be a good fit to have this person in their facility. Think of the interview as if you were actually applying for a job with the facility. There may be an open position that the stu-

dent could fill after completion of the externship. The externship site uses the weeks of externship with the student as a working interview. They want to see how the person interacts with the staff and patients as well as how well the student completes assigned duties. Start thinking about the questions the site may ask and develop a few questions that you will ask during the interview.

Chapter Recap

● The study of anatomy and physiology is the basic starting place for anyone entering the health care field. It is critical that we have an understanding of the main structures and functions of the body.

● The abdomen is divided with imaginary lines into nine regions and four quadrants. These divisions allow for more accurate descriptions of the location of body organs and patient's pain or discomfort.

● The body requires maintenance of homeostasis in order to remain healthy. Negative feedback is required in most situations to bring the body back into balance.

● The integumentary system is one of eleven systems in the body. The other systems include the skeletal, muscular, nervous, endocrine, cardiovascular, lymphatic, respiratory, digestive, urinary, and reproductive systems.

● The skin is the body's major first line of defense against invading microorganisms and protects underlying structures. The skin is also key is helping to maintain body temperature.

● There are many skin conditions and diseases, which may result from bacteria, fungi, viruses, and parasites.

● The most dangerous skin cancer is melanoma. All persons need to avoid the sun's UV rays, which contribute to the development of skin cancer.

Online Resources for Students

Student Resources available on the text's online site include:

● Audio Glossaries

● Animations

● Competency Evaluation Forms

● Videos

● Anatomy & Physiology Module with Heart and Lung Sounds

● Weblinks

● Worksheets

Exercises and Activities

Certification Preparation Questions

1. Chronic skin disease characterized by red flat areas covered with silvery scales.
   a. Urticaria
   b. Eczema
   c. Shingles
   d. Psoriasis

2. The dermis is _____ to the epidermis.
   a. superficial
   b. deep
   c. lateral
   d. medial

3. What type of gland is involved in acne?
   a. Sudoriferous
   b. Sebaceous
   c. Ceruminous
   d. Endocrine

4. Which of the following is not a type of skin lesion?
   a. Pallor
   b. Vesicle
   c. Papule
   d. Laceration

5. Which skin discoloration is caused by an accumulation of bile pigment in the blood?
   a. Pallor
   b. Cyanosis
   c. Jaundice
   d. Carotenemia

6. If a person received burns over both lower extremities and the genital area, what percentage of the body is burned?
   a. 18%
   b. 19%
   c. 27%
   d. 37%

7. Which science studies normal body structure?

   a. Homeostasis
   b. Anatomy
   c. Physiology
   d. Pathology

8. Where is intracellular fluid located?

   a. Between body cells
   b. In blood plasma
   c. In lymph
   d. Inside body cells

9. A plane that divides the body into right and left portions is a:

   a. frontal plane.
   b. transverse plane.
   c. sagittal plane.
   d. horizontal plane.

10. Which cavity contains the mediastinum?

    a. Abdominal
    b. Dorsal
    c. Thoracic
    d. Pelvic

Skeletal and Muscular Systems

Chapter Objectives

- Describe the structure and growth of long bones.
- Identify the major bones of the axial skeleton.
- Identify the major bones of the appendicular skeleton.
- Describe various types of bone disorders and fractures.
- Recognize normal and abnormal curves of the spine.
- Identify the categories of joints and the movement provided by each one.
- Compare the three types of muscle tissue.

- Explain the function of skeletal muscle.
- Name some of the major muscles of the body and describe their location and function.
- Compare isotonic and isometric contractions.
- Describe major muscle disorders.
- Describe diagnostic and treatment methods associated with musculoskeletal disorders.
- Discuss the role of the medical assistant in the orthopedic office.

CAAHEP & ABHES Competencies

CAAHEP

- Describe the structural organization of the human body.
- Identify body systems.
- List the major organs in each body system.
- Describe the normal function of each body system.
- Identify common pathology related to each body system including signs, symptoms, and etiology.
- Analyze pathology for each body system including diagnostic measures and treatment modalities.

ABHES

- List all body systems and their structure and functions.
- Describe common diseases, symptoms, and etiologies as they apply to each system.
- Identify diagnostic and treatment modalities as they relate to each body system.

Chapter Terms

Abduction	Appendicular	Arthroplasty	Articular cartilage
Adduction	Arthrocentesis	Arthroscopy	Atrophy

Axial	Extension	Osseous tissue	Periosteum
Cancellous	Flexion	Ossicles	Plantar flexion
Chondrosarcoma	Fontanelles	Ossification	Pronation
Circumduction	Hyperextension	Osteitis deformans	Rickets
Collagen	Hypertrophy	Osteoblast	Rotation
Cramps	Insertion	Osteoclast	Sesamoid bone
Diaphysis	Inversion	Osteocyte	Spasm
Dislocation	Isometric	Osteogenesis imperfecta	Sprain
Dorsiflexion	Isotonic	Osteomalacia	Strain
Endosteum	Ligaments	Osteomyelitis	Supination
Epiphyseal plates	Medullary cavity	Osteoporosis	Tendons
Eversion	Origin	Osteosarcoma	

Abbreviations

ATP	DJD	OA	RA
DIP	MP	PIP	

Case Study

Hunter, a 7-year-old second grader, was playing on the monkey bars at school and fell to the ground landing on his wrist. He immediately felt pain in his lower arm and wrist. When he went to the school nurse, she put an ice pack on his arm and called his mother to come pick him up from school. His mother immediately took Hunter to their primary care physician to have his arm examined. The doctor ordered an x-ray of his lower arm, wrist, and hand. The x-ray revealed that Hunter had a greenstick fracture of the radius. A short arm cast was applied, and his arm was put into a sling. The doctor requested a follow-up appointment in 2 weeks. The medical assistant provided Hunter's mother with an instruction sheet that included information on cast care and signs or symptoms to watch for that might require immediate medical care.

This chapter presents both the skeletal and muscular systems, which work together allowing the body to move, provide support, and protect vital internal organs. In order for the body to move, the bones and muscles need joints to allow bending.

THE SKELETAL SYSTEM

The human body uses the skeleton as a framework, so the bones must be strong to support and protect the body and the internal structures. The skeletal bones have several functions in the body, some of which may not seem so apparent at first. The bones:

- Provide a framework for the body
- Protect underlying structures such as the brain, spinal cord, heart, and lungs
- Work with the muscles to produce movement
- Store calcium salts, which may be released into the blood when calcium is needed
- Produce blood cells in the red marrow

There are approximately 206 bones in the human skeleton. The skeleton is subdivided into the **axial** skeleton, which includes the bones of the head and torso, and the **appendicular** skeleton, which includes all the bones of the extremities. The word appendicular means pertaining to the appendages. Figure 5-1 shows the axial and appendicular divisions of the skeleton as well as the major bones.

Case Question

Hunter is very upset that he will not be able to play on the monkey bars or play softball for a few weeks. If you are the medical assistant, how would you respond to him?

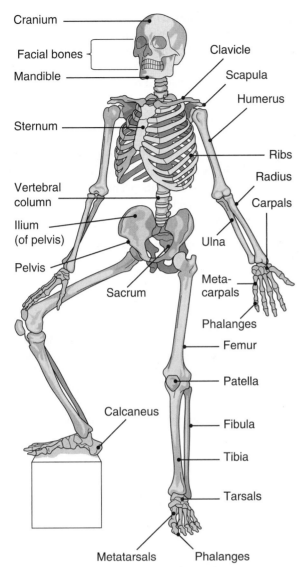

Figure 5-1   Axial and appendicular skeleton. (Reprinted from Cohen BJ. *Memmler's The Human Body in Health and Disease.* 13th ed. Burlington, MA: Jones & Bartlett Learning, LLC; 2014.)

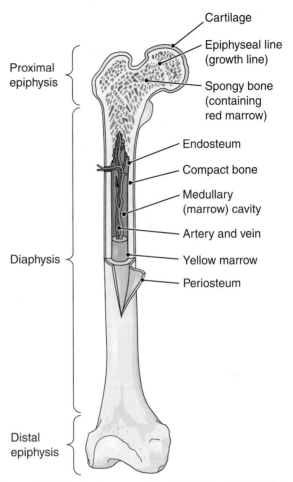

Figure 5-2   Bone diagram. (Reprinted from Cohen BJ. *Memmler's The Human Body in Health and Disease.* 13th ed. Burlington, MA: Jones & Bartlett Learning, LLC; 2014.)

bone is called the epiphysis. There is a proximal end and a distal end of the bone. The proximal end is closer to the midpart of the body and the distal end farther away. For example, the femur's (thigh bone) proximal end is at the hip and the distal end is at the knee. Figure 5-2 is a cutaway diagram of a bone showing the various parts and layers.

Bone Tissue

The bones are made up of living tissue, **osseous tissue**, and have their own blood vessels and nerves. The bone's strength and hardness is due to the matrix between the bone cells. The bones also require **collagen**, a protein substance, which allows the bones to bend slightly and not break or shatter. There are three types of cells within bone tissue:

- **Osteoblasts**—the cells responsible for building bone tissue
- **Osteocytes**—mature bone cells
- **Osteoclasts**—the cells responsible for resorption, the breakdown of bone tissue

The skeletal bones are classified by their shape. There are

- Flat bones—examples include ribs and cranium
- Irregular bones—examples include vertebrae and facial bones
- Short bones—examples include carpals (wrist) and tarsals (ankle)
- Long bones—examples include arms and legs

Parts of the Bone

Long bones are elongate in shape and have a narrow shaft called the **diaphysis**. Through the center of the diaphysis is the **medullary cavity** where the bone marrow is located. The irregularly shaped end of the long

Types of Bone Tissue

There are two types of bone tissue, compact and spongy. Compact bone is hard, dense tissue that makes up the main shaft of long bones. Spongy bone, also known as **cancellous** bone, is found at the ends of the long bones, the epiphyses (pl), and in the lining of the medullary cavity. The bones are covered by a membrane called **periosteum**, except at the joint regions. The **endosteum** lines the bone marrow cavity. Blood vessels within the periosteum help to maintain the bone throughout life. Nerve fibers are also located in this membrane and provide sensations such as pain when there is injury or damage to the bone. Osteoblasts are found in both membranes and are necessary to build, repair, and maintain the bone.

Bone Marrow

There are two kinds of bone marrow, red and yellow. Red marrow is found in the spongy bone at the ends of long bones and at the center of other bones. Blood cells are manufactured in the red marrow. The yellow marrow is primarily made up of fat. During the early periods of development, the long bones of babies and children contain more red marrow to maintain the increased need for new blood cells.

Bone Formation and Regulation

During fetal development, the bones are composed primarily of cartilage. As the fetus develops, cartilage converts to bone during the process of **ossification**. Ossification takes place when the osteoclasts remove the cartilage and the osteoblasts deposit new bone tissue. Once the material has hardened, the cells, osteocytes, continue to maintain the bone matrix. The transformation of cartilage into bone begins at the center of the shaft of the bone and continues to develop toward the ends of the bone. At birth, the ends of long bones have **epiphyseal plates** where continued growth of the bone takes place. When a person reaches approximately 20 years of age, the bones stop growing. After the growing stops, the epiphyseal plate becomes a thin line known as the epiphyseal line. Doctors can evaluate the age of an individual based on the presence of the epiphyseal plate or line shown on x-rays.

Throughout a person's life, the bones are maintained and repaired through a process called resorption. Osteoblasts build up new bone matrix, and osteoclasts clean up the bone tissue by resorbing it. This process is essential when there is a fracture of a bone. The bone will heal and return to the proper shape through the process of resorption.

Formation and resorption relies on the parathyroid hormone produced by the parathyroid glands (posterior to the thyroid gland). This hormone regulates osteoclast activity. The bones also store the majority of the body's calcium supply. Vitamin D, acquired through the diet, is necessary to promote calcium absorption from the intestine. As we age, the bones may lose density due to the slowing of bone tissue renewal. The bones become weaker, and it takes longer to heal injuries.

Bone Markings

Why do bones have various shapes? They need the nooks, depressions, holes, and curves to allow the other structures of the body to attach and allow nerves and blood vessels to pass through. Some major bone markings include the following:

- Projection—outgrowth or protuberance on a bone
- Process—large projection of a bone
- Head—round end of the bone with a slender region below it, the neck (head of the femur)
- Condyle—round projection (epicondyle is a small projection above a condyle)
- Crest—ridge or border (iliac crest of the hip)
- Spine—sharp projection (spine of the shoulder blade)
- Foramen—hole or opening that allows a blood vessel or nerve to pass through
- Sinus—cavity or hollow space (sinuses of the face)
- Fossa—depression on bone surface
- Meatus—passageway or channel (auditory meatus, ear canal)

The Axial Skeleton

The axial skeleton includes the 80 bones of the head and trunk. The word axial refers to the axis or situated on the axis of a structure of the body.

Bones of the Head

The head, referred to as the skull, divides into two parts, the cranium and the facial bones.

Cranium
The cranium is a rounded structure that covers the brain. There are eight individual cranial bones.

- Frontal—forms the forehead, the front of the skull's rook, and the top of the eye orbits
- Parietal—two bones that form most of the top and the side walls of the cranium
- Temporal—two bones that form the sides and the base of the skull
- Ethmoid—fragile bone located between the eyes; the downward extension of this bone forms much of the nasal septum
- Sphenoid—at the base of the skull in front of the temporal bones and forms part of the eye orbit
- Occipital—forms the posterior portion of the skull; the foramen magnum (large hole) is located at the base of the occipital bone and allows passage of the spinal cord from the brain

The cranial bones fuse together with immovable joints called sutures. The more prominent sutures are as follows:

- Coronal suture—joins the frontal bones and two parietal bones
- Squamous suture—joins the temporal bone to the parietal bones
- Lambdoid suture—joins the occipital bone with the parietal bones
- Sagittal suture—joins the two parietal bones on the top of the head

Skull Development

During fetal development, bone formation of the skull is incomplete, which allows the skull to change shape to accommodate the birth canal. The infant has areas of membranes or "soft spots" called **fontanelles**. As the infant grows, the cranial bones will continue to grow and eventually close at about 18 months of age. The delay in this process also allows the brain to grow within the cranium.

Facial Bones

Fourteen bones compose the facial portion of the skull and include the following:

- Mandible—lower jaw bone
- Maxillae (pl)—two bones of the upper jaw bone fused at the midline
- Zygomatic bones—two bones that form the prominences of the cheeks (most pronounced area is called the zygomatic arch)
- Nasal bones—two bones that form the bridge of the nose
- Lacrimal bones—two bones that form the anterior medial wall of the orbital cavity
- Vomer—forms the inferior part of the nasal septum
- Palatine bones—pair of bones that form the posterior part of the hard palate (roof of the mouth)
- Inferior nasal conchae (pl)—two bones that form the side wall of the nasal cavity

Figure 5-3 is a diagram of the cranial and jaw bones of the skull.

There are additional bones in the skull that are not included with the cranium or facial bones. The **ossicles** are three tiny bones in each middle ear. The incus (shaped like an anvil), malleus (shaped like a hammer), and stapes (shaped like a stirrup).

Another tiny bone, the hyoid bone, is located just below the mandible and is a U-shaped bone that attaches the tongue and other muscles.

Bones of the Trunk

The axial skeleton also includes the bones in the trunk of the body, the central portion. The vertebral column (spine) and thorax (chest bones) are found in the trunk.

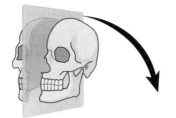
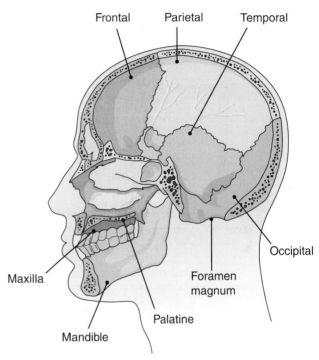

Figure 5-3 Cranial and jaw bones of the skull. (Reprinted from Cohen BJ. *Memmler's The Human Body in Health and Disease*. 13th ed. Burlington, MA: Jones & Bartlett Learning, LLC; 2014.)

Vertebral Column

The spine is the bony support and protective cage for the spinal cord. Figure 5-4 is a diagram of the structure of the vertebral column. The vertebrae are irregularly shaped bones that are smaller at the top of the column and gradually become larger at the lower end of the spine.

The vertebral column is divided into five sections:

- Cervical—7 vertebrae, C1–C7 in the neck region; C1 is the atlas and C2 is the axis
- Thoracic—12 vertebrae, T1–T12 in the thorax (chest) region
- Lumbar—5 vertebrae, L1–L5 in the lower back
- Sacrum—1 vertebrae (5 vertebrae in a child that fuse together)
- Coccyx—1 vertebrae, tailbone (4–5 vertebrae in a child that fuse together)

Each vertebra, other than the axis and atlas, has a body shaped like a drum with a disk of cartilage separating each one. In the center of each vertebra is a hole that provides the opening for the spinal cord to pass through. The spinous

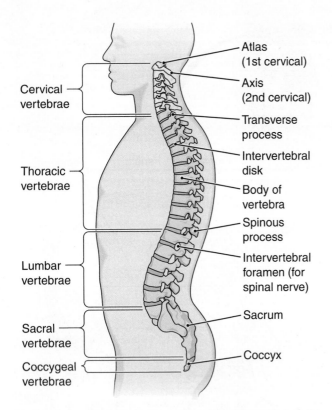

Figure 5-4   Vertebral column. (Reprinted from Cohen BJ. *Memmler's The Human Body in Health and Disease.* 13th ed. Burlington, MA: Jones & Bartlett Learning, LLC; 2014.)

process is the posterior projection, and a transverse process lies on each side of the vertebra. These processes provide a place of attachment of the muscles of the back. There are four curves in the vertebral column that provide the flexibility necessary for balance and movement.

Thoracic Bones

The thorax is formed by the ribs, which attach to the spinal vertebrae in the back and to the sternum in the front of the body. These bones form a cage to protect the vital internal organs of the thorax, primarily the heart and lungs. The upper most portion of the sternum is the manubrium. The collarbone (clavicle) connects on the right and left sides of the manubrium. The largest middle portion of the sternum is the body, and the lowest part of the sternum is the tip called the xiphoid process. It is made of cartilage, not bone.

The 12 pairs of ribs are classified as:

- True ribs—first seven pairs that attach directly to the sternum
- False ribs—five remaining pairs of ribs; attach to cartilage of the rib above
- Floating ribs—last two pairs of false ribs; no anterior attachment to the sternum

Each rib is separated by an intercostal space, which contains muscles, blood vessels, and nerves. Figure 5-5 shows the thoracic bones demonstrating the different types of ribs.

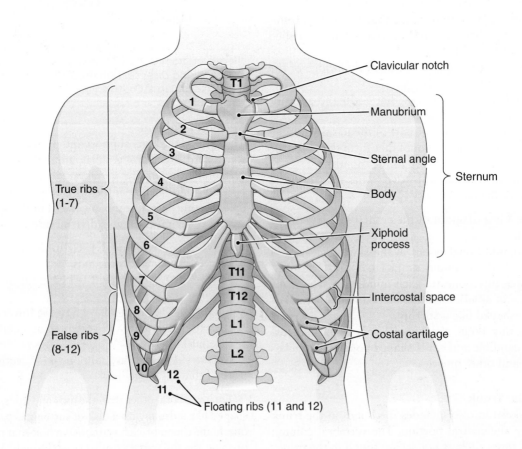

Figure 5-5   Thoracic bones. (Reprinted from Cohen BJ. *Memmler's The Human Body in Health and Disease.* 13th ed. Burlington, MA: Jones & Bartlett Learning, LLC; 2014.)

The Appendicular Skeleton

The term appendicular means pertaining to the append-ages. This skeleton has an upper and lower division. The arms and shoulders are in the upper division, and the legs and hips are in the lower division. There are 126 bones in the appendicular skeleton.

The Upper Division

The upper division includes the shoulder girdle, arms, wrists, hands, and fingers. There are two major bones in the shoulder girdle: the clavicle, commonly called the collar bone, and the scapula, called the shoulder blade. The scapula has a projection, the acromion process, that connects with the clavicle. Inferior to the acromion process is a socket, the glenoid cavity, which is the place where the head of the humerus joins forming a ball and socket joint. This joint allows free movement of the arm. Figure 5-6 is a view of the anterior and posterior shoulder.

The upper arm bone, the humerus, meets the forearm bones, radius and ulna, to form the elbow joint. When standing in anatomical position, the radius is located on the thumb side and the ulna on the little finger side. Below the forearm are the carpals (wrist bones), the metacarpals (bones of the hand), and the phalanges (fingers).

There are 14 phalanges, three in each finger and two in the thumb. The phalanges connect at the joints called the knuckles. In charting patient information, the physician will refer to the joints of the fingers as the **MP** joint, metacarpophalangeal joint, the **PIP** joint, proximal interphalangeal joint, and the **DIP** joint, distal interphalangeal joint. See Figure 5-7 is a detailed diagram of the hand.

The Lower Division

The lower division includes the pelvic girdle (hip), legs, ankles, feet, and toes. The primary bone of the pelvic girdle is the hip bone. This bone begins as three separate

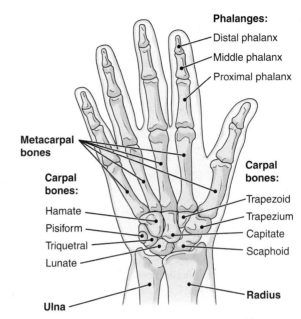

Figure 5-7   Diagram of the hand. (Reprinted from Cohen BJ. *Memmler's The Human Body in Health and Disease.* 13th ed. Burlington, MA: Jones & Bartlett Learning, LLC; 2014.)

bones, which then fuse together to become one continuous bone. The three bones are the ilium, ischium, and pubis. In the anterior part of the pelvis, the hip bones come together as a joint called the pubic symphysis. During pregnancy and childbirth, this joint becomes flexible allowing for the passage of the baby during delivery.

The fused pelvic bones form a socket that allows the head of the femur to fit and form the hip joint. This socket is called the acetabulum. See Figure 5-8 for a diagram of the pelvic bones.

The lower extremity, the leg, has three major bones. The femur, the thigh bone, is the longest and strongest bone in the body. It extends from the hip to the knee. The lower leg, below the knee, consists of the tibia, the shin bone, and the fibula. The tibia is the larger, longer

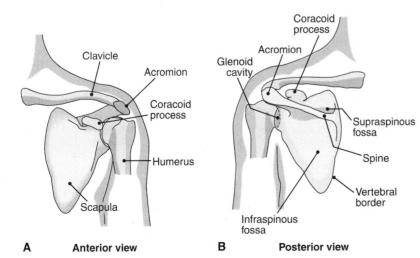

Figure 5-6   Anterior and posterior shoulder. (Reprinted from Cohen BJ. *Memmler's The Human Body in Health and Disease.* 13th ed. Burlington, MA: Jones & Bartlett Learning, LLC; 2014.)

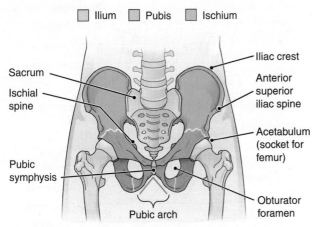

Ilium   Pubis   Ischium

Sacrum
Ischial spine
Pubic symphysis
Pubic arch

Iliac crest
Anterior superior iliac spine
Acetabulum (socket for femur)
Obturator foramen

Figure 5-8 Diagram of pelvic bones. (Reprinted from Cohen BJ. *Memmler's The Human Body in Health and Disease.* 13th ed. Burlington, MA: Jones & Bartlett Learning, LLC; 2014.)

bone. The fibula is slender and lies laterally to the tibia. The patella, kneecap, is a **sesamoid bone** that is held in place by a tendon.

The ankle is formed from the distal end of the tibia and the tarsal bones (ankle bones). The largest tarsal bone is the calcaneus (heel bone). The metatarsal bones form the foot and the phalanges, the toes. There are three phalanges in each toe except the great toe, which has two phalanges.

Study Skill

Repeat, repeat, and repeat again. Repetition is the best way to approach learning a group of items like the bones of the skeleton. One suggestion is to use the diagrams in the textbook as a learning tool. Simply place a piece of paper over the skeletal diagram and cut out part of the paper only to reveal the bones and the lines leading to them. Make sure none of the terms can be seen. Now, on the paper, write the name of each bone next to the line leading to that bone. Spelling counts, so try your best, but always correct any misspelled words. This is a very inexpensive way to learn the skeleton. It also provides a great visual if you are that kind of learner.

 BONE DISORDERS

There are various types of bone disorders categorized by the origin of the disorder. X-rays and laboratory testing are used to diagnose these disorders. The main categories of disorder include the following:

- Metabolic
- Tumors
- Infections
- Structural
- Fractures

Metabolic Disorders

Metabolic problems result from a breakdown of bone tissue due to impaired function of the osteoblasts, cells that build bone tissue, or osteoclasts, cells that breakdown bone tissue, or from a lack of specific minerals or proteins that are required for proper bone matrix. **Osteoporosis** is a condition associated with fragile, porous bones due to a loss of bone mass. This condition will put the person at risk of fractures especially the weight-bearing bones such as the hips and spine. Both men and women can develop osteoporosis merely from the aging process; however, postmenopausal women are at a higher risk for development of osteoporosis when the estrogen levels drop. Although hormone replacement is a treatment for this condition, HRT (hormone replacement therapy) increases the risk of developing breast cancer. Bone growth is also stimulated by weight-bearing exercises such as walking and weight lifting. Bone density testing is important to determine the risk of developing osteoporosis and to monitor the progression of the disorder.

Another metabolic disorder is Paget disease or **osteitis deformans**. This condition causes an increase in bone mass due to overactivity of the osteoblasts in response to excessive osteoclast activity. Basically, bone mass increases due to increased breakdown of bone tissue. It might sound good to have a lot of bone mass, but the quality of the bone is weak and deformed. The bones fracture easily.

Osteomalacia, softening of bones, is due to a lack of calcium in the bones. This condition may stem from a vitamin D deficiency or disease of the liver or kidneys. When osteomalacia occurs in children, it is called **rickets**. Rickets could be related to poor diet or inadequate sunlight, which is required to synthesize the vitamin D.

A more rare metabolic disorder is **osteogenesis imperfecta**, a genetic disorder resulting in defective collagen production. The bones become brittle and break easily. Some children suffer multiple fractures from simple causes, and some fractures are even evident prior to birth.

Tumors

A neoplasm (new growth) is also known as a tumor. Tumors may be benign (noncancerous) or malignant (cancerous). **Osteosarcoma** and **chondrosarcoma** are malignant tumors that develop within the bone (oste/o) or cartilage (chondr/o). Most osteosarcomas develop in a young person's bones, especially around the knee.

Bone Infections

Bone infections are caused from bacteria invading the bone through injury where the skin is broken or through the bloodstream. **Osteomyelitis** is caused by pyogenic bacteria (pus-forming). The infection may remain localized in one area of the bone or spread throughout the bone infecting the marrow and periosteum. Antibiotics are used to treat bone infections and usually have a good outcome for the patient.

Although you may not think tuberculosis is associated with bone infections, TB is able to spread to the bones, usually the bones of the extremities. Pott disease is tuberculosis of the spine. The vertebrae become infected, are weakened, and collapse causing deformity and pressure on the spinal cord.

Structural Diseases

The structural diseases of the bones include abnormal spinal curves. Figure 5-9 shows the three abnormal spinal curves.

These include the following:

- Kyphosis—known as hunchback; an exaggeration of the thoracic spinal curve
- Lordosis—known as swayback; an excessive lumbar curve
- Scoliosis—most common type of abnormal curve; a lateral curvature of the spine

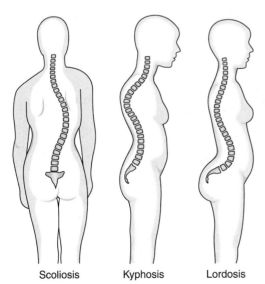

Scoliosis   Kyphosis   Lordosis

Figure 5-9 Abnormal spinal curves. (Reprinted from Cohen BJ. *Memmler's The Human Body in Health and Disease.* 13th ed. Burlington, MA: Jones & Bartlett Learning, LLC; 2014.)

Another type of structural disorder occurs when the maxillary bones (upper jaw) do not fuse during development of the fetus. This malformation results in a condition called cleft palate, an opening in the roof of the mouth. Surgery is used to correct the defect.

Fractures

What is the difference between a broken bone and a fractured bone? Other than the name, there is no difference. The words are interchangeable. A fracture (break) is usually caused from external force placed on the bone. Figure 5-10 shows the various types of bone fractures.

There are different types of fractures including

- Open fracture—a fractured bone that protrudes through the skin creating a visible external wound of the skin
- Closed fracture—a fractured bone without injury to the skin; no external wound
- Greenstick fracture—a partial break in the bone similar to bending a green stick, most common in children
- Impacted fracture—the bone breaks and the broken ends become jammed into each other
- Comminuted fracture—the bone breaks into many pieces, typically seen in a crushing injury
- Spiral fracture—the bone breaks as it twists, like wringing a mop
- Transverse fracture—the bone breaks completely across the bone
- Oblique fracture—the bone breaks at an angle across the bone

Case Question

Hunter, the boy from our case study, asks what the difference is between a broken bone and a fractured bone. How would you explain this to a 7-year-old? If Hunter's mother questioned you about the term greenstick, how would you explain this to her?

There can be dangerous complications involved with a fractured bone. First aid to prevent further injury is a key element in the treatment of an individual with a fractured bone. The fracture needs to be protected by splinting the area "as is." Do not try to align the bone. Leave that to the experts. Since a main function of bones is to provide protection to underlying structures, a fractured rib may puncture vital organs such as the heart or lungs. A fracture of the spine may result in injury to the spinal cord.

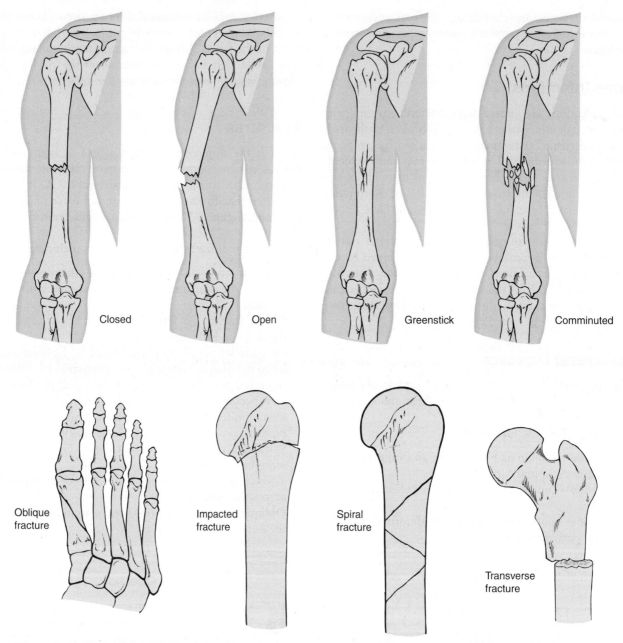

Figure 5-10 Bone fractures. (Reprinted from Kronenberger J, Ledbetter J. *Jones & Bartlett Learning's Comprehensive Medical Assisting.* 5th ed. Burlington, MA: Jones & Bartlett Learning, LLC; 2016.)

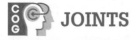 **JOINTS**

A joint is formed by the junction of two or more bones. Also called an articulation, they are initially classified according to the degree of movement allowed by the joint. There are three classifications:

- Synarthrosis—immovable joints; also called fibrous joints, they come together and do not allow any movement; an example is the sutures of the skull
- Amphiarthrosis—slightly movable joints; also referred to as cartilaginous joints; an example is the joint created where the pubic bones join at the symphysis pubis

- Diarthrosis—freely movable joints; most common joint in the body; joint cavity has a synovial lining and the cavity is filled with synovial fluid, which acts as a cushion for the joint; an example is the knee joint

The synovial joints need supporting structures to provide stability to these freely moving joints. **Ligaments** connect bone to bone around synovial joints. They are bands of very dense connective tissue that reinforce the joints. The joints are also are cushioned by a layer of **articular cartilage** located at the ends of the bones. Close to some of the joints are small sacs filled with synovial fluid. These sacs, called bursae (pl), help to reduce the stress around the joints allowing for ease of movement.

Synovial joints are further classified by the type of movement they provide for the body. The movement is based on the body in anatomical position. Figure 5-11 shows the various types of joint movement.

The types of movement are as follows:

- **Flexion**—decreases the angle of the joint; bending the elbow decreases the angle between the upper and lower arm
- **Dorsiflexion**—moving the foot upward toward the body decreasing the angle between the foot and lower leg
  - **Plantar flexion**—opposite of dorsiflexion; bending the foot downward as in standing on the tiptoes; increases the angle between the foot and lower leg
- **Extension**—increases the angle of the joint; straightening of the arm from a flexed position
  - **Hyperextension**—extending a body part beyond the anatomical position; hyperextending the knee when kicking a ball or hyperextending the elbow when throwing a ball
- **Abduction**—moving away from the midline of the body; example is motion when moving the arm straight out to the side
- **Adduction**—moving toward the midline of the body; example is motion when moving the arm toward the body, opposite of abduction
- **Inversion**—turning the sole of the foot inward so the bottom of the foot faces the other foot

- **Eversion**—turning the sole of the foot outward so the bottom of the foot faces away from the body
- **Circumduction**—moving in a circular pattern as when moving the outstretched arm in a circle
- **Rotation**—turning a bone on its own axis; turning the head from side to side to indicate no; the axis and atlas bones allow this movement
- **Supination**—turning the palm of the hand up; forward when in anatomical position
- **Pronation**—turning the palm of the hand down; backward when in anatomical position

The various types of movement require different types of synovial joints. These types include the following:

- Gliding joint—bones slide over each other with little change in the joint angle; example is the joints formed between the wrist and ankle joints
- Hinge joint—bones fit together due to the curves they have; one curves outward, the other inward; example is the elbow and finger joints
- Pivot joint—a bone with a rounded part rests on and fits into another bone with a groove; example is atlas and axis of the spine allowing rotation of the head
- Condyloid joint—the oval part of a bone fits into the concave part of another bone; example is the knuckles where the metacarpals join the proximal phalanges
- Saddle joint—resembles a saddle with one bone sitting on another bone like a person sitting on a saddle;

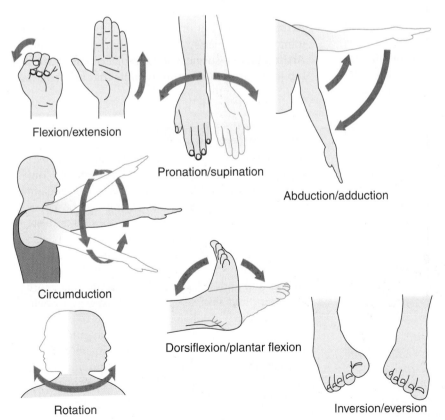

Flexion/extension

Pronation/supination

Abduction/adduction

Circumduction

Dorsiflexion/plantar flexion

Rotation

Inversion/eversion

Figure 5-11 Types of joint movement. (Reprinted from Cohen BJ. *Memmler's The Human Body in Health and Disease.* 13th ed. Burlington, MA: Jones & Bartlett Learning, LLC; 2014.)

example is the thumb where the wrist bone and metacarpal of the thumb come together
- Ball and socket joint—ball-shaped, rounded end of the bone fits into a cup-like depression of another bone; example is hip joint or shoulder joint

Joint Disorders

There are various conditions affecting the joints that may be caused by injury or inflammation. These disorders include the following:

- **Dislocation**—the structures of the joint become deranged. The shoulder is the most common joint to become dislocated.
- **Sprain**—excessive movement of a joint resulting in a rupture or tearing of the ligaments surrounding the joint. The ankle is the most common joint to become sprained. Typically caused from inward turning of the foot.
- Bursitis—inflammation of a bursa. One of the common locations for bursitis is in front of the knee. Also known as "housemaid's knee" because of the effect kneeling has on this area.
- Arthritis—inflammation of a joint
  - Osteoarthritis (**OA**), also known as degenerative joint disease (**DJD**), is a form of arthritis caused from normal wear and tear on joints
  - Rheumatoid arthritis (**RA**), an autoimmune disease and form of arthritis that causes swelling and crippling of the hands and feet; deformation results from the crippling; Figure 5-12 demonstrates the disfiguring effects of rheumatoid arthritis
  - Gout, a type of arthritis caused by a metabolic disturbance; overproduction of uric acid, which accumulates in the joints; most affected joint is the big toe

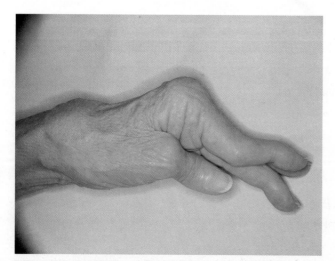

Figure 5-12   Effects of rheumatoid arthritis. (Reprinted from Kronenberger J, Ledbetter J. *Jones & Bartlett Learning's Comprehensive Medical Assisting.* 5th ed. Burlington, MA: Jones & Bartlett Learning, LLC; 2016.)

Disorders of the Spine

The vertebrae of the spine are held together by joints, which are surrounded by ligaments, and muscles, and have an intervertebral disk between them. The spine is subject to numerous disorders that frequently cause back pain, more likely low back pain.

- Herniated disk—the disk between a vertebra protrudes or "slips" out of the normal space and pushes on surrounding nerves; sciatica results from disk pressure on the sciatic nerve
- Strained ligaments of the spine—most commonly located in the lumbosacral joint of the lower back

Taking Care of the Joints

There are joint disorders that may be diagnosed and treated by primary care physicians; however, a referral to an orthopedic specialist may be required for further evaluation and possible invasive assessment of the problem. Orthopedic physicians also specialize in surgical procedures to correct musculoskeletal problems. Physical therapy and medication may be indicated to treat some joint disorders. Procedures that assist in the examination and treatment of the joints include the following:

- **Arthroscopy**—a procedure using an arthroscope (endoscope), a lighted instrument, to examine the inside of a joint; during arthroscopy, ligament replacement and cartilage repair can be made. See Figure 5-13, which is an image of an endoscope used to examine the knee joint.
- **Arthrocentesis**—draining accumulated fluid from a joint cavity; typically caused by injury to the joint
- **Arthroplasty**—surgical joint replacement; knee and hip joints are most common joints that are replaced

Patient Education

Throughout our lifetime, the aging process causes changes to the musculoskeletal system. As our body's metabolism slows, we start to lose calcium necessary to keep the bones strong. As the bones become weaker and more fragile, they are subject to injury including fractures. Muscle tissue is also lost over time, which may affect our balance and reflexes. These changes can all lead to increased risk of falls and injury. As we age, we also become more sedentary and decrease exercise. One way to help maintain the musculoskeletal system is to continue to exercise even for a few minutes a day, and it does not have to be strenuous exercise. Simple walking is great to help maintain the bones and muscles. A well balanced diet is also necessary to provide the nutrients for proper bone and muscle repair.

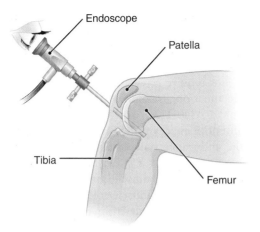

Endoscope

Patella

Tibia

Femur

Figure 5-13 Endoscope exam of knee joint. (Reprinted from Cohen BJ. *Memmler's The Human Body in Health and Disease*. 13th ed. Burlington, MA: Jones & Bartlett Learning, LLC; 2014.)

THE MUSCULAR SYSTEM

The muscular system has three types of muscle tissue: smooth, cardiac, and skeletal muscle. Since you have been introduced to the skeletal system in the first part of this chapter, this section focuses primarily on skeletal muscle. First let's discuss the smooth and cardiac muscle.

Smooth Muscle

This muscle is found in the walls of the hollow body organs such as the blood vessels, digestive system, and the pathways of the respiratory system. It is an involuntary muscle, which means that we do not control the action of this muscle by our conscious thoughts. It is made up of elongated spindle-shaped cells with no striations. This muscle functions automatically using peristalsis, a wave-like motion, to move the substances through the system. Smooth muscle found in the blood vessels can regulate the size or diameter of the vessel by dilating or constricting. An example of the action of smooth muscle is found in the muscular wall of the uterus, which contracts during childbirth. In this case, the uterine muscle contracts from hormonal stimulation.

Cardiac Muscle

Found only in the heart, cardiac muscle is also involuntary and appears striated. Each heartbeat results from the involuntary contraction and relaxation of cardiac muscle. The normal heart beats 60 to 80 times per minute. Cardiac muscle is regulated by nerve stimulation and messages received from the central nervous system (brain and spinal cord).

Skeletal Muscle

This muscle is the only voluntary muscle in the body and relies on the nervous system to provide stimulation to the muscle. We consciously control this muscle. It appears striated having long and cylindrical cells. These are referred to as muscle fibers. Each muscle fiber can contract as a single unit when it is stimulated. This muscle tissue can contract and relax very rapidly allowing body movement.

It is skeletal muscle because these muscles attach to the bones, allowing movement of the joints. Some voluntary, skeletal muscles do not provide joint movement such as those found in the abdominal wall. We can control the function of these muscles, but primarily, they provide support to maintain the body in sitting and standing positions. The facial muscles are another good example of voluntary muscles that allow facial expression but no joint movement.

There are more than 600 skeletal muscles accounting for the largest portion of the body's muscle mass, approximately 40% of our total body weight. The three primary functions of the skeletal muscles are as follows:

- Skeletal movement—the muscles are attached to the bones and shorten or lengthen to cause the bones to move at the joints.
- Support body posture—some of the muscles remain in a steady partial contracted state called muscle tone. This allows the body to maintain posture.
- Produce heat—the muscles generate most of the body's heat necessary to keep it at the normal temperature of 98.6°F. When we are cold, the muscles increase contractions causing us to shiver that produces heat to warm us.

Muscle Tissue

Skeletal muscles are made of fibers bound together into bundles. These bundles are then bound together to form a muscle. Each of these bundles and the muscle has its own covering. The coverings are made up of connective tissue and include the following:

- Endomysium—the innermost layer that covers each muscle fiber
- Perimysium—covers the bundles of muscle fibers called fascicles
- Epimysium—the outermost layer that covers the entire muscle

These tissues merge to form the **tendons**, the dense connective tissues that attach the muscles to bones. Figure 5-14 is an image of a muscle and tendon attached to the bone. It also demonstrates the intricate parts of the muscle structure.

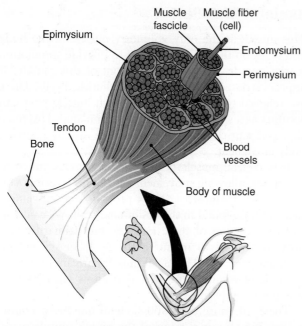

Figure 5-14   Muscle and tendon attached to bone.
(Reprinted from Cohen BJ. *Memmler's The Human Body
in Health and Disease*. 13th ed. Burlington, MA: Jones &
Bartlett Learning, LLC; 2014.)

Muscle Function

Most of us take for granted that our muscles will just
do what we want them to do without giving a second
thought. There are many processes and components
necessary to make them work properly. Let's take a
look at the basics of muscle function. Skeletal muscles
rely on nerve impulses to function and cause them to
contract. Sensory nerve impulses carry messages from
the muscles to the brain and spinal cord where the
messages are interpreted. Then, motor nerve impulses
send messages from the brain and spinal cord back
to the muscles signaling them to contract and cause
movement.

In order for a muscle to shorten and become thicker,
the muscle tissue must have contractibility. The muscle
fibers contain many threads or filaments that are composed of two types of protein that provide the ability of
the muscles to contract. Under a microscope, the protein
actin appears as a light filament and myosin appears
darker. The difference in the appearance of these proteins is what gives skeletal muscle the appearance of
striation.

Muscles also require energy for action. This energy
comes from adenosine triphosphate (**ATP**). Calcium
is also necessary for muscle contraction. It creates the
bridge between actin and myosin so the muscle can
effectively contract.

ATP can be produced through metabolism using oxygen (aerobic) or without oxygen (anaerobic). Aerobic
exercise increases oxygen use and improves muscle

endurance. Exercise such as riding a bike, swimming,
and running requires more endurance. Athletes improve
their ability to generate ATP and get rid of waste products through endurance training. Since anaerobic exercise does not require oxygen to produce ATP, this type
of muscle function uses glucose in the form of glycogen to make ATP. This form of exercise provides the
small amount of energy for short-term vigorous exercise
versus the endurance type of exercise. During anaerobic exercise, lactic acid, a chemical, can accumulate in
the muscles and cause muscle fatigue. When this substance accumulates, the muscle contractibility decreases.
Muscle cramps may occur from the increased muscle
fatigue.

Exercising the Muscles

To ensure that the muscles are well conditioned and
toned, we need to exercise them, so they will adapt
to the increased workload when needed. The type of
exercise affects the change in the muscle. For example,
weight lifting increases the size or bulk of a muscle.
This is referred to as **hypertrophy**. In contrast, endurance training exercises increase the muscle's ability to
withstand lengthy exercise without increasing the size
of the muscle. Male sex hormones have a positive effect
on the building of muscles. This accounts for number of
athletes who have used steroid preparations to increase
the size of their muscles.

One of the main muscles requiring exercise is the
cardiac muscle found in the heart. Routine exercise
strengthens the heart muscle so it can continue to efficiently pump throughout our lifetime. You have probably heard of this type of exercise as "cardio." Because
they routinely exercise, well-conditioned athletes typically have a slower resting heartbeat.

Muscle Contractions

Even when you are sitting or lying down, your muscles
are contracted. This is a condition we refer to as muscle
tone. The muscles are always ready for action when the
nerves stimulate them. When we don't use our muscles,
they become weak and flabby. The body depends on two
types of contractions:

- **Isotonic** contraction—the muscle tension remains
  the same, but it changes in length; the word literally
  means equal or same tension
- **Isometric** contraction—the muscle tension increases,
  but the size remains the same; the word means equal
  or same measure

When you are walking, you are performing both
types of contractions. Isotonic contractions move
you and isometric contractions keep your body in
position.

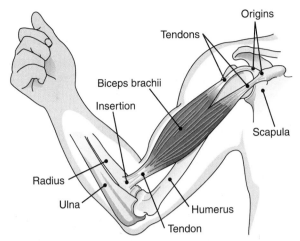

Figure 5-15 Origin and insertion of muscles. (Reprinted from Cohen BJ. *Memmler's The Human Body in Health and Disease.* 13th ed. Burlington, MA: Jones & Bartlett Learning, LLC; 2014.)

More Muscle Movement

There are two ends to the muscle, the **origin** and the ***insertion***. The origin is the less moveable, fixed end of the muscle, and the insertion is the moveable end of the muscle attached to the bone that is moved. Some muscles have more than two points of attachment. At the point of insertion, the muscle divides, and if there are two heads, it will usually begin with the prefix "bi," as in biceps, and if there are three heads of the muscle, the prefix "tri," as in triceps. See Figure 5-15 that illustrates the origin of the biceps muscle of the upper arm and the insertion of the moveable end on the radius bone of the lower arm.

Muscles work together to efficiently move the body. The main muscle that performs is the prime mover. Muscles are identified as an agonist or an antagonist. The agonist performs a specific action, and the antagonist produces an opposite action. When the agonist is working, the antagonist is relaxing.

 ## SKELETAL MUSCLES

The muscles of the body can be grouped together by the region they are located and other characteristics that are used to help identify and remember them. These characteristics include the following:

- Size—within their name, a muscle may have terms such as maximus (large), major (main), minor (lesser), longus (long), or brevis (short) indicating the size of the muscle
- Shape—muscles appear as various shapes such as circular (orbicularis), trapezoidal (trapezius), or triangular (deltoid)
- Location—some muscles are named for the bone that is close to it and include lateral, medial, external, and

internal to designate where it is in relationship to the bone
- Action—muscles are named for the action they provide such as flexor or extensor and adductor or abductor
- Number of heads—a muscle with multiple attachment points will be indicated by the prefixes bi (two), tri (three), and quad (four)
- Fiber direction—the terms rectus (straight) and oblique (angled) are used to describe the direction the muscle is situated in the body

The major skeletal muscles of the body will be presented in the separate tables by region they are located. Look for some of the identifying characteristics as discussed in the previous section. We will start at the top of the body and work our way down to the feet. Refer to Figure 5-16, an anterior view, and Figure 5-17, a posterior view of the body muscles.

Muscles of the Head and Neck

Table 5-1 lists the major muscles of the head and neck. The table also provides the location of each muscle and the basic function. The muscles of the face primarily provide the actions of chewing and facial expressions.

Muscles of the Upper Extremities

The muscles of the upper extremities include the shoulder muscles and those that move the upper arm, forearm, and hand. Table 5-2 lists these muscles and their location and basic function.

Muscles of the Trunk, Abdomen, and Pelvis

The muscles in this group include those that are involved in allowing us to breathe. The muscles of the abdomen and pelvis support internal organs and provide the necessary compression of the abdomen during actions such as coughing, sneezing, urination, childbirth, and elimination. They also include deep muscles located in the back that support the spine and support the body during movement. Table 5-3 lists the major muscles of the trunk, abdomen, and pelvis and their location and basic function.

Muscles of the Lower Extremities, Leg and Foot

The body primarily relies on the muscles of the lower extremities for support, balance, and movement. These muscles are the longest and strongest muscles in the body. Table 5-4 lists the major muscles in this region of the body, their location, and basic function.

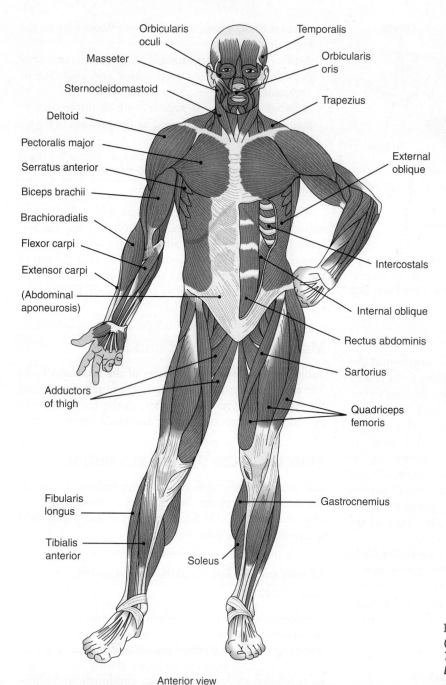

Orbicularis oculi

Masseter

Sternocleidomastoid

Deltoid

Pectoralis major

Serratus anterior

Biceps brachii

Brachioradialis

Flexor carpi

Extensor carpi

(Abdominal aponeurosis)

Adductors of thigh

Fibularis longus

Tibialis anterior

Temporalis

Orbicularis oris

Trapezius

External oblique

Intercostals

Internal oblique

Rectus abdominis

Sartorius

Quadriceps femoris

Gastrocnemius

Soleus

Anterior view

Figure 5-16 Anterior view of muscles. (Reprinted from Cohen BJ. *Memmler's The Human Body in Health and Disease.* 13th ed. Burlington, MA: Jones & Bartlett Learning, LLC; 2014.)

MUSCLE DISORDERS AND INJURIES

The muscular system is subject to problems just like any other body systems. We explore the more common disorders and injuries that affect the muscles. The most common problem would have to be a muscle **spasm**. This is a sudden and involuntary contraction that causes various levels of pain from minor to intense. A spasm can occur in any muscle, not just skeletal muscles. For example, the smooth muscle of the intestinal tract might spasm causing abdominal pain. A seizure can also create a series of skeletal muscle spasms. Muscle **cramps** are more intense contractions usually following exercise or strenuous activity. Muscle cramps can also occur when the body is at rest. We refer to these as a "charley horse," and they usually affect the legs. **Atrophy** is a term used to describe a decrease in size or lack of development. When a muscle begins to atrophy, it will become weak and shrink. A person who is bedridden and not exercising their muscles will begin to experience muscle atrophy. Even the muscles of a limb that has been in a cast for a length of time will experience some level of atrophy. More significant atrophy occurs when there is nerve involvement causing paralysis.

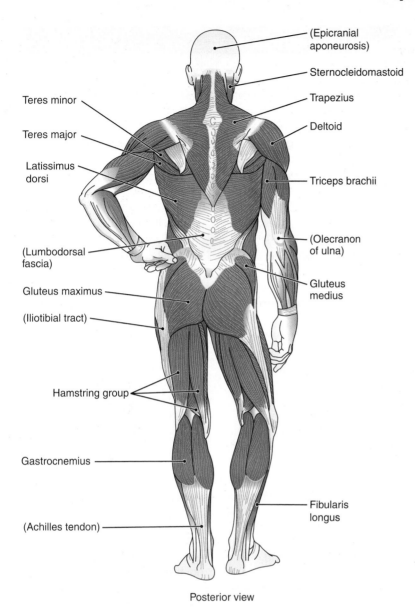

Teres minor

Teres major

Latissimus dorsi

(Lumbodorsal fascia)

Gluteus maximus

(Iliotibial tract)

Hamstring group

Gastrocnemius

(Achilles tendon)

(Epicranial aponeurosis)

Sternocleidomastoid

Trapezius

Deltoid

Triceps brachii

(Olecranon of ulna)

Gluteus medius

Fibularis longus

Posterior view

Figure 5-17 Posterior view of muscles. (Reprinted from Cohen BJ. *Memmler's The Human Body in Health and Disease.* 13th ed. Burlington, MA: Jones & Bartlett Learning, LLC; 2014.)

Table 5-1 Muscles of the Head and Neck

Muscle	Location	Function
Orbicularis oculi	Surrounds the eye	Closing the eye
Orbicularis oris	Surrounds the mouth	Puckering the lips
Buccinator	Fleshy part of the cheek	Chewing and keeping food between the teeth
Temporalis	Above the ear	Close the lower jaw
Masseter	At the angle of the jaw	Aids in chewing
Sternocleidomastoid	Extends from the sternum and clavicle to the mastoid process behind the ear	Turn the head; flex the neck and extend the head

Table 5-2   Muscles of the Upper Extremities, Forearm, and Hand

Muscle	Location	Function
Trapezius	Covers the posterior neck and extends across the posterior shoulder inserting on the clavicle and scapula	Elevates and depresses the scapula
Latissimus dorsi	Originates from the spine in the middle and lower back; covers lower half of the thoracic region forming a portion of the armpit	Adducts the arm and rotates it medially, and extends it
Pectoralis major	Arises from the sternum, upper ribs, and clavicle on either side of the upper chest; inserts into the upper arm bone, humerus	Adducts and rotates the arm
Serratus anterior	Below the axilla (underarm) on the side of the chest; inserts posteriorly on the scapula	Rotates the scapula and pulls it forward, elevates the ribs
Deltoid	Covers the shoulder joint at the top of the arm	Abduction, flexion, extension, and rotation of the humerus at the shoulder joint
Biceps brachii	Anterior arm along the humerus; brachii means arm	Flexes the elbow and supinates the forearm
Brachialis	Deep to the biceps brachii and extends anteriorly over the elbow joint	Flexes the elbow
Brachioradialis	Originates at the distal humerus and inserts on the distal radius (length of the forearm)	Flexes the elbow
Triceps brachii	Originates in the posterior upper arm at the head of the scapula and extends to the lower arm	Extends the elbow
Extensor carpi radialis longus and extensor carpi radialis brevis	Both extend posteriorly from the lower humerus to metacarpal bones; longus to the second metacarpal, brevis to the third metacarpal	Extend and adduct the hand at the wrist joint
Flexor carpi radialis and flexor carpi ulnaris	Both extend anteriorly from the lower humerus to metacarpal bones; radialis (radial bone side) inserts at the second metacarpal; ulnaris (ulnar bone side) inserts at the pisiform (wrist bone) and the fifth metacarpal	Flex and abduct the wrist
Flexor digitorum and extensor digitorum	Both originate at the distal end of the humerus and extend to the phalanges	Flex and extend the fingers but not the thumb

Table 5-3   Muscles of the Trunk, Abdomen, and Pelvis

Muscle	Location	Function
Diaphragm	Dome-shaped muscle that separates the abdomen from the thorax	Contracts to allow inhalation, and relaxes during exhalation
Intercostal	Attached to and filling the spaces between the ribs	Assist to expand the thoracic cavity during respiration
External and internal oblique	Extend from the back (dorsal) around the sides (lateral) to the front (anterior)	Compress the abdominal wall supporting internal structures
Rectus abdominis	Extends from the xiphoid process of the sternum to the pubis symphysis	Flexes the lumbar spine
Levator ani	Floor of the pelvis, extends from the pubis to the sides of the lower part of the sacrum and coccyx	Aids in defecation, bowel elimination
Erector spinae	Group of muscles extending the length of the spine	Flexes and extends the spine

Table 5-4 Muscles of the Lower Extremities, Leg and Foot

Muscle	Location	Function
Gluteus maximus	Extends from the posterior ilium, sacrum, and coccyx to the femur (thigh bone)	Extends, abducts, and laterally rotates the thigh
Gluteus medius	Extends from the lateral ilium to greater trochanter of the femur	Abducts and medially rotates the thigh
Iliopsoas	Extends from the T12–L5 spine to the lesser trochanter of the femur	Flexes the thigh and vertebral column
Adductor longus	Extends from pubis symphysis to the inner aspect of the femur	Adducts, flexes, and medially rotates the thigh
Adductor magnus	Extends from the ischium to the inner aspect of the femur	Adducts, flexes, and laterally rotates the thigh
Gracilis	Extends from the pubis to the upper, medial tibia (crosses over the knee)	Adducts the thigh, flexes the leg at the knee, and medially rotates the leg
Sartorius	Extends from the anterior iliac spine to the medial tibia	Flexes the thigh at the hip and flexes the leg at the knee
Quadriceps femoris includes 4 heads: 1) Rectus femoris 2) Vastus lateralis 3) Vastus medialis 4) Vastus intermedius	Extends from the length of the anterior thigh to the tibia	As a group, these muscles flex the thigh, extend the leg at the knee, and stabilize the patella and knee
Hamstring muscles include 1) Biceps femoris 2) Semimembranosus 3) Semitendinosus	Posterior thigh extending from the ischium and femur to the tibia and fibula	As a group, these muscles flex the leg and extend and rotate the thigh
Gastrocnemius	Major muscle of the calf (posterior lower leg), extends from the distal end of the femur to the calcaneus ankle bone (Achilles tendon attaches the muscle to the heel bone)	Plantar flexion of the foot (standing on tiptoes)
Soleus	Extends from the distal femur to the calcaneus (ankle bone)	Plantar flexion of the foot at the ankle
Tibialis anterior	Anterior to the tibia	Dorsiflexion, lifting foot off the ground
Flexor digitorum longus and extensor digitorum longus	Flexor is in the posterior lower leg, and extensor is in the anterior lower leg	Flex and extend the foot and phalanges (toes)

Muscle injuries due to overstretching muscles will cause a **strain** of the muscle. The muscle tissue will actually tear between the muscle and the attached tendon. Straining a muscle can occur when lifting heavy objects incorrectly or from prolonged poor posture.

Case Question

 Let's go back to Hunter's problem with the fractured radius. When the physician was talking with his mother, he mentioned that Hunter will probably need to be in a cast for 6 to 8 weeks but should not have any muscle atrophy. Why do you think the physician made this determination?

Muscle Diseases

Diseases that affect the muscles leave the muscles very weak and unable to function to provide the body with support and movement. Among these muscle diseases are muscular dystrophy, myasthenia gravis, and myalgia.

Muscular Dystrophy

The term dystrophy means bad development, or in this case, a wasting or deterioration of the muscle. Muscular dystrophy is a general term for a variety of hereditary, progressive degenerative disorders affecting the skeletal muscles. Duchenne muscular dystrophy is a specific type that frequently affects male children. This form of dystrophy results from a protein defect that affects the structure of the muscle fiber. The muscles eventually weaken and paralysis sets in. The cardiac and respiratory muscles are also affected as the disease progresses, leading to death.

Myasthenia Gravis

This muscular condition affects adults and is characterized by muscular fatigue with only minimal exertion. Early symptoms include drooping eyelids. The neurons that supply the muscles are not triggered to contract due to a loss of acetylcholine receptors.

Myalgia

Myalgia is a general term meaning pain in the muscle (myo—muscle, algia—pain). Myositis results when there is inflammation of the muscle tissue. When there is involvement of the connective tissues and the muscles, the term fibrositis is combined with myositis resulting in the diagnosis fibromyositis. This condition causes severe pain, which may be acute or chronic. To relieve the symptoms, anti-inflammatory medications are indicated as well as rest, heat, and massage. Another term associated with these conditions is fibromyalgia. This condition causes diffuse muscle aches, tenderness, and stiffness throughout the body. Although it is difficult to diagnose this condition, it may be associated with an autoimmune disease where the body reacts to its own tissues.

Associated Disorders

Other structures associated with the musculoskeletal system may become injured or diseased. These structures become injured causing pain and inflammation. These conditions include the following:

- Tendonitis—inflammation of the tendon, the structure that attaches the muscle to the bone. Typically occurs when there is overuse of the tendon. The tiny fibers of the muscle tear away from the tendon, and with repeated use of the muscle, tendonitis occurs. For example, tennis elbow from the repeated overuse of the elbow joint; the tendons become inflamed.
- Plantar fasciitis—inflammation of the connective tissue on the bottom of the foot; may be caused from improper posture and obesity
- Shin splints—pain in the anterior area of the tibia (shin bone); may be caused from running on hard surfaces without adequate footwear
- Torticollis—also called wryneck; caused by injury or spasm of muscles of the neck making it painful and difficult to turn the head

In addition to the disorders mentioned above, aging takes its toll on the muscles too. As we age, there is a gradual loss of muscle cells that leads to a decrease in the size of the muscle. Routine exercise is important to delay the aging process that affects the muscles. Something as simple as light weight lifting, resistance exercise, increases muscle strength and function.

ORTHOPEDICS

Patients with musculoskeletal injuries and disorders seek medical care with their primary care physician or may be referred to a specialist in the practice of orthopedics. The field of orthopedics is a very fascinating practice. There is no age limit to the clients who are treated for muscle and bone conditions. Some orthopedic specialists further specialize in the treatment of pediatric patients and others may focus on the aging client. Most orthopedic physicians also perform surgery of the bones and muscles.

As a result of some of the conditions and diseases of the bones, especially fractures, patients will find the need to use crutches to assist in ambulating. The medical assistant will teach the patient how to properly use the crutches to avoid further injury. Figure 5-18 shows a medical assistant fitting a crutch for a patient. Crutches are adjustable, and there should be a two-finger space

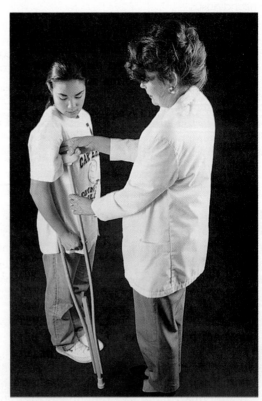

Figure 5-18 Medical assistant fitting crutch. (Reprinted from Kronenberger J, Ledbetter J. *Jones & Bartlett Learning's Comprehensive Medical Assisting.* 5th ed. Burlington, MA: Jones & Bartlett Learning, LLC; 2016.)

between the top of the crutch and the patient's underarm. The hand rest should be adjusted to allow the elbow to slightly flex.

In addition to adjusting the crutches, the medical assistant will instruct the patient how to walk with the crutches so there is weight bearing or non–weight bearing. The physician will determine whether the patient should put any weight on the affected side. Figure 5-19

is a chart showing the correct foot and crutch placement used to achieve the desired gait.

Other health care professionals are involved in the treatment of orthopedic conditions. X-ray technicians are responsible for taking x-rays that will assist the physician in making an accurate diagnosis. Physical therapists are involved in the rehabilitation process assisting patients in strengthening muscles and increasing mobility of joints.

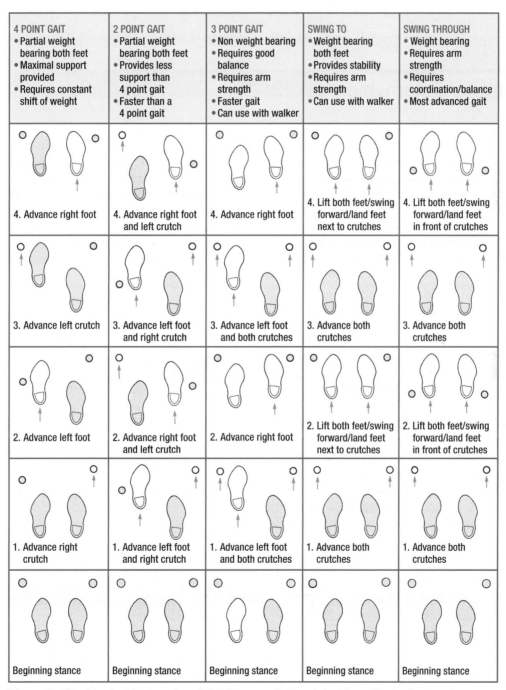

Figure 5-19 Chart of foot and crutch placement. (Reprinted from Kronenberger J, Ledbetter J. *Jones & Bartlett Learning's Comprehensive Medical Assisting.* 5th ed. Burlington, MA: Jones & Bartlett Learning, LLC; 2016.)

Cultural Connection

Acupuncture predates recorded history possibly as far back as 8,000 years. It has been used as a useful tool for pain management that has been practiced and documented in oriental medicine for over 2,000. Chinese physicians developed the philosophy behind acupuncture. It involves the application of needles to specific meridian points in the body. These meridians are the pathways of energy flow through the body. This energy or life force is known as qi or chi (chee).

Acupuncture is a treatment that is becoming more and more popular with Westerners and conventional medical practitioners. It has been found to improve health outcomes and is recommended for the treatment of lower back pain, sports injuries, neck and facial pain, osteoarthritis, and tennis elbow. A benefit of treating with acupuncture is that it is cost-effective and a great alternative to the use of prescribed pain medications.

Preparing for Externship

You may have heard that your attitude determines your altitude. This is a saying that means you can soar higher in your career if you maintain a positive attitude. As you start preparing for your externship, keep in mind that the site might be looking for a new employee and what a great chance for you to audition for that position. It would be great to get your first medical assisting position at your externship. If the site is not hiring, you may want to ask for a letter of recommendation you can use to start your job search. Most medical facilities are eager to assist new graduates with their search for the first job. They may actually have knowledge of other facilities in the area that are hiring. The externship supervisor may be able to introduce you to the facilities that are hiring. In order to secure a position with your externship site or receive a letter of recommendation or introduction to another facility, a positive attitude is critical. This could be one of your most valuable assets and qualities.

Chapter Recap

- There are approximately 206 bones and 600 muscles in the human body that work together to provide support and mobility to the body.
- Bone is made up of living tissue that needs to repair and rebuild itself throughout our life.
- The skeleton is divided into the axial and appendicular skeleton. The axial is the head and trunk bones, and the appendicular is composed of the extremities.
- Bone disorders include those that are caused by metabolic conditions, tumor growth, infection, structural defects, and fractures.

- The joints are critical junctions between bones that allow for movement of the body.
- There are three types of muscle including cardiac, smooth, and skeletal.
- Various types of muscle disorders include muscular dystrophy, myasthenia gravis, and myalgia.
- Exercise is necessary to keep the body's muscle toned and able to support the skeleton.

Online Resources for Students

Student Resources available on the text's online site include:
- Audio Glossaries
- Animations
- Competency Evaluation Forms

- Videos
- Anatomy & Physiology Module with Heart and Lung Sounds
- Weblinks
- Worksheets

Exercises and Activities

Certification Preparation Questions

1. What is the term for a decrease in muscle size, as from disuse?
   a. Strain
   b. Sprain
   c. Atrophy
   d. Dislocation
   e. Hypertrophy

2. Which condition involves the area on the anterior tibia and frequently occurs in runners?
   a. Shin-splints
   b. Fibromyalgia
   c. Myositis
   d. Tendonitis
   e. Torticollis

3. What is an abnormal exaggerated lumbar spinal curve called?
   a. Kyphosis
   b. Lordosis
   c. Osteomyelitis
   d. Scoliosis
   e. Herniation

4. Which type of bone fracture involves one broken side and one bent side?
   a. Open
   b. Impacted
   c. Greenstick
   d. Comminuted
   e. Transverse

5. The main shaft of a bone is called the:
   a. epiphysis.
   b. meatus.
   c. spine.
   d. diaphysis.
   e. fossa.

6. The part of the muscle that is the fixed, immoveable end is the:
   a. tendon.
   b. myofibril.
   c. insertion.
   d. maximus.
   e. origin.

7. What type of fracture involves a break in the bone and the bone protruding through the skin?
   a. Simple
   b. Compound
   c. Impacted
   d. Comminuted
   e. Oblique

8. What condition is associated with fragile, porous bones due to a loss of bone mass?
   a. Myalgia
   b. Osteitis
   c. Osteogenesis
   d. Osteoporosis
   e. Ossification

9. Which of these is a general term for a variety of hereditary, progressive degenerative disorders affecting the skeletal muscles?
   a. Myalgia
   b. Myasthenia gravis
   c. Muscular dystrophy
   d. Fibromyositis
   e. Atrophy

10. Which of these is the group of muscles found in the anterior thigh?
    a. Quadriceps
    b. Hamstrings
    c. Gluteals
    d. Adductors
    e. Abductors

CareTracker Connection

Documenting Clinical Data and Entering a Referral Related to the Musculoskeletal System

 HARRIS CareTracker Activities Related to
CareTracker This Chapter

- Case Study 9: Urgent Care Practicum

Musculoskeletal conditions range from common acute injuries, such as fractures and strains, to complex chronic diseases, such as muscular dystrophy and rheumatoid arthritis. As a medical assistant, you will document patients' complaints, signs and symptoms, and health history; assist with physical examinations, tests, and procedures; enter medication and test orders; and process referrals pertaining to a wide range of musculoskeletal conditions. All of these tasks can be efficiently performed in CareTracker.

Tasks discussed in this chapter that can be performed in CareTracker include the following:

- Documenting the following patient's clinical information related to musculoskeletal conditions:
  - Health history
    - Diseases and conditions
    - Hospitalizations
    - Surgeries and procedures
    - Preventive care
    - Family history
  - Review of systems
  - Physical examination findings
  - Tests and procedures completed during the visit
    - X-rays
    - Computed tomography scans
    - Magnetic resonance imaging scans
    - Electromyograms
    - Bone scans
    - Diagnoses
    - Treatment plan
- Ordering the following related to musculoskeletal conditions:
  - Medications
  - Laboratory tests
  - Diagnostic tests

Many of these tasks are discussed in CareTracker Connection features in other chapters. A task we'll consider here is entering a patient referral to an orthopedic surgeon.

When a condition or disease requires expertise that goes beyond the scope of practice of a primary care physician, the patient may be referred to a specialist, such as an orthopedic surgeon. In CareTracker, you may enter a referral by clicking on the 🖼 icon in the Clinical Toolbar near the top of the screen in the Medical Record (either from the main screen or from within the Progress Note).

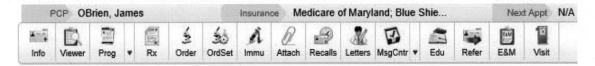

Alternatively, you may click on the 🖼 icon at the bottom of the PLAN tab in the Progress Note.

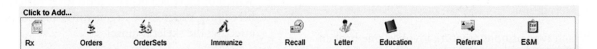

Within the Referral window, you select the referral type (outgoing or incoming), the name of the referring provider, the name of the provider the patient is being referred to, the group and specialty of the referred provider, from and to dates that the referral is good for, the authorization type (visits, amount, or hours), the authorization number (if needed), and the number of visits authorized (if needed). Below is an example of a referral, in which the primary care physician Jim Schroeder is referring a patient to the orthopedic surgeon James O'Brien for a single visit that must occur within 2 months from the date authorized.

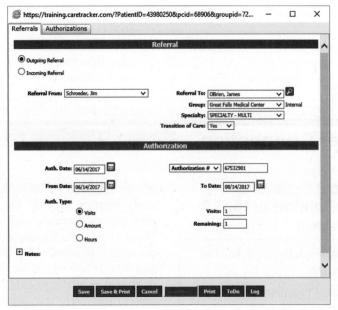

When complete, click on Save & Print, and a printable referral report will appear.

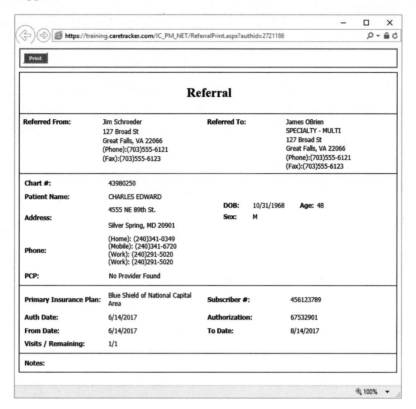

6 Nervous System, Special Senses, and Endocrine System

Chapter Objectives

- Describe the structure of a neuron.
- Describe how neuron fibers are built into a nerve.
- Explain the function of neurotransmitters in synapse transmission.
- Explain the functions of the sympathetic and parasympathetic nervous systems.
- Describe common disorders of the spinal cord and spinal nerves.
- Explain the function of the three meninges.
- Describe the function of cerebrospinal fluid.
- Identify the three subdivisions of the brain stem and the function of each.
- List the 12 cranial nerves.
- Describe disorders that affect the brain and cranial nerves.
- Explain the function of the special senses.
- Describe the major structures of the eye.
- Explain the processes involved in the sense of sight.
- Describe common disorders of the eye and vision.
- Describe the major structures of the ear.
- Explain the processes involved in the sense of hearing.
- Describe common disorders of the ear and hearing.
- Identify the glands of the endocrine system and the hormones they produce.
- Describe the functions of hormones.
- Describe common disorders of the endocrine glands.

CAAHEP & ABHES Competencies

CAAHEP

- Describe structural organization of the human body.
- Identify body systems.
- List major organs in each body system.
- Describe the normal function of each body system.
- Identify common pathology related to each body system including signs, symptoms, and etiology.
- Analyze pathology for each body system including diagnostic measures and treatment modalities.

ABHES

- List all body systems, their structure, and functions.
- Describe common diseases, symptoms, and etiologies as they apply to each system.
- Common diseases, diagnoses, and treatments.
- Identify diagnostic and treatment modalities as they relate to each body system.

Chapter Terms

Acromegaly	Diabetes mellitus	Myelin	Poliomyelitis
Axon	Epinephrine	Myopia	Quadriplegia
Cataract	Gigantism	Nerve	Reflex
Cerebrum	Glaucoma	Neurons	Sciatica
Ceruminosis	Incus	Neuropathy	Seizure
Conjunctivitis	Malleus	Otitis media	Stapes
Dendrite	Meninges	Paraplegia	Synapse

Abbreviations

ACTH	CT	LH	PNS
ADH	CVA	MRI	PRL
ALS	EEG	MS	T1DM
CNS	FSH	MTBI	T2DM
CSF	GH	PET	TSH

Case Study

Alicia, a college student, is attending her first year as a freshman at the state university. It is midterm and she has been really spending a lot of hours studying for her exams. Today, she woke up in her dorm room and didn't really feel well. She felt a little achy and warm and decided to stay in bed for awhile thinking she probably just needed a little rest. She knew other classmates who had been coughing and sneezing but just thought they were coming down with a cold so she figured she had caught a cold from one of them. She fell asleep and when she woke up in a couple of hours, she knew she was running a fever, she had a terrific headache, and her neck felt tight and stiff.

In this chapter, we will explore the nervous system, including the senses, and the endocrine system. Homeostasis is a concept of maintaining body functions within set limits. The nervous, endocrine, and sensory systems play a major role in helping the body maintain homeostatic balance. These body systems are able to act on the changes detected in the external and internal environments and make adjustments in the body.

THE NERVOUS SYSTEM

The nervous system is the main coordination and communication system in the body. The system relies on the brain, spinal cord, and the nerves throughout the body to accomplish these functions. The brain acts as the main communication center interpreting the senses that are transmitted from the body's nerves through the spinal cord to the brain. A **nerve** is composed of a bundle of neuron fibers. It is similar to an electrical cord with numerous wires encased by an insulated covering.

Nervous System Divisions

The nervous system is divided into two parts, the central nervous system (CNS) and the peripheral nervous system (PNS). The **CNS** is comprised of the brain and spinal cord. The **PNS** includes the nerves that lie outside of the CNS. This system includes the cranial nerves, carrying impulses to and from the brain, and the spinal

Case Question

As you read through the chapter, see if you can figure out what might be causing Alicia's symptoms. What should she do?

Central nervous system:

Peripheral nervous system:

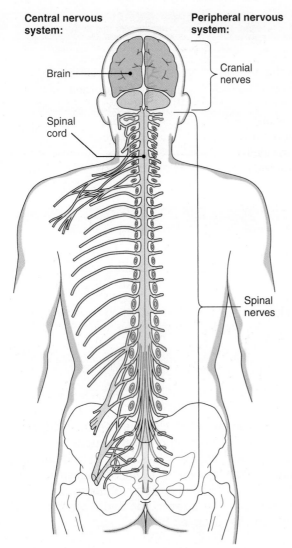

Brain

Spinal cord

Cranial nerves

Spinal nerves

Figure 6-1 Central nervous and peripheral nervous systems. (Reprinted from Cohen BJ. *Memmler's The Human Body in Health and Disease.* 13th ed. Burlington, MA: Jones & Bartlett Learning, LLC; 2014.)

nerves, which carry messages to and from the spinal cord. Figure 6-1 shows the division of the CNS and PNS with the main structures of each system identified.

The Peripheral Nervous System

The PNS is further divided into the somatic nervous system, which is controlled voluntarily and the autonomic nervous system, which functions involuntarily.

- Somatic nervous system—Skeletal muscles act as the effectors responding to the stimuli communicated through the somatic nerves; an example of this action is when your hand is pulled away quickly from a hot stove.
- Autonomic nervous system—Also referred to as the visceral nervous system; the effectors are smooth muscle, cardiac muscle, and glands, which function involuntarily; numerous examples of autonomic action includes the heart functioning without conscious control.

Neurons

The highly specialized cells of the nervous system are called **neurons**. Each neuron has a nucleus and thread-like fibers that extend out from the cell body carrying impulses across the neuron. These fibers are the dendrites and axons.

- **Dendrites**—The neuron fibers that conduct impulses *to* the cell body. They function as the receptors in the nervous system (receive the stimulus).
- **Axons**—The neuron fibers that conduct impulses away from the cell body. Their function is to deliver the impulses from one neuron to another neuron or to a muscle or gland.

See Figure 6-2, which is a neuron with the dendrites, axons, and myelin sheath.

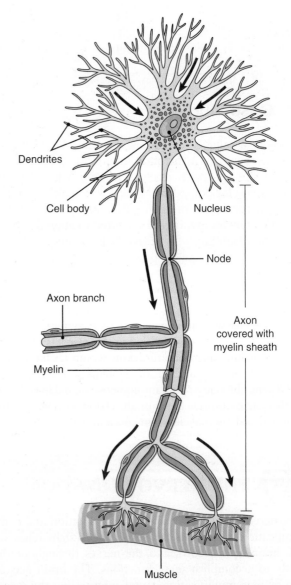

Dendrites

Cell body

Nucleus

Node

Axon branch

Axon covered with myelin sheath

Myelin

Muscle

Figure 6-2 A neuron with dendrite, axon, and myelin. (Reprinted from Cohen BJ. *Memmler's The Human Body in Health and Disease.* 13th ed. Burlington, MA: Jones & Bartlett Learning, LLC; 2014.)

Neurons are also categorized by their function, relaying information to or from the central nervous system. There are three types of neurons including sensory, motor, and interneurons.

- Sensory neurons—Called afferent neurons; they conduct impulses to the spinal cord and brain, for example, when your fingers feel the heat from the hot stove, a signal is carried to the brain through afferent neurons.
- Motor neurons—Called efferent neurons; they conduct impulse from the brain and spinal cord to the muscles and glands (the effectors) where action will take place, for example, when you pull your hand away from the hot stove.
- Interneurons—Called central or association neurons; they conduct impulses within the central nervous system; they help us learn to avoid painful situations and assist during times of immediate response to a stimulus, for example, helping to maintain balance and coordination when responding to a situation.

Myelin Sheath

Myelin is a whitish, fatty substance that covers some of the axons just like the insulation on an electrical cord. This sheath of tissue protects and insulates the axon fiber. In the peripheral nervous system, the myelin is actually cells called Schwann cells, which wrap around the axon. In the peripheral nervous system, Schwann cells are important to help neurons regenerate. In the central nervous system, when the neurons are injured, the damage is usually permanent. Within the CNS, the myelinated axons are called white fibers because of the myelin's color. The section of the brain and spinal cord called white matter is made up of these white fibers. The gray matter is an area of the brain and spinal cord not covered with these myelin fibers.

The Synapse

Neurons rely on impulses that are passed from one to another. The junction for that transmission is the **synapse**. The synapse allows transmission of the impulse from the axon of one neuron to the dendrite of another neuron. In order for the synapse to occur, chemicals called neurotransmitters are required. The most common neurotransmitters are norepinephrine, serotonin, dopamine, and acetylcholine.

There are some synapses controlled not by chemicals but by electrical signals. For example, cardiac muscle is activated by these electrical signals that travel directly from one cell to another causing the heart muscle to contract.

 ## THE SPINAL CORD

The spinal cord is the primary connection between the spinal nerves and the brain. It is located in and protected by the vertebral column. It extends from the upper cervical region to the lumbar region between the first and second lumbar vertebrae. The spinal cord is surrounded by cerebrospinal fluid (**CSF**) that acts as a cushion for protection and carries nutrients and oxygen to the cord. The spinal cord serves as the pathway for the sensory and motor impulses traveling to and from the brain.

 ## SPINAL NERVES

There are 31 pairs of spinal nerves that branch off of the spinal cord. These nerves serve specific areas of the body. The cervical spinal nerves are located in the

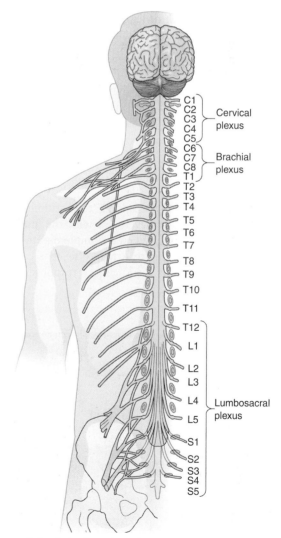

Figure 6-3 Spinal cord and spinal nerves. (Reprinted from Cohen BJ. *Memmler's The Human Body in Health and Disease.* 13th ed. Burlington, MA: Jones & Bartlett Learning, LLC; 2014.)

cervical (neck) region. The spinal nerves serve different regions or structures of the body. The motor function of the nerves as assigned as follows:

- C1–C6: Neck flexor muscles
- C1–T1: Neck extensor muscles
- C3, C4, C5: Supply diaphragm
- C5, C6: Shoulder movement, raise arm, flexion of elbow, external rotation of the arm
- C6, C7: Extends elbow and wrist, pronates wrist
- C7, T1: Flex wrist, supply small muscles of the hand
- T1–T6: Intercostals and trunk above the waist
- T1–L1: Abdominal muscles
- L1–L4: Thigh flexion
- L2, L3, L4: Thigh adduction, extension of the leg at the knee (quadriceps femoris)
- L4, L5, S1: Thigh abduction, flexion of the leg at the knee (hamstrings), dorsiflexion of foot, extension of toes
- L5, S1, S2: Extension of leg at the hip (gluteus maximus), plantar flexion of foot, and flexion of toes

See Figure 6-3, which identifies the location of the spinal nerves.

The spinal nerves also receive messages from sensory neurons located all over the skin except the face and scalp. These skin regions are called dermatomes.

 ## REFLEXES

A **reflex** is an involuntary response to a stimulus. The nervous system is highly developed with the ability to coordinate the responses. When a complete pathway is formed from the stimulus to a response, it is called a reflex arc. An example is the knee-jerk response. When the physician taps the patellar tendon just beneath the patella, the normal response is to move the lower leg forward. The stimulus is the reflex hammer striking the tendon and the response is the movement of the leg. A complete reflex arc occurred from the beginning of the stimulus when a message is sent to the brain, it is interpreted, then a message is returned to the nerve associated with that region and the leg moves. Another basic response is when the eyes are closed when you see an object approaching your eyes. Figure 6-4 demonstrates how the physician examines a patient's tendon reflexes.

 # THE AUTONOMIC NERVOUS SYSTEM

This is the nervous system that acts automatically without conscious awareness. This system regulates the blood vessels, heart muscle, smooth muscle of the internal organs, and the glands. There are two divisions of the autonomic nervous system, the sympathetic and the parasympathetic.

Sympathetic Nervous System

This system acts as an accelerator for the body to meet stressful situations, promoting the fight-or-flight response. This is the response when faced with the decision to stay and fight the enemy or flee from the enemy and run away. When we are faced with an emergency, a stressful situation, or when doing exercise, the sympathetic system affects the following:

- Heart contractions—Increase rate and force
- Blood pressure—Increases in response to constriction of small arteries and more effective heartbeat

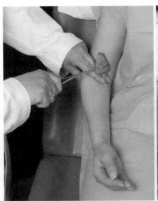 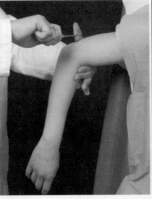 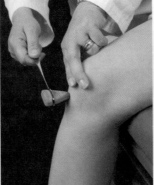 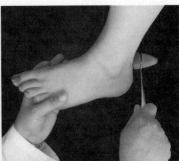

Figure 6-4 Techniques for eliciting major tendon reflexes. **A.** Biceps reflex. **B.** Triceps reflex. **C.** Patellar reflex. **D.** Ankle or achilles reflex. (Reprinted from Kronenberger J, Ledbetter J. *Jones & Bartlett Learning's Comprehensive Medical Assisting.* 5th ed. Burlington, MA: Jones & Bartlett Learning, LLC; 2016.)

- Blood vessels—Dilate to increase blood flow to the skeletal muscles
- Bronchial tubes—Dilate to allow increased respiration, deliver more oxygen, and excrete more carbon dioxide
- Adrenal gland—Increases output of adrenaline, epinephrine, a stimulating hormone. You may have heard the saying "an adrenaline rush."
- Pupil of the eye—Dilates the pupil allowing for increased distance vision

Parasympathetic Nervous System

This system acts as a balance providing the opposite function of the sympathetic nervous system. It is sometimes referred to as the "rest and digest" system. It has the effect on the following:

- Heart rate—Slows the heart rate
- Bronchial tubes—Constrict the tubes, lowering the respiratory rate
- Pupil of the eye—Constriction of the eye
- Digestive and urinary system—Increase urine output and activity of the digestive tract

 THE CRANIAL NERVES

There are 12 pairs of cranial nerves that connect directly to the cerebrum, brainstem, and cervical spinal cord.

They supply the structures of the head and have specific functions. Table 6-1 is a list of the cranial nerves and their function. You will notice that they are labeled using a Roman numeral.

Study Skill

When you need to remember a list of items or structures in anatomy, it is easier if you put together a pneumonic that uses the first letter of each word to make a statement that is easier to remember. You can make your own statement something that is one you will never forget. Here is one used to recall the 12 cranial nerves **O**n **O**ld **O**lympus **T**iny **T**ops **A** **F**in **A**nd **G**erman **V**iewed **A**mber **H**ops.

 THE BRAIN

The brain is a main part of the central nervous system (CNS). It is the control center of the nervous system where information received from the body is interpreted, processed, and coordinated. Our ability to reason, learn, and memorize information takes place in the brain. The brain is located in the cranial cavity and is protected by the skull bones. There are four main regions of the brain:

- **Cerebrum**—Largest part of the brain divided into a right and left hemisphere.

Table 6-1 Cranial Nerves and Their Function

Cranial Nerve	Function
I—Olfactory Nerve	Carries smell impulses from receptors in the nasal mucosa to the brain
II—Optic Nerve	Carries visual impulses from the eye to the brain
III—Oculomotor Nerve	Controls the contraction of most of the eye muscles. These muscles are skeletal muscles and are under voluntary control
IV—Trochlear Nerve	Supplies one eyeball muscle
V—Trigeminal Nerve	Great sensory nerve of the face and head; has three branches that carry general sensory impulses from the eye, the upper jaw, and the lower jaw (muscles of chewing)
VI—Abducens Nerve	Sends motor impulses to an eyeball muscle
VII—Facial Nerve	Controls the muscles of facial expression; includes special sensory fibers for taste; contains secretory fibers to salivary glands and lacrimal glands
VIII—Auditory Nerve	Carries sensory impulses for hearing and equilibrium from the inner ear; formerly called the auditory or acoustic nerve; also called the vestibulocochlear nerve
IX—Glossopharyngeal Nerve	Contains sensory fibers from the tongue (taste) and the pharynx (swallowing)
X—Vagus Nerve	Longest cranial nerve; carries autonomic motor impulses to most of the organs in the thoracic and abdominal cavities, including the muscles and glands of the digestive system; contains somatic motor fibers supplying the larynx
XI—Accessory Nerve	Controls two muscles of the neck, the trapezius and sternocleidomastoid; supplies muscles of the larynx
XII—Hypoglossal Nerve	Carries impulses controlling the tongue muscles

- Diencephalon—In the center of the brain between the hemispheres and above the brain stem; the thalamus and hypothalamus are located there.
- Brain stem—Located in the region between the diencephalon and the spinal cord; has three divisions including the midbrain, pons, and medulla oblongata.
- Cerebellum—Located behind the brainstem; the term cerebellum means little brain.

See Figure 6-5, which demonstrates the major structures of the brain.

Brain and Spinal Cord Protection

Due to the delicate nature of the brain and spinal cord, there are three membranes, the **meninges**, and fluid that surround the structures to help protect and cushion them from injury and trauma. The meninges are:

- Pia mater—Innermost layer; pia means delicate or soft and mater is Latin for mother; holds the blood vessels that supply the oxygen and nutrients to the brain and spinal cord.
- Arachnoid—Middle layer or space that has web-like fibers resembling a spider web.

- Dura mater—Outermost layer; hard, tough layer.

Cerebrospinal fluid (CSF) is a clear liquid that surrounds the brain and spinal cord. It is produced in the ventricles of the brain. In addition to cushioning the brain and spinal cord, it carries nutrients to the cells and transports waste from the cells

Cerebrum

As mentioned earlier, the cerebrum is divided into two hemispheres, and each hemisphere is then divided into four lobes. These lobes are the frontal, parietal, temporal, and occipital. These lie in the region of the skull bones with the same names. Each hemisphere has an outer covering called the cerebral cortex. This is where specific body functions are processed including thought, reasoning, and mental functions.

Each lobe of the cerebrum is assigned a specific function such as these general functions:

- Frontal lobe—Primary motor area providing conscious control of skeletal muscles.
- Parietal lobe—Primary somatosensory area allowing processing of impulses from the skin such as pain and temperature; stores memories so we can interpret

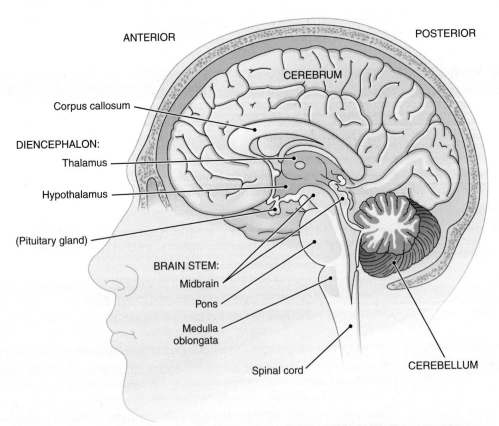

Figure 6-5 Cross-section view of the brain and major components. (Reprinted from Cohen BJ. *Memmler's The Human Body in Health and Disease.* 13th ed. Burlington, MA: Jones & Bartlett Learning, LLC; 2014.)

what we touch identifying hot versus cold and hard and soft.

- Temporal lobe—Auditory reception area detecting sound from the environment; speech recognition is also located in this area.
- Occipital lobe—Visual reception area allowing us to see brightness and color; visual association so we can identify various objects and differentiate a flower from a person

A primary function of the brain is to store volumes of memory. Memory is categorized into short-term memory that allows us to store bits of information for a few seconds or minutes and long-term memory that allows us to recall information at a later time even years later.

Diencephalon

This area of the brain houses the thalamus and hypothalamus. The thalamus is similar to a relay station sending impulses to the particular areas of the cerebral cortex where they will be processed. The hypothalamus helps the body maintain homeostasis by controlling the body temperature, water balance, our sleep pattern, appetite, and some emotions including fear and pleasure.

Brainstem

The structures of the brain stem have very specific responsibilities acting as a connection between the cerebrum and spinal cord:

- Midbrain—Responds to reflexes involving the eye and ear; coordination of eye movement
- Pons—Regulation of respiration and involuntary reflex actions

- Medulla oblongata—Controls muscles of respiration; regulates rate and force of the heartbeat; regulates contraction of smooth muscle of the blood vessels controlling blood flow and blood pressure

The motor function of the cerebral hemispheres is designed to allow contralateral control, which means that motor functions controlled in the right hemisphere will control the left side of the body and those controlled in the left hemisphere will affect function of the right side of the body.

Cerebellum

The primary functions of the cerebellum include assisting with the coordination of voluntary muscles allowing us to maintain our balance and helping us to maintain muscle tone so we are ready to move as needed.

MEDICAL PROCEDURES INVOLVING THE NERVOUS SYSTEM

In order to treat the numerous medical conditions that affect the nervous system structures and function, a physician needs to do testing to determine the cause or root of the problem. Let's explore just a few of the common procedures that you may see ordered by physicians treating patients with abnormal signs and symptoms of the nervous system.

- Lumbar puncture—Also called a spinal tap, is an invasive procedure that involves inserting a needle into the space between vertebrae to withdraw a small amount of cerebrospinal fluid for analysis. The physician is testing for the presence of inflammation or infection. Figure 6-6 shows the positioning of a

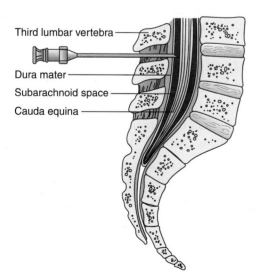
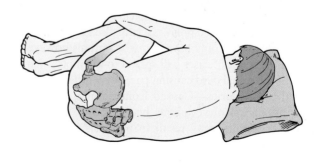

Third lumbar vertebra

Dura mater

Subarachnoid space

Cauda equina

Figure 6-6 Spinal location and patient position used to perform a lumbar puncture. The L3 to L5 spaces are just below the line connecting the anterior and superior iliac spines. (From Taylor C, Lillis CA, LeMone P. *Fundamentals of Nursing*. 2nd ed. Philadelphia, PA: Lippincott; 1993:543.)

patient for a lumbar puncture and the location in the spine where the fluid is extracted.

- **CT** scan—Computed tomography; provides images of the brain and bones, used to visualize abnormalities such as tumors or structural deformity.
- **MRI**—Magnetic resonance imaging; provides more detail of the brain and structures than those visible on the CT scan, used to visualize tumors and hemorrhage.
- **PET** scan—Positron emission tomography; visualizes the brain in action.
- **EEG**—Electroencephalograph is used to measure the electrical activity of the brain, the brain waves; may be used to study sleep disorders.

DISORDERS OF THE NERVOUS SYSTEM

There are many conditions that can affect the structures and function of the nervous system. A general term used to describe any disease of the nervous system is **neuropathy**. More specifically, a patient may have peripheral neuropathy, which is a condition affecting the nerves outside of the central nervous system. The term neuralgia is used as a general term to describe nerve pain and can be an associated symptom with any nerve condition. Here are some of the nervous system disorders affecting the overall body:

- Multiple sclerosis (**MS**)—An autoimmune disease that causes loss of the myelin sheath around the axon; results in a disruption in the nervous system communication process; one of the most common, chronic CNS diseases in young adults, affecting women more than men.
- Amyotrophic lateral sclerosis (**ALS**)—Progressive, degenerative disorder that destroys the motor neurons; muscles waste away (atrophy) and motor control is lost eventually, affecting the ability to talk, swallow, and breathe; often referred to as Lou Gehrig disease, the famous baseball player.
- **Poliomyelitis**—Called polio, is a viral disease of the nervous system; may only have minor symptoms however in small amount of cases will spread to the motor neurons of the spinal cord causing paralysis of the limbs.
- Spinal cord injuries—Caused from trauma, fracture, and dislocation of vertebrae, herniation of vertebral disks, or tumors; may result in paralysis in varying degrees:
  - Monoplegia—Paralysis of one limb
  - **Paraplegia**—Paralysis of both lower limbs
  - Hemiplegia—Paralysis of one side of the body
  - **Quadriplegia**—Paralysis of all four limbs
- **Sciatica**—Compression of the sciatic nerve of the lower back causing pain, numbness, and tingling from the lower back continuing down the leg

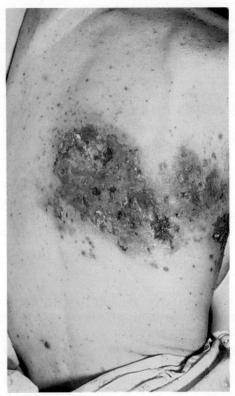

Figure 6-7 Shingles caused by the herpes zoster virus. (Reprinted from Kronenberger J, Ledbetter J. *Jones & Bartlett Learning's Comprehensive Medical Assisting.* 5th ed. Burlington, MA: Jones & Bartlett Learning, LLC; 2016.)

- Bell palsy—Partial facial paralysis caused by inflammation of the VII facial nerve

Herpes zoster, commonly known as shingles, is sometimes associated with disorders of the nervous system because the virus that causes this condition lies dormant along a nerve. The virus, which is the same one that causes chicken pox, becomes reactivated years later and causes intense nerve pain and a severe skin rash. Figure 6-7 is a photo of a person with herpes zoster.

Disorders of the Central Nervous System

In addition to general nervous system disorders, there are some conditions that are more specifically associated with the brain and spinal cord, the CNS.

- **Seizure**—Results from abnormal electrical activity in the brain that might be due to infection, trauma, or high fever; causes uncontrollable muscle contractions.
- Epilepsy—The recurrence of seizures; in most cases, the cause is idiopathic, which means unknown source or origin.
- Meningitis—Infection or inflammation of the meninges usually caused by a virus or bacteria (meningococcus); symptoms include headache, stiff neck, nausea, and vomiting

- Encephalitis—Inflammation of the brain; may be caused from poliovirus, rabies virus, West Nile virus, and HIV
- Hydrocephalus–Abnormal accumulation of cerebrospinal fluid within the brain; caused by congenital deformity, tumors, and hemorrhage
- Stroke—Cerebrovascular accident (**CVA**); caused by a blood clot that blocks blood flow to a specific area of the brain or a ruptured blood vessel resulting in hemorrhage; results in various levels of paralysis and aphasia (loss of speech or communication)
- Concussion—Known as mild traumatic brain injury (**MTBI**); caused by head trauma resulting in symptoms including headache, dizziness, vomiting, and sometimes loss of consciousness
- Cerebral palsy—Caused by brain damage occurring before or during the birth process; results in varying degrees of muscular and speech disorder and paralysis
- Alzheimer disease—Degeneration of the cerebral cortex resulting in gradual intellectual impairment and memory loss
- Parkinson disease—Progressive neurologic condition; causes tremors and rigidity of the limbs and joints

Case Questions

 Remember Alicia, the college student in the case study? Were you able to figure out what might be going on with her? Throughout the day, she continued to get worse and started feeling very nauseated. She went to the college medical clinic where the physician decided to admit her to a local hospital. He ordered a lumbar puncture and immediately started her on an antibiotic.

Why do you think the physician hospitalized Alicia, ordered the spinal tap, and started her on antibiotics?

TREATING THE NERVOUS SYSTEM

Since the nervous system disorders typically involve pain and discomfort, one of the more common treatments is the use of pain medication. A method of administration of pain medication is to deliver it into the epidural space of the spinal region. The injection in this area allows the medication to diffuse into the spinal cord causing an analgesic effect (pain relief). This method is also indicated for use during childbirth and is referred to as an "epidural." Physicians also use a variety of psychoactive drugs that affect the neurotransmitter activity in the brain. They are used to treat depression, anxiety, and obsessive–compulsive disorder.

 ## THE SENSORY SYSTEM

The nervous system is composed of both motor and sensory nerves. This section will focus on those senses that provide us with ways to evaluate and respond to our environment. The body has various types of receptors that respond to the stimuli surrounding us:

- Chemoreceptors—Allow us to detect chemicals in solutions; receptor for taste and smell.
- Photoreceptors—Respond to light; located in the retina of the eye.
- Thermoreceptors—Allow us to detect changes in temperature; most are located in the skin.
- Mechanoreceptors—Allow us to respond to movement such as vibration and pressure; located in the skin; also receptors of hearing and equilibrium in the ear.

General and Special Senses

The body has general senses that include pressure, temperature, pain, and touch. The receptors for these senses are found in the skin and internal organs. The sense of position is determined by receptors found in the muscles, tendons, and joints. The special senses associated with specific areas of the body include:

- Vision—Receptors are in the eye.
- Hearing—Receptors are in the inner ear.
- Equilibrium (balance)—Receptors are in the inner ear.
- Taste—Receptors are in the tongue.
- Smell—Receptors are in the upper nasal cavities.

The Sense of Vision

The eyes provide a window to the world. We perceive more than half of our information from what we see. Since the eyes are so valuable, they need structures to protect them from injury and damage. The bones surrounding the eye that form the orbits of the eyes are the first line of protection. Other protective structures include:

- Eyelids—Upper and lower lids protect the front of the eye, lubricating the eye each time you blink.
- Eyelashes and eyebrows—These structures help keep foreign matter out of the eye catching dust and debris before it can get to the eye.
- Lacrimal glands—Produce tears that bathe the eye and help wash away foreign materials; the lacrimal apparatus is the entire structure that includes the glands and nasolacrimal ducts that cause the tears to run into the nose when there is overproduction.
- Conjunctiva—Lines the inner eyelid and the white of the eye (sclera); provides a layer of lubricating mucus to protect the eye.

There are numerous muscles attached to the eyeball that allow the eyeball to move up, down, side to side, and in a circular field. The eye also requires a variety of nerves to supply specific functions including the optic nerve that carries visual impulses from the photoreceptors in the eye to the brain.

The Eyeball

The eyeball has many structures and layers including the:

- Sclera—Outermost layer of the eyeball that is referred to as the white of the eye
- Cornea—The transparent, colorless, anterior portion of the sclera; the window of the eye
- Choroid—The middle, vascular layer; contains melanin, which absorbs light rays to reduce sun glare
- Ciliary muscle and suspensory ligaments—Control the shape of the lens.
- Iris—Colored ring-like portion of the eye that controls the size of the pupil.
- Pupil—Opening in the center of the iris that becomes larger or smaller allowing more or less light to enter the eye, called dilation.

- Retina—Nerve layer of the inner part of the eyeball; contains the rods and cones.
- Rods and cones—Found in the retinal layer; rods allow differentiation of shades of gray and dim light, cones allow us to see color, and when there is a deficiency in the cones, a person could be color-blind.
- Aqueous humor—A watery fluid that fills the eyeball anterior to the lens and helps maintain the cornea's convex curve.
- Vitreous body—A soft jelly-like substance that fills the space behind the lens; helps maintain the shape of the eyeball.
- Lens—A clear, circular structure made of an elastic material capable of changing shape to accommodate vision.
- Optic disk—Where the optic nerve connects with the retina, called the blind spot.
- Fovea centralis—Area on the retina close to the optic disk where there is the most acute, sharp vision.

See Figure 6-8, a detailed image of the eye and the internal structures.

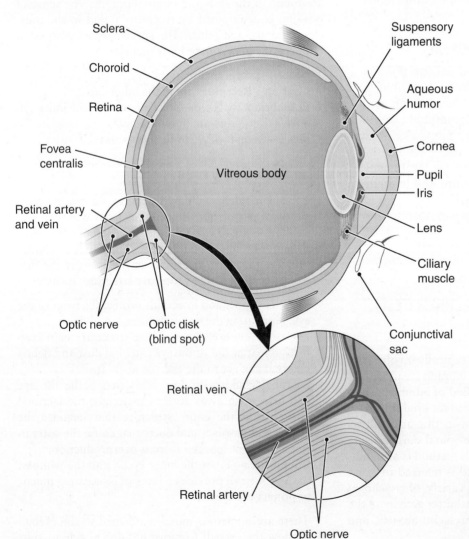

Figure 6-8 Structures of the eyeball. (Reprinted from Cohen BJ. *Memmler's The Human Body in Health and Disease.* 13th ed. Burlington, MA: Jones & Bartlett Learning, LLC; 2014.)

The Process of Vision

There are many structures that the light must pass through and changes in the eye structures that take place in order for us to see. The light rays are bent and changed through a process called refraction. As light rays go through the cornea, lens, and fluids of the eye, the rays bend and are able to focus on the retina. Another process required for vision is accommodation, which is the ability of the lens to change shape and become thicker or thinner. This provides the vision for far and near distances. The ciliary muscle contracts and relaxes to allow the change in the lens.

Problems with the Eye and Vision

There are numerous problems that can occur with the eye and its structures that affect the function of the eye and ability to see images properly. Some of the physical problems that affect the eye include:

- **Conjunctivitis**—Inflammation of the conjunctiva; caused from irritant or pathogen; an acute, contagious type caused by bacteria is referred to as pinkeye.
- Corneal abrasion—Injury to the cornea causing scratches.
- Enucleation—Eyeball removed through surgical procedure; may be result of severe injury to the eyeball.
- **Cataract**—Cloudiness of the lens causing gradual loss of vision; requires surgical replacement of the lens.
- **Glaucoma**—Excessive pressure of the aqueous humor; leads to destruction of some of the optic nerve fibers.
- Retinopathy—Disease of the retina resulting in damage to the blood vessels of the choroid layer; may be directly related to diabetes (diabetic retinopathy)
- Retinal detachment—The retina separates from the choroid layer; requires surgical repair and if untreated will result in blindness.
- Macular degeneration—Deterioration of the fovea centralis region of the retina causing gradual vision loss; typically age related.

Figure 6-9 is a photo of a healthy retina. The blood vessels are normal.

Vision Disorders

There are also many conditions that cause problems with the ability to see properly. These conditions include:

- Night blindness—Difficulty seeing in dim light; due to vitamin A deficiency that provides nutrient to the pigment found in the rods
- Hyperopia—Farsightedness, able to see things at a distance (far away) but not things up close (near)
- **Myopia**—Nearsightedness, able to see things close by (near) but not things far away at a distance
- Presbyopia—Age-related loss of elasticity in the lens causing inability to properly focus on objects
- Astigmatism—Caused by irregularity in the curvature of the cornea or lens; causes distorted vision; may be found in people with myopia or hyperopia
- Strabismus—Condition involving the eye muscles not allowing the eyes to move properly but may cause appearance of cross eyed, the eyes converge toward the nose

See Figure 6-10 to see how the images are not properly reflected on the retina with conditions like myopia and hyperopia. Corrective lenses are required to allow the rays to properly converge on the retina.

Treatment of Eye Conditions

An ophthalmologist is a medical doctor who specializes in the treatment of eye conditions. This doctor is trained to perform eye surgery, prescribe medications for the eye, and perform basic eye examinations. Many people see an optometrist who is not a medical doctor and can examine the eye for visual problems that require corrective lenses. The optician is a trained

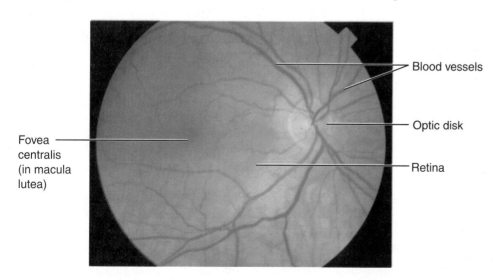

Fovea centralis (in macula lutea)

Blood vessels

Optic disk

Retina

Figure 6-9 A healthy retina. (Reprinted from Cohen BJ. *Memmler's The Human Body in Health and Disease.* 13th ed. Burlington, MA: Jones & Bartlett Learning, LLC; 2014.)

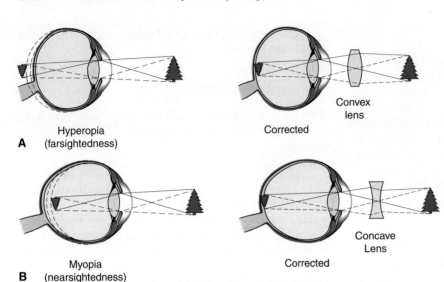

A Hyperopia (farsightedness)

Convex lens

Corrected

B Myopia (nearsightedness)

Concave Lens

Corrected

Figure 6-10   Refraction errors caused by **(A)** myopia (nearsightedness) with concave corrective lens. Hyperopia **(B)** (farsightedness) with convex corrective lens. (Reprinted from Cohen BJ. *Memmler's The Human Body in Health and Disease.* 13th ed. Burlington, MA: Jones & Bartlett Learning, LLC; 2014.)

person who can make lenses and fit eyeglasses. They also instruct in the use of contact lenses. The main instrument used to examine the eyes is an ophthalmoscope. It is used to visualize the back of the eye, the retina. A tonometer is a device used to measure the intraocular pressure to rule out glaucoma. Laser surgical procedures are used to correct vision problems including nearsightedness, farsightedness, and astigmatism.

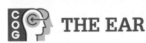 # THE EAR

The ear is the sense organ responsible for hearing and equilibrium (balance). There are three specific areas of the ear, the outer, middle, and inner ear.

Outer Ear

The external portion of the ear that you can see is called the pinna or auricle. The shape of the pinna allows sound waves to be captured and directed into the ear. The external auditory canal is the tube entrance into the ear. It is visible from the outside and extends into the eardrum. Ceruminous glands are located in the canal and secrete a substance called cerumen (earwax). At the end of the external auditory canal is the tympanic membrane, or eardrum. This structure separates the outer ear from the middle ear. The eardrum vibrates when the sound waves enter the ear.

Middle Ear

The middle ear is the space between the outer and inner ear where the ossicles are located. These are three little bones that vibrate and amplify the sound waves. The bones are the **malleus**, shaped like a hammer, **incus** anvil shaped, and **stapes** that looks like a stirrup.

The eustachian tube (auditory tube) connects the middle ear with the pharynx (throat). This tube equalizes pressure within the ear.

Inner Ear

The inner ear is the most complicated part of the ear. It contains the structures that help maintain our equilibrium and balance and serve as a pathway sending impulses to the brain where they are interpreted into sounds (hearing). The inner ear has been described as a labyrinth because of its complex structure. There are three divisions of the inner ear, the vestibule and semicircular canals that contain receptors for equilibrium and the cochlea where the receptors for hearing are located. Within the labyrinth are two fluids, perilymph in the outer portion and endolymph in the inner portion. These fluids are necessary to transmit the sensory impulses.

Figure 6-11 is a diagram of the ear showing the divisions of the outer, middle, and inner ear.

The Process of Hearing

Hearing starts as the sound waves enter the external auditory canal. The waves vibrate the eardrum which activates the ossicles to move. The movement now stimulates the structures within the inner ear triggering the structures to convert the sound waves into nerve impulses, which now travel to the brain through the vestibulocochlear nerve.

Equilibrium and Balance

The receptors for equilibrium and balance are located in the vestibule and the semicircular canals. These receptors are ciliated hair cells that respond to the changes in the position of the head generating nerve impulses that are sent to the brain for interpretation.

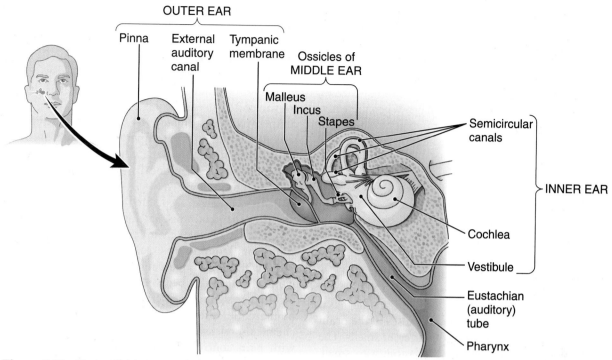

Figure 6-11 Three divisions of the ear: outer, middle, and inner. (Reprinted from Cohen BJ. *Memmler's The Human Body in Health and Disease*. 13th ed. Burlington, MA: Jones & Bartlett Learning, LLC; 2014.)

Disorders of the Ear

Disorders of the ear include infection, hearing loss, and disturbances in equilibrium. Some of the more common disorders include:

- **Ceruminosis**—Impacted ear wax; a buildup of cerumen that becomes hardened in the external auditory canal. To treat this condition, the wax is softened, using warm water or medication, and is rinsed out of the canal.
- **Otitis media**—Infection and inflammation of the middle ear; caused by bacteria or virus and may be a complication of a cold or flu. Figure 6-12 is a photo of an eardrum that is inflamed and bulging due to otitis media.
- Otitis externa—Inflammation of the external auditory canal usually due to bacteria or fungus; also common among swimmers when the canal stays damp with water, known as swimmer's ear.
- Conductive hearing loss—Varying levels of deafness due to inability of the sound waves to travel through the ear. A simple problem might be blockage such as a buildup of earwax not allowing the sound waves to travel past the blocked area. Otosclerosis is a hereditary problem caused when the stapes does not vibrate allowing the sound waves to be conducted.
- Sensorineural hearing loss—Loss of hearing due to the inability of the nerve to properly transmit the impulses to the brain; may be due to excessive use of headphones playing loud music and noises; problems with the cochlea may also cause this type of hearing loss
- Presbycusis—An age-related hearing loss, begins with loss of high-pitched sounds

- Vertigo—Sensation of spinning or that the environment is spinning; caused by stimulation of the receptors that affect the equilibrium and balance; alcohol consumption, certain drugs, and low blood pressure may contribute to the feeling of dizziness or light-headedness.

Treating Ear Conditions

As mentioned earlier, ear wax removal is a way to relive a blockage that may have caused some conduction hearing

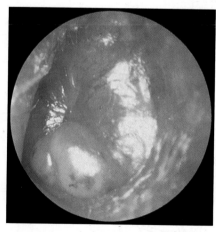

Otitis media

Figure 6-12 A bulging eardrum caused by otitis media. (Reprinted from Kronenberger J, Ledbetter J. *Jones & Bartlett Learning's Comprehensive Medical Assisting*. 5th ed. Burlington, MA: Jones & Bartlett Learning, LLC; 2016.) (From Moore KL, Dalley AF II. *Clinical Oriented Anatomy*. 4th ed. Baltimore, MD: Lippincott Williams & Wilkins; 1999.)

loss. There are several surgical procedures used to relieve ear conditions. A myringotomy, an incision into the tympanic membrane, is a procedure used to relieve pressure in the middle ear due to buildup of pus or fluid. A longer effect for this condition is to place a tympanostomy tube into the eardrum. This allows the pressure to equalize in the middle ear preventing further damage. When there is a problem with the cochlea, a cochlear implant may correct the problem allowing the person to hear certain sounds.

 ## SENSE OF TASTE AND SMELL

Gustation is the sense of taste. The tongue has taste buds located in specific areas that allow us to differentiate five basic tastes. These tastes include sweet (sugar), salty (sodium), sour, bitter, and umami (savory). Olfaction is the sense of smell. The receptor cells are in the nasal cavity. The olfactory nerve delivers impulses to the brain where we can interpret over 10,000 different smells. The sense of taste is closely related to the ability to smell. This is why when you have a cold or stuffy nose, you cannot taste food.

 ## THE OTHER SENSES

The other senses are not specific to a single organ or location but have receptors spread throughout the body. These include receptors for touch, pressure, temperature, position, and pain. The sense of touch relies on receptors primarily located in the skin and hair follicles. The sense of pressure responds to sensory receptors located in the subcutaneous tissues. The ability to sense temperature is due to the free nerve endings that are found in the skin. They respond to varying degrees of heat and cold. Our internal temperature is adjusted by the brain's hypothalamus according to the temperature of the blood. The sense of position, knowing whether we are upright or horizontal, is determined by the receptors known as proprioceptors.

Pain is a sense associated with the nerve endings found in the skin, muscles, joints, and internal organs. The pain may vary from mild to severe. Sometimes stimulants from allergic substances cause these nerve endings to be irritated causing mild to intense itching, which also might become painful. Pain relief might include analgesic medications, such as narcotic and nonnarcotic preparations. Endorphins are natural chemicals released from the brain and are associated with pain control. These chemicals are released during exercise, body massage, and electrical stimulation therapy.

 ## THE ENDOCRINE SYSTEM

The endocrine system consists of a group of glands that secrete hormones. Figure 6-13 shows the location of the endocrine glands in the body.

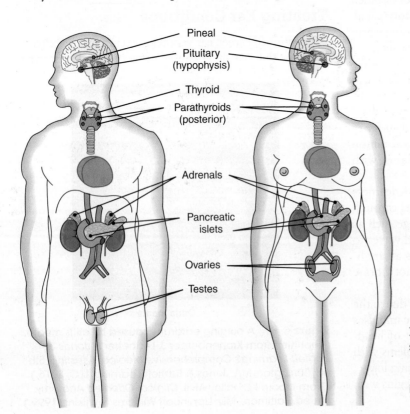

Figure 6-13 Glands of the endocrine system. (Reprinted from Cohen BJ. *Memmler's The Human Body in Health and Disease.* 13th ed. Burlington, MA: Jones & Bartlett Learning, LLC; 2014.)

Each gland specializes in a specific function and secretes a hormone, a regulatory substance. The endocrine system works with the nervous system coordinating functions throughout the body. The endocrine glands secrete their hormones directly into the bloodstream where the hormones travel to the target tissue, the tissue and cells that respond to that hormone. The action of the endocrine glands and the release of their hormones are stimulated by the process of negative feedback. An example is the release of insulin when the blood sugar increases. A hormone may be released following a rhythmic pattern such as how the hormones are released in the female based on the menstrual cycle. Each gland will be introduced listing the hormone(s) produced and their function.

The Pituitary

This gland, also called the hypophysis, is situated beneath the brain and connects with the hypothalamus. The pituitary is divided into anterior and posterior lobes. Each lobe secretes specific hormones that target organs throughout the body. See Figure 6-14 diagram of the anterior and posterior pituitary with all the hormones produced within the pituitary gland.

Anterior Pituitary

Hormones produced and released by the hypothalamus stimulate the anterior pituitary to release the hormones it produces. The anterior pituitary is referred to as the

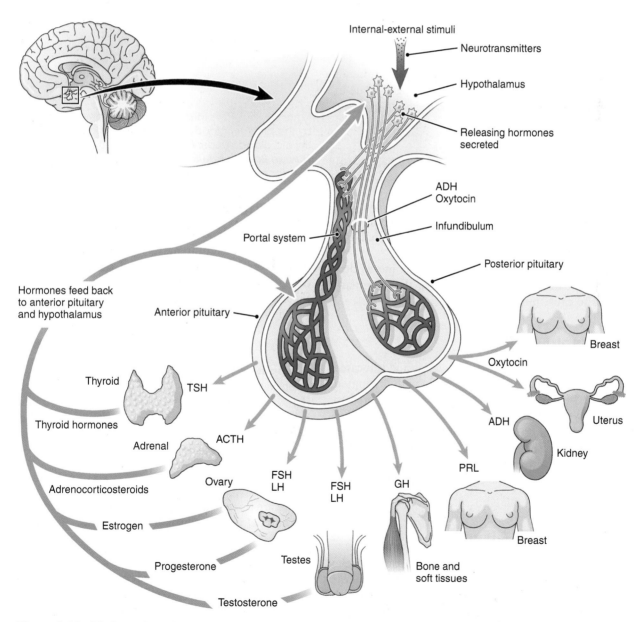

Figure 6-14 Pituitary gland hormones secreted and the organs they affect. (Reprinted from Cohen BJ. *Memmler's The Human Body in Health and Disease.* 13th ed. Burlington, MA: Jones & Bartlett Learning, LLC; 2014.)

master gland because it releases hormones that affect many other glands in the body including the thyroid, gonads, and adrenal glands. The hormones produced by the anterior pituitary include:

- Growth hormone (**GH**)—Somatotropin, promotes growth in the body, specifically size and height during youth
- Thyroid-stimulating hormone (**TSH**)—Stimulates the thyroid gland in the neck to produce thyroid hormones
- Adrenocorticotropic hormone (**ACTH**)—Stimulates hormone production in the adrenal glands, specifically the outer layer called the cortex
- Prolactin hormone (**PRL**)—Stimulates milk production in the breasts
- Follicle-stimulating hormone (**FSH**)—Stimulates the ovary causing development of the follicles, the place where the eggs mature, and also stimulates the testes for the development of sperm cells
- Luteinizing hormone (**LH**)—Causes ovulation in women and promotes production of progesterone in females and testosterone in males

Posterior Pituitary

The posterior pituitary only secretes two hormones; however, they are very critical to the function of the organs they stimulate. The hormones include:

- Antidiuretic hormone (**ADH**)—Stimulates the kidneys to reabsorb water that is lost through the filtration process
- Oxytocin—Stimulates contraction of the uterus during childbirth and the contraction of the mammary glands to cause milk ejection

The Thyroid Gland

This is the largest of the endocrine glands and is located in the neck. It is shaped like a butterfly with a wing on either side of the larynx. The thyroid is stimulated to function by the TSH produced in the anterior pituitary gland. The thyroid produces two hormones that regulate cell metabolism. The hormones are labeled T_3 (triiodothyronine) and T_4 (thyroxine). Figure 6-15 demonstrates the connection between the pituitary gland and the thyroid gland.

The Parathyroid Glands

These are four tiny glands that are embedded in the thyroid gland, two on each side. They secrete parathyroid hormone (PTH), which promotes calcium release from bone tissue increasing the blood calcium level and regulates the amount of calcium the kidneys excrete.

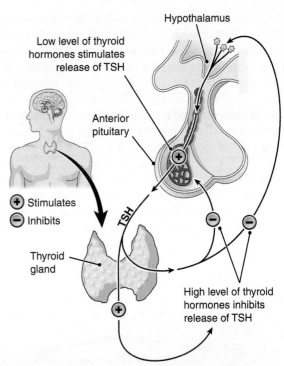

Figure 6-15 Thyroid-stimulating hormone secreted by the pituitary gland stimulates the functioning of the thyroid gland. (Reprinted from Cohen BJ. *Memmler's The Human Body in Health and Disease.* 13th ed. Burlington, MA: Jones & Bartlett Learning, LLC; 2014.)

The Adrenal Glands

These glands are located on top of the kidneys and are also called the suprarenal glands. The glands have an outer layer called the cortex and the inner portion is the medulla. Each area secretes different hormones. Figure 6-16 shows the adrenal gland location and the two divisions, cortex and medulla.

Adrenal Medulla

The primary hormone produced in the adrenal medulla is **epinephrine** (adrenaline). This hormone stimulates the sympathetic nervous system and is a major chemical released for the fight-or-flight response. Some of the effects it causes include a rise in blood pressure, heart rate, and overall metabolic rate of body cells.

Adrenal Cortex

There are three main categories of hormones secreted by the adrenal cortex, which are as follows:

- Glucocorticoids—Maintain blood glucose levels during times of stress; suppress the inflammatory response with a specific hormone called cortisol (hydrocortisone).
- Mineralocorticoids—Regulate electrolyte balance controlling the sodium reabsorption and potassium secretion in the kidney; a major hormone in this group is aldosterone.

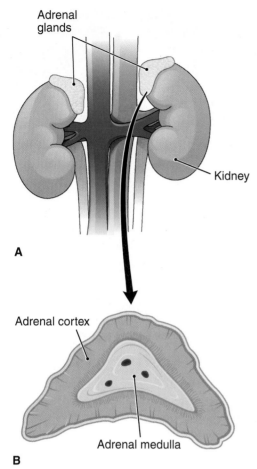

A

B

Figure 6-16 **A.** Adrenal glands located on top of the kidneys. **B.** Cortex and medulla of the adrenal gland. (Reprinted from Cohen BJ. *Memmler's The Human Body in Health and Disease*, 13th ed. Burlington, MA: Jones & Bartlett Learning, LLC; 2014.)

- Androgens—Male sex hormones only secreted in small amount from the adrenal gland but is also secreted in pre- and postmenopausal women; promote bone and muscle growth and stimulate sexual desire.

The Pancreas

The pancreas is both an exocrine and endocrine gland located in the left upper quadrant of the abdomen. The exocrine portion secretes pancreatic juices, through a duct, directly into the small intestine to assist in the breakdown of nutrients. The endocrine portion of the pancreas is found in the islets of Langerhans. These are specialized cells that secrete their hormone directly into the bloodstream. Insulin is the most important hormone secreted with the major responsibility of maintaining glucose balance. Insulin is necessary to transport glucose into the cells where it can be utilized for energy. Figure 6-17 demonstrates what happens to glucose in the body when a person does not have diabetes and when someone does have it. A normal functioning pancreas will produce insulin, which will properly transport glucose into the cells to be used as energy. In a diabetic person, insulin production is decreased and less glucose moved into the cells to be used. This creates the accumulation of glucose in the bloodstream that can adversely affect other organs and structures in the body. One of the areas affected is the retina of the eye where damage is caused to the blood vessels that supply the retina.

The Ovaries

The ovaries are located in the pelvic cavity, one at the end of each fallopian tube. The primary hormone, estrogen, is responsible for the development of secondary, female

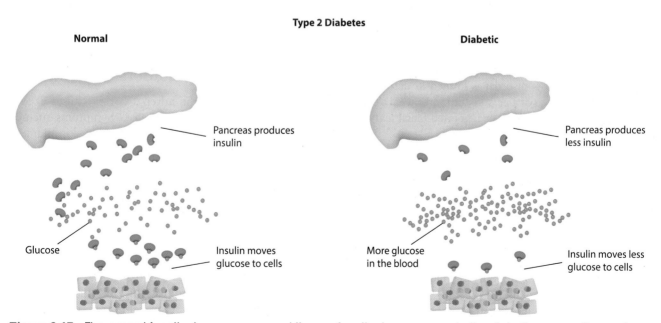

Figure 6-17 The normal functioning pancreas and the nonfunctioning pancreas in the diabetic person. (Image from Shutterstock.com.)

sex characteristics. It also stimulates mammary gland development and the start of the menses. Progesterone is the other hormone produced by the ovaries. It assists in the normal development of pregnancy.

The Testes

The testes are located in the scrotal sac of the male. The hormone testosterone is produced as the male enters puberty. It causes the voice to deepen, facial and body hair to grow, and muscle to develop. Male hormones are classified as androgens.

The Pineal Gland

This tiny gland is located behind the midbrain. It produces the hormone melatonin. More of this hormone is produced during darker periods and less during daylight hours. It regulates our sleep cycle.

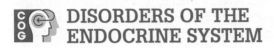

DISORDERS OF THE ENDOCRINE SYSTEM

With so many glands producing these regulating hormones, you can expect to find abnormal conditions associated with the glands in this system. The disorders are typically caused by overproduction of the hormone, hypersecretion, or from underproduction of the hormone, hyposecretion.

Pituitary Gland Disorders

A tumor may develop in any area of the body, but when there is a tumor affecting the pituitary gland, it can produce numerous problems. One of these is a pituitary tumor that stimulates overproduction of the growth hormone. This condition, developing in childhood, is called **gigantism** causing the child to grow abnormally tall. When this occurs in adults, the bones of the face, hands, and feet enlarge. This disorder is known as **acromegaly**. Figure 6-18 is a photo of a person with acromegaly. Notice the very enlarged hands and exaggerated facial features.

Thyroid Gland Disorders

Underproduction of the thyroid hormones results in hypothyroidism, and overproduction of these hormones results in hyperthyroidism. Since the thyroid hormones regulate the body's metabolism, some signs and symptoms of hypothyroidism include a sluggish feeling, dry skin and hair, and weight gain. Just the opposite occurs with hyperthyroidism with symptoms that include weight loss, rapid pulse, sweating, and nervousness. A common type of hyperthyroidism is Graves' disease. This disease causes development of a goiter, enlargement of the thyroid gland. Another symptom is the development of exophthalmos,

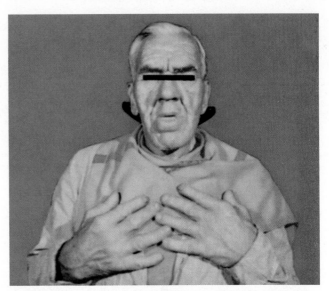

Figure 6-18   Acromegaly showing enlarged extremities and facial features. (From Willis MC. *Medical Terminology: A Programmed Learning Approach to the Language of Health Care.* Baltimore, MD: Lipppincott Williams & Wilkins; 2002.)

swelling of the eyeballs causing an appearance of bulging eyes. Blood tests are used to measure the levels of thyroid hormone in the bloodstream. Treatment of hypothyroidism includes replacement hormone medication.

Parathyroid Gland Disorders

Since the parathyroid hormone affects the calcium levels in the body, too little may cause muscle contractions or spasms called tetany. Too much production of the hormone causes the bones to release too much calcium into the bloodstream. With this condition, it is not uncommon for the person to develop kidney stones since the kidneys are filtering an excessive amount of calcium.

Adrenal Cortex Disorders

Underfunctioning of the adrenal cortex causes a condition known as Addison disease. Symptoms include weakness, loss of muscle tissue, excessive skin pigmentation, and salt and water imbalance. Overfunctioning of the hormone cortisol results in Cushing syndrome with very pronounced symptoms including obesity and a round appearance to the face called "moon face."

Pancreas Disorders

When the islets of Langerhans do not produce enough insulin or the body is not utilizing the insulin properly, Type 2 **diabetes mellitus** (T2DM) develops. It is associated with those who are overweight. It is one of the most common endocrine disorders. Hyperglycemia is the term that means elevated glucose in the blood, a result of insulin deficiency. Patients with diabetes have numerous symptoms including excessive thirst (polydipsia), coronary artery damage, and increased risk for heart disease, diabetic retinopathy, and poor healing of wounds.

Type 1 diabetes mellitus (**T1DM**) occurs before the age of 30 and is less common but severe. The pancreatic cells in the islet of Langerhans are destroyed and unable to produce insulin. When diabetes develops only during pregnancy, it is called gestational diabetes. This type of diabetes usually disappears after the birth.

Diabetes is determined by evaluating blood glucose levels. A single fasting blood test may indicate an initial problem but continued monitoring is required. Diet, exercise, and oral antidiabetic medication are used to treat diabetes. Occasionally, injectable insulin is required to maintain proper glucose levels.

Cultural Connection

The U.S. Department of Health and Human Services, specifically the Indian Health Services Division, stated that American Indians and Alaskan Natives have a 2.2 times higher risk of developing Type 2 Diabetes Mellitus than non-Hispanic whites. It is estimated that 30% of this population has prediabetes and will probably develop diabetes mellitus. The American Diabetes Association has awareness programs that include education and counseling on the ways to avoid developing diabetes. The slogan "Awakening the Spirit" focuses on ways to encourage people to create a healthy pathway in their life.

Preparing for Externship

These chapters on anatomy and physiology include information about the various body systems that may be a special area of practice in the medical field. For example, this chapter discusses the nervous and endocrine systems. A neurologist and endocrinologist are the specialists that treat patients who have disorders of these body systems. Your school will select the externship site assignment. You may find yourself at a specialty medical practice. Prior to starting the externship course, research as much as you can about the typical patients disorders, the procedures performed, and treatments for the various conditions. While doing your research, review the basic medical terms and abbreviations associated with this type of special practice.

Chapter Recap

- The nervous system is comprised of nerve cells called neurons, which form fibers and ultimately build the nerves.
- Chemicals called neurotransmitters are necessary for the nerves to send their signals through a series of synapses.
- The sympathetic and parasympathetic nervous systems have very different and specific functions regulating the functions in the body.
- Numerous diseases and disorders of the nervous system can lead to the inability of organs and muscles to function properly. Some of these conditions cause intense nerve pain and occasionally paralysis of regions of the body.

- The central nervous system that includes the brain and spinal cord relies on the bony vertebrae and meninges for protection and the cerebrospinal fluid to cushion and provides nourishment to the spinal cord.
- The special senses of the body allow us to experience our external and internal environment. These senses include sight, sound, taste, smell, and touch.
- The endocrine glands and the hormones secrete and regulate a majority of the function in the body.
- Hypersecretion and hyposecretion of hormones are the most common reasons for the disorders of the endocrine system.

Online Resources for Students

Student Resources available on the text's online site include:

- Audio Glossaries
- Animations
- Competency Evaluation Forms

- Videos
- Anatomy & Physiology Module with Heart and Lung Sounds
- Weblinks
- Worksheets

Exercises and Activities

Certification Preparation Questions

1. Which of these structures are found in the CNS?

   a. Peripheral nerves
   b. Brain and spinal cord
   c. Midbrain and visceral nerves
   d. Sympathetic nerves
   e. Somatic nerves and cerebellum

2. Which of these is the whitish covering over the axons?

   a. Meninges
   b. Synapse
   c. Myelin
   d. Neurons
   e. Gray matter

3. Which of these is NOT an effect of the sympathetic nervous system?

   a. Constricts blood vessels
   b. Dilates bronchial tubes
   c. Dilates pupils
   d. Increases blood pressure
   e. Raises heart rate

4. Which of these is used to measure the electrical activity of the brain?

   a. PET
   b. LP
   c. MRI
   d. CT
   e. EEG

5. The abbreviation MTBI refers to a condition that has another term which is:

   a. stroke.
   b. concussion.
   c. epilepsy.
   d. meningitis.
   e. hydrocephalus.

6. Excessive pressure of the aqueous humor causes:

   a. cataracts.
   b. glaucoma.
   c. myopia.
   d. retinopathy.
   e. corneal abrasion.

7. The pinna is located:

   a. in the middle ear.
   b. behind the eardrum.
   c. at the opening of the outer ear.
   d. in the inner ear.
   e. inside the cochlea.

8. Which of these is produced in the pituitary and stimulates the production of hormone in the adrenal cortex?

   a. FSH
   b. TSH
   c. ACTH
   d. GH
   e. LH

9. Epinephrine is produced in the:

   a. thyroid gland.
   b. pancreas.
   c. adrenal gland.
   d. parathyroid gland.
   e. posterior pituitary.

10. A condition occurring in adults that causes enlargement of the hands and facial features is:

    a. gigantism.
    b. hypothyroidism.
    c. goiter.
    d. Addison disease.
    e. acromegaly.

Internet Resource

For more information on brain disorders caused from injury to the brain, visit the Web site for the Brain Injury Association of America at www.biausa.org

7 Digestive System and Nutrition

Chapter Objectives

- Describe the function of the digestive system.
- List the organs of the digestive tract and describe their specific function.
- List the accessory organs of digestion and describe how they assist the digestive system.
- Explain the process of absorption in the digestive system.
- Explain the purpose of bile.
- Describe the muscular contraction of the digestive system.
- Describe common disorders of the digestive tract and the accessory organs.
- Describe the roles of minerals and vitamins in the body.
- Explain the use of protein, carbohydrates, and fats in the body.
- Compare saturated and unsaturated fats.
- Describe common nutritional disorders.

CAAHEP & ABHES Competencies

CAAHEP

- Describe structural organization of the human body.
- Identify body systems.
- List major organs in each body system.
- Describe the normal function of each body system.
- Identify common pathology related to each body system including signs, symptoms, and etiology.
- Analyze pathology for each body system including diagnostic measures and treatment modalities.

ABHES

- List all body systems, their structure, and functions.
- Describe common diseases, symptoms, and etiologies as they apply to each system.
- Identify diagnostic and treatment modalities as they relate to each body system.

Chapter Terms

Anorexia	Cirrhosis	Hepatitis	Parotitis
Appendicitis	Defecation	Ingestion	Peristalsis
Chyme	Diverticulosis	Mastication	Ulcerative colitis
Cholecystectomy	Endoscopy	Nausea	Villi
Cholelithiasis	Gastritis	Oral thrush	Vomiting

Abbreviations

BMR	HBV	IBD	LES
GERD	HCL	IBS	LDL
GI			

Case Study

Mary Ann Gibson is a 14-year-old and a new patient of the clinic. She recently relocated to this area with her family. When the family moved, she had to leave behind her friends that she has gone to school with since first grade. She is entering the new high school as a freshman this year. She is accompanied by her mother who is concerned that

Mary Ann is losing weight although she seems to have a good appetite and eats regularly. Mary Ann is reluctant to step on the scale to obtain her height and weight. Rosa, the medical assistant, continues to escort her to the examination room. Mary Ann asks Rosa quietly if she can see the doctor without her mother in the room.

In this chapter, we will explore the digestive system including the organs of digestion and the accessory organs that are necessary for proper digestion of food. We will examine how nutrition is processed in the digestive tract for use by the body cells.

 ## THE DIGESTIVE SYSTEM

The primary function of the digestive system is to process the nutrients from the foods we eat into usable nutrients that supply each body cell with the energy necessary to perform specific actions in the body. Digestion, absorption, and elimination are the major processes that take place in the digestive tract. Digestion is the process of breaking down the nutrients into simple chemicals that can be used by the body cells. Absorption is the transfer of these chemicals from the digestive tract to the blood in the circulatory system where they will be transported to the body cells. Products that cannot be digested are eliminated as waste material.

The gastrointestinal (**GI**) tract, also called the alimentary canal, is a hollow passageway that begins at the mouth and ends at the anus where waste products are

eliminated. The accessory organs that are not actually part of the canal are the salivary glands, liver, and pancreas. They supply the necessary substances that further help to break down the food into chemicals that the body can use. Figure 7-1 is a diagram of the entire GI tract from the mouth to the anus.

 ## THE MOUTH

The oral cavity is the first part of the alimentary canal. The mouth has many structures that initially start the digestive process. The process of taking food into the mouth is called **ingestion**. The teeth, tongue, cheeks, and lips help in this process. **Mastication** is the process of chewing the food. The teeth grind the food and the tongue, cheeks, and lips hold the food in the mouth and move the food around. There are different shapes of the teeth allowing different

Case Question

 How would you handle Mary Ann's request if you were the medical assistant?

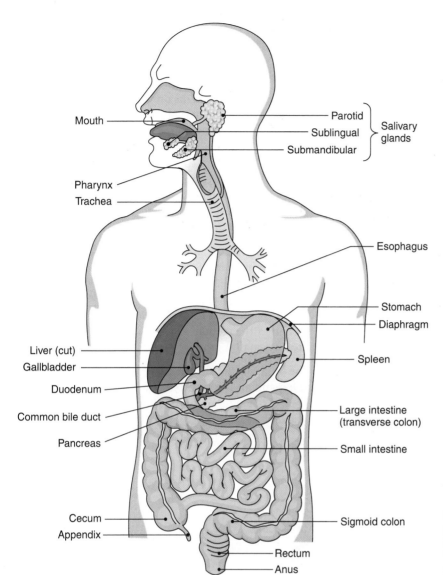

Figure 7-1 The digestive system. (Reprinted from Cohen BJ. *Memmler's The Human Body in Health and Disease.* 13th ed. Burlington, MA: Jones & Bartlett Learning, LLC; 2014.)

functions in breaking down the food. The incisors are cutting teeth. The cuspids (canines) are used for gripping and tearing food, and the molars are used for grinding.

The tongue has taste buds that allow us to recognize the difference between sweet, sour, bitter, and salty. The food mixes with saliva, the secretion from the salivary glands. There are three pairs of salivary glands that contribute this secretion:

- Parotid—at the back of the mouth in front of the ear; these become inflamed when someone has the mumps.
- Submandibular—beneath the lower jawbone, mandible.
- Sublingual—under the tongue.

Figure 7-2 is a diagram of the location of the salivary glands.

Now, it is time to swallow the food through the process called deglutition.

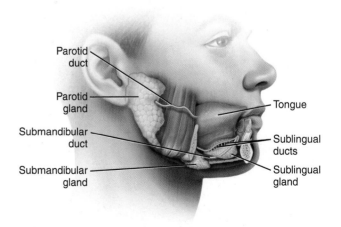

Figure 7-2 Salivary glands. (Reprinted from Cohen BJ. *Memmler's The Human Body in Health and Disease.* 13th ed. Burlington, MA: Jones & Bartlett Learning, LLC; 2014.)

The Pharynx

We commonly know the pharynx as the throat. There are three sections of the pharynx:

- Nasopharynx—upper part of the pharynx at the back of the nose
- Oropharynx—middle section of the pharynx that is visible when the mouth is open
- Laryngopharynx—lower part of the pharynx that lies above the larynx (voice box)

When the food moves from the mouth to the pharynx, it is now called a bolus, a small bit of food that has been chewed, mixed with saliva, and now is ready for the stomach.

The Esophagus

The esophagus extends from the pharynx to the stomach. It is a muscular structure about 10 inches long. The bolus of food is not changed but is lubricated with mucus produced by the lining of the esophagus. This structure is made of smooth muscle, which uses peristalsis to move the food along down to the stomach. The esophagus passes through the diaphragm through an opening called the esophageal hiatus.

This is a common place for hernia formation, which we will discuss later.

The Stomach

The stomach is located in the upper, left part of the abdominal cavity. It is a muscular organ that continues grinding the food and missing it with the digestive juices secreted in the stomach. The stomach has a greater and lesser curvature, which shapes the stomach. The uppermost rounded part of the stomach is the fundus. The lower end of the stomach leading to the small intestine is the pylorus.

The stomach has two sphincter muscles, which regulate the size of an opening:

- Lower esophageal sphincter (**LES**)—also called the cardiac sphincter because of its location close to the heart. This sphincter controls the flow of food from the esophagus into the stomach.
- Pyloric sphincter—this sphincter muscle is located at the end of the stomach and regulates the flow of food into the small intestine.

The lining of the stomach has folds called rugae. The folds expand allowing the stomach to enlarge as we eat. Figure 7-3 is a diagram of the stomach and demonstrates the rugae.

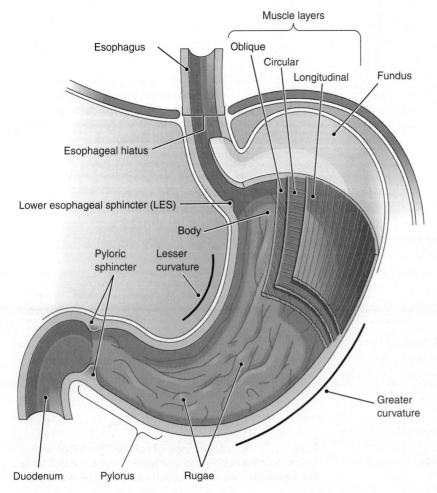

Figure 7-3 Stomach. (Reprinted from Cohen BJ. *Memmler's The Human Body in Health and Disease.* 13th ed. Burlington, MA: Jones & Bartlett Learning, LLC; 2014.)

The stomach produces gastric juices that are used to further dissolve the bolus of food into a liquid form that can be more easily absorbed into the bloodstream. These gastric juices are:

- Hydrochloric acid (HCL)—an extremely strong acid that breaks down protein and destroys foreign organisms. HCL production starts prior to food entering the stomach. This is done so when the food does enter the stomach it immediately starts breaking it down.
- Pepsin—an enzyme that combines with the HCL to turn the bolus into a semiliquid.

The semiliquid formed from the HCL, pepsin, and the bolus of food is now called chyme. It is ready to enter into the small intestine.

Small Intestine

This is the longest part of the digestive tract at approximately 20 feet. There are three sections of the small intestine:

- Duodenum
- Jejunum
- Ileum

The mucous lining of the small intestine secretes mucus that will protect the intestine from the strong acid chyme. Carbohydrates and proteins undergo a final digestive process in the small intestine. The liver and pancreas secretions are now added to the contents of the small intestine. Most of the nutrients and water will be absorbed in the small intestine. These substances are absorbed through the villi and microvilli found on the mucosal lining of the small intestine. **Villi** are finger-like projections and microvilli are smaller microscopic projections. They both provide significantly increased surface area for absorption of the nutrients and water as those substances travel through the intestine.

Large Intestine

The next part of the alimentary canal is the large intestine. It is approximately 5 foot long and much wider than the small intestine. The large intestine begins in the lower right region of the abdomen with a structure called the cecum, a pouch. The small and large intestines are separated by a valve called the ileocecal valve (ileum + cecum). This valve permits food to enter the large intestine from the small intestine and then closes so nothing can flow backward. A small finger-like projection is found at the base of the cecum. This is the vermiform appendix that we just usually call the appendix. The remaining parts of the large intestine include:

- Ascending colon—the portion that extends up the right side of the abdomen from the cecum to the transverse colon.

- Transverse colon—extends across the abdomen from the right side to the left side lying below the liver, stomach, and spleen.
- Descending colon—extends downward from the transverse colon to the sigmoid colon.
- Sigmoid colon—the end of the colon that forms an "S" shape as it approaches the rectum.
- Rectum—the part of the alimentary canal that stores the indigestible food before it is eliminated from the body.
- Anal canal and anus—the final portion of the alimentary canal that leads to the outside of the body; the anus is a sphincter muscle that controls the expulsion of the waste from the body.

The large intestine is responsible for reabsorbing water and forming the waste material into a substance called feces or stool. **Peristalsis** is the rhythmic action of moving this material through the large intestine. **Defecation** is the term used for the process of eliminating the waste from the body. The anal sphincter allows voluntary control over this process. Bacteria, normally found in the colon, produce vitamin k, necessary for proper clotting. The bacteria do not cause disease, unless allowed to enter other areas of the body through contamination.

The Peritoneum

Although the peritoneum is not considered to be an organ, it contains the organs of the abdominal cavity. It is a serous membrane that lines the cavity and covers the organs. There are two layers, the parietal and the visceral. The parietal peritoneum lines the wall of the cavity and the visceral peritoneum covers the organs. Two other structures that are subdivisions of the peritoneum are the mesentery and the omentum, greater and lesser. The mesentery attaches from the posterior abdominal wall to the small intestine. The greater omentum extends from the stomach into the pelvic cavity and up the transverse colon. The lesser omentum, which is smaller, extends between the stomach and the liver.

 THE ACCESSORY ORGANS

The digestive tract needs the assistance of the accessory organs and their secretions in order to carry out the process of digestion. In the mouth, the salivary glands provide the first secretion, saliva. This substance moistens the food and begins the process of digestion. From there as the food travels through the alimentary canal, the liver, gallbladder, and pancreas add secretions to help complete the process.

The Liver

Located in the upper right quadrant of the abdomen below the diaphragm, the liver is the largest accessory organ. Blood is delivered to the liver through the hepatic

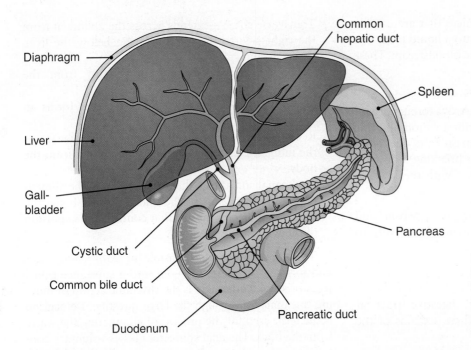

Common hepatic duct
Diaphragm
Spleen
Liver
Gall-bladder
Cystic duct
Pancreas
Common bile duct
Pancreatic duct
Duodenum

Figure 7-4 Accessory organs of the digestive system. (Reprinted from Cohen BJ. *Memmler's The Human Body in Health and Disease.* 13th ed. Burlington, MA: Jones & Bartlett Learning, LLC; 2014.)

artery. This vessel carries oxygen-rich blood to the liver. Blood is also delivered through the hepatic venous portal system. This system of veins carries blood from the gastrointestinal tract with a lower concentration of oxygen. This blood will be filtered by the liver, one of the main functions of this organ. Once filtered, some of the blood will be transported to the kidneys to be filtered for elimination of waste products from the body. The liver has several functions:

- Stores glycogen, a form of glucose for use when the glucose level needs to be restored
- Produces blood plasma proteins, such as albumin, globulins, and clotting factors
- Produces bile—essential for metabolizing fats
- Destroys old red blood cells and eliminates the by-product called bilirubin (bilirubin is the substance that gives color to stool)
- Stores iron and vitamins
- Detoxifies chemicals and metabolizes drugs including alcohol
- Converts waste products for excretion by the kidneys; an example is urea, a waste product of protein metabolism

The Gallbladder

A primary function of the liver is to produce bile necessary to breakdown fats. When bile leaves the liver, it is carried through ducts to the gallbladder where it is stored until it is needed. The common hepatic (liver) duct joins with the cystic (gallbladder) duct to form the common bile duct. Bile flows through the common bile duct and empties into the duodenum where the process of fat breakdown takes place.

The Pancreas

The pancreas is located in the upper left quadrant of the abdomen behind the stomach. It is an endocrine and exocrine gland. The endocrine portion secretes insulin directly into the bloodstream. We are interested in the exocrine function of the pancreas. This gland produces enzymes that are secreted into pancreatic ducts, which connect with the bile duct and lead to the small intestine. These enzymes digest fats, carbohydrates, and fats. The pancreas also releases sodium bicarbonate, which neutralizes the acidic contents of the small intestine. See Figure 7-4 showing the location of the accessory organs of the digestive system.

END-TO-END PROCESS

Now that we have explored the organs of the digestive tract, let's recap the process from beginning to end.

Digestion

After taking food into the mouth, the teeth chew the food into smaller pieces and saliva mixes with the food to make it soft and moist and easier to swallow. The digestive process has now begun. From the mouth, the food travels down the esophagus and into the stomach. Here, it will mix with hydrochloric acid and enzymes. The food mixes and further breaks down into a semiliquid substance called **chyme**. The chyme moves through the pyloric sphincter of the stomach into the duodenum of the small intestine. While in the small intestine, bile from the liver and pancreatic secretions are added to the chyme causing further digestion of the food we ate. Now we are ready for the absorption process.

Absorption

The products of digestion are ready to be absorbed into the bloodstream. Most of the absorption will take place in through the villi of the small intestine. These tiny structures have minute blood vessels and capillaries supplying them where the absorption takes place. Most of the fat will not be absorbed into the bloodstream but will be absorbed into the lymphatic system through the permeable membrane. The lymphatic vessels carry lymph fluid with the fat droplets to the veins close to the heart. The fat will eventually be moved through the blood to the liver for processing. In the large intestine, the bacterial action produces vitamin K and some B vitamins, which are absorbed from the large intestine.

Mechanism of Controlling Digestion

The nervous system plays a major role in regulating or controlling digestion. The sympathetic system decreases activity in the digestive tract and the parasympathetic system stimulates or increases activity. You may recall from the discussion of the sympathetic system that stress has an effect on the function of this system. Digestive disturbances may be more frequent during times of stress. Our senses act to stimulate our digestive system into action. When you smell food, for example a hot cinnamon roll fresh out of the oven, your mouth will start watering getting ready with saliva to mix with the first bite you take. Sometimes, the very thought of something good to eat will start stimulating the digestive process into action. After the saliva production, the stomach starts secreting its juices getting ready to receive the food from the mouth. From there, the intestines are stimulated to get ready to receive the chyme from the stomach. Throughout the process, the nerve impulses regulate the rate of flow through the digestive system.

Mechanism of Controlling Appetite and Hunger

Hunger and appetite differ in that hunger is the need for food and appetite is a desire for food but not necessarily the need for it. We develop hunger and appetites based on factors such as our emotional state and force of habit. When we say we are hungry for a specific food, we are drawing off our memory of that food. The hypothalamus regulates our sensation of hunger telling us when we are hungry and when we have had enough to eat. As we eat and fill the digestive tract, this too signals our body to stop consuming food therefore decreasing our hunger.

We eat because we are hungry or have an appetite, but we need to eat to provide energy for our body to function properly. The metabolic rate relates to overall energy requirements. It is the rate that cellular respiration converts nutrients into ATP, necessary for cell function. Metabolic rate changes from person to person. Age, body composition, gender, activity, and thyroid function can all affect the metabolic rate. The basal metabolic rate, **BMR**, is the calculation of the amount of energy needed to minimally maintain life functions. As we begin to look at nutrition requirements, it is important to understand what a calorie is. A kilocalorie is the amount of heat needed to raise 1 kg of water 1 degree centigrade. Calorie is the simple term used to describe a kilocalorie.

 NUTRITION

Proper nutrition is critical to the overall health of our cells. Let's begin by looking at the three basic nutritional needs, proteins, carbohydrates, and fats. Most nutritional guidelines recommend that our daily intake should be 15% to 20% from protein, 55% to 60% from carbohydrates, and 30% or less from fats. These values are based on a normal, healthy individual who participates in a moderate exercise plan. Diets are altered to meet the needs of the individual. For example, a diabetic patient may want to increase the protein and decrease the carbohydrate amounts.

Carbohydrates

Carbohydrates are a primary source of energy digested into simple sugar before they are absorbed into the bloodstream. The liver converts them into glucose as a usable form of energy. If the body does not need the immediate supply of glucose, the liver converts the glucose into glucagon, which is stored until needed. If there is an overabundance of glucose and glucagon, it then converts to fat and is stored in the liver and in adipose tissue (fatty tissue). Carbohydrates are found in fresh fruits, vegetables, and whole grains. There may be limited amounts of carbohydrates in beans and nuts. Carbohydrates are also in desserts and foods with added sugar. These types of carbohydrates should be limited in the daily diet since they add little nutritional value.

Fats

Fats are another critical nutrient; however, not all fat is the same. Fats give the body energy to work properly; however, it is harmful to eat too many. The body uses carbohydrates for initial energy and then depends on calories from fat. Fats help absorb vitamins A, D, E, and K, which are the fat-soluble vitamins. A benefit of fat stored in the body is that it insulates us and protects some organs. Fat has 9 calories per gram, compared to 4 calories per gram provided by proteins and carbohydrates. Essential fatty acids are necessary for brain development and blood clotting, but the body cannot manufacture these. We need to include some fat in the daily diet to ensure we are getting the essential fatty acids, which are linoleic and linolenic acid.

Saturated and Unsaturated Fatty Acids

Saturated fats are responsible for increasing the low-density lipids (**LDL**), the bad cholesterol. A person with a high LDL will be at a greater risk for heart attack and stroke. Saturated fats are primarily found in animal products such as butter, cheese, and whole milk. Saturated fats are those that are solid when at room temperature. They increase the cholesterol buildup in arteries leading to clogged and blocked arteries.

Unsaturated fats can help lower the LDL cholesterol. These fats are in a liquid form when at room temperature. There are monounsaturated fats such as olive and canola oil and polyunsaturated fats including safflower, corn, and soy oil.

Trans-fatty acids are a type of fat that form when vegetable oil hardens. This process is called hydrogenation. These fats are frequently used in foods to keep them fresh for a longer time. These fats can raise LDL cholesterol levels in the blood and should be limited in the daily diet.

Proteins

Proteins are necessary in the body to build, strengthen, and repair cells and tissues. They are involved in muscle contractions and movement. Protein is not stored in the body the same as carbohydrates and fats. When more protein is available in the body than required, it is broken down for energy or will be converted to triglycerides. When protein is diminished in the diet, the body will use the structural proteins found in muscle tissue. Carbohydrates and fats are used for energy before proteins so are called protein-sparing nutrients. Protein foods should be part of the daily diet since they are not stored in the body. Proteins are found in animal products and some plants. All of the essential amino acids are found in animal protein. Amino acids are the building blocks of protein. Most of the plant proteins lack one or more of the essential amino acids. Vegetarians that do not eat any animal protein must obtain the necessary amino acids by combining vegetables and grains to ensure that they receive all the essential amino acids.

Minerals and Vitamins

Minerals and vitamins are equally essential to the body as proteins, carbohydrates, and fats. Minerals are necessary for many functions including fluid balance and blood clotting. Vitamins are essential for metabolism. Vitamins are classified as water soluble or fat soluble.

The B vitamins and vitamin C are water soluble, which means that they are dissolved in the body fluid and not stored in the body so are used on a daily basis then need to be replaced regularly with the food we eat. The fat-soluble vitamins A, D, E, and K are stored in fat and used as needed. An overabundance of these vitamins may lead to a toxic condition so should be taken in large doses. Essential vitamins and their basic function include:

- Vitamin A—needed for healthy mucus membranes, skin and eye pigments
- Vitamin B_6—helps form red blood cells
- Vitamin B_{12}—necessary for metabolism and maintain central nervous system
- Vitamin C—an antioxidant that promotes healthy teeth and gums, promotes wound healing
- Vitamin D—helps the body absorb calcium for healthy teeth and bones; the sunshine vitamin since it is produced by the body by being in the sun
- Vitamin E—formation of red blood cells and helps body use vitamin K
- Vitamin K—necessary for coagulation of blood cells
- Biotin—metabolism of proteins and carbohydrates
- Niacin—helps maintain healthy skin and nerves
- Folate—formation of red blood cells
- Pantothenic acid—metabolism of food
- Riboflavin—body growth and production of red blood cells
- Thiamine—helps body cells change carbohydrates into energy

There are minerals that the body needs in larger amounts that include calcium, phosphorus, magnesium, sodium, potassium, chloride, and sulfur. Also, there are trace minerals found in smaller amounts that include iron, manganese, copper, iodine, zinc, cobalt, fluoride, and selenium.

 DISORDERS OF THE DIGESTIVE SYSTEM

The digestive system has many structures that can become diseased and not function properly. The organs can become infected, have structural problems, or malfunction due to dietary issues. We will examine some of the conditions that affect the digestive system including the accessory organs.

Mouth and Teeth

When there is a problem in the mouth with the soft tissue, gums, tongue, or the teeth, it may hinder our ability to eat certain foods, which might affect our intake of nutrition. When we have problems in this area, we avoid eating specific foods. For example, if there is a sore in the mouth, we usually avoid sour foods such as citrus, which will cause more pain or discomfort. If there are missing or decayed teeth (dental caries), we may avoid foods that require more chewing. Other conditions that affect the mouth are gingivitis, gum infection, and periodontitis, a more serious condition of gum disease that if untreated may lead to tooth loss. These conditions are treated with proper dental hygiene. A fungal infection that affects the mouth is caused by the yeast organism *Candida albicans*. It is commonly called **oral thrush** and might develop following antibiotic therapy killing normal bacteria found in the mouth. The normal bacteria prevent the growth of this fungus.

Parotitis is inflammation of the parotid glands located in the back of the mouth. Mumps is a viral, contagious infection of the parotid glands. When young males are affected during or after puberty, they are at risk of becoming sterile because this virus may attack the testicles.

Disorders of the Esophagus and Stomach

The esophagus and stomach are the next organs where food travels once it leaves the mouth. As the food enters the stomach, it passes through the esophageal sphincter. There are disorders that affect the area where these two organs join. The common disorders of these organs are:

- Hiatal hernia—weakened area of the diaphragm allowing the stomach to protrude upward causing the hernia; symptoms include pain following meals and frequent gastritis; surgical repair of the hernia may be needed. Figure 7-5 demonstrates a hiatal hernia.
- Gastric reflux—stomach acid flows back into the lower end of the esophagus; chronic reflux is called

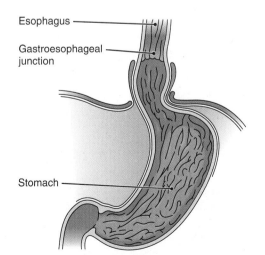

Esophagus
Gastroesophageal junction
Stomach

Figure 7-5 Hiatal hernia. A weakness in the diaphragm allows a portion of the stomach to protrude upward through that muscle. (Reprinted from Cohen BJ. *Memmler's The Human Body in Health and Disease.* 13th ed. Burlington, MA: Jones & Bartlett Learning, LLC; 2014.)

GERD, gastroesophageal reflux disease; treated with antacids and medication that decreases the production of hydrochloric acid in the stomach.
- **Gastritis**—any inflammation of the stomach lining that develops from numerous causes including bacteria, overuse of drugs like aspirin, and chronic use of alcohol and cigarette smoking.
- Stomach ulcer—erosion of the lining of the stomach typically due to chronic gastritis; *Helicobacter pylori* is the bacteria that reside in the mucous coating of the stomach and stimulates HCL production leading to the development of stomach ulcers; peptic ulcer is found in the esophagus and stomach or may develop in the duodenum and is then called a duodenal ulcer.
- Stomach cancer—develops in the lining of the stomach; adenocarcinoma is one type usually resulting from long history of indigestion, which is the most important warning sign of stomach cancer.

Nausea and vomiting are not diseases of the stomach however are symptoms associated with the disorders of the stomach. **Vomiting** is the process of expelling the stomach contents through the mouth. **Nausea** is a feeling of queasiness that usually precedes vomiting. Nausea and vomiting can be caused by stomach inflammation, motion sickness, medications (chemotherapy drugs), and pregnancy.

Intestinal and Abdominal Disorders

Beyond the stomach are the intestines, which also can develop diseases and conditions that may affect the further breakdown and absorption of the nutrients our body needs. Among these disorders are:

- Peritonitis—inflammation of the peritoneum, the lining of the abdomen and organs; may be localized or generalized; a ruptured appendix might cause generalized peritonitis.
- **Appendicitis**—inflammation of the appendix due to infection or obstruction; symptoms include nausea, vomiting, and localized pain in the right lower quadrant of the abdomen; treatment is to surgically remove the appendix (appendectomy).
- Inflammatory bowel disease (IBD)—generalized inflammation of the intestine causing pain, diarrhea, rectal bleeding, and occasionally weight loss; two types include:
  - Crohn disease—an autoimmune disease causing inflammation of the distal end of the small intestine
  - **Ulcerative colitis**—inflammation and ulceration of the colon and rectum
- Celiac disease—inability to tolerate gluten, protein found in wheat, rye, and barley; causes inflammation that damages or destroys the intestinal villi; symptoms similar to IBD and may include constipation and bloating after eating foods with gluten

- Irritable bowel syndrome (**IBS**)—GI disorder that causes constipation or diarrhea and pain; usually due to stress
- **Diverticulosis**—development of large numbers of diverticula, small pouches in the wall of the intestine; inflammation of these is called diverticulitis; may be caused from low fiber in the diet (Fig. 7-6)
- Intestinal obstruction—blockage of the intestine; may be caused from twisting of the intestine or from slipping of part of the intestine into an adjacent part of the intestine (intussusception)
- Hemorrhoids—varicose veins of the rectum; cause pain and bleeding
- Colon cancer—malignant tumor of the colon or rectum; may arise from benign polyps in the lining of the colon

Terms used to describe digestive disorders include enteritis, intestinal inflammation and gastroenteritis, and inflammation of both the stomach and intestines. These are general terms usually used to describe disorders until the actual or absolute cause can be determined. Diarrhea, frequent watery bowel movements, is usually one of the symptoms of inflammation. Diarrhea can be caused from contaminated food or water, viral and bacterial infections, and as a result of other diseases of the GI tract. The primary concern with diarrhea is the loss of fluid, which leads to dehydration. Physicians may request a stool specimen to aid in determining the cause of the diarrhea.

Constipation is also a symptom that accompanies some disorders. Constipation is caused by hard stools or difficulty moving the bowels. Certain medications may cause constipation as well as a decrease in the amount of fiber in the diet, which will help with regularity. Laxatives and enemas are used to soften and loosen the stool for elimination (defecation).

Endoscopy is the use of a lighted scope to visualize the gastrointestinal tract. Gastroscopy is used to examine the stomach, and colonoscopy is a procedure used to examine the colon. Prior to performing these exams, the physician may order an occult (hidden) blood test of the stool to determine if there is any blood in the stool that is not visible with the naked eye. A positive test indicates that there is a source of bleeding in the intestine that needs to be investigated.

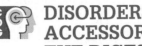 DISORDERS OF THE ACCESSORY ORGANS OF THE DIGESTIVE SYSTEM

We cannot overlook the disorders that affect the liver, gallbladder, and pancreas. When these organs are diseased or not functioning well, digestion and absorption can be affected.

The Liver

Cirrhosis of the liver is a chronic disease, commonly caused by excessive alcohol consumption. The disease causes the healthy liver cells to become inactive and replaced with scar tissue. When this occurs, the normal blood flow into the liver is obstructed causing accumulation of blood in other areas of the GI tract. Varicose veins develop due to the increased pressure within the vessels. These veins may rupture causing hemorrhage and possibly death from sudden bleeding.

Jaundice is a visible symptom of liver malfunction. Signs of this condition include a yellowish color to the white of the eyes and skin, and the stool will become pale, chalky in color due to lack of bilirubin. Figure 7-7 is a photo of a patient's eye showing the yellowish coloration to the sclera.

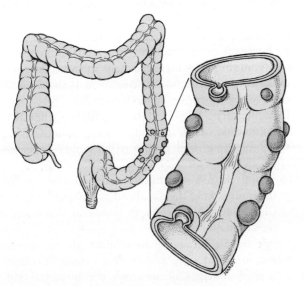

Figure 7-6 Diverticula of the colon. (Reprinted with permission from Neil Hardy, Westpoint, CT.)

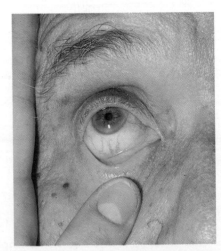

Figure 7-7 A patient with jaundice. (From Bickley LS, Szilagyi P. *Bates' Guide to Physical Examination and History Taking.* 8th ed. Philadelphia, PA: Lippincott Williams & Wilkins; 2003.)

Bilirubin is a byproduct of blood cell destruction, a function of the liver. Bilirubin is normally excreted in the bile. When the liver is not functioning properly, bilirubin may be blocked from reaching the bile ducts. Bilirubin levels in the blood will then be elevated.

Hepatitis is inflammation of the liver that may be caused by drugs, infection, or alcohol consumption. There are different types of hepatitis caused by a virus and named with the letter A through E.

- Hepatitis A (HAV)—transmitted through contaminated food and water and contact with fecal matter; food workers who do not use frequent, proper hand hygiene can spread hepatitis A through food preparation and service.
- Hepatitis B (**HBV**)—transmitted through blood or body fluids but may also be spread through fecal contamination; health care workers are usually required to have the hepatitis B vaccine to help prevent contracting the disease from contaminated needles and blood and body fluids.
- Hepatitis C (HCV)—primarily transmitted through infected blood; may also be through sexual transmission.
- Hepatitis D (HDV)—transmitted by direct blood exchange with those infected with hepatitis B.
- Hepatitis E (HEV)—transmitted by fecal contamination of water.

Most hepatitis patients recover well, but some forms of hepatitis may lead to liver cancer. Liver cancer may not originate in the liver but is the result of metastasis of cancer from another area of the body. For example, a patient may have pancreatic or intestinal cancer, which is the primary source. Cancer cells are carried to the liver through the blood.

The Gallbladder

The gallbladder stores bile until the body needs it for metabolism of fat. One of the more common conditions is that stones will form from the bile. This condition known as **cholelithiasis** will cause the development of stones that may become large enough to block the bile ducts. When this occurs, it may lead to inflammation of the gallbladder, cholecystitis. Surgery may be required to remove the stones or in some cases the entire gallbladder. The removal of the gallbladder is called **cholecystectomy**. Figure 7-8 is a photo of a gallbladder that was removed due to numerous gallstones.

The Pancreas

Pancreatitis is inflammation of the pancreas, which may be caused from a blockage in the pancreatic ducts that supply the pancreatic enzymes to the small intestine. The enzymes back up into the pancreas causing damage to

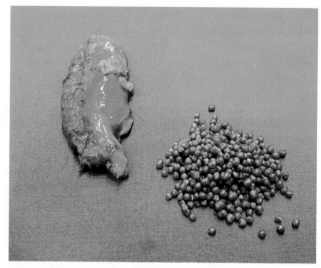

Figure 7-8 Gallstones from surgically removed gallbladder. (Image from Shutterstock.com.)

the pancreas. This will result in malabsorption of the nutrients in the small intestine that would have been broken down by the enzymes. Acute pancreatitis will usually have a short duration; however, if chronic, it is a risk factor for development of pancreatic cancer.

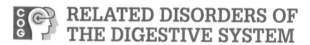

RELATED DISORDERS OF THE DIGESTIVE SYSTEM

There are other conditions not directly related to a specific organ of the digestive tract but may affect the body's nutrition and absorption of nutrients. Malnutrition simply means bad nutrition. Something is probably missing from the diet or is not able to be absorbed into the body. It could be caused from not eating enough or not eating the right foods that will supply the necessary nutrition to keep us healthy. Kwashiorkor is a condition when there is a serious shortage of protein in the diet and is frequently seen in impoverished areas of the world where the food supply is limited. Most significant visible symptom is the accumulation of fluid in the abdomen (ascites) causing it to bulge. In some countries where this is more prevalent, it is the primary cause of death for children under age five.

Weight control is a problem faced by many in countries where food is abundant and good food choices are replaced by processed foods that are high in fat and sugar. Overweight is also prevalent in persons who have a more sedentary lifestyles. Childhood obesity has been a concern for years with the increase in fast food available and decreased activity due to more technology engaging the children rather than physical activity. It is no surprise that there is also an increase in diseases involving the cardiovascular system and specific conditions such as diabetes. Figure 7-9 is the MyPyramid guide that

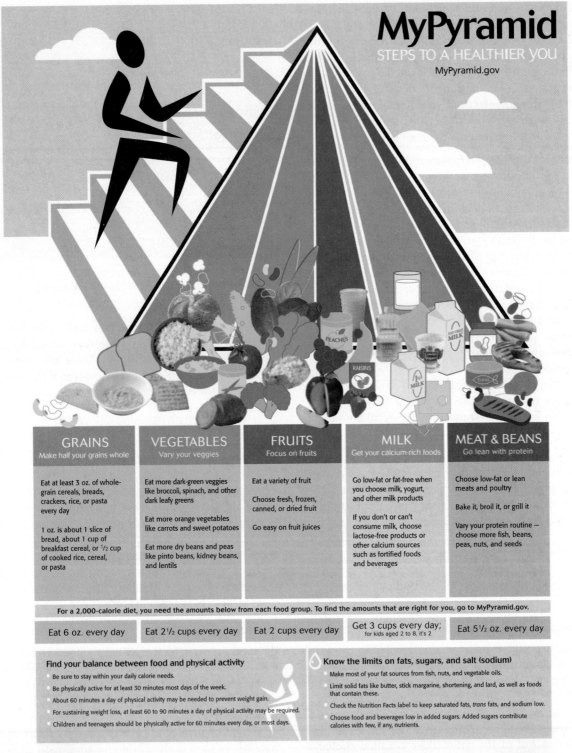

Figure 7-9 MyPyramid guide based on a 2,000-calorie diet. (Reprinted from Kronenberger J, Ledbetter J. *Jones & Bartlett Learning's Comprehensive Medical Assisting.* 5th ed. Burlington, MA: Jones & Bartlett Learning, LLC; 2016.)

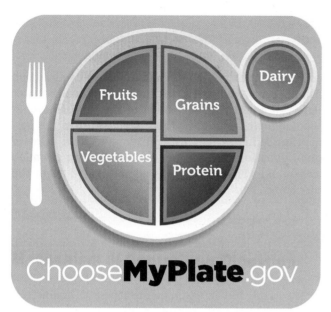

Figure 7-10   MyPlate icon. The plate shows the recommended proportion of each food category in the diet. (Reprinted from Kronenberger J, Ledbetter J. *Jones & Bartlett Learning's Comprehensive Medical Assisting*, 5th ed. Burlington, MA: Jones & Bartlett Learning, LLC; 2016.)

was developed by the U.S. Department of Agriculture. This image was established by the USDA in 2005 and serves as a guide to the proper nutrition we need in our diets.

In 2011, the USDA added ChooseMyPlate, which is easier to visualize and shows the distribution of the five food groups on a plate. See Figure 7-10, which is the image of ChooseMyPlate.

Cultural Connection

The American Indian community has a very high incidence of type 2 diabetes among its population. The Centers for Disease Control (CDC) stated that Native American youth ages 10 to 19 have a higher rate of developing diabetes than other ethnic and racial groups. There are reasons that contribute to this including the more sedentary lifestyle and poor diet decisions. The CDC partnered with Indian communities throughout the United States to set up projects encouraging these populations to reclaim their traditional foods and adopt the healthy lifestyle that includes increased physical activity. Traditionally, Native Americans grew an abundant supply of fresh vegetables and relied on the bounty of Mother Earth to sustain a healthy lifestyle. For more information about these projects, visit the CDC Web site and Native American Diabetic Projects.

Underweight may not be quite as common as overweight, but there are those who struggle gaining weight or maintaining a healthy weight for their stature. **Anorexia**, chronic loss of appetite, is the more common cause of underweight. Causes of anorexia may be physical or mental. Certain medications may cause a loss of appetite as well as acute illnesses like gastrointestinal infections. Anorexia nervosa is a psychological problem in which the person starves themselves. The person with this problem perceives that they are overweight and is attempting to lose weight through not eating. Bulimia is a similar problem as anorexia however the person eats food then forces vomiting to get the food out before it can be digested and absorbed. It is called a binge and purge syndrome. Anorexia and bulimia lead to many physical problems other than just weight loss. Over a long period of time, the person experiences muscle loss, cardiac irregularities, and erosion of the esophagus from the repeated vomiting. In serious cases, these disorders may lead to death.

Study Skill

To study the digestive system, it might be helpful to build a roadmap. Use a large sheet of paper, start at the mouth, and draw a highway the leads to the end of the digestive tract. For each structure along the road, build a city that lists the function of the organ or structure, how the structure contributes to the digestion of food, and what happens when it malfunctions. This exercise will give you a great visual to study from. Make it colorful and full of animation.

Case Question

Remember the case study patient, Mary Ann? Her mother is in the waiting room and Mary Ann is having her blood drawn for a complete metabolic panel. While she and Rosa are alone, she shares that she has been vomiting quite a bit lately and wants to know if this will cause any problems with her stomach. She said the doctor asked her if she if purposely vomiting. If you were the medical assistant how would you explain to her why the doctor was asking her that question?

BMI is the body mass index. It calculates the height and weight of an individual to determine the body fat. The standard says that an individual with <18.5 BMI is considered underweight and >30 BMI is overweight.

Food allergy is another related problem that can affect our nutrition. Some of the more common food allergies are related to wheat (gluten), shellfish, eggs, milk (lactose), and nuts (peanuts). An allergic reaction can cause symptoms like hives, wheezing, and GI discomfort. For those with more sensitivity to the allergen, anaphylactic shock may occur, which can lead to death.

Preparing for Externship

You should treat your externship as a job, but remember that you are still a student. The externship does not pay students for hours worked at the site. Some students adopt the attitude that if they are not paid they do not need to apply 100% of their effort each day. This is a negative approach to the externship. You should always strive to give your best in all you do. Think of the patients that you work with and the coworkers that rely on you. You need to be assertive asking what you can do to help everyone. Be prepared to be on your feet most of the time. Students who do not appear to be alert and busy give the perception of being lazy or uninterested. Ask a lot of good questions and be involved observing as much as you can. There is always something to do in the medical office.

Chapter Recap

- The digestive system includes the structures of the mouth, esophagus, stomach, small and large intestine, rectum, and anus.
- Accessory organs that support the digestive process include the liver, gallbladder, and pancreas.
- The digestive process requires substances to help breakdown the food into usable nutrients that can be absorbed into the bloodstream. These include saliva, hydrochloric acid, bile, and pancreatic enzymes.
- Minerals and vitamins are essential to the function of the body. Vitamins are primarily responsible for assisting in metabolism and the manufacture of red blood cells.
- Disorders and diseases of the digestive organs can affect the overall health of the body due to the inability of nutrients to get into the body cells. These include infections, organ malfunction and defects, and lack of enzyme secretion for the breakdown of nutrients for absorption.
- Protein, carbohydrates, and fats are necessary in the daily diet in order to provide the proper nutrition for healthy body cells. These nutrients are required for cell production and repair and energy for adequate functioning of the cells.

Online Resources for Students

Student Resources available on the text's online site include:
- Audio Glossaries
- Animations
- Competency Evaluation Forms
- Videos
- Anatomy & Physiology Module with Heart and Lung Sounds
- Weblinks
- Worksheets

Exercises and Activities

Certification Preparation Questions

1. Which of these is the substance produced in the stomach that breaks down protein and destroys foreign organisms?
   a. Vitamin K
   b. Chyme
   c. Hydrochloric acid
   d. Bile
   e. Pepsin

2. Which of these are the three sections of the small intestine in the order they are located?
   a. Duodenum, ileum, jejunum
   b. Ileum, sigmoid, jejunum
   c. Jejunum, duodenum, ileum
   d. Sigmoid, ileum, duodenum
   e. Duodenum, jejunum, ileum

3. The term used for the surgical removal of the gallbladder is:

    a. colectomy.
    b. colectomy.
    c. cholecystotomy.
    d. cholecystectomy.
    e. cholehepatectomy.

4. Which of these are fat-soluble vitamins?

    a. A, B, C
    b. B, C, D
    c. E, D, K
    d. B, C, E
    e. A, D, B

5. Which of these is a condition associated with excessive alcohol consumption and causes healthy liver cells to be replaced with scar tissue?

    a. Jaundice
    b. Cirrhosis
    c. Hepatitis A
    d. Hepatitis C
    e. Celiac disease

6. Which of these is a condition caused by inflammation of small pouches in the intestine?

    a. Crohn disease
    b. Celiac disease
    c. Cirrhosis
    d. Diverticulitis
    e. Peritonitis

7. A hiatal hernia is located

    a. At the junction of the small and large intestine
    b. Between the stomach and the pylorus
    c. At the distal end of the small intestine
    d. At the junction of the esophagus and stomach
    e. At the point where the descending colon becomes the sigmoid colon

8. Which of these statements describes cholelithiasis?

    a. It is inflammation of the gallbladder.
    b. It is the development of gallstones in the gallbladder.
    c. It is inflammation of the liver and gallbladder.
    d. It is blockage of the bile ducts leading from the liver to the gallbladder.
    e. It is the surgical removal of the gallbladder.

9. GERD is a condition that involves the:

    a. stomach and esophagus.
    b. stomach and pylorus.
    c. duodenum and pylorus.
    d. ileum and ascending colon.
    e. descending colon and sigmoid colon.

10. Mastication is a term meaning the process of:

    a. elimination of waste products from the body.
    b. changing food into chyme.
    c. chewing food into smaller pieces.
    d. moving digested food through the intestines.
    e. swallowing a bolus of food.

CareTracker Connection

Documenting Clinical Data and Ordering Laboratory Tests Related to the Digestive System and Nutrition

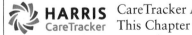 CareTracker Activities Related to This Chapter
- Case Study 8: Gerontology Patient Practicum

Although many factors that affect our health are beyond our control—such as genetics, age, race, and sociocultural values and norms—some can significantly influence in our day-to-day choices. One of the biggest health choices we make is what we put in our mouths. Many diseases and conditions, not just of the gastrointestinal system but of the body as a whole, are strongly associated with our diet. As a medical assistant, you will be responsible for gathering and entering much gastrointestinal- and nutrition-related patient information in the form

of complaints, signs and symptoms, history of disease, examination findings, laboratory and diagnostic test results, diagnoses, and treatments. CareTracker facilitates all of these tasks.

Tasks discussed in this chapter that can be performed in CareTracker include the following:

- Documenting the following patient clinical information related to gastrointestinal conditions and nutrition:
  - Health history
    - Diseases and conditions
    - Hospitalizations
    - Alcohol use
    - Caffeine use
    - Surgeries and procedures
    - Preventive care
    - Family history
  - Review of systems
  - Physical examination findings

- Tests and procedures completed during the visit
  - Lipid panel
  - Fecal occult blood
- Diagnoses
- Treatment plan
  - BMI follow-up plan documented
  - Nutrition counseling
  - Dietary consultation order
  - Colonoscopy
  - Air contrast barium enema
  - Sigmoidoscopy
  - Fecal analysis
  - High fiber
  - Healthy diet
  - Low cholesterol
  - Lose weight
  - Junk-free
  - Gain weight
- Ordering the following related to gastrointestinal conditions and nutrition:
  - Medications
  - Laboratory tests
  - Diagnostic tests

Many of these tasks are discussed in CareTracker Connection features in other chapters. A task we'll consider here is ordering a laboratory test.

Once the primary care provider has finished examining the patient and diagnosed any conditions present, he or she may ask you, the medical assistant, to enter a medication prescription or order a laboratory or diagnostic test related to the diagnosis. To order a laboratory test, you first click on the ⚕ icon in the Clinical Toolbar near the top of the screen in the Medical Record (either from the main screen or from within the Progress Note).

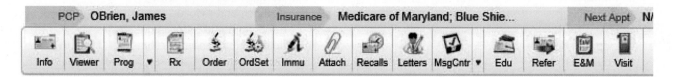

Alternatively, you may click on the ⚕ icon at the bottom of the PLAN tab in the Progress Note.

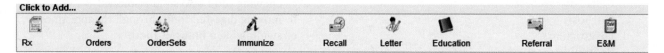

Within the Order window, you may select Lab as the Order Type. The ordering physician and facility may be selected from drop-down menus in these fields, as can the diagnosis associated with the test being ordered. In the example below, for instance, the order for a comprehensive metabolic panel (CMP) is related to the patient's diagnosis of acute intestinal obstruction. The due date, collection date and time, requested time of day to receive the test results, and the frequency of the test may also be selected. The test itself may be selected from the list of preloaded tests or searched for in CareTracker's database of tests using the search field. The selected test or tests appear in the Tests Summary field below. The urgency and fasting status can be entered to the right. Below is an example of a completed order for a laboratory test.

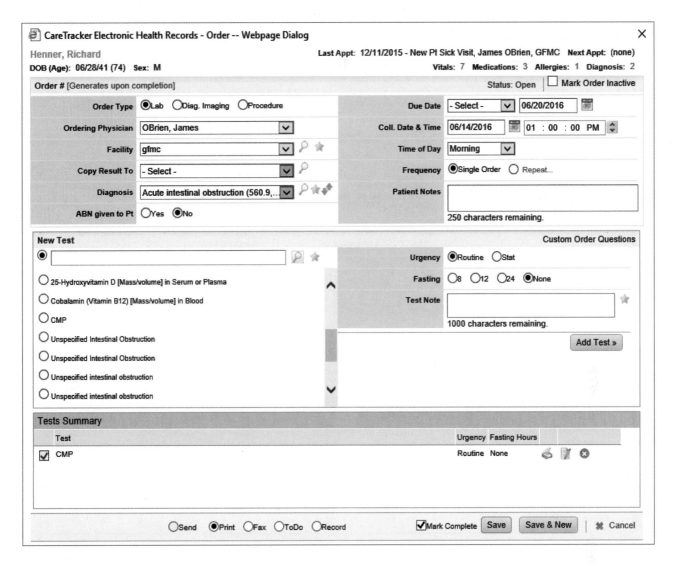

Once you have completed the order, click on Save, and a printable copy of the order will appear.

https://training.caretracker.com/CT_NET/CL/PrintLabOrder.aspx?PatientID=43979167&orderID=...   —   ☐   ✕

https://training.caretracker.com/CT_NET/CL/PrintLabOrder.aspx?PatientID=43979167&orderID=1094583&returnvalue=08

Order #1094583   Order Date 6/14/2016 | Due Date 6/20/2016

Patient Name	Pt ID	Gender	DOB	Address	Phone	Insurance	Subscriber #	Policy Holder
Henner, Richard ,43979167	2389 Jingle Bell Ct., Beltsville, MD 20705	Medicare of Maryland	789456126	
Male, 6/28/1941	(301) 598-2229	Richard Henner
		Blue Shield of National Capital Area	
		B687532	Richard Henner

Facility	Send Copy of Results to	Diagnosis
gfmc		(560.9)
ｧ , ｨ		
Ordering Physician		**Patient Notes**
James OBrien, MD, NPI: 0000000006		
127 Broad Street, Great Falls, VA 22066		
Ph: (703) 555-6121, Fax: (703) 555-6123		**Collection Time of Day**
		Morning

Physicians and non-physician practitioners should only order those laboratory tests that are medically necessary for the diagnosis or treatment of a patient. Before ordering tests, please consider carefully whether the tests are justified and justifiable for the diagnosis or treatment of the specific patient. Please note that Medicare generally does not cover routine screening tests.

Tests Ordered

#	Test	Test #	Urgency	Test Notes	Ask On Order Entry
1	CMP		Routine		

James OBrien, MD
Ordering Physician

Internet Resources

<u>www.choosemyplate.gov</u> U.S. Department of Agriculture—investigate this Web site for additional information on nutrition and dietary plans.

<u>www.cdc.gov</u> Center for Disease Control, Native American Diabetic Projects—access this site for additional information on the federal diabetic programs established for Native Americans.

8 Cardiovascular and Respiratory Systems

Chapter Objectives

- Describe the function of the cardiovascular system.
- Describe the chambers of the heart and their function.
- Describe the location and function of the valves of the heart.
- Describe the three tissue layers of the heart wall.
- List the structures of the vascular system.
- Briefly describe blood circulation through the myocardium.
- Describe the cardiac cycle.
- Name and locate the components of the heart's conduction system.
- Define common terms that describe variations in heart rates.
- Identify common types of heart disease.
- List risk factors for coronary artery disease.
- List common diagnostic exams used to detect cardiovascular disorders.
- Describe common approaches to the treatment of heart disease.
- List the different types of blood vessels.
- List common disorders of the circulatory system.
- Explain the process of respiration and the factors that control respiration.
- Name and describe all the structures of the respiratory system.
- Discuss the processes of internal and external gas exchange.
- Explain the process for the transportation of oxygen and carbon dioxide in the blood.
- List common types of respiratory disorders.
- List the common procedures and treatments used for respiratory diseases.

CAAHEP & ABHES Competencies

CAAHEP

- Describe structural organization of the human body.
- Identify body systems.
- List major organs in each body system.
- Describe the normal function of each body system.
- Identify common pathology related to each body system including signs, symptoms, and etiology.
- Analyze pathology for each body system including diagnostic measures and treatment modalities.

ABHES

- List all body systems, their structure, and functions.
- Describe common diseases, symptoms, and etiologies as they apply to each system.
- Identify diagnostic and treatment modalities as they relate to each body system.

Chapter Terms

Aneurysm	Catheterization	Hypertension	Pericardium
Apex	Coronary angiography	Hypotension	Plaque
Arrhythmia	Coronary	Ischemia	–pnea
Arteriosclerosis	Deoxygenated	Mediastinum	Semilunar valve
Atherosclerosis	Diastole	Murmur	Sinus rhythm
Atrioventricular valve	Dysrhythmia	Myocarditis	Spirometer
Bradycardia	Endocardium	Myocardium	Stenosis
Bronchodilators	Effusion	Necrosis	Systole
Bronchoscope	Epicarditis	Oxygenated	Tachycardia
Carbaminohemoglobin	Epicardium	Oxyhemoglobin	Thrombosis
Cardiologist	Epistaxis	Pericarditis	

Abbreviations

ARDS	CO_2	NSR	PVC
AV	CPR	O_2	RSV
bpm	CT	PAC	SA
CABG	ECG/EKG	PAT	TB
COPD	MI	PTCA	URI

Case Study

Mr. Hoffman is a 54-year-old patient who arrives at Dr. Ashton's office because he has been short of breath, quite fatigued, and experiencing dizziness. As the receptionist is checking in Mr. Hoffman, she notices that he is holding his chest and is sweating. She immediately calls for Dr. Ashton's medi-

cal assistant, Carlos, to escort Mr. Hoffman to an examination room. Once in the exam room, Carlos obtains a pulse, respiration, and blood pressure on Mr. Hoffman, which are P 100, R 22, and BP 160/94.

Carlos immediately notifies Dr. Ashton of Mr. Hoffman's vital signs and condition.

In this chapter, we will explore the cardiovascular and respiratory systems. The heart and lungs work together in concert to keep the blood flowing through the body carrying oxygen to the body cells and removing carbon dioxide.

 ## THE CARDIOVASCULAR SYSTEM

The cardiovascular system includes the heart and the blood vessels. The heart pumps the blood, which travels through the blood vessels. One of the main functions of the blood is to carry oxygen to the body cells and return carbon dioxide to the lungs to be exhaled by the body. The system of blood vessels is also referred to as the circulatory system since their function is to provide circulation throughout the body. It is a one-way system with the blood traveling only in one direction.

 ## THE HEART

The heart begins beating when the fetus is developing in the womb and stops when we die. During that time, it beats continuously approximately 70 to 80 beats per minute. The rate can increase or decrease depending on the body's need for additional oxygen and nutrients. As you start to explore the structures of the heart, refer to

Case Question

 If you are Dr. Ashton's medical assistant, how would you reassure Mr. Hoffman if he is extremely worried about his condition?

Figure 8-1, which shows the heart and major blood vessels leading in and out of the heart. Notice the right side is blue and the left side red indicating oxygen-rich blood flows through this side.

Heart Structure

The adult heart is approximately the size of a fist. It is located slightly to the left of the midline of the body in the **mediastinum**, which is in the central area of the chest cavity. The lower, rounded area of the heart is called the **apex**. The heart is a hollow organ with three layers:

- **Endocardium**—the innermost lining of the heart covering the inside of the heart chambers and heart valves
- **Myocardium**—the muscular layer of the heart (cardiac muscle)
- **Epicardium**—the outermost layer, which also serves as the visceral (organ) layer of the pericardium

Chambers of the Heart

The heart is a double-sided pump receiving deoxygenated blood from the body into the right side and pumping oxygenated blood back out to the body from the left side. **Oxygenated** blood is blood that is rich in oxygen,

and **deoxygenated** blood has less oxygen and will return to the lungs to pick up more oxygen. The heart is divided into four chambers with each one having a function in the circulation of blood through the heart. The chambers include the following:

- Right atrium—upper chamber that receives deoxygenated blood from body
- Right ventricle—lower chamber that receives blood from the right atrium and pumps it to the lungs
- Left atrium—upper chamber that receives oxygenated blood from the lungs
- Left ventricle—lower chamber that receives blood from the left atrium and pumps it out to the body

The right and left chambers are separated by a wall called the septum. Specifically, the interatrial septum separates the atria and the interventricular septum separates the ventricles. The walls are primarily made up of myocardium, heart muscle.

Heart Valves

The function of the heart valves is to ensure that blood continues to flow in one direction and not backflow. The heart valves separating the atria and ventricles are called the **atrioventricular valves** (**AV**). The valves that allow

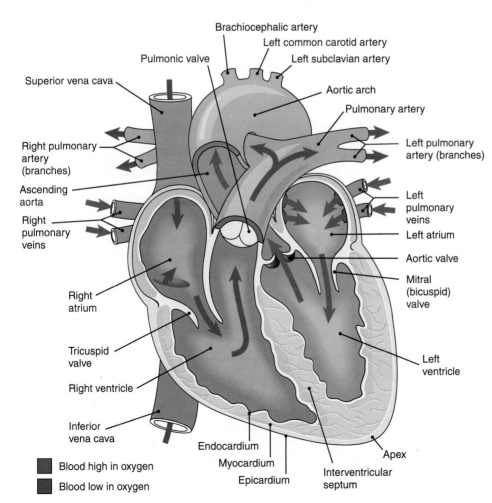

Figure 8-1 Heart and blood vessels. The right heart has blood low in oxygen; the left heart has blood high in oxygen. The *arrows* show the direction of blood flow through the heart. (Reprinted from Cohen BJ. *Memmler's The Human Body in Health and Disease.* 13th ed. Burlington, MA: Jones & Bartlett Learning, LLC; 2014.)

blood to exit the heart into major blood vessels are called **semilunar valves** because they resemble a half-moon shape. Each valve is named separately.

- Tricuspid valve—has three (tri) cusps or flaps, also called the right atrioventricular valve (AV) allowing blood flow from the right atrium into the right ventricle
- Mitral valve—has two cusps, also called the bicuspid valve and left atrioventricular valve (AV) allowing blood to flow from the left atrium into the left ventricle
- Pulmonary valve—a semilunar valve that allows blood flow from the right ventricle into the pulmonary blood vessels leading to the lungs
- Aortic valve—a semilunar valve that allows blood flow from the left ventricle to the aorta then to the body

The Pericardium

The heart is enclosed in a fibrous sac called the **pericardium**. It has two serous layers, the parietal layer that lines the pericardial sac and a visceral layer (epicardium) that adheres to the surface of the heart. Pericardial fluid is found between the outer fibrous sac and the serous lining. This fluid acts as a lubricant allowing the heart to move freely with each beat, reducing friction.

The Myocardium

Now that we have an overview of the heart structures, let's go back and focus on the heart muscle, the myocardium. Cardiac muscle is involuntary; it contracts without conscious thought. The muscle cells are tightly joined with adjacent cells with specialized membrane proteins. These allow the electrical impulses to travel between the cells. These impulses are required for the heart to be stimulated to beat.

Myocardium Blood Supply

The blood flowing through the heart does not provide the oxygen and nutrient to the myocardium. The myocardium has its own blood vessels, the coronary blood vessels. The term **coronary** comes from the word crown, which is how the vessels encircle the heart. The coronary vessels branch off of the aorta as it exits the heart carrying oxygenated blood to the body.

Heart Function

The heart is the pump that keeps the blood flowing throughout the body. The chambers of the heart contract and relax. When the upper chambers, the atria, are contracting, the lower chambers, the ventricles, are relaxing. The active, contracting phase is called **systole**, and the resting, relaxing phase is known as **diastole**. Each heartbeat consists of a systole and diastole. This is referred to

as a cardiac cycle. As the atria relax, blood is allowed to fill the atria. This happens when the ventricles are contracting to empty the blood in preparation of receiving blood from the atria on the next beat. Cardiac output is the amount of blood pumped by each ventricle in 1 minute. During exercise, the cardiac output increases as much as two to four times greater than at rest.

The Conduction System of the Heart

As mentioned earlier, the heart muscle functions by electrical stimulation that travels from cell to cell. The heart muscle has structures called nodes that generate the electrical activity. The nodes conduct the electricity throughout the heart muscle causing contraction. Figure 8-2 shows the components of the conduction system of the heart.

The structures of the conduction system include the following:

- Sinoatrial (**SA**) node—located in the upper wall of the right atrium; called the pacemaker of the heart because it sets the rate of heart contractions
- Atrioventricular (**AV**) node—located in the septum between the atria at the bottom of the right atrium
- Atrioventricular (AV) bundle—also called the bundle of His, is located at the top of the septum between the ventricles
- Right and left bundle branches—fibers imbedded down both sides of the septum between the ventricles
- Purkinje fibers—network of fibers that branch throughout the myocardium

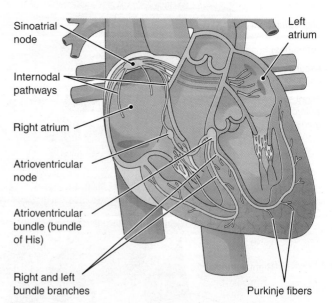

Sinoatrial node

Internodal pathways

Right atrium

Atrioventricular node

Atrioventricular bundle (bundle of His)

Right and left bundle branches

Left atrium

Purkinje fibers

Figure 8-2 Electrical conduction of the heart. (Reprinted from Cohen BJ. *Memmler's The Human Body in Health and Disease.* 13th ed. Burlington, MA: Jones & Bartlett Learning, LLC; 2014.)

A heartbeat starts with the SA node generating an electrical impulse, which travels to the AV node and then to the bundle of His. The impulse travels down the right and left bundle branches and then to the Purkinje fibers initiating the contraction of the heart. A normal heart rhythm is called **sinus rhythm**. There are many factors that can affect the heart's rate. The nervous system responds to changes in the body, which may affect the heart rate. For example, stress and excitement will cause an increase in the heart rate, and when the body is at rest, the heart rate will be lower. Terms used to describe variations in heart rate are as follows:

- **Bradycardia**—slow heart rate of <60 beats per minute (**bpm**) but usually will not drop below 50 bpm.
- **Tachycardia**—rapid heart rate of more than 100 bpm, which is normal during exercise.
- Sinus arrhythmia—a variable heart rate due to changes in the rate and depth of respirations, which is considered a normal occurrence.
- Premature ventricular contraction (PVC)—a ventricular contraction that starts with the Purkinje fibers rather than the SA node. It is felt as a palpitation or skipped beat, which might be caused by caffeine or stress.

Diagnostic Heart Exams

In order to determine the health of the heart, the physician begins by listening to the heart sounds and rhythm with a stethoscope. In addition to heart rate variables, there may be abnormal heart sounds. One of the abnormal sounds is a **murmur** caused by a faulty heart valve that fails to close tightly and blood leaks back. Another sound is caused from a narrowing of the valve opening called a **stenosis**.

Electrocardiograph (ECG or EKG)

The ECG is used to record the electrical activity of the heart. This procedure is discussed in the chapter on Diagnostic Testing. The ECG traces the activity of the heart indicating any myocardial problems that might affect the conduction and cardiac cycle of the heart. The procedure utilizes sensors or electrodes placed on the patient's skin on the arms, legs, and specific locations on the chest. The electrical activity is picked up by the sensors, sent to the electrocardiograph machine, and shows as waves on the ECG tracing. The waves are identified by the letters P, Q, R, S, T, and U. Each heartbeat is represented by a complex of these letters, which correspond to a specific function of the heart including the following:

- P wave—this wave represents the contraction of the atria, depolarization.
- P-R interval—the electrical activity of the atria as they pump out blood.

- R wave—measures electrical activity through the left ventricle of the heart.
- QRS complex—electrical activity of the ventricles as they pump out blood to the body.
- S-T segment—time period between the end of the contraction of the ventricles and the beginning of the period when the ventricles are resting.
- T wave—the resting period of the heart before the next cardiac cycle begins.
- U wave—extra wave sometimes seen after the T wave in someone whose heart has a slow recovery time possibly due to low potassium level or other metabolic problem.

A **cardiologist**, a heart specialist, uses the ECG to monitor changes in the waves and intervals to determine heart injury and arrhythmias.

Invasive Cardiac Procedures

When it is determined that a patient has heart disease or injury, there are procedures that might be performed to identify the location and extent of the damage. Some procedures are also used to identify and prevent heart disease. Heart **catheterization** is an invasive procedure used to diagnose or treat conditions affecting circulation in the coronary arteries. A catheter, a flexible tube, is inserted into a blood vessel either in the arm or in the groin. The catheter is guided to the heart while a fluoroscope, an instrument for examining using x-rays, shows the path of the catheter and any abnormalities. Blood samples and pressure measurements can be obtained during this procedure.

When indicated, **coronary angiography** may also be performed during catheterization. A dye is injected into the coronary arteries to highlight any vessel damage or blockage. Computerized tomography (CT) may also be used to visualize the coronary arteries.

Ultrasound, high-frequency sound waves, can also be used to detect abnormalities in the heart and vessels. The sound waves are emitted from the ultrasound device and are directed at the heart. As the sound wave echoes bounce off the heart structures, the echoes are traced on an electronic instrument and recorded on film. This procedure called echocardiography provides an immediate view of the heart activity. It is a noninvasive procedure but allows the examiner to witness the actual function of the heart.

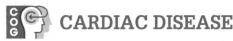 **CARDIAC DISEASE**

Heart and circulatory diseases cause damage to the heart structures and blood vessels. This includes structural defects, inflammation, valve malfunctions, and abnormal rhythms.

Heart Inflammation

As with other structures and organs of the body, the heart can become inflamed and infected. Heart inflammation can be caused by bacteria, viruses, autoimmune diseases, and toxins. Specific medical terms are used to describe the location of the inflammation. When the three layers of the heart are involved, the terms include the following:

- **Pericarditis**—inflammation of the sac around the heart
- **Myocarditis**—inflammation of the heart muscle, which could lead to **necrosis** (death of tissue) of the area of heart muscle affected
- **Endocarditis**—inflammation of the lining of the heart, which may involve the valves since they are covered by the endocardium

Rhythm Abnormalities of the Heart

Arrhythmia, also called **dysrhythmia**, is the term used to describe an abnormal heart rhythm. An arrhythmia is caused by a dysfunction within the conduction system of the heart. Two main types of arrhythmia include a flutter, which is an extremely fast heartbeat that may be up to 300 times a minute. The rate is fast, but the contractions are coordinated, not erratic. Fibrillation describes a very rapid rate; however, the contractions are uncoordinated. Fibrillation may involve the upper chambers, the atria or the lower chambers, the ventricles, or both. Although atrial fibrillation is a problem, the ventricles are responsible for the forceful systole of the heart so ventricular fibrillation is a more serious condition. A defibrillator is used to correct fibrillation. It is a device that delivers a very strong electrical current to convert the fibrillation into a normal rhythm. You may have seen one of these devices in public areas for use in case of emergency. Physician offices have a defibrillator on the office crash cart.

Heart block is a condition when there is an interruption of the electrical impulse. The normal pacemaker of the heart, the SA node, may be defective and unable to generate a normal impulse. Heart block may be caused from damage to the heart muscle due to prior infections, heart attack, and the aging process. Table 8-1 lists the types of arrhythmias, symptoms, and possible causes.

Congenital Heart Disease

Conditions that are present at birth are termed congenital and may be the result of defects developing while the fetus is growing in the womb. As the heart and blood

Table 8-1 Heart Arrhythmias

Type of Arrhythmia	Indications and Symptoms	Possible Causes and Consequences
Sinus tachycardia	Abnormally rapid heartbeat (100–180 bpm) resulting in decreased ventricular filling and low blood pressure	Dehydration, extreme anxiety, heart failure, or hemorrhage can also result from intense exercise
Sinus bradycardia	Abnormally slow heartbeat (<60 bpm), but with a normal rhythm	Can result from myocardial infarction or certain medications (such as digoxin); is also often seen in well-conditioned athletes
Paroxysmal atrial tachycardia (**PAT**)	Sudden, temporary onset of a heartbeat of 180–250 bpm, often accompanied by patient weakness and the feeling of a pounding or fluttering in the chest	Extreme anxiety or stress, excessive stimulants (such as nicotine or caffeine); also can have no known cause
Premature atrial contraction (**PAC**)	An electrical impulse starts in the heart before the next expected beat; patient may complain of feeling an "extra" or "skipped" beat	Thyroid disease, heart disease, central nervous system imbalances, stress, or excessive use of stimulants
Premature ventricular contraction (**PVC**)	Ventricles contract before the next expected beat; patient may complain of feeling an "extra" or "skipped" beat; can be more serious than PAC	Electrolyte imbalances, caffeine or other stimulants, anxiety or stress; may also be a sign of pulmonary disease or an injured or diseased heart
Ventricular tachycardia (V tach)	Heart rate exceeds 100 bpm with 3 or more PVCs per minute; results in decreased cardiac output; patient may complain of pressure and the feeling that the heart is "beating out of my chest"	Similar to causes of PVCs; the longer V tach lasts, the more serious it is because cardiac output drops and the blood supply to organs is decreased; unchecked V tach can lead to V fibrillation
Ventricular fibrillation (V fib)	Ventricles begin twitching, making the heart's pumping action ineffective and stopping the circulation of blood	The most serious of all arrhythmias; death will result if not immediately treated with CPR, a defibrillator, or cardiac drugs

vessels are being formed, there are some defects that may result in malfunction of the structures. Some of the congenital conditions include:

- Foramen ovale—small hole in the interatrial septum allowing blood to flow directly from the right atrium into the left atrium before it has traveled to the lungs to pick up oxygen (hole in the heart).
- Ductus arteriosus—which by the name means a duct (blood vessel) between arteries that connects the pulmonary artery and the aorta; instead of blood leaving the heart in the pulmonary artery going to the lungs for oxygenation, blood flows into the aorta.
- Ventricular septal defect—opening in the interventricular septum allowing blood to flow from the left side of the heart into the right side.
- Coarctation of the aorta—the aortic arch is narrowed restricting blood flow out of the heart.
- Tetralogy of Fallot—a combination of defects that includes pulmonary artery stenosis (narrowing), interventricular septal defect, aortic displacement to the right, and right ventricular hypertrophy (overdevelopment, increased size); commonly called a "blue baby" due to severe cyanosis (lack of oxygen).

Most of the congenital defects correct on their own, or heart surgery is indicated for more serious conditions.

Heart Conditions and Disorders

There are numerous heart diseases, conditions, and disorders that affect the structures of the heart causing malfunctions.

Valve Malfunction

As discussed earlier, the valves in the heart have one function, which is to keep the blood flowing in one direction.

Valves can narrow reducing the amount of blood flow to the next chamber or vessel. This condition is called valvular stenosis. A valve may not close properly allowing backflow of blood. This condition is referred to as valvular insufficiency. Valves can become damaged and ineffective due to inflammation and infections that attack the heart's endocardial layer. Rheumatic heart disease results from a streptococcal infection, rheumatic fever. The mitral valve is the most commonly affected valve due to this infection. The valve loses some of the flexibility and thickens not allowing it to open and close properly.

Coronary Artery Disease

The coronary arteries are the vessels that supply the heart muscle with their blood supply. When they become diseased, the blood flow to the myocardium is affected. **Atherosclerosis** is a condition caused by a buildup of **plaque** (fatty deposits). The space inside the vessels becomes narrow leading to decreased blood flow. The lack of blood supply is called **ischemia**. The inside of the vessel becomes rough causing a higher risk for blood clot formation, **thrombosis**. Figure 8-3 shows how the coronary vessel becomes affected with atherosclerosis.

Angina pectoris can also be caused from coronary artery disease. The patient experiences chest pain that may radiate into the jaw, neck, and upper back. It is frequently confused with heartburn. Medication (nitroglycerin) is used to help open the vessels allowing better blood flow.

Myocardial Infarction

Commonly known as a heart attack, myocardial infarction (**MI**) is caused from obstruction of blood flow to the myocardium. The portion of the heart that does

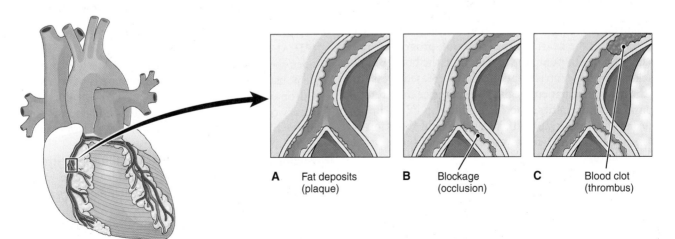

| A | Fat deposits (plaque) | B | Blockage (occlusion) | C | Blood clot (thrombus) |

Figure 8-3 Coronary atherosclerosis. **A.** Fat deposits (plaque) narrow an artery, leading to ischemia (lack of blood supply). **B.** Plaque causes blockage (occlusion) of a vessel. **C.** Formation of a blood clot (thrombus) in a vessel leads to myocardial infarction (MI). (Reprinted from Cohen BJ. *Memmler's The Human Body in Health and Disease.* 13th ed. Burlington, MA: Jones & Bartlett Learning, LLC, 2014.)

not receive blood will begin the process of necrosis (tissue death). It is critical that the patient recognize the signs and symptoms and seek immediate attention. If untreated, many people die from heart attack within the first hour from the onset of symptoms. Symptoms of MI can include the sudden onset of chest pain, radiating pain to the left arm and jaw, shortness of breath, sweating, nausea, and anxiousness. The heart's electrical activity is also affected, causing it to stop beating. At this point, **CPR** (cardiopulmonary resuscitation) is indicated. Defibrillation may also be indicated. Drugs are also administered to dissolve the clots.

Case Questions

 Let's see how Mr. Hoffman is doing. He is lying on the examination table and appears to be a little more comfortable. After Dr. Ashton examined him, he asked Carlos, the medical assistant, to give Mr. Hoffman nitroglycerin and to do an electrocardiogram. The ECG shows that Mr. Hoffman still has tachycardia, but his ECG shows that his heart is in normal sinus rhythm (**NSR**). Mr. Hoffman says he is feeling much better. Dr. Ashton asks Carlos to set up an appointment for Mr. Hoffman to see the cardiologist who has a practice in the same medical building. Why do you think the physician wants Mr. Hoffman to see the cardiologist?

What examinations will the cardiologist probably perform on Mr. Hoffman?

Heart Failure

This condition occurs when the heart cannot pump efficiently and it is failing. It may occur from disorders such as damage to the heart and valve malfunction, which put stress on the heart. As the condition progresses, the heart is unable to pump the blood out to the body. Blood backs up in the ventricles and causes increased pressure in the heart. The patient begins to experience fluid retention in the extremities, and fluid builds up in the lungs causing shortness of breath. When the fluid retention is present, physicians refer to the condition as congestive heart failure.

 ## TREATING HEART DISEASE

When patients are diagnosed with heart conditions and disease, the primary care physician will often refer the patient to a cardiologist, heart specialist, for a full evaluation, treatment, and monitoring of the condition.

Heart Medications

Patients with heart disease typically require medication to help strengthen the heart, decrease fluid retention, lower blood pressure, and lower cholesterol. These are some of the medications used to treat heart conditions:

- Statin drugs—lower cholesterol and inhibit the liver manufacture of cholesterol
- Anticoagulants—prevent clot formation; aspirin may be used on a daily basis when recommended by the physician
- Digitalis—strengthens heart muscle contractions
- Beta-blockers—reduce the rate and strength of heart contractions
- Antiarrhythmic agents—regulate the rate and rhythm of the heartbeat
- Calcium-channel blockers—dilate vessels and control the force of heart contractions
- Thrombolytics—dissolve blood clots (thrombus)

Pacemakers

The SA node is the pacemaker of the heart generating the heartbeats and keeping them regular and normal. When the SA node fails, a mechanical device, an artificial pacemaker, is implanted to take over this function. The pacemaker is an electric, battery-operated device that supplies impulses to the heart. The device is implanted under the skin in the upper left side of the chest. A wire from the pacemaker is placed in the heart muscle.

Heart Surgery

In some cases, it might be necessary to correct heart problems with surgery. Patients may be placed on a heart–lung machine during surgery allowing the blood to bypass the heart yet still be circulated to the body supplying oxygen. Types of heart surgery include the following:

- Percutaneous transluminal coronary angioplasty (**PTCA**)—catheter with balloon inserted into a vessel to open the lumen of an atherosclerotic vessel. Figure 8-4 demonstrates how the PTCA procedure is performed.
- Coronary artery bypass graft (**CABG**)—healthy segments of blood vessels are used to bypass coronary artery obstructions, and a section of vein from the leg is usually used.
- Angioplasty—a balloon is inserted into the restricted artery and inflated increasing the size of the lumen (inside opening) of the artery, which increases blood flow through the artery.
- Stent—a small tube inserted in the blood vessel to keep it open.
- Coronary atherectomy—removal of plaque from the walls of the coronary arteries.
- Heart transplant—surgical replacement of the heart and sometimes the lungs using a compatible donated heart.

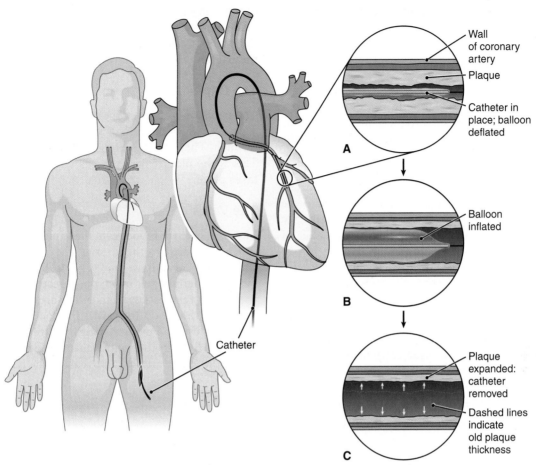

Figure 8-4 Coronary angioplasty. **A.** A guide catheter is threaded into the coronary artery. **B.** A balloon catheter is inserted through the occlusion and inflated. **C.** The balloon is inflated and deflated until plaque is flattened and the vessel is opened. (Reprinted from Cohen BJ. *Memmler's The Human Body in Health and Disease*. 13th ed. Burlington, MA: Jones & Bartlett Learning, LLC, 2014.)

Obviously, the best way to avoid these heart surgeries is to keep your heart healthy. There are some risk factors for heart disease that cannot be managed that include age, gender, heredity, and body type. There are many things that we can change or modify to help avoid the risk of heart disease. These include not smoking, maintaining physical activity, managing weight control, and watching the diet. Diets should be lower in saturated fats and sodium. Diseases such as hypertension and diabetes also may put someone at a greater risk to develop heart disease.

THE CIRCULATORY SYSTEM

Now that we have examined the heart, its function, and disorders, let's take a look at the blood vessels that carry the blood throughout the body. The blood vessels include the following:

- Arteries—carry blood away from the heart
- Arterioles—smaller divisions of the arteries

- Capillaries—smallest vessels and the place where the exchange of gasses and nutrients takes place, connect the arterioles and the venules
- Venules—smaller divisions of the veins
- Veins—carry blood back to the heart from the venules

There are two subdivisions of the circulatory system, one that delivers blood to the lungs, the pulmonary circuit, and the systemic circuit that carries blood to the rest of the body tissues.

Pulmonary Circuit

This circulatory system delivers blood to the lungs to become oxygenated and leave some carbon dioxide, which will be eliminated from the body through respirations. Blood that has returned to the heart from the body is low in oxygen and will leave the right ventricle to be transported to the lungs in the pulmonary arteries. This is the only place where arteries that always carry blood away from the heart are carrying deoxygenated blood. In the lungs, the gas exchange takes place and the blood returns to the heart in the pulmonary veins, the only veins in the body that carry oxygenated blood.

Systemic Circuit

This subdivision of the circulatory system supplies oxygen and nutrients to the body tissues and carries carbon dioxide and waste products away from the tissues. Blood leaves the heart in the largest artery, the aorta. It travels throughout the body from the arteries to the arterioles, through the capillaries, into the venules and then the veins. Blood finally returns to the heart in the superior vena cava, from the upper body, and the inferior vena cava from the lower part of the body. See Figure 8-5, which shows the how the closed circuit of the cardiovascular system keeps blood flowing in one direction. You can also see how the oxygenated blood is supplied by the lungs and sent to the body to give up the oxygen, becoming deoxygenated blood.

The Arteries

The arteries have thicker walls to carry the blood under greater pressure as it leaves the heart and starts the process of circulation. The walls of the arteries are elastic making them easier to enlarge to accommodate the changes in pressure. The middle layer of the arteries is made up of smooth muscle, which is involuntary, working without conscious control. The blood flows from the arteries into the arterioles and then to the capillaries.

The Capillaries

The capillaries connect the arterioles and the venules. They are only wide enough for a single blood cell to pass through. They are the thinnest with only one cell layer. This is the place where the gas and nutrient exchange takes place.

The Veins

The venules carry blood from the capillaries to the veins. When compared to the arteries, the veins have thinner walls. They also have one-way valves only allowing blood to continue to flow in one direction. The pressure within the veins is less than in the arteries. The valves help push the blood forward so it does not flow back. Table 8-2 lists the major arteries and veins of the body and Table 8-3 lists the major veins. See Figure 8-6, which shows the major arteries and veins of the body.

Blood Flow

The blood vessels are able to change their internal diameter to regulate the blood flow. Vasodilation is the increase in the diameter allowing more blood to flow through, and vasoconstriction is a decrease in the diameter causing the blood flow to decrease. These changes are regulated by the autonomic nervous system from signals sent by the medulla of the brainstem. When the blood leaves the heart in the arteries, it is pushed through the circulatory system under greater pressure than the amount found in the veins. The veins need help pushing the blood through the system back to the heart. The body relies on gravity to assist with some of this function. The contraction of the skeletal muscles also aids in pushing the blood through the veins. As mentioned earlier, the veins have valves that also keep the blood flowing without backflow.

Another mechanism that helps venous blood flow is breathing. The movement of the diaphragm helps the blood in the abdomen and thorax to return to the heart. Physical inactivity can cause blood to pool in the lower extremities. The arteries are used to measure the pulse rate. When an artery is pressed against a bone, a pulse is felt. The most common site for taking a pulse is the radial artery located on the thumb side of the posterior wrist. The pulse is counted for a full minute and should be between 60 and 80 beats per minute in a healthy adult at rest. The quality of the pulse is also noted. It can be strong or weak and may be regular or irregular in rhythm. Blood pressure is also measured as the force exerted by the blood against the walls of the arteries.

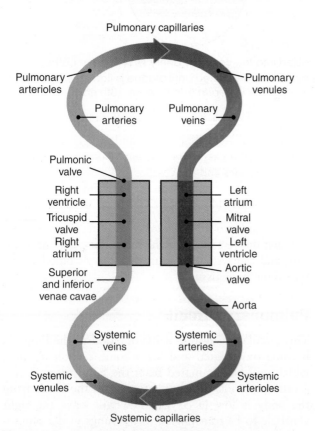

Figure 8-5 Circulation throughout the body. (Reprinted from Cohen BJ. *Memmler's The Human Body in Health and Disease.* 13th ed. Burlington, MA: Jones & Bartlett Learning, LLC; 2014.)

Table 8-2　Major Arteries

Aorta	Exits the heart and includes the ascending aorta, aortic arch, thoracic aorta, and abdominal aorta
Right and left coronary arteries	Branch off the aorta and lead to the right and left sides of the heart supplying the myocardium with blood
Brachiocephalic artery	Supplies the arm and the head on the right side
Right subclavian artery	Extends under the right clavicle and collar bone and supplies the right upper arm and brain
Right common carotid artery	Supplies the right side of the neck, head, and brain
Left common carotid artery	Supplies the left side of the neck and the head
Left subclavian artery	Supplies the left upper extremity and part of the brain
Vertebral artery	Located in the cervical vertebrae supplying blood to the posterior brain
Axillary artery	Under the arm, armpit
Brachial artery	Supplies the upper arm
Radial artery	Supplies the forearm and wrist on the lateral or thumb side of the arm
Ulnar artery	Supplies the forearm and wrist on the medial or little finger side into the hand
Intercostal arteries	9–10 pairs of arteries between the ribs and the chest wall
Left gastric artery	Supplies the stomach
Splenic artery	Supplies the spleen
Hepatic artery	Supplies the liver
Superior and inferior mesenteric arteries	Supply the small and large intestines
Superior and inferior phrenic arteries	Supply the diaphragm
Renal arteries	Supply blood to the kidneys
Ovarian arteries	Supply reproductive organs of the female, ovaries
Testicular arteries	Supply the sex glands of the male, testicles
Lumbar arteries	Supply the muscles of the abdominal wall
Common iliac arteries (internal and external iliac arteries)	Supply the urinary bladder, rectum, and reproductive organs except the gonads (testicles and ovaries)
Femoral artery	Supplies the thigh
Popliteal artery	Extends from lower thigh behind the knee
Tibial arteries (anterior and posterior)	Supply the lower leg and feet
Dorsalis pedis	Terminal end of the tibial artery supplies the feet

Table 8-3　Major Veins

Superior vena cava	Veins of head, neck, upper extremities, and chest drain the blood into this vein
Jugular veins	Drain from the head and neck
Subclavian veins	Drain from beneath the clavicle and upper arm
Cephalic veins	Drain from the head
Brachial, basilic, and median cubital veins	Drain from the upper and mid arm
Radial and ulnar veins	Returns blood from the forearm and wrist
Inferior vena cava	Veins below the diaphragm drain their blood into this vein to return to the heart
Common iliac veins (external and internal)	Return blood from the groin area
Lumbar veins	Return blood from the lower lumbar and spinal cord
Gonadal veins (ovarian and testicular)	Return blood from the ovaries and testicles
Renal veins	Return blood from the kidneys
Hepatic veins	Return blood from the liver
Saphenous veins	Return blood from the lower extremities and are the body's longest veins
Femoral vein	Returns blood from the thigh
Popliteal vein	Returns blood from the midleg behind the knee
Anterior and posterior tibial veins	Return blood from the lower leg and feet

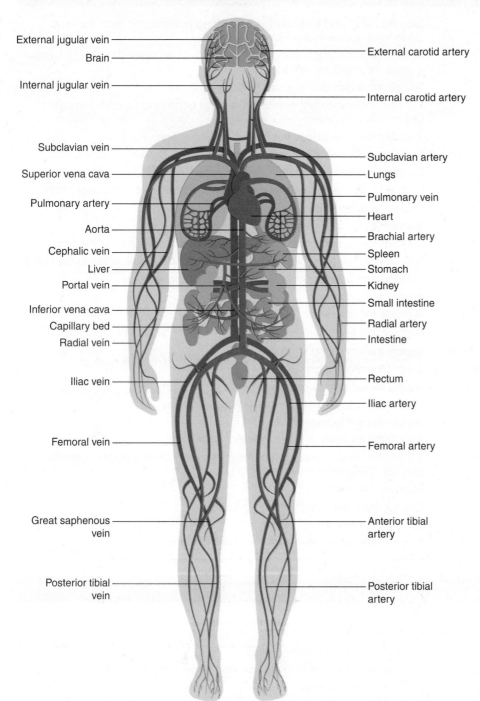

External jugular vein

Brain

Internal jugular vein

Subclavian vein

Superior vena cava

Pulmonary artery

Aorta

Cephalic vein

Liver

Portal vein

Inferior vena cava

Capillary bed

Radial vein

Iliac vein

Femoral vein

Great saphenous vein

Posterior tibial vein

External carotid artery

Internal carotid artery

Subclavian artery

Lungs

Pulmonary vein

Heart

Brachial artery

Spleen

Stomach

Kidney

Small intestine

Radial artery

Intestine

Rectum

Iliac artery

Femoral artery

Anterior tibial artery

Posterior tibial artery

Figure 8-6 Major arteries and veins of the body. (Image from Shutterstock.com.)

 # CIRCULATORY DISORDERS

High blood pressure, **hypertension,** and low blood pressure, **hypotension,** are conditions that are detected by measuring the pressure within the arteries; however, they may be due to underlying conditions not associated with disease of the arteries. Some of the conditions that affect the arteries and veins include the following:

- **Arteriosclerosis**—hardening of the arteries caused by loss of elasticity of the arterial wall, a buildup of scar tissue, and irregular thickening of the walls

- Atherosclerosis—fatty (plaque) buildup on the walls of the arteries; leads to development of blood clots and puts a patient at high risk for heart attack and stroke
- **Aneurysm**—bulging or ballooning sac of a vessel due to weakness in the wall of the vessel; it may be congenital or due to damage of the vessel; undiagnosed, it may rupture and be life threatening due to the hemorrhage
- Hemorrhage—the term literally means bursting forth of blood, and blood flows out of the blood vessels; may be internal or external
- Thrombosis—formation of a blood clot in a blood vessel; embolism is a moving blood clot traveling in the vessel

- Phlebitis—inflammation of a vein; thrombophlebitis is inflammation of the vein due to a blood clot in the vein
- Varicose veins—also called varices are swollen, gnarled veins that do not work effectively moving blood; typically occurring in the lower extremities; in the rectum, they are called hemorrhoids

When there is a lack of blood flow to an area of the body, the tissues may begin to die resulting in gangrene when the dead tissue is invaded by bacteria. This is a common problem for diabetic patients' lower extremities and feet. Treatment for arterial problems includes a surgical treatment called endarterectomy, removing the blood vessel's lining that is damaged from atherosclerosis. A common place for this procedure is the carotid arteries, which can open up more blood flow to the head and brain.

 ## THE RESPIRATORY SYSTEM

The heart and lungs work together to provide the body with the nutrients and oxygen to maintain the health of the body's tissues. Respiration is the process of taking in air from the environment and delivering the oxygen portion to the body cells. Carbon dioxide, a waste product of cell metabolism, is transported to the lungs to be exhaled during respiration. There are two types of respiration:

- External respiration—the exchange of the oxygen (O_2) and carbon dioxide (CO_2) in the alveoli of the lungs with the blood
- Internal respiration—the exchange of the oxygen (O_2) and carbon dioxide (CO_2) at the cellular level in the body, the body tissues

Respirations are measured as one inhalation and one exhalation and should average 12 to 20 per minute.

Case Question

 The patient in the case study asks Carlos, the medical assistant, since he is short of breath, why he is being referred to a heart doctor and not a lung specialist. If you were the medical assistant, how would you respond to the patient?

 ## THE RESPIRATORY SYSTEM STRUCTURE

The respiratory system is basically a pathway that conducts air in and out of the lungs. The structures are divided into the upper respiratory and lower respiratory systems. We will explore the structures from the nose through to the alveoli. Figure 8-7 shows the structures and location of the respiratory system.

The Nasal Cavities

The nasal cavities include two nostrils (nares), which are separated by a dividing wall, the septum. The nose acts as an air conditioner for the air we breathe, moistening, warming, and filtering it before it is delivered to the lungs. To assist with these functions, mucous membranes secrete fluid to moisten it, and cilia (hairs) filter the dust particles. As the air is moved through the nose, it becomes warmer. Although some people are mouth breathers, it is recommended that we only breathe through the nose allowing these functions to take place. The nose also provides us the process of smelling.

The Pharynx

The pharynx is what we refer to as the throat. It carries the air to the respiratory tract and also serves the function of carrying food and liquids to the esophagus and the digestive tract. It does not change the air as it travels through the pharynx. There are three divisions of the pharynx:

- Nasopharynx—the section immediately behind the nasal cavity
- Oropharynx—located in the back of the mouth
- Laryngopharynx—lowest section of the pharynx as it approaches the larynx

The Larynx

The larynx is called the voice box. It connects the pharynx with the trachea. The larynx is composed of hyaline cartilage. In the upper part of the larynx are vocal cords, or folds, which vibrate as air passes over them. As the length and tension of the folds change, the pitch of sound is regulated. The volume of sound is regulated by the amount of air that passes over the vocal cords. A small flap of cartilage, the epiglottis, lies over the larynx closing when swallowing. This protects the respiratory system from food or liquids from entering the respiratory structures beyond the larynx. Occasionally, materials may be inhaled or aspirated into the respiratory tract when the epiglottis is open while talking when eating or drinking.

The Trachea

The trachea is also called the windpipe. It extends from the larynx to the bronchi. The trachea is constructed of C-shaped cartilage, which keeps the trachea open. When the airway above the trachea is blocked or

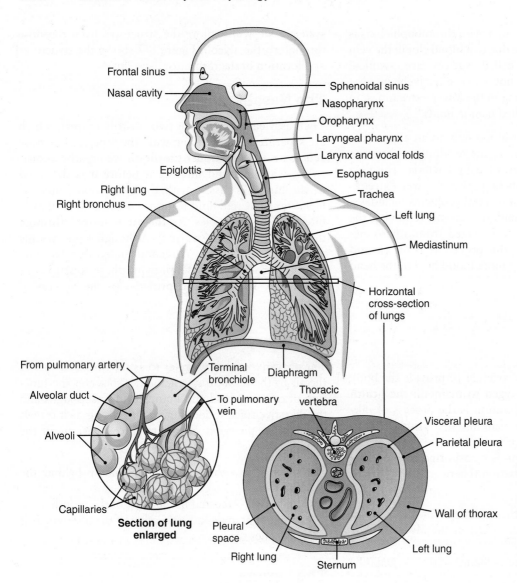

Figure 8-7 labels: Frontal sinus, Nasal cavity, Sphenoidal sinus, Nasopharynx, Oropharynx, Laryngeal pharynx, Larynx and vocal folds, Epiglottis, Esophagus, Right lung, Trachea, Right bronchus, Left lung, Mediastinum, Horizontal cross-section of lungs, From pulmonary artery, Terminal bronchiole, Diaphragm, Alveolar duct, To pulmonary vein, Thoracic vertebra, Alveoli, Visceral pleura, Parietal pleura, Capillaries, Wall of thorax, **Section of lung enlarged**, Pleural space, Right lung, Left lung, Sternum

Figure 8-7 Respiratory system. (Reprinted from Cohen BJ. *Memmler's The Human Body in Health and Disease.* 13th ed. Burlington, MA: Jones & Bartlett Learning, LLC; 2014.)

artificial respiration is required, a tracheostomy (surgical opening) is performed to place an airway tube in place. Figure 8-8 shows a patient with a tracheostomy.

The Bronchi

At the end of the trachea the tube divides into the right and left bronchi, the airways that enter the lungs. These structures are made from cartilage rings to stabilize and keep the airways open. The right bronchus (singular) is larger than the left bronchus because it needs to supply air to the right lung, which is larger than the left lung.

The Lungs

The right and left lungs are located in the thoracic cavity. The right lung has three lobes, and the left lung has two lobes. The reason for the smaller left lung is to pro-

vide space on the left side to accommodate the heart. The lung lobes on the right are the superior, middle, and inferior, and on the left side the lobes are only the superior and inferior. Each bronchus branches off to provide an individual branch to each lobe of the lungs. These are called the secondary bronchi. The bronchi gradually become smaller leading into the bronchioles. As the bronchioles branch out into the lobes of the lungs, they start resembling the branches on a tree. The bronchioles, made up of smooth muscle, are controlled by the autonomic nervous system, which is involuntary.

The Alveoli

At the end of the bronchial tree are the clusters of tiny air sacs called alveoli. They resemble clusters of grapes on the vine. This is the location of the external gas exchange. There are approximately 300 million alveoli in the body. The alveoli are covered with blood capillaries. As the pulmonary arteries deliver blood to the

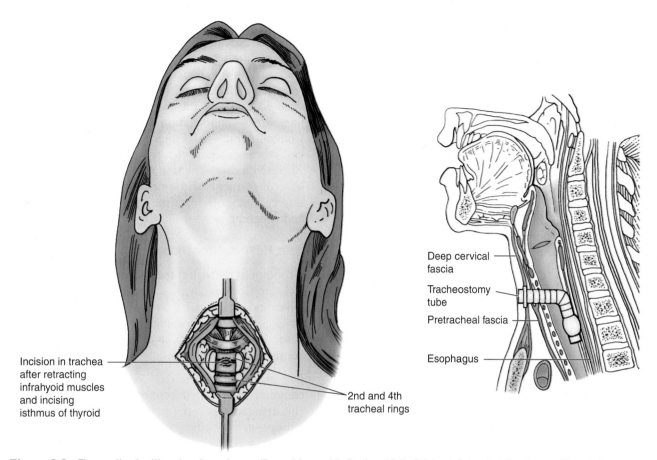

Incision in trachea after retracting infrahyoid muscles and incising isthmus of thyroid

2nd and 4th tracheal rings

Deep cervical fascia

Tracheostomy tube

Pretracheal fascia

Esophagus

Figure 8-8   The patient with a tracheostomy. (From Moore KL, Dalley AF II. *Clinical Oriented Anatomy*. 4th ed. Baltimore, MD: Lippincott Williams & Wilkins; 1999.)

lungs, the deoxygenated blood picks up oxygen and gives up carbon dioxide. The oxygenated blood is sent back to the heart to be distributed throughout the body. The carbon dioxide is eliminated from the body during respiration.

The Pleura

The lungs are covered with a double sac called the pleura. The parietal layer of the sac is attached to the chest wall of the thoracic cavity and the visceral layer attaches to the lung surface. There is a space between the two layers, the pleural space that contains a fluid that lubricates the membranes. This is similar to the pericardial sac that surrounds the heart. The space with fluid allows the lungs to freely move with each breath expanding and contracting. As we inhale, the diaphragm is pushed downward allowing the lungs to fill with air. With expiration, the diaphragm relaxes and pushes upward allowing air to be exhaled.

Transporting the Gasses

Oxyhemoglobin and carbaminohemoglobin are the terms used when describing the transport of oxygen and carbon dioxide throughout the body. The red blood cells contain a protein called hemoglobin, which is the necessary ingredient for the transport of oxygen and carbon dioxide. The binding of the oxygen with the hemoglobin is called **oxyhemoglobin**, and when carbon dioxide combines with hemoglobin, it is **carbaminohemoglobin**. When a person has a condition that causes a decrease in the number of red blood cells, it may affect the transport of these gasses throughout the body. A patient with chronic or severe anemia may have symptoms including shortness of breath, fatigue, and blueness of the extremities, cyanosis.

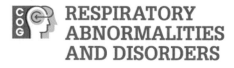

RESPIRATORY ABNORMALITIES AND DISORDERS

As we have discovered with every other body system, the respiratory system is also subject to injury, inflammation, infection, and disease. Since this system is responsible for the critical gasses for the body cells to function, a lack of oxygen to the cells will occasionally result in life-threatening situations.

Breathing Abnormalities

The terms used to describe abnormal respirations usually end in the word **-pnea**, which refers to breathing. Here is a list of terms that are symptoms of an underlying disease or condition:

- Hyperpnea—an increase in the depth and rate of breathing, for example, during exercise
- Hypopnea—a decrease in the rate and depth of breathing
- Tachypnea—an excessive rate of breathing, also as in exercise
- Apnea—lack of breathing but is a temporary condition as in sleep apnea
- Dyspnea—difficult or labored breathing
- Orthopnea—difficulty breathing relieved by sitting up
- Cheyne-Stokes—alternating periods of apnea and rhythmic variation in the depth of breaths, seen in critically ill patients and those near death
- Hyperventilation—rate and depth increase above normal levels; may be seen during panic attack, anxiety, and stress
- Cyanosis—bluish color of skin, typically the extremities and lips, due to insufficient amount of oxygen in the blood
- Hypoxia—also called anoxia, lower than normal oxygen level in the tissues

Respiratory Disorders

The respiratory tract is one of the more common portals of entry for disease-causing organisms to infect the body. It is easy to breathe in these airborne organisms. The environment in the mouth and nose provides a warm, moist place for the growth of bacteria. From the nose, bacteria can travel to the pharynx, larynx, trachea, and into the lungs. Middle ear infections are also associated with upper respiratory infections (**URI**) because of the connection of the eustachian tube and the pharynx.

Upper Respiratory Disorders

The upper respiratory structures include the sinuses, nose, pharynx, and larynx. Here are some common problems that affect the upper respiratory system.

- Sinusitis—infection of the paranasal sinuses located in the skull bones in the area of the nose; causes pain in the facial area around the eyes, congestion of the nasal passages, and postnasal drip
- Deviated septum—an unequal size of the right and left nasal passages usually due to the way the septum divides them
- **Epistaxis**—commonly known as a nosebleed; may be due to injury or trauma to the nose, infection, or drying of the mucous membranes; most stop on their own with pressure on the nostrils (pinching); however, nasal packing may be indicated to stop a persistent nosebleed
- Pharyngitis—inflammation or infection in the pharynx, also called a sore throat; may be caused by the streptococcal bacteria, commonly called strep throat
- Laryngitis—inflammation or infection in the larynx
- Common cold—viral infection that is highly contagious through air droplets from sneezing and coughing
- Allergic rhinitis—reaction to allergens including pollens, dust, mold, and animal dander causing itchy, watery discharge from the eyes and nose, sneezing, and coughing

Lower Respiratory Disorders

The conditions that affect the lower respiratory tract can cause more serious illness and complications. When it involves and infection, it may start with the upper respiratory structures but then migrate to the lower parts and into the lungs. Some of the conditions that affect the lower tract are as follows:

- **RSV**—respiratory syncytial virus; one of the most common causes of infections in infants and young children and may result in pneumonia
- Croup—usually affects children under 3 years of age and is associated with infections; airway constriction results in a wheezing, barking cough; humidifying the air may relieve the symptoms
- Influenza—also called the flu, is an acute contagious viral disease that causes cough, weakness, aches; vaccines have been effective in protecting people from the virus
- Pneumonia—viral or bacterial infection causing inflammation of the lungs and fluid buildup in the air spaces; main types of pneumonia are as follows:
  - Lobar pneumonia—affects an entire lobe of the lung
  - Bronchopneumonia—infection is spread throughout the lung
- Tuberculosis (**TB**)—infection caused by the bacillus, *Mycobacterium tuberculosis*; usually grows in the lungs; however, it may be found in the lymph nodes or carried to other parts of the body through the blood
- Asthma—inflammation of the airways causing smooth muscle spasm and narrowing of the passageways; excessive mucus is produced; causes wheezing when breathing and dyspnea; may be related to allergy but patients might also be sensitive to fumes, tobacco smoke, and cold air, which can trigger attacks
- Chronic obstructive pulmonary disease (**COPD**)—a general term used for several associated lung disorders including emphysema and chronic bronchitis; major cause of developing COPD is cigarette smoking
- Chronic bronchitis—inflammation of the lining of the bronchial tubes; causes coughing with heavy mucus or phlegm production

- Emphysema—an irreversible condition in which there is dilation and destruction of the alveoli; oxygen is decreased and carbon dioxide builds up due to inability to properly exhale; air is trapped in the lungs
- Acute respiratory distress syndrome (**ARDS**)—sudden onset of inflammation resulting from injury or infection; causes might include aspiration of stomach contents, lung trauma, and embolism or tumors resulting in airway obstruction
- Atelectasis—partial or complete collapse of a lung or portion of a lung
- Surfactant deficiency disorder—lack of production of surfactant, substance that facilitates lung expansion; premature babies of <35 weeks' gestation are at risk of this condition; however, they are treated with injections of injected with synthetic surfactant

Cultural Connection

Asthma affects individuals throughout the world in various cultures and ethnicity. Among different cultures, there are many "home remedies" that have been passed down through generations and are still being used to alleviate symptoms of respiratory illness. Some of these preparations are herbal products that have mucolytic, anti-inflammatory, and bronchodilation properties. It is important that patients are questioned about any home treatments that they may be using as these may interact or exaggerate the effect in the body when combined with prescription medications. This information will help the physician provide the safe and appropriate medication for asthma patients. Examples of these herbs include Puerto Rican families that use chamomile and eucalyptus tea, East Indian use of Indian gooseberry and frankincense, the Chinese use of ginkgo biloba and Ma-huang (ephedra), and the European communities that use mustard, horseradish, elderberry, primrose, rose hips, and thyme. The medical assistant needs to make sure to include these home remedies in the patient intake information.

There are some disorders that only affect the pleura, the sac covering the lungs. These conditions include the following:

- Pleurisy—inflammation of the pleura, which is a complication of a lung infection or pneumonia; sticky substance is produced that causes the pleura surfaces to rub together resulting in pain and an increase in pleural fluid
- Pneumothorax—accumulation of air in the pleural space; may be due to puncture wound of the chest wall
- Hemothorax—accumulation of blood in the pleural space; may be due to chest wound with hemorrhage

Cancer of the Respiratory System

The respiratory system structures may develop cancerous tumors with the most common sites found in the larynx and the lungs.

Lung Cancer

Men and women are at both at risk of developing lung cancer. It is the most common cancer-related death. The main cause of lung cancer is cigarette smoking. There is also significant evidence that breathing in secondhand smoke may also lead to lung cancer. There are also many carcinogenic agents, such as asbestos, in the environment that may be the cause of developing this form of cancer.

Larynx Cancer

Cancer of the voice box may be linked to drinking alcohol and cigarette smoking. Symptoms include sore throat and hoarseness. Although the cure rate is high, additional treatment may be required including partial or total removal of the larynx. Without the larynx, patients are required to use a mechanical device in order to talk.

Study Skill

It is never too early to start learning the most common medications ordered to treat the diseases and conditions that affect the body systems. To start this project, access the Internet to locate one of the various Web sites that provides this information. These are usually titled as "Top" number of ordered drugs, for example, "Top 100 Drugs" or "Top 200 Drugs." The information typically includes the generic drug name, brand name, and the drug classification (bronchodilator, steroid, antibiotic). The information you gather can be put onto index cards or organized by classification on a table processed in the computer.

Treatment of Respiratory Disorders

There are many treatments used in managing respiratory conditions. Infections are typically treated with antibiotics, and narrowed airways are relaxed and dilated with the use of inhaled **bronchodilators**. Steroid medication is also indicated to help reduce inflammation. Oxygen is a medication that you may not think about but is used to supply more oxygen to patients who are experiencing a shortage. Oxygen therapy is sometimes used constantly by patients with COPD. They require it around the clock, when awake and during sleep hours. In the physician's office, the medical assistant will use a pulse oximeter to measure the pulse rate and oxygen levels

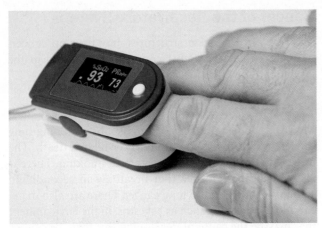

Figure 8-9   A pulse oximeter is used to measure the pulse rate and oxygen levels. (Image from Shutterstock.com.)

of the patient. Figure 8-9 is an example of this small device, which is put on a finger and a digital reading is displayed.

Asthma is a common illness that requires both bronchodilators and steroids. Also, patients are to avoid the things that trigger their asthma attacks. Patients with emphysema use the same medications as do asthmatic patients. The primary goal is to reduce inflammation and open up the air passages.

Testing for tuberculosis is a common procedure for medical assistants to perform. It is accomplished through intradermal skin testing. Once the skin test is confirmed as positive, a chest x-ray and sputum testing are performed to confirm active disease. The TB organism is resistant to many antibiotics, so the treatment of tuberculosis usually requires the use of a combination of several drugs over a period of 6 to 18 months.

In order to initially diagnose respiratory conditions or monitor the progress of a disorder, the physician will perform testing of the patient's breathing with a device called a **spirometer**. This machine can measure and record the volume of air moved with each inhalation and expiration. The physician will evaluate the patient's lung capacity including the total lung capacity, forced expiratory volume and tidal volume, and the amount of normal air moved in and out without effort.

When a visual examination of the inside of the lungs is indicated, a **bronchoscope** is used. It is a flexible fiberoptic instrument passed through the mouth and pharynx, through the larynx and trachea into the bronchi. The physician can see the condition of the bronchial tissues, examine the area for inflammation, and take tissue samples.

Invasive Respiratory Procedures

Some respiratory conditions require more invasive procedures. Some of these procedures include the following:

- Thoracentesis—insertion of a needle into the pleural space to remove fluid; used to treat **effusion**, accumulation of fluid as a result of fluid leaking into a space
- Tracheotomy—incision into the trachea to create an airway opening; a tube is inserted for breathing
- Pneumonectomy—surgical removal of a lung or lobectomy to remove only a lobe of a lung

The ultimate type of treatment of a respiratory emergency is to deliver CPR, cardiopulmonary resuscitation, to a person who is not breathing and has no heartbeat. Artificial respiration is used when the person is not breathing but does have a heartbeat. It is critical for medical assistants to learn CPR and maintain certification to stay current with new techniques.

In summary, the best way to protect your cardiovascular and respiratory health is to refrain from smoking, exercise, and maintain an ideal weight making good diet choices.

Preparing for Externship

The externship course is your time to apply the knowledge you learned in the classroom. You will probably admit that there was a lot of information. How are you going to remember everything especially when the site may have specific way of doing a particular procedure? The key is to jot down notes from the first day on the site. For example, if you are working in a respiratory specialty office, there may be medications routinely ordered to treat lung conditions. Write down the name of the drugs and some of the common doses the physicians order. You will gradually become more familiar with the treatments used in that practice and help you better understand the charting entries. Writing down reminder notes each day is not enough. You need to review your notes each day and make sure you understand the information you wrote. Formulate questions to ask the staff the next day for those areas that you are unclear or uncertain.

Chapter Recap

- The cardiovascular system includes the heart, which pumps the blood, and the blood vessels that carry the blood with oxygen and nutrients throughout the body. They also transport carbon dioxide and waste products for elimination from the body.
- The heart has chambers and valves that allow it to pump oxygenated and deoxygenated blood without mixing it as well as keeping the blood flowing in one direction.
- The blood vessels include arteries, arterioles, capillaries, venules, and veins. The coronary vessels supply the myocardial muscle of the heart with blood
- The heart has an electrical conduction system that generates the heartbeat. Normal sinus rhythm occurs when the heart is healthy; however, there are variations to the heartbeat and heart rate called arrhythmias.

- The heart may develop conditions that are related to infections, structural defects, and abnormalities of the electrical system.
- There are many conditions that affect the blood vessels that affect the ability of the blood to flow properly throughout the body.
- Prevention is one of the best ways to maintain heart and circulatory health. The heart is a muscle and needs exercise just like other muscles in the body. Low-fat diets are essential to help keep cholesterol levels normal.
- The lungs work together with the cardiopulmonary system to supply the body's cells with the nourishment and oxygen necessary for cell health and repair.
- Respiratory disorders include infection, structural defects, inflammation, and cancer.

Online Resources for Students

Student Resources available on the text's online site include:
- Audio Glossaries
- Animations
- Competency Evaluation Forms

- Videos
- Anatomy & Physiology Module with Heart and Lung Sounds
- Weblinks
- Worksheets

Exercises and Activities

Certification Preparation Questions

1. Which of these represents the correct sequence or order of blood vessels as blood flows through the circulatory system?
   a. Artery, venule, capillary
   b. Vein, venule, arteriole
   c. Venule, vein, capillary
   d. Artery, arteriole, capillary
   e. Capillary, venule, arteriole

2. Which of these procedures is the insertion of a balloon into an artery to open the size of the lumen?
   a. Angioplasty
   b. Arthrectomy
   c. Bypass graft
   d. Defibrillation
   e. Angiography

3. Which of these represents the contraction of the atria?
   a. P wave
   b. R wave
   c. T wave
   d. QRS complex
   e. S-T segment

4. The pacemaker of the heart is the:
   a. AV node.
   b. AV bundle.
   c. bundle of HIS.
   d. SA node.
   e. Purkinje fibers.

5. Arteriosclerosis is:
   a. the fatty buildup in an artery.
   b. bulging of an artery.
   c. the death of tissue.
   d. hardening of the arteries.
   e. an embolism in an artery.

6. Which of these is the term used for the collapse of the lung?

    a. Lobectomy
    b. Pleurisy
    c. Emphysema
    d. Pneumonia
    e. Atelectasis

7. Structures associated with the upper respiratory system include the:

    a. sinuses and trachea.
    b. trachea and larynx.
    c. pharynx and trachea.
    d. pharynx and larynx.
    e. larynx and bronchi.

8. Which of the following is a term used for difficult, labored breathing that is relieved by sitting up?

    a. Tachypnea
    b. Dyspnea
    c. Hypoxia
    d. Apnea
    e. Orthopnea

9. Medication that dissolves blood clots is:

    a. digitalis.
    b. antiarrhythmics.
    c. statins.
    d. thrombolytics.
    e. beta-blockers.

10. The procedure used to remove pleural fluid to treat effusion is a:

    a. thoracocentesis.
    b. bronchoscopy.
    c. pneumonectomy.
    d. pleurisy.
    e. pneumothorax.

 ## CareTracker Connection

Documenting Diagnoses and Other Clinical Data Related to the Cardiovascular and Respiratory Systems

 HARRIS CareTracker Activities Related to
CareTracker This Chapter
• Case Study 7: Cardiovascular Patient Practicum

Cardiovascular disease is the number one cause of death in the United States and affects the daily lives of millions. Consequently, medical assistants and other health care professionals enter untold gigabytes of cardiovascular-related data each year in the form of health histories, examination and test findings, diagnoses, and treatment plans. Accurately capturing this information in an orderly, efficient, and consistent manner can be a challenge. Fortunately, electronic health record applications, such as CareTracker, greatly facilitate this task by providing detailed, integrated data-entry fields for all areas and systems of the body, including cardiovascular and respiratory.

Tasks discussed in this chapter that can be performed in CareTracker include the following:

• Documenting the following patient clinical information related to cardiovascular and respiratory conditions:
  ○ Health history
    ○ Diseases and conditions

  ○ Hospitalizations
  ○ Tobacco assessment
  ○ Exercise habits
  ○ Surgeries and procedures
  ○ Preventive care
  ○ Family history
  ○ Review of systems
  ○ Physical examination findings
  ○ Tests and procedures completed during the visit
    ○ Electrocardiogram
    ○ Imaging studies
  ○ Diagnoses
  ○ Treatment plan
    ○ Electrocardiogram
    ○ Echocardiogram
    ○ Holter monitor
    ○ Angiography
    ○ Cardiac stress test
    ○ Cardiac rehab
• Ordering the following related to cardiovascular and respiratory conditions:
  ○ Medications
  ○ Laboratory tests
  ○ Diagnostic tests

Many of these tasks are discussed in CareTracker Connection features in other chapters. A task we'll consider here is entering data related to the cardiovascular system.

The entry of system-specific data typically begins with the patient's health and family histories. As you can see below, the General Medical History section of the History application of CareTracker features many different cardiovascular diseases.

GENERAL MEDICAL HISTORY +/- Clear All

Y N Alcoholism	Y N Depression	Y N Kidney Infections
Y N Allergies/Hayfever	Y N DM Type 1	Y N Kidney stone
Y N Anemia	Y N DM Type 2	Y N Migraine
Y N Anxiety	Y N Epilepsy	Y N Multiple Sclerosis
Y N Asthma	Y N Fracture	Y N Obesity
☑ N Atrial Fibrillation	Y N Gastric ulcer	☑ N Old MI
Y N Blood Transfusions	Y N Gastrointestinal Disease	Y N Osteoarthritis
☑ N CAD	Y N GERD	Y N Osteoporosis
Y N Cancer	Y N Gestational Diabetes	Y N Pneumonia
☑ N Cardiac Pacer	Y N Glaucoma	Y N Progressive Neurological Disord
☑ N Cardiovascular Disease	☑ N Heart Murmur	Y N Pulmonary Disease
☑ N CHF	Y N Hepatitis	☑ N Rheumatic Fever
Y N Cirrhosis	☑ N High Cholesterol	Y N Rheumatoid Arthritis
Y N Colitis	☑ N Hyperlipidemia	Y N STD
Y N COPD	☑ N Hypertension	Y N Terminal Illness
Y N CRF	Y N Hyperthyroidism	Y N Thyroid Disease
Y N Crohn's disease	Y N Hypothyroidism	☑ N TIA
☑ N CVA	Y N Joint Pain	Y N Tuberculosis

The General Family History section likewise provides many selections related to cardiovascular disease.

Findings details windows allow even more detailed information to be recorded.

GENERAL FAMILY HISTORY +/- Clear All

☐ Adopted	☐ Denial of any knowledge of significant family history	
☐ Unknown Paternal Hx	☐ Unknown Maternal Hx	
Y N Alcoholism	Y N Congenital Anomaly	☑ N Hypertension
Y N Anemia	Y N COPD	Y N Hypothyroidism
Y N Anxiety	Y N Crohn's Disease	Y N Kidney Disease
Y N Asthma	Y N Depression	Y N Liver Disease
Y N Birth Defects	Y N Diabetes	Y N Multiple Births
☑ N CAD	Y N Epilepsy	Y N Osteoarthritis
☑ N Cardiovascular Disease	Y N GERD	Y N Osteoporosis
☑ N CHF	☑ N Hypercholesterolemia	Y N Pulmonary Diseas
Cancer [select] ▼	☑ N Hyperlipidemia	☑ N Stroke

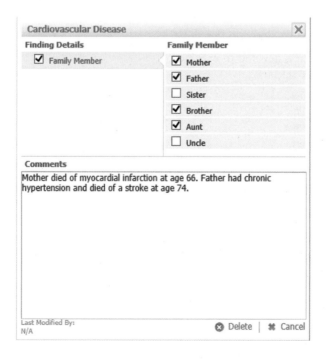

All data entered into the History application in CareTracker appear in the HX (history) tab of the patient's Progress Note. The primary care provider can then enter additional patient data gathered during the physical examination into the ROS (review of systems), PE (physical examination), TESTS PROC (tests and procedures), DX (diagnoses), and PLAN (treatment plan) tabs of the Progress Note. On the DX tab, below, note that you can select a preloaded diagnosis from the template form or search for and select the diagnosis, using either a description or an ICD code, using the search feature.

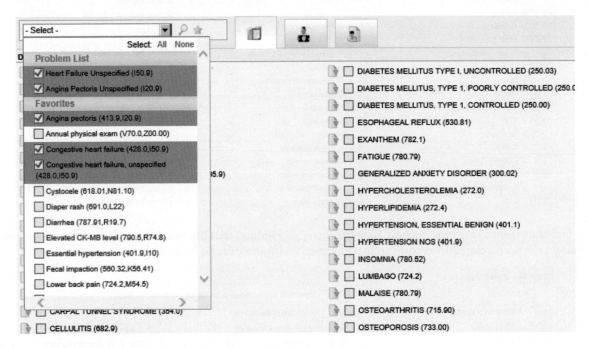

All selected diagnoses are summarized at the bottom of the DX tab.

	Diagnosis	ICD Code	PL	OS
☑	**Today's Selected Diagnosis**			
☑	Angina pectoris	413.9, I20.9	☐	
☑	Heart failure	428.9, I50.9	☐	

The PLAN tab features a section devoted to cardiac-related interventions that may be selected.

Cardiac Related Plan Items

☑ Electrocardiogram   ☐ Echocardiogram

☐ Holter monitor   ☐ Angiography

☑ Cardiac Stress Test   ☐ Cardiac Rehab

The ⬚ and ⬚ applications allow you to enter cardiovascular-related medication prescriptions and laboratory/diagnostic orders, respectively.

9 Urinary and Reproductive Systems

Chapter Objectives

- List the urinary system organs and the function of each.
- Explain the kidney's role in maintaining homeostasis.
- Describe the function of the nephron.
- Explain the process of urine formation.
- Explain the process of urination.
- Discuss various types of urinary system disorders.
- Explain the purpose of renal dialysis.
- List the organs of the male and female reproductive systems.
- Describe the function of the male and female reproductive organs.
- Describe a spermatozoon and describe the function of semen.
- Identify the hormones that regulate the male and female reproductive organs.
- Discuss various types of male and female reproductive system disorders.
- Explain the changes during and after menopause.
- Describe the process of fertilization.
- Explain the main process of fetal development.
- List the stages of labor.

CAAHEP & ABHES Competencies

CAAHEP

- Describe structural organization of the human body.
- Identify body systems.
- List major organs in each body system.
- Describe the normal function of each body system.
- Identify common pathology related to each body system including signs, symptoms, and etiology.
- Analyze pathology for each body system including diagnostic measures and treatment modalities.

ABHES

- List all body systems, their structure, and functions.
- Describe common diseases, symptoms, and etiologies as they apply to each system.
- Identify diagnostic and treatment modalities as they relate to each body system.

Chapter Terms

Abortion	Endometrium	Hydronephrosis	Pyuria
Cesarean section	Enuresis	Incontinence	Uremia
Cryptorchidism	Episiotomy	Lithotripsy	Ureterocele
Cystitis	Excretory	Mammogram	Urethritis
Dialysis	Glomerulonephritis	Micturition	Viable
Dysmenorrhea	Glycosuria	Ovulation	
Endometriosis	Hematuria	Pyelonephritis	

Abbreviations

ADH	FSH	LMP	STI
BPH	HPV	PID	TAH
EDC	HRT	PMS	UTI
ESWL	LH	PSA	

Case Study

Ms. Williams, a patient who was treated a month ago for a urinary tract infection, is returning to see the physician because she continues to have pain with urination and a sense of urgency to urinate frequently. During her first visit, the physician ordered an antibiotic and instructed her to drink plenty of water. As the medical assistant, Robin, is preparing Ms. Williams to see the physician, the patient asks Robin if it is normal to still have an infection.

 THE URINARY SYSTEM

The urinary system is another vital system in the body that helps to maintain homeostasis by regulating fluid and electrolyte balance. The urinary system is also called the **excretory** system. The major structures of the urinary system include the following:

- Kidneys—two kidneys, one on the right and one on the left side, filter the waste products from the blood and balance fluids by eliminating excess water.
- Ureters—one leading from each kidney; serve as tubes to transport the urine from the kidneys to the bladder.
- Urinary bladder—collects and holds the urine until it is excreted from the body.
- Urethra—tube that transports the urine from the bladder to the outside of the body.

Figure 9-1 shows the major structures of the urinary system.

The Kidneys

The kidneys are located in the upper abdomen behind the peritoneum (retroperitoneal). They are at the level of the lower thoracic and upper lumbar region. The right kidney is slightly lower than the left one because of the location of the liver on the right side. Each kidney is wrapped in a membrane of fibrous connective tissue called the renal capsule. A protective layer of fat (adipose) also surrounds each kidney. The inner portion of the kidney is called the renal medulla. This is the location of the functional area of the kidney. The kidney resembles the shape of a kidney bean and is approximately the size of a fist. On the inner curve of the kidney, the

Case Question

 What can Robin say to the patient that will reassure her?

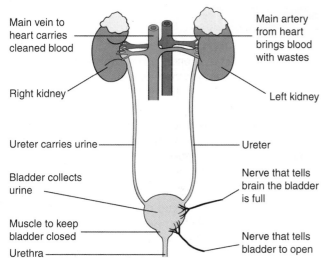

Figure 9-1 Major structures of the urinary system. (Image from Shutterstock.com.)

renal vein and renal artery connect with the kidney. The renal artery branching off the abdominal aorta carries blood to the kidney for filtering. The renal vein returns blood to the inferior vena cava and back to the heart. In the renal medulla, the urine is formed and flows into the region shaped like a funnel, the renal pelvis.

The Nephrons

The nephron is the microscopic, functional unit of the kidney and the structure that actually produces the urine. Each kidney has approximately 1 million nephrons.

The nephron receives blood into the capillary system at the glomerular capsule, called the Bowman capsule. From there, the blood is further filtered in the tiny renal tubules. The tubules have specific areas where the fluid is transformed into urine. The tubule structure begins with the proximal convoluted tubule, the nephron loop, called the loop of Henle, and then ends at the distal convoluted tubule. The glomerulus is supplied with blood from the afferent arteriole and leaves through the efferent arteriole. Figure 9-2 shows the main structures of the nephron.

Study Skill

The terms afferent and efferent are used in describing structures in body systems. It is easy to remember that afferent starts with an "a" and can be associated with the word arriving. The word efferent starts with "e" and can remind you with the word exiting. So in the nephron, the afferent arteriole is arriving to the glomerulus and the efferent arteriole is exiting.

The Ureters

The two ureters are muscular tubes that connect the kidneys with the bladder. They do not change the composition of the urine as it is transported from the kidney to the bladder. The ureters connect to the bladder on the posterior side of the bladder. They have a one-way valve so urine does not flow back once it is

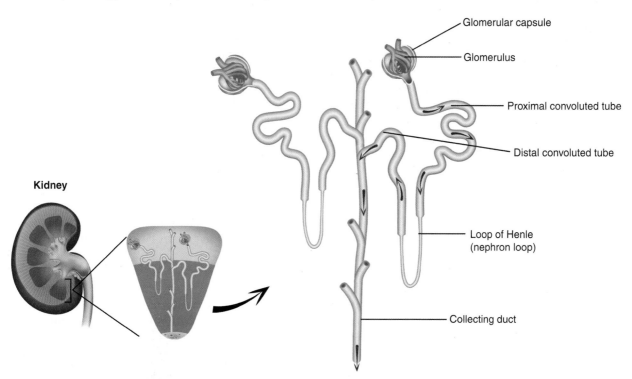

Figure 9-2 The structure of a nephron. (Image from Shutterstock.com.)

in the bladder. Urine flows downward out of the kidney assisted by gravity; however, the smooth muscle also uses peristaltic motion to move the urine along the tubes.

The Urinary Bladder

The bladder is a temporary holding or storage sac for the urine. It is located behind the pubic symphysis. When the bladder is empty, the inside has folds called rugae. The rugae allow for expansion of the bladder as it fills with urine. It is a smooth muscle that is capable of stretching. The bladder can hold about one-half liter of urine when moderately full.

The Urethra

The urethra is the tube that leads from the bladder to the outside of the body. Its only function is to transport the urine. It does not change the composition of the urine. In the female, it is short, approximately 1½ inches, and opens at the urinary meatus anterior to the vaginal opening. In the male, the urethra extends through the length of the penis. It carries urine and also acts as a transport tube for semen with spermatozoa.

Kidney Function and Urine Production

The kidneys are responsible for several functions including the following:

- Elimination of waste and toxins; one of the waste products is urea, nitrogen waste that is a by-product of amino acid metabolism.
- Maintaining homeostasis of body fluids—control water and sodium (salt) balance.
- Production of hormones—produce erythropoietin, which encourages red cell production in the bone marrow.
- Regulation of blood pressure—renin, an enzyme, affects the filtration and reabsorption of sodium helping to regulate the blood pressure.

Urine Production

The primary function of the kidneys is to eliminate waste products and excess fluid from the body; however, it is a very delicate balance to ensure that too much fluid is not excreted. The kidneys are constantly filtering blood, as much as 180 L of plasma (liquid part of the blood) each day. Almost 99% of the filtrate is reabsorbed back into the blood, which leaves about 1.5 to 2 L of urine produced each day. Substances that are reabsorbed are put back into the circulatory system. Any substances that are not reabsorbed are excreted in the urine.

An antidiuretic hormone (**ADH**) is released by the posterior pituitary gland and controls the reabsorption of water. The ADH affects the ability of the collecting duct in the nephron to reabsorb the water. This protects the body from too much water loss through the kidneys.

Urine

The chapter that presents urinalysis will provide greater detail about the composition of normal and abnormal urine and the laboratory examination of urine. Urine is 95% water, and the rest of it is dissolved solids and gases. Normal urine contains nitrogenous waste products, electrolytes, and a pigment, urochrome, a substance that gives the urine its yellow color. The color of the urine can change from ingestion of specific foods, such as beets, certain vitamins, and some drugs.

Abnormal substances in the urine include the following:

- Glucose—**glycosuria** or glucosuria, usually indicates diabetes mellitus
- Albumin (protein)—albuminuria; this protein passes through the nephron instead of being reabsorbed into the blood; caused by damage in the glomerulus
- Blood (RBC)—**hematuria**, indicates injury or disease in the urinary system
- Blood Cells (WBC)—indicates possible infection in the bladder or kidneys; when pus is present, it is called **pyuria**
- Ketones—ketonuria, result from the breakdown of fat, usually seen in diabetes mellitus and starvation when the body is using the fat reserve for energy

Urine can also be examined for the presence of drugs and hormones and may be cultured to determine the type of bacteria that might be causing an infection.

Urination

Now that the urine has formed, it needs to be eliminated from the body. Urination is also called **micturition**. Voiding is a term used to describe the process of expelling the urine. The bladder has two sphincter muscles that regulate the retention and excretion of urine. An internal, involuntary sphincter is located near the bladder where the urethra exits and an external, voluntary sphincter is a muscle formed by the pelvic muscles. The process of urination involves nerve impulses sent from receptors in the bladder to the spinal cord and then the brain. The bladder wall contracts as the urethral sphincters relax allowing the urine to flow out of the bladder.

Urinary Incontinence

Incontinence refers to an involuntary loss of urine, which may result from a nerve disorder, malfunction of the bladder, or weakness of the muscles in the pelvis. Incontinence may occur during certain types of activity that put stress on the bladder such as coughing, sneezing, lifting heavy objects, and while exercising. An overactive bladder results when the person perceives that the bladder is full and loses control of the contractions. **Enuresis** is another form of involuntary urination usually occurring at night. We know it as bedwetting.

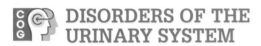

DISORDERS OF THE URINARY SYSTEM

As with the other body systems, the urinary tract from the kidneys to the urethra can be affected by infections, structural problems, and cancer. The medical assistant may encounter patients with symptoms associated with these conditions, which include pain with urination, abdominal pain, fever, and increased or decreased urine output.

Structural and Blockage Disorders

When there is a problem with a blocked passageway in the urinary system, it can cause the urine to be retained in the kidney or bladder. **Hydronephrosis** is the term used to describe the accumulation of fluid in the kidney.

Unresolved, this condition can leave the kidney permanently damaged. Physicians need to determine where the blockage is located and open the blocked area. The most common cause of an obstruction is renal calculi, known as a kidney stone. These are made of substances that are found in the blood but are filtered out instead of staying in the blood. The most common substances are uric acid and calcium salts. These stones can be very small and pass easily with the urine through the urinary tract or may be so large that they remain in the renal pelvis of the kidney, unable to pass through the ureter. Most people experience intense pain trying to pass the stone. The formation of kidney stones might be due to dehydration and urinary tract infections (**UTIs**). Younger men usually have a higher incidence of development of kidney stones than do women. If kidney stones cannot be passed, a procedure called **lithotripsy**, extracorporeal shock wave lithotripsy (**ESWL**), can be used to crush the stones into small pieces that are able to be passed through the urinary tract. Figure 9-3 demonstrates how the process of lithotripsy works.

Another type of treatment is surgical removal of the stones using a laparoscopic technique. A small incision is made for insertion of the endoscope, and instruments are used to remove the stones.

The urinary tract can also have structural defects that may affect the ability to produce urine or eliminate it from the body. Some of these conditions include the following:

- Congenital abnormalities—renal hypoplasia, underdeveloped or abnormally small kidneys; renal dysplasia, the nephrons are malformed and unable to adequately filter the blood and produce urine.
- **Ureterocele**—a type of herniation of the ureter as it enters the bladder.
- Hypospadias—in the male, the urethral opening is on the underside of the penis instead of the end of the penis.

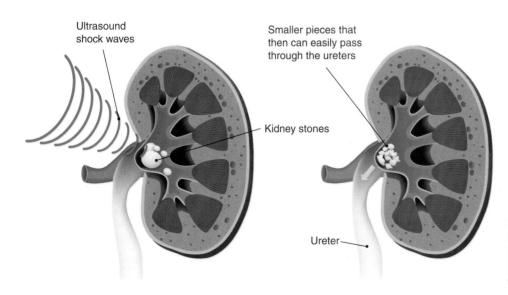

Figure 9-3 Extracorporeal shock wave lithotripsy (ESWL) for kidney stones. (Image from Shutterstock.com.)

Infection and Inflammation Disorders

Urinary tract infections (UTIs) are probably the most common condition affecting the urinary tract. The system may become contaminated with bacteria or might be the result of underlying conditions that cause retention of urine. Most UTIs begin at the urethra typically caused from contamination and are frequently a problem affecting females due to the shorter urethra in the female. The contamination may come from the *Escherichia coli* bacteria found in the bowel. **Urethritis**, inflammation of the urethra, migrates from the urethra to other structures in the urinary tract. Most of the infections respond well to antibiotic therapy. These infections include the following:

- **Cystitis**—inflammation of the bladder due to infection and retention of urine in the bladder; may be caused by enlarged prostate in men; symptoms include burning with urination and urgency and frequency of urination.
- **Pyelonephritis**—inflammation of the renal pelvis lower portion of the kidney; may be a chronic condition due to persistent or multiple bacterial infections. See Figure 9-4, which shows the location and effects of pyelonephritis.
- **Glomerulonephritis**—frequently diagnosed in children following strep throat infection; the antibodies formed in response to the streptococci bacteria remain in the glomerulus causing damage to the structures; the malfunctioning glomeruli cause increased protein and red blood cells in the urine, albuminuria and hematuria.

Case Study

The patient Ms. Williams finished her appointment with the physician and now is instructed by Robin, the medical assistant, to obtain a sterile urine specimen. The physician has ordered a urine culture and sensitivity. Ms. Williams inquires about the urine test and is upset that she has to have another urine test.

Case Questions

 How can Robin explain to the patient that a urine C&S is different from the routine urine test performed when she was seen a month ago?

Why would the physician need a culture and sensitivity?

Benign and Malignant Tumors

The urinary tract is also susceptible to the development of growths that may be cancerous or noncancerous. They can develop in the bladder or kidney. When the growth is a malignant tumor in the kidney, there may not be any treatment other than removal of the kidney. Bladder tumors are more frequently found in

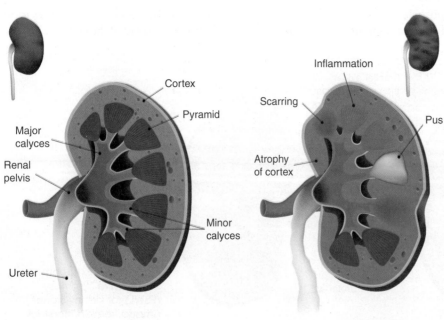

Normal kidney

Cortex
Pyramid
Major calyces
Renal pelvis
Minor calyces
Ureter

Pyelonephritis

Inflammation
Scarring
Pus
Atrophy of cortex

Figure 9-4 Pyelonephritis. (Image from Shutterstock.com.)

men over the age of 50. These also may be benign or malignant.

In order to visualize the inside of the bladder, a cystoscope is used. It is a lighted endoscope that is inserted through the urethra into the bladder. After the growth is identified, it can be surgically removed, and if malignant, radiation or chemotherapy may be indicated. If the bladder has suffered too much damage or involvement, removal of the bladder is required, a cystectomy. In this case, the ureters are rerouted to the small intestine.

Other Urinary System Disorders

There are several other specific disorders of the urinary tract that include the following:

- Polycystic kidney disease—genetic disorder resulting in development of fluid-filled sacs (cysts) in the kidney; the sacs put pressure on the nephrons causing renal failure, which results in the need for renal dialysis and kidney transplant.
- Kidney (renal) failure—kidneys fail to function properly.
- Acute renal failure—may be a complication of a serious illness or due to toxins entering the body.
- Chronic renal failure—loss of nephrons over a period of time.

With renal failure, usually chronic type, there are associated symptoms including the following:

- Edema—accumulation of fluid in the tissues; the kidneys lose the ability to filter excess water.
- **Uremia**—excess of nitrogen waste substances in the blood; the kidneys lose the ability to properly filter the blood.
- Dehydration—excessive fluid loss; the kidneys lose the ability to concentrate the urine and filter too much water out of the body.

In addition to the above symptoms, patients may develop hypertension due to the water retention and electrolyte imbalance. Anemia may also be present due to the kidney's inability to produce the hormone necessary to activate red blood cell production in the bone marrow.

Kidney Treatments

After confirmation of a diagnosis of a kidney disorder, there may be a need for more aggressive treatments to help resolve the condition, these include the following:

- **Dialysis**—also called hemodialysis; it uses a dialysis machine to filter the blood; patients may have a fistula that connects their blood vessel to the machine's filtering system. Figure 9-5 is a diagram of a fistula in a dialysis patient's arm. Notice the exit for the blood

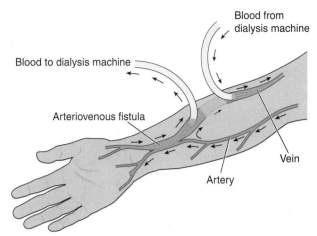

Figure 9-5 Fistula in a dialysis patient's arm. (Image from Shutterstock.com.)

to leave the body for the machine and the reentry of the blood from the machine after it has been filtered.

- Kidney transplant—removing the affected kidney and replacing it with a donor kidney; many patients have had a family member donate one of their kidneys; this is a better way to ensure a good tissue match.

 ## THE REPRODUCTIVE SYSTEM

The reproductive system is located in close proximity to the urinary system. There are primary and accessory organs. The primary male sex glands are the testes, and the female glands are the ovaries. Another term for sex glands is gonads. We will examine the male and female reproductive systems separately.

 ## MALE REPRODUCTIVE SYSTEM

The male reproductive system produces the sperm and delivers it to the female in order to fertilize the female ova (eggs) resulting in reproduction of the human species. Figure 9-6 is a diagram of the major structures of the male reproductive system.

The Testes

The testes are the male gonads (sex glands). They are located in the scrotum, an external sac between the thighs. Prior to birth, the testes are formed in the abdomen and then normally descend into the scrotum through the inguinal canal. They are suspended into the scrotum

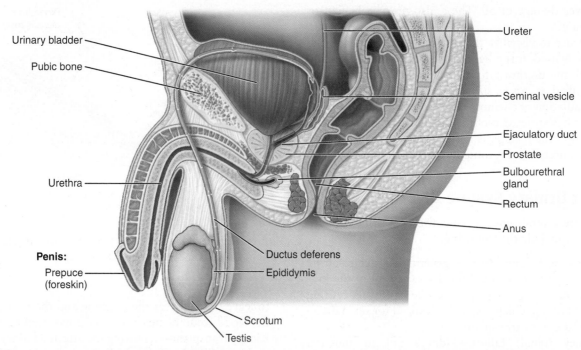

Figure 9-6 Male reproductive system. (Reprinted from Cohen BJ. *Memmler's The Human Body in Health and Disease.* 13th ed. Burlington, MA: Jones & Bartlett Learning, LLC; 2014.)

by the spermatic cord. The scrotal sac provides a good environment, out of the abdomen, where the testes are maintained at an ideal temperature for the production and maturing of the sperm. In the testis are seminiferous tubules where the sperm are nourished and develop. Also, the testes secrete testosterone, the male hormone.

Spermatozoa

Males begin to produce sperm during puberty. This is a constant process, which begins to decrease as the male approaches 40 years of age. Some men continue to produce sperm as late as 70 to 90 years of age.

Each sperm has a head, midsection, and a tail. The head, the acrosome, contains enzymes that help the sperm to penetrate the female egg. The midsection contains mitochondria, also necessary to provide energy for the sperm's movement. The flagellum (tail) is used to propel the sperm as it swims in the semen headed for the female egg. See Figure 9-7, a diagram of a single spermatozoa.

Male Accessory Organs

The testes are the primary reproductive organs; however, there are additional structures necessary to support the process of reproduction transferring the sperm to the female body. After the sperm are produced in the testis (singular), the sperm are delivered to the epididymis, a coiled tube, where they will mature and become very motile section capable of the long journey from the

male body to the female. The sperm travel from the epididymis to the vas deferens, a long tube that leads to the seminal vesicle, then to the ejaculatory duct where they finally empty into the urethra. The urethra from the bladder serves two functions, to transport urine and semen with sperm.

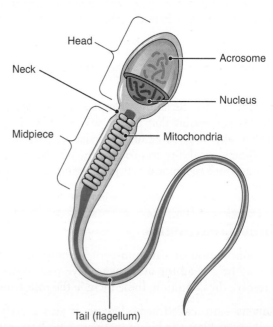

Figure 9-7 Spermatozoa. (Reprinted from Cohen BJ. *Memmler's The Human Body in Health and Disease.* 13th ed. Burlington, MA: Jones & Bartlett Learning, LLC; 2014.)

Semen

Although semen is not an accessory organ, it is required for the transport of the sperm. It is necessary to nourish the sperm and protect it from the acidic environment of the male urethra and female vaginal canal. It has an alkaline pH of 7.2 to 7.8 (7.0 is neutral, neither acidic nor alkaline). The seminal vesicles produce a large part of the semen's volume, which is made up of simple sugar and other substances.

Prostate Gland

The prostate gland is located inferior to the urinary bladder. The urethra from the bladder is surrounded by the prostate. Imagine a donut, the prostate gland, and the urethra going through the donut hole. The prostate gland also secretes an alkaline substance that is added to the semen. The gland is muscular allowing it to assist in the ejaculation of the sperm from the body. Below the prostate gland are two small organs called the bulbourethral glands (Cowper glands). These glands secrete a substance that lubricates the urethra and tip of the penis during sexual stimulation.

The Penis

The urethra extends through the length of the penis and carries urine and semen. During sexual arousal, blood fills the spongy tissue of the penis causing it to become erect (erection). At the end of the penis, there is a loose fold of skin called the foreskin, also known as the prepuce. A circumcision is the surgical removal of the foreskin. It is typically performed on infants for cultural or religious reasons but also thought to improve cleanliness of the penis and promote disease prevention.

Cultural Connection

There are many cultural rituals surrounding the birth of a baby; however, one of the more recognized is the circumcision of a male infant. Even though many Jews may not follow all the parts of Judaism, circumcision is almost always observed. The Brit Milah, the Covenant of Circumcision, is the celebration of the circumcision when the actual procedure is performed on the 8th day of the child's life. The circumcision, surgical removal of the foreskin of the penis, is performed by a mohel (the circumciser), a Jew who is educated in Jewish law and surgical techniques. A regular physician does not qualify to perform the Brit Milah unless he or she is also religiously qualified. Even though circumcision is performed as a Jewish rite, non-Jewish men are frequently circumcised because of the hygienic benefits. Also, circumcised males have a lower risk of certain cancers.

The erect penis is better able to deliver the semen with sperm into the female vagina through a process called ejaculation, the forceful expulsion of semen through the urethra. When this occurs, an involuntary sphincter near the bladder closes so that urine cannot be released. It only takes one sperm to fertilize the female ovum; however, there can be as many as 50 to 150 million sperm in 1 mL of semen.

Male Hormones

Hormones are substances that stimulate processes and changes in the body. The male reproductive system functions under the control of two hormones:

- **FSH**—follicle-stimulating hormone to promote the formation of sperm.
- **LH**—luteinizing hormone produces testosterone and development of the sperm.

Testosterone

Testosterone is produced in the testes and is responsible for development of sperm and maintenance of the male reproductive system, but one of the primary functions is the development of secondary sex characteristics. These include development of the body with more muscle tissue, broader shoulders, deepening of the voice, and body hair growth.

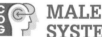 ## MALE REPRODUCTIVE SYSTEM DISORDERS

The structures of the male reproductive system can become infected and inflamed, may be deformed from birth or through injury, and are subject to developing tumors. Table 9-1 is a list of the more common disorders affecting the male reproductive system.

Cancer of Male Reproductive System

The most common location of cancer in the male is in the prostate gland and the testicle.

Prostate Gland Cancer

Cancer of the prostate gland usually affects males over 50 years of age. The prostate gland is located below the bladder and surrounds the urethra. The physician examines the prostate by palpating the gland during a rectal examination. If a nodule is detected, further investigation of the gland is recommended to determine if there is a problem with the prostate including cancer. The physician will order a blood test to check the **PSA** level, prostate-specific antigen. The PSA is a protein that

Table 9-1 Male Reproductive System Disorders

Cryptorchidism	Undescended testicle; could result in infertility if uncorrected; usually requires surgical correction
Testicular torsion	Testis rotates in the scrotum; the spermatic cord twists interfering with the blood supply.
Phimosis	Foreskin of the penis is tight and cannot be drawn back; surgical correction with circumcision
Inguinal hernia	Weakened area of the abdominal wall allows part of the small intestine to pass through the inguinal canal into the scrotum; typically results from heavy lifting that puts excess stress on the weakened area; surgical repair required to correct problem
Epididymitis	Inflammation of the epididymis; may be caused by a bacterial infection, including sexually transmitted infections (**STIs**), such as gonorrhea or chlamydia
Prostatitis	Inflammation of the prostate gland; may be caused by infection or injury to the prostate
Orchitis	Inflammation of the testis; may be caused from other infected area of the reproductive structures and following an infection from the virus that causes mumps
Genital herpes	Common sexually transmitted infection (STI), formerly STD, sexually transmitted disease; caused by a virus characterized by blisters in the genital region
Syphilis	Caused by a spirochete, *Treponema pallidum*; STI that causes genital ulcers
Erectile dysfunction	Inability to obtain or maintain an erection; affects men of any age, but higher incidence with age
Benign prostatic hyperplasia (**BPH**)	Nonmalignant prostate enlargement; the gland enlarges putting pressure on the urethra, interfering with urination. Treatment includes medication to shrink the prostate, surgical removal of the prostate, or reducing the urethral obstruction by implanting a stent. Figure 9-8 is a comparison of a healthy prostate gland and one that has enlarged around the urethra

increases when there is cancer in the prostate gland. The risk factors for prostate cancer include the patient's age, family history and high-fat diet. The cure rate for prostate cancer is good. Treatments include radiation therapy, surgical removal of the prostate, or hormone therapy.

Testicular Cancer

This type of cancer typically affects young to middle-aged adults. As with other cancers, early detection is the key to a good prognosis and outcome. Testicular self-examination is recommended for all young men and is part of the regular physical examination by a health care

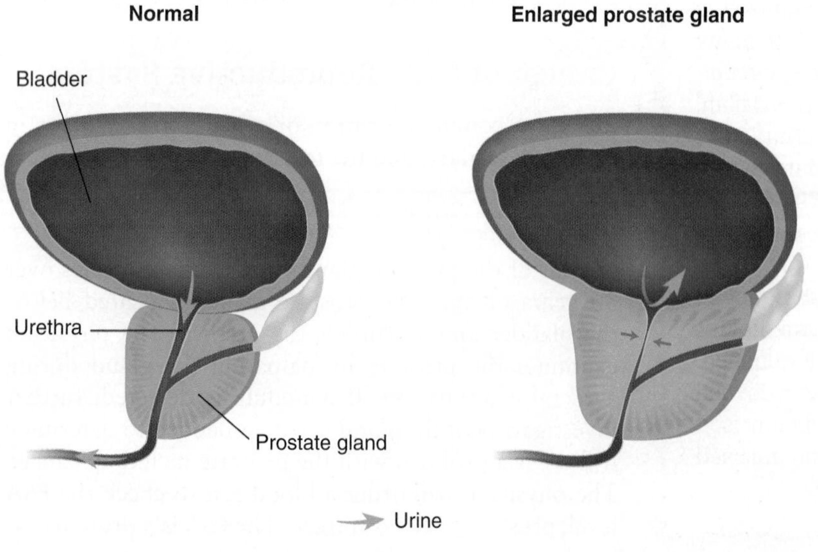

Figure 9-8 Benign prostatic hyperplasia. (Image from Shutterstock.com.)

provider. In the event that a testicle would need to be removed, sperm banking is recommended to preserve sperm for future fertilization.

THE FEMALE REPRODUCTIVE SYSTEM

The female reproductive system consists of the primary glands or gonads, the ovaries where the ova are matured and several accessory organs. Figure 9-9 is a diagram of the major female reproductive structures.

The Ovaries

The right and left ovaries are located in the pelvic cavity near the end of the fallopian tubes. Females are born with all the ova (eggs) they will ever produce. In the newborn, there are more than a million immature follicles containing the eggs, which will begin to develop as the female enters puberty. Then each month during the female cycle, an individual ovum will mature. During puberty, the follicles begin to develop and mature the ova. Each month of a female's reproductive years, a follicle will release a mature egg ready for fertilization.

Female Reproductive Accessory Organs

The organs that support the female reproductive system include the uterus, uterine tubes (fallopian tubes), and vagina. The female breasts are also included in these organs since they support the further nourishment of the newborn.

The Uterus

The uterus is a muscular organ that serves only one function, to allow a fetus to develop. It is located in the pelvic cavity between the bladder and the rectum. The upper

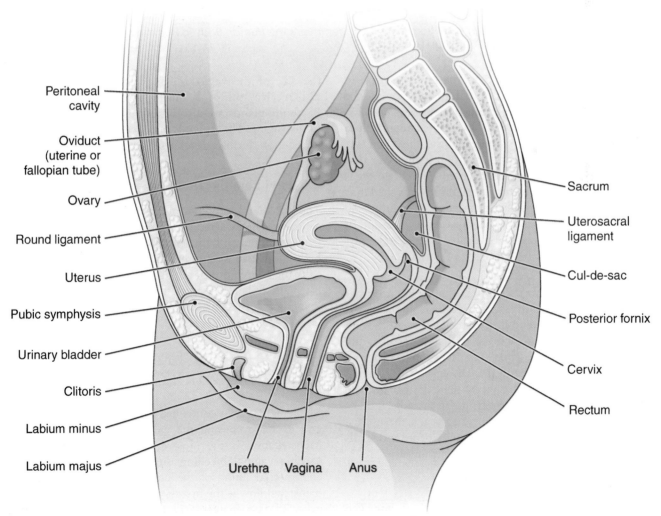

Figure 9-9 Female reproductive system. (Reprinted from Kronenberger J, Ledbetter J. *Jones & Bartlett Learning's Comprehensive Medical Assisting.* 5th ed. Burlington, MA: Jones & Bartlett Learning, LLC; 2016.)

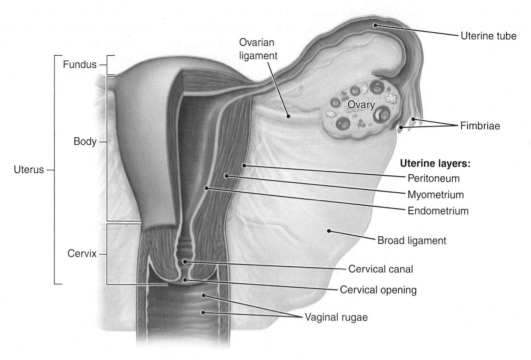

Frontal view

Figure 9-10 Anterior uterus. (Reprinted from Cohen BJ. *Memmler's The Human Body in Health and Disease.* 13th ed. Burlington, MA: Jones & Bartlett Learning, LLC; 2014.)

region of the uterus is the body. The lower portion of the uterus narrows toward the inferior end becoming the cervix (neck). The superior, rounded part of the uterus is the fundus. The uterus has three layers, the **endometrium** (inner), the myometrium (muscular, middle), and the perimetrium (outer). The endometrium is the layer that prepares to receive the fertilized egg; however, if no egg is implanted on the endometrial layer, the layer is shed during the monthly cycle called menstruation. Figure 9-10 is an anterior view of the uterus showing the location of the fundus, body, cervix, and the three layers.

The Uterine Tubes

These tubes, known as the fallopian tubes, are approximately 5 inches long and extend laterally from the uterus to an area where they end close to the ovaries. At the end of each tube is a small extension that looks like tiny fingers called fimbriae. These extensions collect the egg as it is released from the ovary. The egg is then carried down the uterine tube assisted by the cilia that line the tube. From the time the egg starts down the tube, it takes approximately 5 days for the egg to reach the uterus. This provides enough time for sperm to locate and fertilize the egg so it can be implanted on the uterus.

The Vagina

The vagina is a muscular tube about 3 inches long. The cervix of the uterus is visible at the uppermost part of the vagina. The vagina has rugae (folds) that enlarge

the size of the vagina during childbirth. The vagina also receives the penis during sexual intercourse. The Bartholin glands are also found just above the opening of the vagina. These glands produce mucus that provides lubrication during intercourse.

External Female Genitalia

The vulva and perineum make up the external female genitalia. The external region includes the labia majora, labia minora, and the clitoris, a small organ that is highly sensitive to stimulation. The perineum is technically the entire floor of the pelvic cavity; in the female, it is usually only referring to the area between the vaginal opening and the anus.

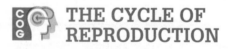

THE CYCLE OF REPRODUCTION

The female cycle is controlled by hormones that increase and decrease causing the various stages of the cycle. Menstruation is the most common part of the cycle causing vaginal bleeding due to the shedding of the endometrial lining of the uterus. The first day of the menstrual flow is the first day of the cycle, which occurs every 28 days on average; however, some women have a cycle length between 22 and 45 days. Figure 9-11 shows the typical 28-day menstrual cycle.

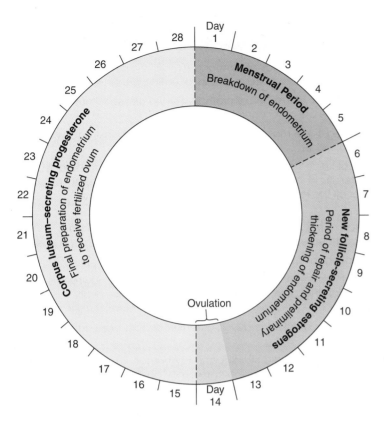

Figure 9-11 Menstruation cycle. (Reprinted from Cohen BJ, Wood DL. *Memmler's The Human Body in Health and Disease.* 11th ed. Burlington, MA: Jones & Bartlett Learning, LLC; 2009, with permission.)

Ovulation

Ovulation is the process of releasing an egg from the ovary follicle. There are two phases to the process:

- Preovulatory phase—also known as the follicular phase; it is stimulated by follicle-stimulating hormone (FSH) produced in the pituitary gland; causes growth and maturing of the follicle; estrogen is also released causing the endometrium to prepare for a fertilized egg.
- Postovulatory phase—also known as the luteal phase; it is stimulated by luteinizing hormone (LH); the follicle ruptures and the egg is released, ovulation; LH also promotes the transformation of the follicle into the corpus luteum, which secretes progesterone, a hormone necessary to help the fertilized ovum survive.

Menstruation

During an average cycle of 28 days, ovulation usually occurs on the 14th day, and then if fertilization did not occur, the menstrual flow starts 2 weeks later. Menstruation, also called menses, is the shedding of the lining of the uterus, the endometrium causing bleeding. An average menstrual cycle lasts from 2 to 6 days with an average of 4 to 5 days.

Menopause

Menopause occurs when menstruation no longer takes place. Women can begin to experience symptoms of menopause in their mid 40s or 50s. The ovaries gradually begin to decrease their function during this time. Since the ovaries are no longer functioning, there is a decrease in the amount of estrogen and progesterone causing changes to take place in the female reproductive organs. They begin to atrophy, and the vaginal canal becomes dryer and more sensitive due to the lack of mucus production. Although menopause is a normal occurrence in all women, it brings about varying effects or symptoms. Some of these include hot flashes, anxiety, and insomnia. Some physicians may suggest hormone replacement therapy (**HRT**) to help manage these symptoms. HRT may have benefits; however, it also increases the risk of breast cancer and development of blood clots.

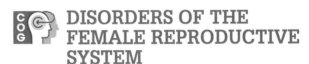

DISORDERS OF THE FEMALE REPRODUCTIVE SYSTEM

The female reproductive organs are subject to conditions including infections, menstrual disorders, and cancer. Table 9-2 provides information about some of the most common conditions affecting the female organs.

Table 9-2 Female Reproductive System Disorders

Amenorrhea	Absence of menstrual flow; may be due to lack of hormone stimulation, psychological disorders, and women who are very athletic or have dietary or eating disorders
Dysmenorrhea	Painful or difficult menstruation related with muscular cramping of the uterus; in most women, there is no known cause unless there are other conditions present such as endometriosis
Abnormal uterine bleeding (symptom)	Menorrhagia is excessive bleeding; there may be other than during the menstrual cycle; these may indicate underlying disease
Endometriosis	Condition when the endometrial tissue grows outside the uterus, attaching to the ovaries, peritoneum, or pelvic organs; results in inflammation that may require surgical removal of the uterus (hysterectomy) or all the reproductive organs (**TAH**), total abdominal hysterectomy
Premenstrual syndrome (**PMS**)	Occurs 1 to 2 wk before the start of the menstrual period; symptoms include bloating, headache, fatigue, irritability, and depression usually due to the changes in hormone levels.
Vaginitis	Any inflammation of the vaginal canal; may be caused from bacteria, yeast, or parasite
Ovarian cysts	Small ovarian fluid-filled sac that forms from the corpus luteum; causes pain; however, may rupture causing severe abdominal pain; may require surgery to remove ovary (oophorectomy)
Genital warts	Caused by **HPV**, human papillomavirus; linked to development of cancer in the reproductive organs
Sexually transmitted infections (STI)	Includes gonorrhea, genital herpes, chlamydia, syphilis, and HIV, human immunodeficiency virus; these infections may lead to infertility or, in some cases, may pass from the mother to the fetus
Salpingitis	In the female, inflammation of the uterine (fallopian) tubes usually caused from gonorrhea or chlamydia
Pelvic inflammatory disease (**PID**)	Infection, occasionally caused from multiple bacterial organisms, invades the reproductive organs and into the pelvic cavity sometimes involving the peritoneum; also may result in infertility
Fibroids	Tumors of the uterus that are usually benign; may enlarge putting pressure on surrounding structures; some fibroids may be surgically removed; however, a hysterectomy may be necessary
Endometrial cancer	Typically affects women during or after menopause; may be due to high levels of estrogen through HRT; cancer is determined by tissue biopsy
Ovarian cancer	Cancer of the ovary that might result from ovarian cysts; vague symptoms make this type of cancer difficult to detect
Cervical cancer	Cancer of the cervix that is linked to HPV infection; the virus is sexually transmitted, so sexual activity at an early age and with multiple partners may contribute to the development of this cancer; a vaccine against HPV is recommended for females from 11 to 12 y of age

 # CARING FOR THE FEMALE REPRODUCTIVE SYSTEM

The female reproductive organs sometimes need the attention of a gynecologist, a specialist that cares for women's disorders. One of the most common procedures performed by the gynecologist is a pap smear, Papanicolaou test, named after the inventor and Greek physician, Georgios Papanikolaou. The procedure involves collection of cells from the cervix for microscopic examination. This is the earliest way to detect the presence of cancer cells. All women are encouraged to start annual testing when they become sexually active or as soon as 18 years of age.

Infertility

Several of the disorders of the female reproductive system may contribute to infertility, which is the inability to achieve pregnancy. The diagnosis is not determined until after at least 1 year of unprotected, regular sexual intercourse. Either the male or female, or both, may have a problem that is the cause of the infertility. In the male, it could be due to oligospermia, low sperm count. This condition could be due to infections causing blockage to the ducts, exposure to x-rays, or even excessive heat to the area such as a hot tub. The female who is infertile may also have a history of infections or other abnormalities of the reproductive organs that contribute to the infertile environment. STI are commonly the cause of the development of scar tissue that blocks the fallopian tubes.

Birth Control

Birth control is the process of preventing pregnancy until it is desired. Contraception is the termed used to describe an artificial method to prevent the fertilization of the egg and implantation on the uterine wall. There are several methods of birth control that include the following:

- Surgical sterilization—in the female, tubal ligation, and in the male, vasectomy; these procedures interrupt the fallopian tube (female) or the vas deferens (male) by severing them or cauterizing the ducts.
- Hormone contraception—delivered to the body by pill, injection, skin patch, or implant; interferes with the maturation of the follicle and development of the egg, preventing ovulation.
- Morning after pill—RU-486 (mifepristone) is an emergency contraceptive pill that is taken within several hours of intercourse; forces the uterus to shed its lining and release the fertilized egg; it has been referred to as the "abortion pill."
- Condom—a sheath that fits over the penis or into the vagina designed to act as a barrier for semen to enter the female; also used as a means to protect from transfer of STI between partners.
- Abstinence—voluntarily withholding from sexual intercourse in an effort to avoid pregnancy; probably not the most reliable method of birth control.

PREGNANCY AND CHILDBIRTH

So we have looked at both the male and female reproductive systems, and if all systems are working properly, a pregnancy may occur. Now let's see how the pregnancy develops with the fertilization of the egg through the birth of the baby. The normal time of gestation, period of development, is 280 days, or 40 weeks from the first day of the woman's last menstrual period (**LMP**). The due date is called the estimated date of confinement (**EDC**). When a woman is pregnant, she will usually seek medical care from an obstetrician, a specialist who oversees pregnancy, prenatal, delivery, and postnatal periods.

Getting Pregnant

The natural first step in becoming pregnant is the deposit of semen in the vagina by the male. Millions of sperm are in the semen and their goal is to travel (swim) to the egg and fertilize it. The egg cell (oocyte) needs to be present in the fallopian tube where the sperm will surround it. Only one sperm will be allowed to puncture through the cell wall and fertilize it. The head of the sperm uses the enzymes to dissolve the coating around the egg. Once the sperm and the egg unite, the single cell is called a zygote, which has the 46 required human chromosomes. The zygote now makes it way down the uterine tube toward the uterus where it will implant and begin to develop. After implantation on the uterine wall, it is called an embryo.

After implantation, human chorionic gonadotropin (hCG) is produced for about 12 weeks. This is the substance that is the indicator for pregnancy tests. The urine pregnancy tests used in the physician's office and the home kits check for hCG in the urine. At the beginning of the 3rd month of pregnancy, the embryo is now called the fetus. There are two supporting structures for the fetus:

- Placenta—an organ composed of a spongy network of blood-filled areas and capillaries that provide nourishment, respiration, and excretion for the fetus; gases are exchanged, nutrients supplied, and waste products eliminated.
- Umbilical cord—the connection of the fetus to the placenta; this is the blood supply for the fetus.

The Developing Fetus

The pregnancy is divided into equal 3 month segments called trimesters. By the end of the 2nd month of pregnancy, the embryo has started to develop the heart, brain, nervous system, and limb buds. The heartbeat is detectable by the end of the first month, and it is the most sensitive to harmful substances, smoking and drinking being among the primary ones. Miscarriage, the loss of an embryo or fetus, more frequently occurs during this time. The fetus is contained within a sac of fluid called the amniotic sac. At birth, this sac ruptures and the amniotic fluid is released. We say that the mother's "water broke." Figure 9-12 is a picture of a full-term pregnancy with developed fetus ready for delivery.

The Pregnant Mother

One of the first symptoms that a pregnant woman may experience is nausea and vomiting. There are hormonal changes taking place, and now the pregnancy needs to supply all the required nourishment and oxygen to the developing fetus as well as provide for the elimination of the waste products. The mother's body metabolism changes to accommodate the growing fetus for these organs:

- Heart—increased blood supply pumped to the fetus
- Kidneys—increased kidney function to excrete wastes from the fetus
- Lungs—increased oxygen intake and elimination of carbon dioxide
- Digestive—increased nutrients during pregnancy and milk production following birth

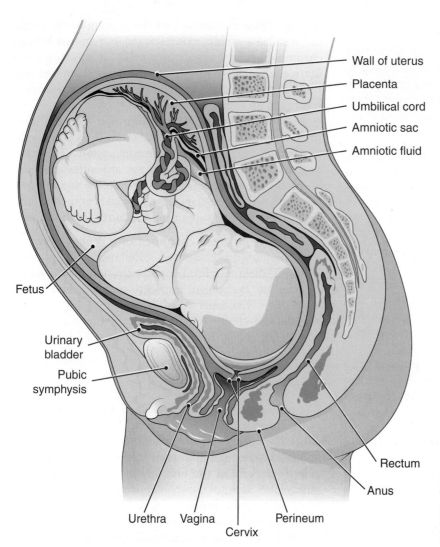

Wall of uterus
Placenta
Umbilical cord
Amniotic sac
Amniotic fluid

Fetus

Urinary bladder

Pubic symphysis

Rectum

Anus

Urethra   Vagina   Perineum

Cervix

Figure 9-12   Full-term fetus. (Reprinted from Cohen BJ. *Memmler's The Human Body in Health and Disease*. 13th ed. Burlington, MA: Jones & Bartlett Learning, LLC; 2014.)

As the pregnancy progresses, the mother may also start to experience frequent urination and occasionally constipation. Throughout the pregnancy, the obstetrician may perform an ultrasound to study the progression of the fetus, the fetal age, and location of the placenta. Ultrasonography is a safe, painless, noninvasive procedure that uses reflected high-frequency sound waves to provide an image of the soft tissue on the monitor. It is also possible to determine some fetal abnormalities and defects.

The Birth of the Baby

The mother and baby work in concert to accomplish the delivery of the baby. The first event that initiates a normal delivery is the contraction of the uterus, which involves the following:

- Uterine contractions begin as the uterine muscles stimulate prostaglandins, hormone-like substances that affect smooth muscle contraction.
- The baby stimulates release of the hormone oxytocin by putting pressure on the cervix further stimulating uterine contractions; this is an example of positive

feedback, amplifying stimulation to accomplish a temporary goal.
- The baby's adrenal cortex affects a decrease in the mother's progesterone and thus an increase in estrogen, which stimulates uterine contractions.

The uterine contractions signal the beginning of labor, which has four stages:

- First stage—regular uterine contractions causing the cervix to become thinner; also, rupture of the amniotic sac of fluid.
- Second stage—complete dilation of the cervix and delivery of the baby through the birth canal; should be delivered head first.
- Third stage—delivery of the placenta, the afterbirth.
- Fourth stage—bleeding is controlled by contraction of the uterine muscles acting to close the blood vessels where the placenta was located.

During the delivery, it may be necessary for the obstetrician, or health care provider, to perform an **episiotomy**. This is a procedure that involves making a small incision between the vagina and the anus to increase the size of the delivery area, avoiding tearing the vaginal opening. After the final stage of labor, the incision is sutured.

If there is a concern for the mother or baby completing a normal vaginal delivery, a **cesarean section** (C-section) may be performed. This involves a surgical incision made in the abdominal wall and uterus to remove the baby. The decision to perform a C-section may be due to the abnormal position of the fetus with the buttocks presenting first, not the head, or if the fetus is too large to safely deliver through the vaginal canal. A woman may start to have premature labor causing risk to the fetus. C-section also ensures a speedy delivery, taking only a few minutes.

Multiple Births

Occasionally, a pregnancy will produce more than one baby. Multiple births include twins, two babies; triplets, three babies; quadruplets, four babies; and quintuplets, five babies. Many of the multiple births have resulted from the use of fertility drugs. There have been multiple births that result in more than five babies; however, these are not very common and are extremely high risk for the life of the mother and the babies. Since twins are the most common multiple birth scenario, there are two types of twins:

- Fraternal twins—different individuals result from fertilization of two different eggs and by two different sperm; each fetus has a placenta and amniotic sac.

- Identical twins—always the same sex and have the same traits (appear alike); develop from a single egg and sperm; however, during development, the embryo separates into two units; there is a single placenta but a separate umbilical cord for each fetus.

Pregnancy Conditions

There is joy at the birth of a healthy, bouncing baby; however, there are also situations and conditions that may lead to complications. The initial health and condition of a newborn is determined by an Apgar score. The infant is graded on its respiration, heart rate, color, and responses to stimulation. A maximum Apgar score is 10, and babies with a low Apgar require immediate medical attention. Table 9-3 lists some of the terms used during pregnancy and the various situations encountered.

The Female Breasts

Following the delivery of the infant, the mother will experience changes in the breasts as they prepare to nurse the baby. The mammary glands, in the breasts, provide the nourishment for the baby. The mammary glands are composed of several lobes, which secrete the milk through the lactiferous ducts. The first amount of milk that is secreted is very thin, watery liquid called colostrum. The most nutritious milk will not be available for several days following the birth. Most pediatricians, baby doctors, will recommend nursing

Table 9-3	Pregnancy Conditions
Term infant	Infant born at full gestation period of 37–42 wk
Live birth	Infant delivered and able to breathe unassisted and has heartbeat
Preterm	Infant born prior to 37 wk; called premature and usually weighs <5 pounds; may have breathing problems; the term **viable** means able to live outside the uterus
Spontaneous abortion	Also known as a miscarriage; occurs naturally; however, may be the result of chromosome abnormalities or maternal diseases including infections and chronic disorders (diabetes); **abortion** is a general term that means the loss of the embryo or fetus prior to week 20 of the pregnancy
Induced abortion	A deliberate interruption of the pregnancy
Stillbirth	Death of the baby after 24 wk but before birth; intrauterine means the fetus died while in the uterus
Ectopic pregnancy	Develops outside the uterine cavity; most common location is in the uterine tube (tubal pregnancy); the tube will eventually rupture if not surgically removed; more prevalent in women with history of PID and endometriosis
Placenta previa	Placenta attaches too close to the internal opening of the cervix; risk of premature detachment of the placenta risking the fetal blood and oxygen supply
Abruptio placentae	Premature separation of the placenta from the uterine wall causing hemorrhage; may require termination of the pregnancy
Gestational diabetes mellitus	Diagnosis of diabetes only during pregnancy; most return to normal following the delivery; however, some women may go onto develop type 2 diabetes
Preeclampsia	Also known as pregnancy-induced hypertension (PIH); later in the pregnancy, the mother experiences high blood pressure and proteinuria (protein in the urine)
Postpartum depression	A psychologic condition that occurs within the first year following childbirth; may be due to hormonal changes and stress of the new family

an infant for the first few weeks to months because of the immune properties (antibodies) of the mother's milk that are passed on to the baby. Nursing an infant also ensures bonding between the mother and the infant.

Breast Disorders

One of the most common types of cancer occurring in women is breast cancer. The common factors that increase the chances of developing breast cancer is the age of the women, over 40 years of age, family history, and long-term use of hormones. A growth in the breast may be benign or malignant, so all masses should be investigated. A **mammogram** is an x-ray study of the breast and will detect even small growths. A physician may want to perform a needle biopsy of the growth to collect cells for microscopic examination. Treatment of breast cancer includes radiation and chemotherapy and surgical removal of

the lump or the entire breast (mastectomy). Mastitis, inflammation of the breast, is also a condition caused by an infection. The mammary glands become infected and painful. Antibiotics are used to treat this condition.

Study Skill

As an educator, I frequently ask students if they studied for an exam and 9 times of 10, I get the answer "yes, I studied for hours." Research has shown that students do better retaining information when they study in blocks of time usually no more than 1 hour at a time. Make a study schedule and stick to it. Organize a study location and try to do your studying in that same location, around the same time. This plan helps you build a good study habit. Good habits usually equal success.

Preparing for Externship

As you approach your externship, keep your eye on the "prize." In this case, the prize is successful completion of the externship and on to graduation. Don't let anything interfere with your ability to be successful during the externship course. Sometimes there are issues that arise that are caused by personality conflicts. Even though the medical office accepts extern students, not all the office staff may be excited about the prospect of having a student in the office for a few weeks. When a student is in the office, the other medical assistants may feel burdened by the responsibility of watching over the new student. You can be more assertive asking what you can do to assist everyone

and not seem like extra work for the staff. There may be a staff member who feels threatened about losing his or her job to a new employee. That new employee just might be you. If there is a specific incident that causes conflict between you and a staff member, do not argue and make the matter worse. Talk with your school instructor or externship coordinator about the situation and the best way to handle it. When a negative situation arises, a student may ask to be moved to a new extern site but that is not the best solution. Try to find a way to resolve the conflict. You cannot always avoid a situation and run away from it. Become the professional and work toward a win–win result.

Chapter Recap

- The urinary system is another vital system in the body, which helps to maintain homeostasis by regulating fluid and electrolyte balance.
- The nephron is the microscopic, functional unit of the kidney and the structure that actually produces the urine.
- The kidneys are constantly filtering blood, as much as 180 L of plasma (liquid part of the blood) each day.
- Urine is 95% water, and the rest of it is dissolved solids and gases.
- The urinary tract from the kidneys to the urethra can be affected by infections, structural problems, and cancer; however, urinary tract infections (UTIs) are probably the most common condition affecting the urinary tract.
- The male reproductive system produces the sperm and delivers it to the female in order to fertilize the

female ova (eggs) resulting in reproduction of the human species.
- The testes are the male gonads (sex glands), and the ovaries are the female gonads.
- The male and female may experience infertility due to infections or underlying diseases that alter the ability of the organs to function properly.
- Both the male and female reproductive organs are at risk to the development of various types of cancer.
- During pregnancy, there are many conditions that can affect the development of the fetus to term.
- The mother's breasts are the primary accessory organs that support the infant in the early stages of development after delivery.

Online Resources for Students

Student Resources available on the text's online site include:
- Audio Glossaries
- Animations
- Competency Evaluation Forms
- Videos
- Anatomy & Physiology Module with Heart and Lung Sounds
- Weblinks
- Worksheets

Exercises and Activities

Certification Preparation Questions

1. Which of these is necessary for controlling the reabsorption of water in the kidney?
   a. ADH
   b. FSH
   c. HRT
   d. hCG
   e. LH

2. Which of these terms is associated with a urinary infection?
   a. Albuminuria
   b. Ketonuria
   c. Pyuria
   d. Glycosuria
   e. Anuria

3. What condition is associated with the buildup of nitrogenous waste in the blood?
   a. Enuresis
   b. Edema
   c. Anuria
   d. Nocturemia
   e. Uremia

4. Which of these is the functional unit of the kidney?
   a. Renal pelvis
   b. Medulla
   c. Nephron
   d. Cortex
   e. Loop of Henle

5. The term used to describe the location of the kidneys is:
   a. medioperitoneal.
   b. anteroperitoneal.
   c. subthoracic.
   d. retroperitoneal.
   e. suprapubic.

6. Which of these is a condition of having an undescended testicle?
   a. Phimosis
   b. Cryptorchidism
   c. Testicular torsion
   d. Epididymitis
   e. Orchitis

7. BPH is a condition that involves enlargement of the:
   a. penis.
   b. testis.
   c. prostate.
   d. epididymis.
   e. bulbourethral glands.

8. Which term is used to describe painful or difficult menstruation?
   a. Amenorrhea
   b. Dysmenorrhea
   c. Menorrhagia
   d. Menopause
   e. Premenstrual syndrome

9. Which term is used to describe the condition when there is growth of uterine lining outside the uterus?
   a. Vaginitis
   b. Salpingitis
   c. Cervicitis
   d. Fibroids
   e. Endometriosis

10. Which abbreviation is used to express the due date of the baby?
    a. EDC
    b. FSH
    c. HRT
    d. LMP
    e. hCG

Section III

Administrative Medical Assistant Skills

10 Appointments and Schedules

Chapter Objectives

- Relate the basics of appointment scheduling and management.
- Describe the systems used for scheduling appointments.
- Identify the factors that affect appointment scheduling.
- Follow a set of steps to schedule new patients and return visits.
- Specify three ways to remind patients of appointments.
- Explain how to triage patient emergencies, acutely ill patients, and walk-ins.
- Understand how to handle late patients, delays, cancellations, and missed appointments.
- Schedule inpatient and outpatient admissions and procedures.
- Make referral and consultation appointments with other physicians.
- Follow third-party guidelines to schedule tests and other procedures.
- Schedule hospital admissions for patients.

CAAHEP & ABHES Competencies

CAAHEP

- Discuss pros and cons of various types of appointment management systems.
- Describe scheduling guidelines.
- Recognize office policies and protocols for handling appointments.
- Identify critical information required for scheduling patient admissions and/or procedures.
- Manage appointment schedule, using established priorities.
- Schedule patient admissions and/or procedures.

ABHES

- Apply scheduling principles.
- Scheduling of in- and outpatient procedures.
- Understand procedures for hospital admission and procedures.

Chapter Terms

Acute
Chronic
Clustering
Constellation of
    symptoms

Consultation
Double-booking
Fixed scheduling
Itinerary
Matrix

Modified wave scheduling
Precertification
Preferred provider
Referral
Streaming

Third-party payers
Wave scheduling

Abbreviations

CPE
EMS

ER
NPT (NP)

OV
STAT

Case Study

Matthew McNeil, a new patient (**NPT**), is calling your clinic to schedule an appointment. As Judy Simmons, medical assistant, questions Mr. McNeil about the purpose of the visit, she learns that he was referred by Dr. Linda Jones for treatment of his hypertension. He would like an appointment this week.

Patients call the office for a variety of appointments. You are probably familiar with some of them. Patients may require same-day appointments for acute illness or minor injury; others may be calling for routine care appointments, such as annual physicals or diabetic maintenance, weeks to months from today. Additionally, there may be times when patients call with an urgent or even emergency situation. You must handle such calls with calm professionalism. Your clinic may have protocols to follow utilizing basic guidelines. If you are handling an urgent or emergency case, first find out what the issue or concern is and then obtain a phone number and location. You can continue to evaluate the situation after you have the critical information (phone number and location). If the situation is a true life-threatening emergency, try to keep the patient or caller on the line while you activate **EMS** (9-1-1). If the situation is urgent, try to schedule the patient as soon as possible that day. Many clinics leave open time slots during the day for urgent need cases.

 BASICS OF APPOINTMENT SCHEDULING AND MANAGEMENT

The key to an efficiently run clinic lies in your hands. No medical clinic can run smoothly without a good system for scheduling appointments. The medical assistant must utilize care when scheduling to insure that an appropriate amount of time is reserved and that necessary equipment or rooms are available. For example, if your clinic maintains one set of surgical instruments you would need to schedule your surgical procedures to allow adequate time for cleaning and sterilization of the instruments. If someone were to schedule back-to-back surgeries, the equipment would not be ready and a serious delay would occur. You'll learn more about effective scheduling practices and ways to avoid time-wasting problems in this chapter. Of course, every office will have emergencies, delays, and unexpected schedule changes. In this chapter, you'll also learn how to manage these challenges in an efficient and professional manner.

 APPOINTMENT SCHEDULING SYSTEMS

There are two ways of scheduling appointments for patients: manual or computerized.

Case Question

If the medical assistant is not familiar with that doctor's name, how should she ask the patient about the doctor?

- In a manual system, each patient's appointment is handwritten into an appointment book using a pencil or pen.
- In a computerized system, a medical software program is used to schedule patients into an electronic appointment book that is stored on the computer.

The method you use may depend on the size of the practice and preference of the physicians/managers. A large medical practice will have many providers who see patients by appointment. These providers could include physicians, physicians' assistants, nurse practitioners, physical therapists, and other health care professionals.

Determining the best system for your clinic will require looking at all the factors. For example, are you the only person responsible for scheduling or is there a team of schedulers? After exploring the factors and the needs of the clinic, select the system that will work best for your situation.

Manual Scheduling

Some clinics may schedule all appointments manually, even if the other systems used in the office are computerized. As previously discussed, this method will require the use of an appointment book.

The Appointment Book

To schedule patients in a manual system, the first thing you'll need is an appointment book. This book will contain enough pages to record all patient appointments over a set length of time—usually a year. You may want to see a full week of appointments across the book's two facing pages when the book is open. You may prefer an appointment book with pages that show 1 day at a time.

Some appointment books even have a different page color for each day of the week. You would find this feature helpful if you had to flip forward in the book 3 weeks to make an appointment on a Wednesday, for instance.

If you work in a clinic with more than one provider, an appointment book with a page for each day is usually preferred. Each page will have a column for each provider. If your office requires a lot of patient information when scheduling, the book pages should be large enough to contain all the information.

In some offices, each doctor has their own appointment book. Appointment books come in many different colors, and each physician can have a specific color.

Appointment Book Standards

Any appointment book should meet these standards:

- The book should be divided into units of time that are appropriate for your office. Some offices may schedule patients every 10 minutes. Other offices may prefer 15-minute or 20-minute intervals.

- The book should lie flat on your desk when you're using it. It should be easy to put back into its storage space when not in use.
- Each appointment space should be large enough for you to write in all the information your office requires. This should include at least the patient's name, phone number, and the reason for the visit.

The Matrix

Before scheduling appointments, you'll need to set up a **matrix**. You do this by blocking out the times providers are not available for appointments. Some of these times—such as lunch, for instance—may be the same every day. Other times providers are not available may repeat on the same day each week—meetings, for instance. You should insure that the schedule reflects the times that your physicians are available to see the patient. Never assume that everyone knows the physician's schedule as this could result in patients being scheduled for times when a provider is not available. When creating a matrix, it is also helpful to block out hours that the office is closed. For example, if on Wednesdays your clinic is open from 7:00 AM to noon, you would block off from noon to the end of the day.

You'll have to block out other times, too, on a case-by-case basis, for vacations, business meetings, and so on. It's also a good idea to block off time in each provider's schedule as "catch-up" time for urgent or emergency appointments and delays.

The appointment system or book is important for more than just scheduling appointments. Along with the notes in a patient's chart, it provides evidence of a patient's office visits. It also shows changes such as missed and rescheduled appointments. That information could help protect a physician in legal disputes like those you read about in the chapter on Law and Ethics. The medical assistant is responsible for insuring that the appointment book is professionally maintained including the accuracy of its content. Figure 10-1 shows a typical page from a manual appointment scheduling book with the matrix built.

Case Question

If the patient in the case study says the only time he can come for an appointment time is at noon when the office is closed for the lunch break, how should the medical assistant handle this situation?

Computerized Scheduling

Most software packages available for medical office management include a system for appointment scheduling. Using a computer to create schedules is helpful because it

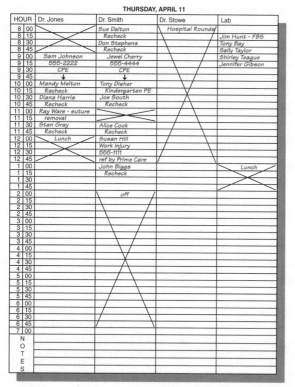

HOUR	Dr. Jones	Dr. Smith	Dr. Stowe	Lab
8 00		Sue Dalton	Hospital Rounds	
8 15		Recheck		Jim Hunt - FBS
8 30		Don Stephens		Tony Bay
8 45		Recheck		Sally Taylor
9 00	Sam Johnson	Jewel Cherry		Shirley Teague
9 15	555-2222	555-4444		Jennifer Gibson
9 30	CPE	CPE		
9 45	↓	↓		
10 00	Mandy Melton	Tony Disher		
10 15	Recheck	Kindergarten PE		
10 30	Diana Harris	Joe South		
10 45	Recheck	Recheck		
11 00	Ray Ware - suture			
11 15	removal			
11 30	Stan Gray	Alice Cook		
11 45	Recheck	Recheck		
12 00	Lunch	Susan Hill		
12 15		Work Injury		
12 30		555-1111		
12 45		ref by Prime Care		
1 00		John Biggs		Lunch
1 15		Recheck		
1 30				
1 45				
2 00		off		
2 15				
2 30				
2 45				
3 00				
3 15				
3 30				
3 45				
4 00				
4 15				
4 30				
4 45				
5 00				
5 15				
5 30				
5 45				
6 00				
6 15				
6 30				
6 45				
7 00				
NOTES				

Figure 10-1 Sample page from manual appointment book. (Reprinted from Kronenberger J, Ledbetter J. *Jones & Bartlett Learning's Comprehensive Medical Assisting.* 5th ed. Burlington, MA: Jones & Bartlett Learning, LLC; 2016.)

saves time. For example, you only have to enter routine information for a matrix one time—such as lunch every day at noon, hospital rounds on Tuesdays from 9:00 AM to 11:00 AM, and so on. You can also add a patient appointment, add a patient to the waiting list, and view the calendar or search for available times with just one click. Leaving catch-up time in the schedule makes it easy for you to fit in last-minute appointments and emergency visits.

To use the search feature, all you have to do is enter the date. The computer then shows the schedule for that day. Times available for appointments will be highlighted. A computerized system also makes scheduling for multiple physicians easy; you simply enter the physician's name or code and their schedule will be viewable. Additionally, visits could be assigned codes designating specific time allowance; for example, an NPV (new patient visit) would block more time than an RPV (routine established patient visit). Additional codes could be assigned based on the practice specialty. See Figure 10-2, which is a screenshot of a section of a computer-generated appointment schedule.

FACTORS THAT AFFECT SCHEDULING

There's much more to scheduling appointments than just matching patients to time slots and hoping everything

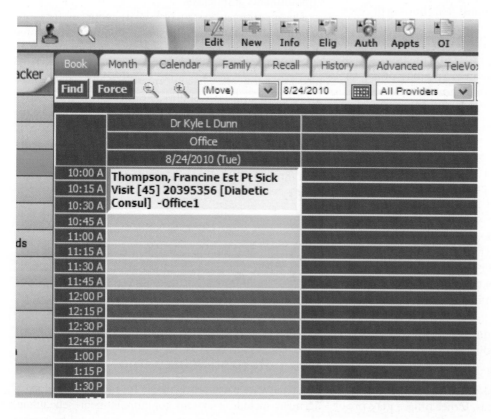

Figure 10-2 A computer-generated appointment schedule. (Courtesy of Harris CareTracker.)

goes smoothly. Before you make an appointment, you should review the schedule and do the following:

- Evaluate the patient's needs.
- Respect the physician's needs.
- Consider the office's limitations.

The Patient's Needs

Most of the calls received are to make appointments and will be routine. Some patients, however, may be shy, anxious, embarrassed, or fearful about their medical problem. You can assist them best by maintaining a polite, friendly, and professional attitude. Here are some questions you should ask the patient when scheduling an appointment:

- Why do you wish to see the physician?
- Is the problem **acute** (a sudden onset) or **chronic** (long-standing)?
- How long have you had the symptoms?
- How severe are the symptoms?
- When is the best time for you to come to the office? (Try to meet the patient's time requests, if you can; however, don't overload the schedule.)
- Do you have any special needs, such as community van services, that we should keep in mind when making your appointment? (Some community van services operate only during certain hours.)
- Do you need to see other office staff while you're here?
- Does your insurance provider have any requirements that we should know about?

When scheduling an office visit (**OV**), it is also a great opportunity to collect insurance information to verify that the clinic participates in the patient's plan. Explanation of the clinic's payment requirements should also be reviewed so that the patient is prepared.

The Provider's Needs

Patients should be scheduled according to the guidelines set by the physician/office manager. These guidelines should be reviewed periodically to insure their effectiveness. If providers consistently fall behind in their schedule, a time allotment review is in order. Learning your provider's work patterns and habits allows you to control the schedule more efficiently.

The physician's schedule should also allow time for completion of other tasks. You may need to allow time for the physician to:

- Receive and return phone calls
- Review lab reports and other test results
- Dictate chart notes and letters
- Meet with other physicians
- Meet with representatives from drug companies and medical suppliers
- Visit hospital patients admitted by the physician

Remember to keep these items in mind when creating your matrix. Not all physicians will need time to handle all of the tasks listed, so you will need to learn which items apply to your physician. Physicians on the staff at a teaching hospital may require extra time for clinic conferences and other teaching duties. You should incorporate time for each of the items utilized into your matrix.

In your position as a medical assistant, you can have a positive effect on the provider's schedule. Clinical duties performed by you, such as removal of sutures or administration of injections, give the physician more time to see patients.

You should ask the physician their preference in handling unscheduled office visitors who are not patients. For example, the physician may want to be told immediately if another physician comes to the office. Staff persons may be asked to meet with sales representatives who drop by unexpectedly. If the physician wants to meet with the person, ask them to schedule an appointment when the physician can meet with them. Also, sales and pharmaceutical representatives will drop in frequently with information about new products and samples. Know your office's policy on handling sales calls.

Physical Facilities

The office's available facilities will also affect how you manage the appointment schedule. For example:

- How many providers are there?
- How many examination rooms are there?
- Is more than one set of instruments available, or must the same instruments be sterilized between procedures?
- How long does a procedure normally take?

You wouldn't schedule two patients for a sigmoidoscopy at the same time if there were only one room equipped for the procedure. Nor would you want to schedule the second patient 15 minutes if the procedure requires 30 minutes to complete.

 TYPES OF SCHEDULING

Most offices use some type of structured appointment system for scheduling visits. Patients are assigned a specific time on the schedule and allowed a set period for care. You'll probably use one of these methods for scheduling appointments:

- Fixed scheduling
- Streaming
- Double-booking
- Wave and modified wave
- Clustering

Methods can also be combined. To help schedule appointments effectively, get to know all of the procedures the office staff performs.

Fixed Scheduling

You'll probably use some form of fixed scheduling. In fixed scheduling, each hour usually is divided into four 15-minute appointment slots. This is still the most common method of scheduling appointments. But if you don't do it well, fixed scheduling can have several disadvantages.

- The patient may need more time than you scheduled. You can help prevent this by finding out the patient's needs before you make the appointment. Knowing why the patient is coming to see the physician will tell you how many issues the physician must deal with. Then you can assign the number of time slots you think the patient will need. This practice is called **streaming**.
- *Patients who are late can disrupt the schedule by backing up the day's flow.* One way you can handle this is to schedule patients with a history of lateness toward the end of the day. You also can tell such patients to arrive 15 or 30 minutes before their actual scheduled time.
- *Patients who don't show up for their appointments can cause problems by wasting providers' time.* You can use double-booking to avoid this problem.

How Much Time to Allow

A number of things can influence how much time you should allow for a patient's appointment. Factors, as previously discussed, include the number exam rooms, number of providers and equipment needs. Here are a few typical services and approximately how much time you should give for each:

- Complete physical examination: 1 hour
- School physical: 30 minutes
- Recheck: 15 minutes
- Dressing change: 10 minutes
- Blood pressure check: 5 minutes
- Patient teaching: 30 minutes to 1 hour

Streaming

Streaming patients helps reduce schedule backups as well as gaps in time. You assign appointment lengths based on patients' needs. For example, you might give a patient coming in for a complete physical an hour-long appointment—that is, four 15-minute time slots. A patient in for a blood pressure check would get just one time slot, or 15 minutes. And you might even double-book that time slot.

Double-Booking

When you double-book, you schedule two patients in the same time slot with the same physician. One sees the physician while the other goes for tests or is served by another applied health professional. Then they switch. When you use this method, the appointment slot isn't completely empty if one of the patients doesn't show up.

Wave Scheduling

Many offices use a form of **wave scheduling** or change it in some way to fit their special needs. With wave scheduling, you schedule several patients for the same time. For example, you would give all patients to be seen in an hour the same appointment time, for instance, 11:00 AM. Then, the physician takes the hour seeing these patients in the order they arrived.

The advantage of this system is that the physician isn't hurried to see patients at specific times. The disadvantage is that some patients may have long waits.

Modified Wave

The wave method has been modified, or changed, in many ways. One change is to fill the first half of each hour with one major appointment, such as a physical examination. In the second half hour, you would schedule three or four brief recheck or follow-up visits.

Here's another way you can use modified wave scheduling.

- Schedule half the number of patients the physician can see in an hour for the beginning of the hour.
- Schedule a third of the number of patients the physician can see in an hour at 20 minutes past the hour.
- Schedule the rest of the hour's patients at 40 minutes past the hour.

Table A	
1:00	*Larry Jones 555-4321 headaches*
1:15	
1:30	*Frank Ness 555-1234 follow-up*
1:45	*Rick Smith 555-8976 cast removal*
	Nancy Wilson 555-7681 recheck throat
	Peter Paulson 555-9919 BP check

Table B	
1:00	*Frank Ness 555-1234 follow-up*
	Dorothy Close 555-4321 CPE
	Larry Jones 555-3124 headaches
1:20	*Rick Smith 555-8976 cast removal*
	Nancy Wilson 555-7861 recheck throat
1:40	*Peter Paulson 555-9919 BP check*

The appointment schedules shown in Tables A and B are two methods of modified wave scheduling. Note that one patient seen in method B could not be scheduled using method A. That's because a complete physical examination (**CPE**) is a major appointment, and method A allows only one major appointment per hour.

Clustering

Clustering is the practice of grouping patients with similar problems or needs. Some medical offices reserve certain times or days for certain activities, such as physical examinations or other activities. For example, a pediatrician's office might have you schedule vaccinations only on certain days of the week. If you're working in an OB-GYN practice, the physicians might see pregnant patients in the mornings and other patients in the afternoons.

Remembering Appointment Types

You can use the name of each type of appointment to help remember how it works.

- **Fixed scheduling:** Something that is "fixed" is stuck or attached to one place. In this method, patients are attached or stuck into one appointment slot.
- **Double-booking:** Double means two. In this case, two patients are given the same appointment slot.
- Streaming: Like rivers, some streams are long and others are short. When patients are streamed, their appointment times are of different lengths too.
- Wave: Picture all patients arriving at once, as if they were being swept into the office on a big ocean wave.
- Clustering: A "cluster" is things of the same kind that are bunched together. In clustering, patients with similar needs are seen in the same time period—bunched together in a "cluster."

Another use of clustering is that you might schedule certain tests, such as sigmoidoscopies, only at certain times of the week. Clustering has several advantages.

- It makes the best use of special equipment.
- Patients with similar problems can be educated at the same time.
- The schedule is easier to manage.
- It makes the use of staff time more efficient.

You can combine clustering with fixed scheduling, wave scheduling, or modified wave. You also can combine double-booking with this and other forms of scheduling.

 SCHEDULING GUIDELINES

Some patients will call for appointments. Others will schedule their appointments in person. Whatever the method, you should always be professional, pleasant, and helpful.

Leave a few open appointment times in the morning and again in the afternoon. Late arrivals and other delays often will upset the schedule. These open time slots can help the schedule "catch up" again. They also create time for emergencies, last-minute appointments, or walk-in patients.

Cultural Connection

When scheduling a new patient, you should ask the patient's native language and determine if an interpreter is needed. Communication is the key in quality patient care. A family member may be making the appointment for the patient, so you can ask if there will be someone accompanying the patient to the appointment. When communicating with patients who are not comfortable with the English language, speak slowly, not loudly. Remember, this person may have a hard time understanding the language but is not hard of hearing. Although it may be accepted in the United States to refer to someone by their first name, in most countries it is respectful to always use the person's last name when addressing them.

Appointments for New Patients

Most appointments for new patients are made by telephone. You must have very good communication with the patient at this time. It's critical that you record the patient's information accurately.

Case Question

 Recall the case study, Mr. McNeil is an NPT referred by another physician for treatment of his HTN. What critical information should be collected from Mr. McNeil at the time he makes his appointment?

It is likely that your office will have its own procedures for making new patient appointments. Some offices might even have you follow a script to make sure it's done right. Critical information includes patient's legal name (correct spelling), patient's preferred name (if different from legal name), billing address, date of birth (DOB), social security number, (SSN), insurance information, referring physician's name (if applies), and reason for the visit. It is extremely important that insurance information be verified to insure that your practice participates in the patient's plan. You will also need to determine if an insurance referral is required.

If there's enough time before the appointment, mail or e-mail an office brochure and new patient forms to the patient. The patient can complete the forms and bring them in at the appointment. It saves time if the form doesn't have to be filled out at the office.

Appointments for Established Patients

The physician may tell a patient to return for a follow-up visit. Most return appointments are made before the patient leaves the office. Always write the patient's phone number on the appointment schedule. Emergencies happen, and schedule changes are easier if the patient's phone number is handy.

 ## THE DAILY SCHEDULE

In most offices, you'll be asked to prepare a daily schedule of appointments. You can use computer-scheduling software to print out these schedules.

Make a schedule for each provider with copies for other staff members. Place the next day's schedule on the physician's desk before he or she leaves for the day. Give next week's schedule to the physician before leaving on Friday.

You should include the following information on these schedules:

- Next day's patient appointments
- Physician's hospital rounds
- Physician's surgery schedule
- Professional or business meetings
- Personal appointments that are on the schedule

If you work in an office that uses computer scheduling, you may need to create and print a weekly schedule as well. Many offices create a weekly schedule in case of a computer "crash" that erases important information. If you have a weekly schedule printed, you will still have a fairly accurate record of appointments. The schedule may change as the day progresses. Remember to give everyone any corrected copies of the schedule that you distribute.

 ## PATIENT REMINDERS

Patients are less likely to miss an appointment when they are reminded of it. Medical offices use appointment cards, telephone calls, emails, and mailed cards to help patients remember upcoming visits. When calling patients, use the term "confirming" as opposed to "reminding." Patients could be offended by the fact that you are calling to remind them of an appointment as it could imply that they are forgetful. Confirming implies that you are just insuring that your records are correct.

Appointment Cards

You should give the patient a card showing his or her next appointment when they leave the office. Figure 10-3 demonstrates the receptionist assisting a patient by providing a reminder card for her next appointment.

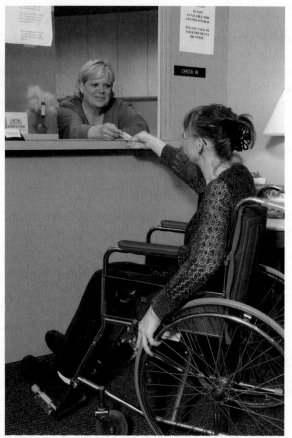

Figure 10-3 An appointment card will help the patient remember his or her appointment and reduce no-shows. (Reprinted from Kronenberger J, Ledbetter J. *Jones & Bartlett Learning's Comprehensive Medical Assisting.* 5th ed. Burlington, MA: Jones & Bartlett Learning, LLC; 2016.)

The card should have the following information on it:

- The patient's name
- The day, date, and time of the next visit
- The physician's name and phone number

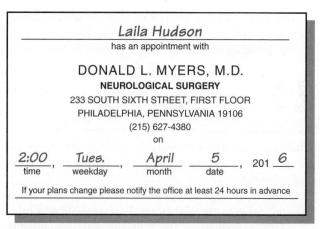

Figure 10-4 Sample appointment reminder card. (Reprinted from Kronenberger J, Ledbetter J. *Jones & Bartlett Learning's Comprehensive Medical Assisting.* 5th ed. Burlington, MA: Jones & Bartlett Learning, LLC; 2016.)

Figure 10-4 is an example of a typical appointment card or reminder card.

Computer-scheduling software also can print appointment cards for you. If you write them by hand, use ink that can't be erased. If the patient needs a series of appointments, try to make them for the same time and on the same day of the week. If there's space on the card, you could list the whole series of appointments on it. But it's probably better to give the patient a card for his/her next visit only. Just give him/her a new card after each visit. Handing out all the cards for a series of visits can lead to confusion and lost cards.

Telephone Reminders

Patients also should receive a telephone reminder or confirmation call 1 or 2 days before their appointment. Some computer scheduling software will call patients automatically with a recorded reminder message.

Whether you make the call or whether it's made by computer, call only the patient's home number. Don't call a work number unless the patient asks you to do so. Document the patient's preferences in the chart so everyone in the office can see this information. Federal privacy laws allow you to leave an appointment reminder message on a patient's answering machine or with whoever answers their home phone. But it's still a good idea to ask the patient if that is okay. You should ask at the time you make the appointment.

Don't leave a message on a patient's work phone or with a coworker, even if the patient has asked you to call her there. Leaving a message at work isn't a good idea. It raises privacy concerns that usually don't exist when you make reminder calls to the patient's home.

Don't ever include the reason for the visit in a reminder message. If a person answers the phone and wants more information, politely decline to give it. Tell the person that patient privacy issues don't allow you to answer the question.

Sample Telephone Reminder

Your reminder call should be brief. Simply state your name, your office, and the date and time of the appointment. For example, you might say:

- "This is Ms. Palmer from Dr. Reid's office. I'm calling to confirm your appointment for tomorrow, Thursday, February 10, at 3:30 PM."
- Unless the patient has a question, just say, "Thank you and goodbye."
- You should write "confirmed," "left message," or "no answer" on the appointment schedule to show the results of each call.

Recorded messages left by the computer should have the same basic content. They should include a call-back number if the patient can't keep the appointment. Include a callback number when you leave a reminder message, too.

Reminder Cards

Your office may send reminder cards or letters instead of making phone calls. These cards also can be used for patients who don't want phone reminders. You should mail the reminder card at least a week before the appointment date.

Some offices use reminder cards to alert patients that it's time for some annual exam, such as a Pap smear, mammogram, prostate exam, or complete physical. For privacy reasons, however, the reminder card should never state the kind of exam. It should have a general message printed on it. Here's an example:

"According to our records, you are due for your annual visit. Please call the office and we will be glad to make an appointment for you."

For privacy reasons, some patients may want their reminder cards mailed inside an envelope. This is a reasonable request, and you should provide this method of sending. You also should accommodate a patient who wants the card mailed to a place other than his home. Write only the appointment date and time on the reminder card, never the reason for the visit. Remember, you have no way of knowing who will see the card after it's been mailed.

Reminder calls and cards help patients remember their appointments. If they need to cancel or reschedule, you may be able to fill that slot with another patient. Keep a list of names and phone numbers of patients who have asked to be called if an earlier appointment becomes available. You might call this a cancellation list, a waiting list, or a move-up list in your office. Many computerized scheduling systems offer a waiting list option.

 ## ADAPTING THE SCHEDULE

It will be an unusual day in the office if everything goes according to plan. Often, patients will be late for appointments or even miss them altogether. Providers may experience delays. Patients who don't have appointments may call the office with emergencies. You may have to adjust the appointment schedule when these things happen.

Emergencies

When a patient calls with an emergency, first find out whether the problem can be treated in the office. Every office should have a policy for evaluating emergency calls.

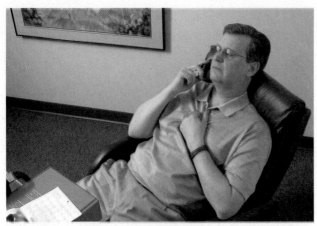

Figure 10-5 When a patient calls from home with a possible heart attack, you will call 9-1-1. (Reprinted from Kronenberger J, Ledbetter J. *Jones & Bartlett Learning's Comprehensive Medical Assisting.* 4th ed. Burlington, MA: Jones & Bartlett Learning, LLC; 2013.)

Sending Patients to the ER

Follow your office policy, but in general, you should put through to the office nurse or physician any caller who complains of these symptoms:

- Chest pain
- Shortness of breath
- Loss of consciousness
- Severe bleeding

Figure 10-5 shows a patient calling the office from his home. This patient will need emergency care.

Most likely, patients with these symptoms need to be seen in a hospital emergency room (**ER**).

Seen in the Office

Here are some typical symptoms that would require the patient to be seen in the office the same day. Again, the policy in your office will be the final word on how to handle these cases.

- Severe vomiting for more than 2 days
- High fever for more than 2 days
- Severe headache with neck stiffness
- Abdominal pain with symptoms of appendicitis
- Wounds that don't require a trip to the ER

Study Skill

Repetition is a great way to instill information into your memory. Repeatedly write words that are new to you. Once you have mastered the word, practice writing the word with its definition. Soon, you will be able to recognize and understand words or terms that were once strange to you and not part of your vocabulary. This is especially important to help you learn medical terms and names of drugs.

Constellation of Symptoms

When certain symptoms occur together, it can signal a specific problem. Such a group of complaints is called a **constellation of symptoms**. Keep the following in mind:

- Severe pain in the lower right abdomen, nausea, and fever is the constellation of symptoms for appendicitis.
- Chest pain, shortness of breath, arm or neck pain, and nausea and/or vomiting is the constellation of symptoms for a heart attack.
- Severe headache, dizziness, trouble speaking or seeing, and numbness or weakness of the face, arm, or leg is the constellation of symptoms for a stroke.

If a patient needs to be seen the same day and no appointments are available, you can adapt the schedule in three possible ways:

- Work in the patient between existing appointments. This will result in delays for patients with appointments that follow, but the emergency may need to be addressed immediately.
- Schedule the patient in an open slot you have created as catch-up time in the schedule. Keep in mind that some emergencies may require quicker attention.
- Schedule the patient into a filled time slot, and then call that person and reschedule his or her appointment. Explain that an emergency requires you to do this. This may not be a good alternative, however, if the emergency patient needs to be seen quickly.

Acutely Ill Patients

You'll also receive calls from patients who are seriously ill but don't have a true emergency. These patients need to be seen as soon as possible, but not necessarily that very day. You should triage these calls in this way:

- Get as much information about the patient's problem as you can. Write a note containing this information. This will help the physician decide when the patient should be seen.
- Place the patient's chart with the note in the place the physician has chosen for such calls.
- Tell the patient you'll call back as soon as the physician makes a decision.

Once again, your office policy will determine how calls like this are handled. Here are some examples of complaints from patients who need to be seen soon, although not necessarily that very day.

- Severe sore throat
- Severe back pain
- Burning and/or painful urination
- Headache lasting more than 3 days
- Jaundice that has appeared in the last week

- Severe respiratory symptoms of more than a week
- Severe rash lasting more than 3 days
- Heart palpitations for more than 2 days

If the physician wants to see the patient, he will tell you how soon. You can adjust the schedule using the same system you use to work in emergency patients.

Acutely ill patients don't need to be seen as quickly, however. So if you must cancel a scheduled appointment to work in an acutely ill patient, try not to do it for the same day. This is because you might not be able to reach the patient you're cancelling in time. You do not want that person showing up in the office only to find that her appointment was cancelled. But if you cancel an appointment for the next day, you can call the patient's home and leave a message that she'll probably get.

Most importantly, remember that the physician or the triage nurse always should make the final decision when adjusting the schedule for an emergency.

Other Schedule Busters

Other events that will require you to adapt the schedule may be more common.

Walk-In Patients

Walk-ins are patients who come to the office without an appointment. Your office may have a procedure for handling these patients. But in general, you must first find out why the patient has come in. If it's an emergency, the patient should be seen immediately. Otherwise, have the patient sit in the waiting room while you tell the physician. The physician can then decide whether to see the patient or ask him to make an appointment.

If the physician is going to see the patient, explain that you'll work him in as soon as possible. When the patient leaves after being seen, apologize for the delay. Suggest that he make an appointment next time.

The Late Patient

Patients who are late can cause problems in the schedule for the rest of the day. You should remind the patient gently but firmly that she was late and tell her the physician is with another patient. Offer the patient the choice of waiting or rescheduling the appointment.

Some offices have a policy requiring that patients who are more than 15 minutes late be rescheduled. Of course, late patients may not always be a problem. If the physician is running behind, a late patient may have arrived before it's his turn to be seen.

One thing you might do is schedule patients who have a habit of being late toward the end of the day. That way, their lateness will affect the day's schedule less. Also, you can ask patients to call the office if they know they are going to be late.

Always call patients with a history of being late to remind them of their appointment. You should do this even if it's not normally office policy to make appointment reminders by phone.

Case Question

Recall our case study, Matt McNeil was a new patient to our office. Since that time, he has been scheduling routine follow-up appointments. Unfortunately, he has arrived so late to his last three appointments you have had to cancel and reschedule his appointments. Currently, Mr. McNeil is calling to request an afternoon appointment, what is the best way to handle this situation?

Perhaps the best way to handle this situation is to first explain that he has been late to the last three late afternoon appointments and has had to reschedule. You could suggest an appointment earlier in the day. Unfortunately, patients don't always realize how much they affect the physician's schedule when they arrive hours after their appointed time.

The No-Show Patient

A no-show occurs when a patient misses an appointment and doesn't call the office ahead of time. When this happens, try to call the patient to find out why the appointment was missed. Then, try to reschedule the patient for another day. It's essential that information about no-shows be documented in the chart as well as on the daily schedule. Use red ink when marking a no-show on the daily schedule and the patient's chart.

You should make notes in the patient's record of all actions involving missed appointments. Copies of any letters sent to the patient should be included in the chart too.

The information in both the appointment schedule and patient's chart must look the same. This is vital information for legal issues as well as for the patient's welfare.

If you cannot reach the patient by phone, send a card asking him to call the office to reschedule. Write in the patient's chart that the appointment was missed. Also, note if you rescheduled the appointment or mailed a card for the patient to reschedule.

Tell the physician about patients who continually miss appointments. She may want to call the patient or send a letter of concern for the patient's welfare. This is especially true for patients who are seriously ill. In extreme cases, the physician may want to end the relationship with the patient.

Cancelled Appointments

Here's what to do when a patient cancels an appointment.

- Ask the patient why she is cancelling.
- Mark the cancellation on the appointment schedule.
- Note the cancellation and the reason in the patient's chart.
- Offer to reschedule the appointment at another time.

If the physician is seeing the patient for a continuing medical concern, make sure the patient understands the importance of rescheduling. The patient may say she'll call later to reschedule. Make a note to yourself to check on the callback in a few days.

If a patient cancels and you have a full schedule, no action is needed. But if the schedule is light, use your wait list to try to fill the opening.

Documenting Missed Appointments

You should note missed appointments, whether they're cancellations or no-shows, in the patient's record. Also, include a summary of the reason for the missed appointment. Here is an example of a note in a patient's chart:

Mrs. Parrish was called regarding missing scheduled appointment for today at 9:30 AM. Patient said she forgot about the appointment. Appointment was rescheduled for 10/15/07 at 10:00 AM. Patient was advised of the need to have regular prenatal checkups. Patient verbalized understanding. Dr. Wong was notified that appointment was missed and rescheduled.—Noreen Brooks, CMA

Office Cancellations

The office may have to cancel patients' appointments if the doctor is ill, has an emergency, or takes personal time off. Patients don't need to be told the specific reason for the physician's absence. Cancellation by the office should be noted in a patient's record too. Here are some guidelines to follow:

- *If you have advance notice*: Write a letter to patients with appointments you must cancel. Simply state that the physician will be away from the office and will return by a certain date. Ask the patient to call the office to reschedule. Remember to place a copy of the letter in the patient's chart.
- *If you must cancel on the day of the appointment*: Call the patient. Explain that the physician has been called out of the office unexpectedly. Try to reschedule the appointment while the patient is still on the phone.
- *If the patient arrives before you can contact him*: Apologize and politely explain the situation. Most patients understand this situation.

When the physician won't be available for a long time, another physician must cover the practice or be on call. If a substitute physician is employed, office appointments won't be disrupted.

You also should have a list of the names and addresses of physicians who are on call to see patients. Give this information to patients you must cancel, if your office policy allows it.

When the Schedule Doesn't Work

You've been doing everything right. You follow office procedures for scheduling new and established patients. You remind patients of their appointments. You're using scheduling strategies with frequently late patients, and you try hard to fill slots created by cancellations. You expect that some days will not run smoothly. But the schedule seems in chaos almost every day, and you just can't figure out why.

This situation is a case where a study might help. Here's what to do:

- Look at the schedule over the past 2 or 3 months.
- List all the patients seen, when they arrived, how long they spent with the physician, and when they left the office.

Your study might show that many patients are arriving late or that not enough time is being allowed for certain procedures. Perhaps too many staff members are allowed to make patient appointments. Maybe a physician who is frequently late is part of the problem.

Some problems may never be solved completely. But if you can identify them, you often can make changes so their effects will be less severe.

The Physician Has Been Delayed

Sometimes, the physician will arrive late to the office. If his appointment hours have not yet started, call patients with early appointments. Give them the choice of coming in later or on another day.

If patients are waiting, tell them at once that the physician has been delayed. Also tell them how long the delay is expected to be. Ask if they want to wait or reschedule for another time. If patients reschedule, be sure to note the reason in their chart.

APPOINTMENTS WITH OTHER PROVIDERS

The physician may want a patient to see another doctor, perhaps a specialist in another field of medicine. The patient also may need to be sent to another office or facility for testing or to be admitted to the hospital. In each case, you may need to make the appointment with the other provider.

Third-Party Payers

When making an outside appointment, you must first be sure it meets the requirements of **third-party payers.** These are the insurance companies, HMOs, and other health care plans that pay patients' medical bills. You should know that managed-care companies, such as HMOs, have guidelines for sending patients to other providers. The requirements are called **precertification.** This means the insurer must approve the appointment in advance.

Call the phone number on the patient's insurance card before making these kinds of appointments:

- Sending the patient to another physician
- Scheduling certain tests or procedures
- Admitting the patient to the hospital (This only applies to admissions that are *not* emergencies.)

The third-party payer may require completion of a referral form. See Figure 10-6, a sample referral form.

The Preferred Provider

Be sure the provider you're calling is a **preferred provider** for the patient's health care plan. These are physicians,

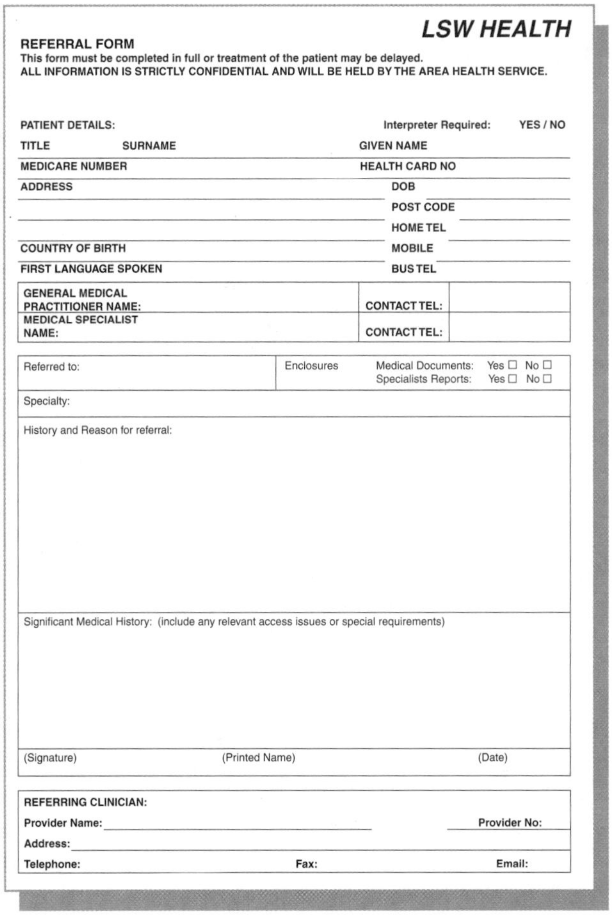

LSW HEALTH

REFERRAL FORM

This form must be completed in full or treatment of the patient may be delayed.

ALL INFORMATION IS STRICTLY CONFIDENTIAL AND WILL BE HELD BY THE AREA HEALTH SERVICE.

PATIENT DETAILS: Interpreter Required: YES / NO

TITLE SURNAME GIVEN NAME

MEDICARE NUMBER HEALTH CARD NO

ADDRESS DOB

POST CODE

HOME TEL

COUNTRY OF BIRTH MOBILE

FIRST LANGUAGE SPOKEN BUS TEL

GENERAL MEDICAL PRACTITIONER NAME:	CONTACT TEL:
MEDICAL SPECIALIST NAME:	CONTACT TEL:

Referred to: Enclosures Medical Documents: Yes ☐ No ☐ Specialists Reports: Yes ☐ No ☐

Specialty:

History and Reason for referral:

Significant Medical History: (include any relevant access issues or special requirements)

(Signature) (Printed Name) (Date)

REFERRING CLINICIAN:

Provider Name: Provider No:

Address:

Telephone: Fax: Email:

Figure 10-6 Sample referral form. (Reprinted from Kronenberger J, Ledbetter J. *Jones & Bartlett Learning's Comprehensive Medical Assisting*. 5th ed. Burlington, MA: Jones & Bartlett Learning, LLC; 2016.)

hospitals, and others that are in the plan's approved network of providers.

Unless you send the patient to a preferred provider, the plan's payment will be less. Also, if a referral, test, or hospitalization requires precertification and you don't have it, the health care plan may not pay at all. In each case, both the patient and your employer could suffer financial losses.

Consultations and Referrals

Sometimes, the physician will want you to schedule a consultation or a referral for a patient. You need to know the difference between the two. In a **consultation,** the physician wants another physician's opinion about the patient. The second physician reviews the patient's records and usually examines the patient. He then recommends treatment. In a **referral,** the patient's care and treatment is actually transferred to the other physician.

Precertification

A health care plan will want certain information before granting approval to send a patient to another provider. Each plan will be different. But in general, you should have this information ready when you call a patient's plan for approval:

- The information on the patient's plan ID card
- The patient's name, address, phone number, and age
- If the patient is a family member of the insured, her relationship to the insured
- The name, address, and phone number of the provider asking for the approval
- The name, address, and phone number of the provider to whom the patient will be sent
- The patient's diagnosis or symptoms
- The type of care being sought
- If the patient is being admitted to a hospital, the name, address, and phone number of the hospital

You will need to get the health care plan's approval first, unless the patient is being sent as an emergency case. In that case, you should call for approval as soon as you can.

- In a consultation, the patient's physician carries out the treatment, not the other physician. One required part of a consultation is a consultation letter or report from the consultant to the primary care physician.
- In a referral, the patient's care and treatment is actually transferred to the other physician.

In some cases, the patient will want to make his own appointment with the other physician. If so, ask the patient to call you when the appointment is made. Write the date and time the patient gives you in the patient's chart.

Diagnostic Tests

A physician in your office may want to send a patient to another facility for testing. You'll make some of these appointments while the patient is still in the office. This is especially true for labs tests and x-rays. Check with the patient for any scheduling conflicts she might have.

Types of Testing

Some of the tests you might send a patient out for are as follows:

- Laboratory tests (mainly blood tests)
- Radiology (x-rays)
- Computed tomography (CT scans)
- Magnetic resonance imaging (MRIs)
- Nuclear medicine studies

Testing Results

Find out exactly what test or tests the physician wants and how soon she needs the results. Give the patient a lab or x-ray referral slip with the requested tests marked on it. Be sure to tell the provider if the results are needed **STAT**, which means immediately. Also, give the patient a slip with the outside facility's name, address, and phone number and the date and time of his appointment.

Some tests may require advance preparation by the patient. Tell him what he must do, and also give him written instructions. Be sure he understands the importance of following them.

Write the appointment time and date and the name of the outside facility on the patient's chart. Also, put a reminder note in your appointment schedule to check for when the test results are back. Some tests, such as CT scans and MRIs, may require precertification by the patient's health plan.

Scheduling Surgery

You also may have to schedule procedures in a hospital operating room or an outpatient surgery facility. You may have to get precertification for these from the patient's health care plan too. When scheduling surgeries, you'll need to follow these additional steps as well.

- Tell the surgical facility the exact procedure, the type of anesthesia required, and the time needed. The physician will provide this information. Also, give the facility any other information and instructions your physician provides.
- Provide the patient's age, health care plan, and the plan's approval number for the surgery.
- Give patients going to the hospital a preadmission form, if you have a supply from the hospital in your office, or give instructions on how to complete online registration.

- Be sure to follow the policies of the hospital or outpatient facility about preadmission testing. These may include blood tests, x-rays, and a donation of the patient's own blood in advance.
- List all the appointment dates, times, and places the patient needs to go. Give this list to the patient. Make sure the patient understands where to go, when, and what will happen in each place.
- Finally, write the name of the surgical facility and the date and time the surgery is scheduled in the patient's chart. You may need to arrange for hospital admission by providing this information to the hospital admitting department.

THE PHYSICIAN'S SCHEDULE

Your scheduling duties will extend to the physicians in the office as well as the patients. You probably will help manage the physician's professional schedule. This includes allowing time in the appointment schedule for the physician's other professional activities. It also may involve making travel arrangements for the physician.

Managing the Physician's Time

You are already helping manage the physician's time when you create the matrix for the appointment schedule. The matrix sets time aside for the physician's activities outside the office, including surgeries and hospital rounds.

Another duty may be to screen visitors for the physician:

- Pharmaceutical sales representatives can be a valuable resource for a physician. They provide information about new drugs that are available. Ask the physician for a list of pharmaceutical sales reps he wants to see. This probably will depend on the physician's specialty. A cardiologist and a psychiatrist would not be interested in the same kinds of drugs, for instance.
- Medical suppliers are another valuable source of information. But which suppliers are worth seeing also depends on the physician's specialty. For example, an internal medicine doctor wouldn't want to spend time with a supplier of artificial hips and knees.
- Office suppliers and suppliers of medical forms usually meet with the office manager. They should not be allowed to take up the physician's time unless she wants to see them. The same is true of insurance salespeople.
- Community leaders and fundraisers may arrive to ask for the physician's support for some local project. Your medical office probably has a general policy for handling them. Find out if the physician wishes to be notified of these types of visitors. Bluntly refusing

to help is not good for community relations. Instead, you might tell them of the physician's current community activities. If appropriate, explain that he cannot take on any more at this time.

Making Travel Arrangements

Many physicians attend professional meetings and educational conferences to keep current in their field. You may have to make arrangements for physicians in your office to attend such events.

Create a one-page travel profile for each physician. Here's the information you'll need:

- The names and phone numbers of travel agents the physician prefers.
- The airline(s) on which the physician likes to travel. Include his frequent flier number(s), preferred class (e.g., first class or coach), seating preference (e.g., aisle or window seat), and ticket preference (paper ticket or ticketless travel).
- Rental car preferences, including the rental company and type of car preferred (compact, standard, SUV, luxury, etc.).
- Preferred hotel accommodations, including price range, bed size, and features (swimming pool, restaurant, fitness facility, etc.).
- The physician's or office's credit card number(s).

When the physician tells you that she wishes to attend a certain conference, complete the registration form as soon as possible. Once you have confirmed the physician is registered, make the travel arrangements. You may do this through a travel agent, or you might make the reservations yourself using the Internet. In either case, use the information from the physician's travel profile to arrange a flight, hotel, and, if needed, a rental car.

If you use a travel agent, he will provide an **itinerary**. This is a detailed plan of the trip. You will need at least three copies of the itinerary.

- Give the first copy to the physician to carry on the trip.
- The second copy is for the physician to leave with his family.
- Keep the third copy in the office, in case you need to contact the physician.

Being Your Own Online Travel Agent

If you make the travel arrangements using the Internet, you will have to prepare the itinerary yourself. Here's what you should include:

- Air travel: the date of the flight, airport, airline, flight and seat number, and departure and arrival times. Unless the flight is nonstop, do the same for the connecting flight(s). You also will need to provide this information for the return trip.
- Rental car: the rental company's name and phone number, reservation confirmation number, and type of car reserved.
- Hotel: the name and address, phone number, reservation confirmation number, and dates of the stay.
- Meeting or conference: name, location address and phone number, room number, and registration confirmation number.

Be sure to get confirmation numbers when making hotel and rental car reservations. If the physician is flying with a paper ticket, check it when it arrives. The dates, flight numbers, and times should match those on the itinerary you prepared.

Put two copies of the itinerary, a copy of the conference registration form, and the ticket (or airline email for ticketless travel) into an envelope and give it to the physician. Then, all that's left is to wish her a good trip!

Procedure 10-1   Making Appointments for New Patients

Follow these steps when making an appointment for a new patient:

1. Obtain the patient's full name, address, day and evening phone numbers, reason for the visit, and name of who referred the patient. This information helps you determine how soon and for how long the patient will need to be seen.

2. Explain the office's payment policy. Ask the patient to bring insurance information to the office. Patients cannot be expected to make any required payments unless they are aware of the policy. You should also verify insurance to determine whether your office participates in their plan.

3. Make sure the patient knows where the office is located. Give directions if needed. This helps patients arrive on time.

4. Ask the patient if it's acceptable to call them at home or work. Some patients don't want medically related messages left on voicemail or with a coworker.

5. Double-check your appointment book or computer screen to make sure you have recorded the appointment for the correct date and time. Mistakes can cause overbooking, angry patients, and irritated physicians and staff.

6. Before hanging up, confirm the day, date, and time of the appointment with the patient. Repeating this information ensures that no mistakes or misunderstandings have occurred.

7. If another physician referred the patient, make a note to contact the referring physician's office for copies of the patient's records. This will give the physician information about the patient that he needs. It also may eliminate the need to repeat some tests.

Procedure 10-2   Making Appointments for Established Patients

Follow these steps to schedule a return appointment.

1. Find out the reason for the return visit. If a specific test is to be done, check the schedule to see when the equipment is available. This will help you offer a good date and time.

2. Offer the patient a specific date and time. If the patient doesn't agree, offer one or two other dates and times. Just asking the patient, "When would you like to return?" can create indecision in the patient.

3. Enter the patient's name and telephone contact number in the appointment book or the computer. Also, confirm their current insurance to verify that they are still with a participating plan. Having this information with the appointment makes it easier to call the patient if you have to cancel or reschedule it.

4. Place the information on an appointment card and give it to the patient. Repeat aloud to the patient the day, date, and time of the appointment as you hand over the card. This step helps the patient remember the appointment.

5. Double-check your record of the appointment to be sure you have not made an error. Appointment errors waste time for everyone, including the patient, staff, and physician.

6. End your conversation with a pleasant word and smile. Your friendliness will feel good to a patient who may be anxious about having to return to the physician.

Procedure 10-3 | Making Appointments for Patients in Other Facilities

The steps for arranging referrals, testing and other procedures, or hospitalization are much the same. Follow these guidelines when making arrangements:

1. Make certain that the requirements of the patient's health care plan are met. Many health plans require that referrals to specialists, hospital admissions, certain diagnostic tests, and surgical procedures be approved in advance. The phone numbers to call will be printed on the patient's insurance card.

2. Refer to the preferred provider list for the patient's health care plan and call a provider on this list. Many plans have lists of approved physicians, hospitals, and other facilities that patients must use. If there's more than one approved provider, let the patient choose from the list if she wishes.

3. Have the following information available when you call the provider:
   - The name and phone number of your office and physician
   - The patient's name, address, and phone number
   - The reason the patient is being sent to the other provider
   - How urgent it is that the patient be seen

   - The approval number from the patient's health care plan if precertification is required.

   This information allows the other provider to serve the patient's needs.

4. Record the following information in the patient's chart when you make the call:
   - The date and time of the call
   - The name of the person you spoke with.

   You need this record to document the patient's care.

5. Ask the person you're calling to notify you if the patient doesn't keep the appointment. If this happens, tell the physician and record the missed appointment in the patient's chart. This information also helps document the patient's care.

6. Write the following on office stationery and give or mail it to the patient:
   - The name, address, and phone number of the place you are sending the patient
   - The date and time of the patient's appointment at this place

This gives the patient a reminder so the appointment will be kept.

Preparing for Externship

During the externship course, you should keep a daily journal. A journal is like a personal diary. Journaling is a way to do self-reflection about your attitude and performance at the externship site. Your school may require a journal, but if not, keep one anyway. Use a small notebook and use at least one page for each day on the site. Each day, record the procedures you participated with and recall how you could have performed each one. Also, write down new terms and abbreviations you encounter each day. Research each of these so you will know them the next time you see or hear them. Each day, write down your strength and challenge you had. An example of strengths might be receiving a compliment about the way you interacted with a patient. Weaknesses might include the need to improve technique when performing specific tasks. This is an area that as a student you need to accept constructive criticism.

Chapter Recap

- A medical office needs a good and well-managed appointment system to run smoothly and efficiently.
- Scheduling systems include manual ones that use appointment books and computerized ones that use special software.
- Computerized systems make it easier to meet the scheduling needs of patients and providers and to produce updated daily schedules.
- The number of providers, a facility's size, and the services it offers all influence the scheduling system and methods that work best.
- Methods used to schedule appointments include fixed, double-booking, streaming, clustering, wave, and modified wave.
- Scheduling appointments for new and returning patients requires meeting both the patient's and the provider's needs.
- Appointment cards, phone reminders, and reminder cards make patients less likely to miss their appointments.
- On many days, emergencies, delays, late patients, walk-ins, cancellations, and no-shows will require schedule adjustments.
- Some health care plans may place special requirements on sending the patients they cover to other providers.
- Extra steps may be needed when scheduling patients for certain tests, surgical procedures, or hospital admissions.
- In addition to scheduling appointments, you also may help with organizing the physician's schedule and travel plans.

Online Resources for Students

Student Resources available on the text's online site include:
- Audio Glossaries
- Animations
- Competency Evaluation Forms
- Videos
- Anatomy & Physiology Module with Heart and Lung Sounds
- Weblinks
- Worksheets

Exercises and Activities

Certification Preparation Questions

1. Which of the following would best represent a third-party payer?
   a. Patient's parent paying for services
   b. Friend paying for a patient's services
   c. Insurance company
   d. Patient being seen by three different providers
   e. Patient being seen at a free clinic

2. The term precertification means:
   a. the insurance company guarantees to pay for the service/procedure.
   b. the insurance company approves the service/procedure but does not guarantee payment.
   c. the insurance company has verified coverage for the patient.
   d. the facility performing the procedure/service is certified in for the testing to be performed.
   e. the person performing the procedure/service is in the process of certifying his or her skills.

3. Constellation of symptoms is best described as:
   a. a collection of random symptoms.
   b. symptoms that occur only at a specific time of night.
   c. certain symptoms occurring together that signal a particular condition.
   d. symptoms randomly occurring together without reason.
   e. a group of symptoms that never occur together.

4. Which of the following best explains a consultation?
   a. A consultation is when a physician asks another physician to assist in the managing of a patient's case.
   b. A consultation is when a physician refers the care of a patient to another doctor.
   c. A consultation is when a physician talks with his or her patient about their routine care.
   d. A consultation occurs only when a patient is in the hospital.
   e. A consultation can only occur if the patient requires surgery.

5. The term double-booking, in scheduling, means:
   a. to assign an amount of time to an appointment based on the type/reason for appointment.
   b. to allow the same amount of time for every appointment regardless of type/reason.
   c. when a group of patients are scheduled for the same block of time and are seen in order of arrival.
   d. when patients are scheduled on a particular day of the week based on the reason/type of appointment.
   e. when two patients are given the same appointment time.

6. The term STAT means:
   a. as soon as possible.
   b. sometime today.
   c. within 48 hours.
   d. immediately.
   e. as directed.

7. What is a preferred provider?
   a. Physician/provider that the patient prefers over others in the plan
   b. Physician/provider who does NOT participate in a particular insurance plan
   c. Physician/provider who is preferred by the referring physician
   d. Physician/provider who participates in a particular insurance plan
   e. Physician/provider who is preferred by the referring hospital

8. The term streaming, in appointment scheduling, means:
   a. to assign an amount of time to an appointment based on the type/reason for appointment.
   b. to allow the same amount of time for every appointment regardless of type/reason.
   c. when a group of patients are scheduled for the same block of time and are seen in order of arrival.
   d. when patients are scheduled on a particular day of the week based on the reason/type of appointment.
   e. when two patients are given the same appointment time.

9. When scheduling a patient the minimum information you need is:
   a. name, address, and phone number.
   b. name, address, and reason for the visit.
   c. name, address, and insurance information.
   d. name, phone number, and reason for the visit.
   e. name, phone number, and insurance information.

10. The abbreviation NPT stands for:
   a. next patient time.
   b. new patient time.
   c. new provider today.
   d. next patient.
   e. new patient.

CareTracker Connection

Appointments and Scheduling

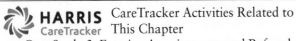 CareTracker Activities Related to This Chapter
- Case Study 3: Entering Appointments and Referrals

One of the greatest challenges medical assistants face is effectively managing the schedule of the medical office. Busy health care providers with unexpected schedule changes and patients who show up late or not at all can keep you scrambling to maintain order and sanity. Computerized appointment scheduling systems, such as the one included in CareTracker, can be a lifesaver.

Tasks discussed in this chapter that can be performed in CareTracker include the following:

- Creating templates for various types of appointments
- Checking provider and resource availability

- Preparing a daily schedule of appointments for each provider
- Scheduling patient appointments of various types
- Double-booking patient appointments
- Rescheduling patient appointments
- Cancelling patient appointments
- Adding a patient to the wait list
- Scheduling consultations and referrals
- Scheduling the use of resources, such as meeting rooms or equipment
- Recalling patient appointments

A task we'll consider here is scheduling a sick visit for an established patient.

When a patient calls the medical office requesting an appointment with a health care provider, the first step is to check that provider's schedule for the day in question. In CareTracker, this involves opening the Scheduling module and entering the desired date and provider. The corresponding schedule will then be displayed.

Book	Month	Calendar	Family	Recall	History	Advanced	TeleVox

| Find | Force | 🔍 | 🔍 | (Move) ▾ | 6/9/2017 | 🗓 | Damien White ▾ | GFMC ▾ | 1 Day ▾ | Go |

	Damien White			
	GFMC			
	6/9/2017 (Fri)			
8:00 A				8:00 A
8:15 A				8:15 A
8:30 A				8:30 A
8:45 A				8:45 A
9:00 A				9:00 A
9:15 A				9:15 A
9:30 A				9:30 A
9:45 A				9:45 A
10:00 A				10:00 A
10:15 A				10:15 A
10:30 A				10:30 A
10:45 A				10:45 A
11:00 A				11:00 A

To book an appointment, you then click in the field next to an available time slot, and the Book Appointment window will appear. You select the appropriate appointment type, select the patient's chief complaint, and add any relevant notes.

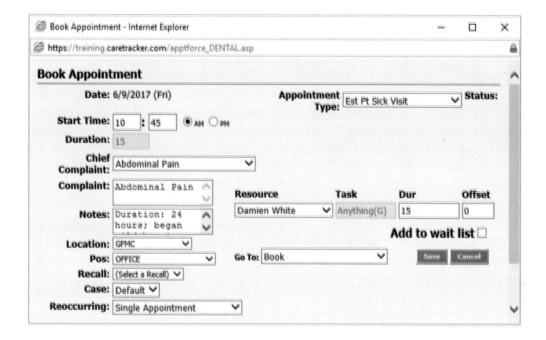

Once you save the appointment, it will appear on the schedule.

11 Medical Documentation

Chapter Objectives

- List information contained in a medical record.
- Establish and maintain the medical record.
- Contrast the ways in which medical records can be organized.
- Discuss security of medical records.
- Explain how to make entries in a patient's medical record.
- Describe how to make corrections in medical records.
- Document appropriately.
- Explain proper access and use of medical records.

CAAHEP & ABHES Competencies

CAAHEP

- Define types of information contained in the patient's medical record.
- Identify methods of organizing the patient's medical record.
- Identify equipment and supplies needed to create, maintain, and store medical records.
- Describe filing indexing rules.
- Differentiate between electronic medical records (EMR) and a practice management system.
- Create a patient's medical record.
- Organize a patient's medical record.
- File patient medical records.
- Utilize an EMR.
- Input patient data utilizing a practice management system.
- Explain the importance of data backup.
- Explain meaningful use as it applies to EMR.

ABHES

- Utilize electronic medical records (EMR) and practice management systems.
- Comply with federal, state, and local laws relating to exchange of information.
- Describe elements of meaningful use and reports generated.
- Demonstrate understanding of records management.

Chapter terms

Active records
Assessment
Closed records
Consultation reports

Database
Flow sheet
Inactive records
Narrative style

Numeric filing systems
Objective
Progress note
Radiographic reports

Secondary records
Subject filing
Subjective
Worker's compensation

Abbreviations

CC
EHR
EMR

FMH
HPI
POMR

PMH
ROS
SH

SOAP
SOMR

Case Study

Matthew McNeil came into the office today for follow-up after passing a kidney stone. A week ago, he went to the emergency room where he was treated and advised to follow up with his primary physician. During his visit, Mary, his medical assistant had to leave the room to get a blood pressure cuff. Mary, knowing she would be right back, left the computer open to Mr. McNeil's chart. Matthew saw the record open and began reading in his chart. He remembered that his wife had been in recently and was awaiting lab result so he decided to search her name. He located his wife's chart and her laboratory results. Mary returned to the room to find Mr. McNeil on the computer viewing his wife's laboratory results. Mary reported this incident to the office compliance officer, who in turned called Mrs. McNeil to report the details of the occurrence. Mary had to attend additional compliance training to insure such events do not occur in the future.

Working with patients' medical records is one of the most important jobs you'll have as a medical assistant. A fair amount of your time will be spent entering notes, documenting procedures, and scanning documents into the patient's record. A medical record is a form of communication as well as a legal document. It provides confidential information about a patient's health to those qualified to access it while also serving as evidence of the care the patient has received. Good medical records are vital to the smooth operation of any medical office. Physicians and other staff must be able to access a patient's chart quickly while insuring the information is protected. In this chapter, you'll learn how to organize and maintain patient records. You'll also learn about managing medical records systems.

MEDICAL RECORDS

Medical records are a critical part of health care. A patient's electronic medical record can be referred to as an **EMR** (electronic medical record), **EHR** (electronic health record), or patient's chart. This record contains the history of a patient's involvement with your office. It's the official record of the following things:

- The physician's evaluation of the patient's health
- Treatments carried out on the patient
- Changes in the patient's medical condition
- Communication between the patient and the staff

Information contained within the record is confidential and can't be shared with others unless the patient has signed an authorization to release the information. Medical records have other uses, too. For example, they can be valuable for research, in creating quality improvement (QI) programs, and for patient education.

Case Question

If you were Mary's supervisor, how would you approach Mary about this situation?

Information from medical records also helps the government protect the public's health as well as plan for future health care needs.

Patients must authorize the release of any information from their medical record. See Figure 11-1, a sample release form.

Southern Arundel OBGYN
3008 Pryson Avenue, Severn, Maryland 21140
Privacy Official: Jessica Pyrtle, CMA
Telephone: 410-966-2100

Authorization for Use or Disclosure of Health Information

Patient Name: _____
[print or type]

Patient's Date of Birth: _____ Patient's Identification/Chart No.: _____

I hereby authorize the use and disclosure of individually identifiable health information relating to me as described below:

Specific Description of the Information to be Used or Disclosed Including (If Practicable) the Dates of Service(s) Related to Such Information: _____

_____

The above information will be called "Authorized Information" throughout the rest of this form.

Persons or Class of Persons Authorized to Make the Use or Disclosure of Authorized Information:

_____

_____

Persons or Class of Persons to Whom the Use or Disclosure of Authorized Information May be Made:

_____

_____

Authorized Information will be used and/or disclosed for the following purposes:
[ ] At the request of the individual (check box if applicable)
[ ] Other *(Please list each purpose of the use(s) or disclosure(s) in the space provided.)*:

_____

_____

• I understand that if the person or entity receiving Authorized Information is not a health plan or health care provider covered by federal privacy regulations, the authorized information may be re-disclosed by the recipient and may no longer be protected by federal or state law.

• I understand that I may revoke this authorization at any time by notifying _____ [NAME OF PRACTICE] in writing. However, if I choose to do so, I understand that my revocation will not affect any actions taken by _____ [NAME OF PRACTICE] before receiving my revocation.

• I understand that I may refuse to sign this authorization and that my refusal to sign in no way affects my treatment, payment, enrollment in a health plan, or eligibility for benefits.
  [ALTERNATIVE, IF APPLICABLE: I understand that _____ [NAME OF PRACTICE] may require me to sign an authorization prior to receiving research-related treatment or treatment solely for the purpose of creating health information for another party and that _____ [NAME OF PRACTICE] will not provide such research-related treatment unless I provide this authorization. **NOTE:** If this provision is applicable, the third party for whom the information is being created must be listed under "Persons or Class of Persons to Whom the Use or Disclosure of Authorized Information May be Made." Also, the purpose for which the information is to be created and disclosed must be listed under "Authorized Information will be Used or Disclosed for the Following Purposes."

• [FOR MARKETING AUTHORIZATIONS ONLY, IF APPLICABLE] I understand that the person or entity I am authorizing to use and/or disclose Authorized Information for marketing purposes may receive either direct or indirect compensation for doing so.

This authorization expires at the earlier of _____ **OR the date the following event occurs:** _____

_____
[describe event or write "not applicable"]

Signature of Patient or Patient's Personal Representative: _____ Date: _____

For Personal Representative of the Patient (if applicable): _____

Print Name of Personal Representative: _____

Describe Personal Representative Relationship/Authority to Act for the Individual (parent, guardian, etc.): _____

_____

Figure 11-1   A sample Notice of Privacy Practices required by HIPAA. (Reprinted from Kronenberger J, Ledbetter J. *Jones & Bartlett Learning's Comprehensive Medical Assisting.* 5th ed. Burlington, MA: Jones & Bartlett Learning, LLC; 2016.)

Medical Record Security

You will deal with medical records nearly every day—documenting, adding lab reports and other items, and so on. Patients' charts must meet certain legal and ethical standards. So must your work with them. Access to medical records must be limited. Only authorized individuals involved in the care of the patient should access a patient's record.

Case Questions

Matthew McNeil, the patient from the case study, was seen looking at his wife's medical record. Is it permissible for family members to view records of other family members? What would happen if he saw records of other patients? Would this also be a problem? How can the medical staff ensure that patients and visitors do not have access to the practice computers and patient medical records? If you were the medical assistant in this situation, how would you approach the patient when he was caught viewing the computer screen?

The information contained in your office medical records must be:

- Easy for appropriate individuals to retrieve
- Organized
- Accurate and complete
- Secure

Security of medical records is a very serious matter. You must have a system in place that insures that only authorized individuals have access to a record. In addition, audits should be routinely performed to insure the information being accessed is appropriate and necessary. Your office must offer a secure and private way for individuals to file a compliancy complaint. These complaints must be investigated, documented, and resolved as quickly as possible. Steps to prevent future issues should be implemented to avoid additional compliancy problems. Remember, just because you have access to medical records, it doesn't mean that you can access records anytime you choose. Access must be limited to only what is needed to provide proper care to the patient. For example, accessing a friend or family member's file for information (even if it is for them) is not authorized use. Most offices have policies that prohibit employees from accessing records of family members or friends in an effort to avoid such situations. Figure 11-2 shows two types of authorization forms for the release of information.

I, _____, give my permission for _____ to release information generated in my medical record between the dates of _____ and _____ to _____.

Signature _____ Date _____
Witness _____ Date _____

Or

I, _____, give my permission for _____ to release information in my medical record regarding the care and treatment of _____ to _____.

Signature _____ Date _____
Witness _____ Date _____

Figure 11-2 A proper authorization for release of information. (Reprinted from Kronenberger J, Ledbetter J. *Jones & Bartlett Learning's Comprehensive Medical Assisting.* 5th ed. Burlington, MA: Jones & Bartlett Learning, LLC; 2016.)

Information Found in the Medical Record

A medical record contains two basic types of information:

1. Personal information includes the patient's name, address, telephone number, date of birth, social security number, emergency contacts, employment, and insurance. Many offices also include a copy of the patient's health insurance card and photo identifier.
2. Clinical information is the information about the patient's health, medical conditions, and treatment.

The history and physical (H&P) portion of the chart contains the following five vital items for each office evaluations:

- Chief complaint (**CC**)—the patient's explanation of why he came to see the doctor, usually stated in the patient's own words, in quotation marks
- History of present illness (**HPI**)—the patient's complaint stated in medical terms, with times and details
- Medical history—includes family medical history (**FMH**), a review of major illnesses of parents and grandparents, aunts and uncles, and brothers and sisters; past medical history (**PMH**), patient's major illnesses, surgeries, and hospitalizations; and social

history (**SH**), patient's dietary habits as well as smoking, drinking, and drug habits

- Review of systems (**ROS**)—an examination of the body systems to look for problems not yet identified
- Diagnosis or medical impression—the physician's opinion of the patient's medical problems

Figure 11-3 is a sample of documentation and the organized format used. This style makes the information easy to find and identify.

Medical records are frequently divided into categories as a means of organizing the information held within. Views of an electronic medical record can frequently be adjusted to accommodate individual or office preferences or needs. Views can include problem-oriented medical records (**POMR**) and source-oriented medical records (**SOMR**). Regardless of the view of the following, information will be held within a medical record:

- **Progress notes**—a record of what happened each time the patient was seen, including phone calls and prescription refills. The progress notes usually begin with the patient's H&P information.
- **Radiographic reports**—reports of x-rays, CT scans, MRIs, and similar studies that were done in the office or at another facility.
- Laboratory results—copies of the results of any tests done at the office or at an outside facility. Examples might include blood work and electrocardiographs (EKGs).
- **Consultation reports**—reports from other physicians with whom the patient's physician asked to consult about the patient.
- Medication administration—a record of the medicines the patient was given or prescribed. Some offices use a separate sheet for any injections and other medication the patient received in the office.
- All correspondence—copies of any letters or memos the office sent about the patient, copies of any letters from the patient, and correspondence from other physicians.

- Miscellaneous—consent forms and the HIPAA privacy notice signed by the patient, as well as copies of any patient instructions regarding end-of-life decisions. These might include organ donation forms, a living will, and a power of attorney for health care.
- **Secondary records**—records received from another physician, hospital, or other source. This information is for review only and is not available for release from your office.

Organization of Information within Medical Records

There are two main organizational methods used for medical records:

- Problem-oriented medical record (POMR) organizes information by the patient's problem. This is a good method for physicians who treat patients for a variety of problems.
- Source-oriented medical record (SOMR) files all items according to their source. For example, all lab reports are in one session of the record, and all radiology results are in another.

Whichever method your office uses, one thing doesn't change, the order. The most recent information always appears first in each section. In other words, most recent findings or events are on top or first. This creates a reverse order to the information. The farther back you go in each section of a patient's record, the older the information is.

POMR Organization

Family practices, pediatricians, and others who treat a variety of problems often use this method of organizing records. The patient's medical problems are listed in the first section of the record. As each problem arises, it is added to the list and given a number. All charting about that problem elsewhere in the record is given the same number. When the problem no longer exists, it is recorded in the progress notes, and an *X* is marked next to the problem on the problem list.

A POMR is divided into sections:

1. **Database**—the patient's information, which includes this information in the chart:
   - The patient's chief complaint
   - The present illness
   - The patient's medical history
   - Review of systems
   - Physical examination
   - Lab reports
2. Problem list—includes every past, present, and future problem the patient has that requires evaluation.
3. Treatment plan—includes the workups, tests, and treatment each problem has required.

Jamie Williams

08/18/16	*Office Visit*
Vitals:	*BP 110/68, P 80, T 98.6*
CC:	*Patient states: "I hurt my left arm when I fell off my horse yesterday." Has been taking Tylenol with some relief.*
HISTORY OF PRESENT ILLNESS:	*Patient's left arm is edematous. Deformity noted. Left radial pulse present. Able to move fingers on left hand. Nail beds on left hand pink and warm to touch.*
	Tonya Swain, RMA

Figure 11-3 EMR entry sample.

4. Progress notes—records of patient contacts that are numbered and grouped together. Some physicians may prefer to group these notes to relate to each numbered problem on the chart's problem list. Others might place them in chronological order.

SOMR Organization

Items in an SOMR are grouped by the type of service, not by the problem to which they're related. So, for example, all the x-ray reports are filed in one group, with the most recent report first, and so on.

Each office's classification system may differ. But the major groupings in an SOMR generally include the following:

- Progress notes
- Lab results
- Radiography reports
- Patient education

This approach to organizing charts is the most common method used to organize records. It is most often used by specialists as they tend treat a narrower range of problems.

Patient Education

Regardless of the format of a patient's record, it is important that they have access and understanding of the information contained within it. Many practices are offering (and encouraging) patients' access to their medical information through special portals. This allows patients to view radiology reports, laboratory results, and other information. Keep in mind that this system does not give the patient access to the entire medical record but rather elements of the records. Additionally, many of the systems allow patients to communicate with their physician electronically using their portal as well. To use their portal, the patient must first receive an access number granted by their medical office. Then, they can log into the system to build an account with a password that they select. Web portals are a great way for patients to access information and communicate with your office. Remember, when communicating using the portal, all transmissions are confidential and should be treated as privileged communication. Take time to insure that all communication is professionally written and concise. If information seems complex or has the potential of being misunderstood, another means of communicating the information, whether in person or by phone, should be used.

DOCUMENTATION AND THE EMR

The **SOAP** (subjective, objective, assessment, plan) format is one of the most common methods of documenting patient visits. The SOAP format is made up of four parts:

- The **subjective** part is the direct statement or description from the patient telling about his or her own condition. These notes should show the patient's exact words using actual quotations. For example, "I've been vomiting all night and have had diarrhea for the past 2 days. The last thing I was able to eat was crackers at dinner time last night."
- The **objective** part includes information the medical assistant and physician observe about the patient. It can include test results and vital signs. For example, "The patient appears weak, pale, and slightly dehydrated and has lost three pounds since her last visit."
- The **assessment** portion is the diagnosis made by the physician.
- The plan is a description of what should be done including any necessary diagnostic tests, treatments that will be given, and when the patient should follow up with the physician, if at all. For example, "Stool culture, CBC with diff, BRAT diet, and Imodium for the next 48 hours. Call office if symptoms worsen; return to office if patient not well by the end of the week."

Figure 11-4 shows a typical SOAP format, which is commonly used for documentation of patient care.

Progress Notes

A chart's progress notes record each contact with a patient—whether by phone, mail, e-mail, or in person—and briefly summarize what happened. All notes are electronically stamped with date, time, and signature of person entering the information.

Medical History Forms

Medical offices use these types of forms to get medical and personal information from a new patient before she sees the physician. Many offices mail these forms to patients before their first appointment. The patient then brings the completed form to the appointment. This process has several advantages:

- The patient has time to think carefully about and answer the questions.
- The patient can gather information about the family medical history.
- The medical office receives a more accurate and complete patient medical history.

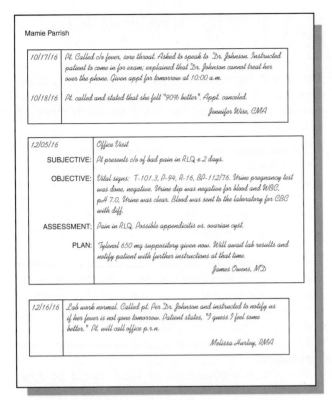

Mamie Parrish

10/17/16	Pt. Called c/o fever, sore throat. Asked to speak to Dr. Johnson. Instructed patient to come in for exam; explained that Dr. Johnson cannot treat her over the phone. Given appt for tomorrow at 10:00 a.m.
10/18/16	Pt. called and stated that she felt "90% better". Appt. canceled.
	Jennifer Wise, CMA

12/05/16	Office Visit
SUBJECTIVE:	Pt presents c/o of bad pain in RLQ x 2 days.
OBJECTIVE:	Vital signs: T-101.3, P-94, R-16, BP-112/76. Urine pregnancy test was done, negative. Urine dip was negative for blood and WBC, pH 7.0. Urine was clear. Blood was sent to the laboratory for CBC with diff.
ASSESSMENT:	Pain in RLQ. Possible appendicitis vs. ovarian cyst.
PLAN:	Tylenol 650 mg suppository given now. Will await lab results and notify patient with further instructions at that time.
	James Owens, MD

| 12/16/16 | Lab work normal. Called pt. Per Dr. Johnson and instructed to notify us if her fever is not gone tomorrow. Patient states, "I guess I feel some better." Pt. will call office p.r.n. |
| | Melissa Hurley, RMA |

Figure 11-4 Sample SOAP notes. (Reprinted from Kronenberger J, Ledbetter J. *Jones & Bartlett Learning's Comprehensive Medical Assisting.* 5th ed. Burlington, MA: Jones & Bartlett Learning, LLC; 2016.)

In an EMR, the information from this form is keyed or scanned into the patient's chart. The completed form is then shredded to protect the privacy of the patient's information.

Flow Sheets

A **flow sheet** is a form that allows information to be recorded in a table or on a graph. An office may use several types of flow sheets. They are generally designed for a specific use, such as charting vital signs or tracking prescribed medications. They are also often color coded. The graph on which to record a child's height and weight at each visit might be pink for girls and blue for boys, for example.

Flow sheets are very useful forms to have in a record, as described below:

- Limit the need for long notes explaining the information.
- Eliminate the need to search through notes in the record to find the information.
- Provide all the information at once. This makes it easier to spot any changes over time.

In an EMR, the software can create the flow sheet; all you have to do is enter the information. The computer automatically puts it on the graph or table.

 MAINTAINING RECORDS

A huge amount of paperwork comes into the typical medical office each day. This includes the following:

- Radiology reports
- Laboratory test results
- Other test results
- Hospital records
- Notes from other physicians
- Insurance information

All this material must be sorted and scanned into the right patient's chart. You will need to verify the patient information and then scan documents not already received electronically.

 WORKERS COMPENSATION RECORDS

From time to time, a current patient will seek treatment for an injury or illness he got on the job. These services should be maintained in special area of the patient record. In a workers' compensation case, you must keep separate medical and financial records for the patient. **Workers' compensation** is health insurance that the law requires employers to have for workers who suffer job-related injuries.

Unless the injury is life threatening, you must first have approval from the patient's employer to treat the patient and bill for workers' compensation. (You'll read more about getting this approval in Chapter 14, Health Insurance and Claims) Be sure to write the name of the person who authorizes treatment in the patient's medical record. Also chart any additional information you receive that relates to the approval process. In workers' compensation cases, the employer's workers' compensation insurer can review any information pertaining to the injury or illness, even if the patient opposes it. However, they are not entitled to any other information within the patient's record, only information directly related to care resulting from the injury/illness.

 MAKING ENTRIES IN MEDICAL RECORDS

A patient's medical record is a legal document. It can be presented in court as evidence in a malpractice suit. The entries the office staff makes in a chart can help win a lawsuit—or prevent one altogether—if they are:

- Accurate and complete
- Clear enough to be read easily
- Timely, written at the time of the event

On the other hand, if charting is inaccurate, incomplete, or improperly done, it can raise questions about what actually happened. This might cause a health care provider to lose a malpractice suit. Always remember, if it's not documented, it didn't happen. Any communication with a patient should be accurately recorded.

Proper Use of Abbreviations in Charting

It's common to see abbreviations in charting entries. Using them saves writing time and space. Your office should have a list of standard abbreviations. Table 11-1 shows some abbreviations that are used commonly in charting.

Be careful how you use abbreviations. Errors in patient care could result if you use a wrong abbreviation, or one that has an unclear meaning, in the chart.

Also, always use the standard abbreviations instead of making up your own. Remember, following these procedures is vital because the medical record is a legal document.

Study Skill

Sometimes, finding the right time to study is the biggest obstacle you will encounter. A great way to insure that you have time to devote to your studies is to schedule it into your day. Consider scheduling 30 minutes to an hour each day as devoted school work time. Make sure you share with family and friends the time you select so they know you are unavailable during that time. Utilize this time to review your notes, study for exams, and work on assignments. At first, it might be a challenge to hold yourself to the new schedule; however, once you get into the routine, it seems completely normal.

Phone Calls

Any phone calls made to or about patients must be recorded in their individual records. Calls include the following:

- Pharmacy calls for new prescriptions or refills. It is important to chart the name of the medication, dosage, directions, quantity, and last refill.

Table 11-1 Abbreviations Used in Charting

Abbreviation	Meaning	Abbreviation	Meaning
p	Before	NKDA	No known drug allergies
Abd	Abdomen	noct.	Nocturnal
ant.	Anterior	$\bar{p}$	After
AP	Anteroposterior	p.c.	After a meal
Apt	Appointment	PE	Physical examination
Ax	Axillary	p.r.n.	As needed
b.i.d.	Twice a day	pt.	Patient
BP	Blood pressure	q.i.d.	Four times a day
$\bar{c}$	With	R	Right
CC	Chief complaint	R/O	Rule out
c/o	Complains of	RLE	Right lower extremity
CPE, CPX	Complete physical exam	RLQ	Right lower quadrant
Cx	Cancelled	RUE	Right upper extremity
D/C	Discontinue	RUQ	Right upper quadrant
F	Fahrenheit	R/S	Rescheduled
Fx	Fracture	$\bar{s}$	Without
h.s.	Bedtime (hour of sleep)	SOB	Shortness of breath
Hx	History	Spec	Specimen
L	Left	s/p	After (status post)
LLE	Left lower extremity	STAT	Immediately
LLQ	Left lower quadrant	t.i.d.	Three times a day
LUE	Left upper extremity	TPR	Temperature, pulse, respiration
LUQ	Left upper quadrant		

- Laboratory results from the lab to the physician or recommendations from the physician to the patient. Be sure to note core values along with the patient results. Also note any questions or concerns the patient may have.

Timely Charting

As you already know, information in the patient record is recorded in chronological order. The most recent entries should always be first. This is one reason why you should record contacts with patients soon after they take place. Another reason is the events will still be fresh in your mind. The EMR system automatically date and time stamps all entries. If you wait, someone might write another, later event in the record. Also, you might forget the details of the encounter.

Charting Communications from Patients

Phone calls from patients are usually charted in **narrative style**, meaning that it is written out as you would speak. Document the conversation immediately. Include the following information in your note:

- What the patient requested or said
- What you said and the actions you took

E-mails from patients should be electronically entered in the chart. Any replies to the patient should only occur using the portal. This will insure the communication is entered into the medical record.

MANAGING MEDICAL RECORDS

Good management of an office's electronic medical records requires five basic things.

1. Properly and accurately create the records for new patients.
2. Scan new items in patients' records accurately and in a timely manner.
3. Properly and accurately enter information regarding care.
4. Maintain the security and confidentiality of records.
5. Utilize a secure method of backing up all records.

Classifications of Medical Records

Patients' records are classified into three categories:

- Active records
- Inactive records
- Closed records

Active Records

Active records are the records of patients who have been seen recently or within the past 3 years.

Inactive Records

Inactive records are the records of patients who have not been seen in 3 or more years. Such patients have not terminated their care nor has their care been terminated so they are welcome to return to see the physician at any point. However, patients who have not been seen in 3 or more years are considered to be new patients.

Closed Records

Closed records are the charts of patients who have ended their relationship with the physician. Here are the main reasons you would classify a patient's chart as closed:

- The patient has moved away.
- The physician–patient relationship has been terminated by letter.
- The patient has elected to change providers
- The patient has died.

Closed records should be removed from active files and archived in the system.

Record Retention

All patient records should be kept permanently, but they don't all have to be kept in the active system. Closed records can be archived within the system. All patient records should be easily accessible. This will allow for access either should the need arise to provide information to aid in the patient's care or should it be needed for legal reasons.

EMR and Ethical Responsibility

A well-known celebrity comes to your office for visit. During the visit, you assist in the care of the patient. You review the patient's current illness, past medical, social, and family history. As with any patient, this information is confidential and privileged and thus can't be shared with anyone. Even the mention that this person was seen in the office is a breach. Care must be taken to insure that you never release any information, knowingly or unknowingly, about any patient.

FILING SYSTEMS

The two main systems used to file and retrieve medical records are as follows:

- Alphabetical filing system
- Numeric (number) filing systems

Most EMR systems utilize both systems allowing you to search for records using either the numeric record number or the patient's name.

Alphabetic Filing

This method of organizing medical records places them in alphabetical order by patients' last names. If two or more patients have the same last name, the system orders them alphabetically by their first names, and so on.

Numeric Filing

Numeric filing systems usually assign a six-digit number to each patient also referred to as a medical record number (MRN). Utilizing an MRN in communication can be more secure and accurate. It eliminates the need to say the patient's name and reduces the risk of misspelling.

Numeric systems have a couple of advantages over the alphabetical system:

- It makes no difference if two or more patients have the same name, such as John Smith. Each John Smith will be assigned a different MRN. Helping to reduce the risk of entering information into the wrong record.
- The results of tests for HIV and AIDS are strictly confidential. Use numbers instead of names to identify the test record of patients to add privacy. This feature has helped make numeric filing systems more popular in laboratory environments.

Cultural Connection

There are some specific populations that are at higher risk for HIV. The CDC reports that young black males, aged 13 to 24, engaging in sexual activity with other males demonstrated the highest occurrence of new cases in 2010. Many offices now include questions on their social history forms regarding sexual activity. This information is both private and confidential. You may be called upon to provide patient education to individuals at risk for HIV or other sexually transmitted illnesses. Regardless of your personal opinion or views, you must present information professionally and without bias.

Other Filing Systems

Your office will have more files than just patient charts. Some examples of other records include the following:

- Employee personnel files
- Inventories of equipment and supplies
- Records of past supply orders
- Accounts payable
- Insurance records
- Catalogs from suppliers

Your office will likely use a system of **subject filing** for keeping such records. This is a system in which records are grouped alphabetically according to their subject—insurance, medications, referrals, and so on. Here are some other filing systems you might see or use.

- Geographic filing—documents are grouped alphabetically according to location, such as state, county, or city. This method is often used in case studies or research projects.
- Chronological filing—documents are grouped in the order of their date, such as year or month. This system is frequently used for accounts payable.

Preparing for Externship

You should approach your externship just as if you are an actual employee of the medical office. Your actions should reflect everything that an employer would expect from any employee. Show up for work on time and give your all each day. Some students adopt the attitude that since they are not receiving pay for this experience, they don't have to apply much effort. Not true. This time above all else is your opportunity to shine and show everyone what a great employee you can be. Your professional behavior will be evaluated by the extern site preceptor. You are not expected to be perfect; however, you need to have an attitude of willingness. You need to be willing to accept all tasks assigned even though you may not like all of them. At the beginning of the externship, most sites assign students basic tasks to help them get acclimated to the site. You will probably shadow another employee the first few days so you can get familiar with the flow of the office. Do not get discouraged thinking that this is all you will be doing. Many offices are just trying to see how you handle the smaller basic tasks before they assign more responsibilities.

Chapter Recap

- Medical records are legal documents that should be complete and accurate.
- All encounters with a patient are documented in their record.
- Security of all patient health information should be a top priority.
- Patient records can be organized using POMR or SOMR format.
- There are three types of patient records: active, inactive, and closed.
- All records should be backed up to a secure location.
- There are two main types of filing systems for medical records: alphabetic and numeric.
- Other files in the office that require filing include employee records, payroll, purchasing invoices, and insurance records.
- Geographic filing systems are frequently used for research.
- Accounts payable are organized using a chronological filing system.

Online Resources for Students

Student Resources available on the text's online site include:
- Audio Glossaries
- Animations
- Competency Evaluation Forms
- Videos
- Anatomy & Physiology Module with Heart and Lung Sounds
- Weblinks
- Worksheets

Exercises and Activities

Certification Preparation Questions

1. Which of the following demonstrates a medical record security practice?
   a. Leaving a medical record open for the patient to view, as it is their record
   b. Turning off the computer screen when walking away from the system
   c. Pressing the window and "L" key to lock the system
   d. Allowing another medical assistant to use your password when they forget theirs
   e. Sharing the names of famous athletes that come to your office to help build the practice

2. Which of the following individuals meets the "meaningful use" standard for entering laboratory orders into patient records?
   a. Any employee working in the office
   b. Only employees in the laboratory
   c. Only the physician
   d. Credentialed medical assistants (RMA or CMA)
   e. Any medical assistant in the office

3. Personal information, in a medical record, includes which of the following?
   a. Social Security Number
   b. Chief complaint
   c. History of present illness
   d. Social history
   e. Laboratory results

4. Medical records organized by department or source of information is referred to as:
   a. source-organized medical record.
   b. problem-organized medical records.
   c. departmentalized medical records.
   d. source-oriented medical records.
   e. problem-oriented medical records.

5. Information that can be obtained only from the patient would be recorded under:
   a. plan.
   b. subjective.
   c. assessment.
   d. objective.
   e. treatment.

6. When documenting in the medical record, information observed by the physician or medical assistant should be entered as:

   a. plan.
   b. subjective.
   c. assessment.
   d. objective.
   e. treatment.

7. If a patient smokes 3 packs of cigarettes a day, where would you note this in the medical record?

   a. Past medical history
   b. History of present illness
   c. Family history
   d. Surgical history
   e. Social history

8. The medical records of a deceased patient would be classified as what type of record?

   a. Inactive
   b. Closed
   c. Active
   d. Deactivated
   e. Dead

9. If files are stored by the medical record number (MRN), what type of "filing" system would this be referred to as?

   a. Numeric
   b. Alphabetical
   c. Geographic
   d. Subject
   e. Chronological

10. If filing records or reports based on the location or region of occurrence this would be referred to as what type of filing system?

    a. Numeric
    b. Alphabetic
    c. Geographic
    d. Subject
    e. Chronological

 ## CareTracker Connection

Patient Medical Records and Documentation

 HARRIS CareTracker Activities Related to
CareTracker This Chapter
● Case Study 2: Entering Patient Demographic and Insurance Information

Managing patients' medical records is a critical responsibility of the medical assistant. An electronic medical record system, such as CareTracker, makes performing this task much easier and more efficient.

Tasks discussed in this chapter that can be performed in CareTracker include the following:

● Creating patient medical records
● Documenting patient personal information
● Documenting the following patient clinical information:
  ○ Chief complaint
  ○ History of present illness
  ○ Medical history
  ○ Review of systems
  ○ Laboratory results
  ○ Diagnosis or medical impression
  ○ Treatment plan
  ○ Progress notes
  ○ Medication administration
  ○ Patient education
● Documenting workers' compensation cases
● Documenting communication with patients
● Managing patient medical records

Many of these tasks are discussed in CareTracker Connection features in other chapters. A task we'll consider here is entering patient demographic and insurance information.

If a patient is new to a medical practice, one of the first responsibilities you'll have is to gather the patient's personal information. This includes name, home and billing addresses, phone number(s), e-mail address, date of birth, Social Security Number, gender, and marital status.

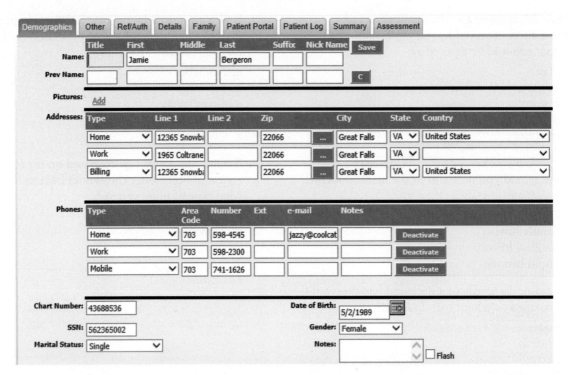

To ensure proper billing and payment, it is also imperative to collect the patient's insurance information, if applicable, including the name and address of the insurance company; name of the plan; subscriber, group, and member numbers; eligibility from and to dates; and copayment amount.

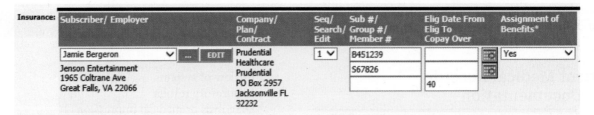

If the patient is employed, you must also collect employment information, including the name and address of the employer, occupation, start and end dates, and work phone number and e-mail.

In addition to gathering this data initially, it is also your responsibility to regularly check in with the patient regarding any changes in this information and to update the medical record accordingly.

Culture Connection Resource

http://www.cdc.gov/nchhstp/newsroom/docs/HIVFactSheets/TodaysEpidemic-508.pdf

http://www.cdc.gov/nchhstp/newsroom/docs/HIVFactSheets/TodaysEpidemic-508.pdf

12 Medical Insurance Coding

Chapter Objectives

- Explain what coding is and why it is used.
- Describe the relationship between diagnostic coding, procedural coding, and reimbursement.
- Describe how the ICD-10-CM is organized.
- List the steps in identifying a proper diagnostic code.
- Name the common errors in diagnostic coding.
- Perform diagnostic coding.
- Describe how the CPT-4 is organized and used.
- Summarize the factors that determine which E/M code to assign a patient visit.

- Understand HCPCS codes and surgical packages.
- Perform procedural coding.
- Demonstrate understanding of upcoding and downcoding.
- Determine medical necessity as it applies to coding.
- Understand the importance of communication with medical providers to ensure accurate code selection.

CAAHEP & ABHES Competencies

CAAHEP

- Describe how to use the most current procedural coding system.
- Describe how to use the most current diagnostic coding classification system.
- Describe how to use the most current HCPCS level II coding system.
- Discuss the effects of upcoding and downcoding.
- Define medical necessity as it applies to procedural and diagnostic coding.

- Perform procedural coding.
- Perform diagnostic coding.
- Utilize medical necessity guidelines.
- Utilize tactful communication skills with medical providers to ensure accurate code selection.

ABHES

- Perform diagnostic and procedural coding.

Chapter Terms

Alphanumeric	Etiology	Medical necessity	Subsequent encounter
Bundled	Global surgical follow-up	Modifiers	Sequela
Comorbidity	Initial encounter	Physical status modifier	Unbundled
Diagnostic codes	Key components	Procedure codes	Unbundling
Downcoding	Late effects	Primary diagnosis	Upcoding

Abbreviations

CMS	HCPCS	ICD-10-CM	OIG
CPT-4	HIPAA	NCHS	WHO
E/M			

Case Study

Jessica McNeil's mother brought her to the office today for her prekindergarten physical examination. During her visit, the doctor ordered two immunizations (DPT and IPV) and a hemoglobin test that you performed. As the medical assistant, you need to complete the coding information.

Medical coding is the translation of a written diagnosis or procedure into an alphanumeric code, the use of numbers and letters. This process can be a complex task, as it requires accuracy, medical knowledge, and careful attention to detail.

Coding is one of the most important jobs you may do as medical assistant. The codes you use to describe a patient's diagnosis and treatment will determine what the patient's health insurance plan will pay. If the codes you assign are incorrect or incomplete, there may be a reduction, delay, or denial of the payment amount to the provider. Since most of a medical office's income generally comes from insurance, proper coding is critical. The information in this chapter will introduce you to the process of billing services rendered to the patient and coding them for submission to the insurance company.

MEDICAL CODING

Medical coding replaces verbal descriptions of diseases, injuries, conditions, and services with **alphanumeric** codes, those made up of letters and numbers. These codes make medical information more standard, or uniform, than written descriptions. Medicare, Medicaid, and other health care plans require providers to use them.

HIPAA, Health Insurance Portability and Accountability Act, requires the use of ICD codes when processing insurance claims. There are two types of codes:

- **Diagnostic codes**—These codes are used to identify the reason the patient is seeking care. These codes come from the International Classification of Diseases, Tenth Revision, Clinical Modification, **ICD-10-CM.** This book has recently undergone a major update allowing more detail when assigning codes.
- **Procedure codes**—These codes describe services provided to the patient. Most services are located in the fourth edition of Current Procedural Terminology (**CPT-4**); however, some codes are in the HCPCS book. The Healthcare Common Procedure Coding System (**HCPCS**) book is used to code for supplies and/or services not listed in the CPT book. HCPCS codes are important, yet frequently forgotten, codes.

Case Questions

 If you discover that the insurance company does not reimburse for the hemoglobin test, how would you inform the patient's mother? What would you say if the mother became angry?

For example, when giving an injection, the code for the administration of the injection is located in the CPT book; however, this does not include the medication. The medication code is listed in the HCPCS book.

There are many benefits of coding, such as:

- Ensuring that all health care providers report the same conditions and procedures in exactly the same way.
- Collecting accurate of health information and statistics.
- Performing medical reviews or medical chart audits is easier. Medical chart audits can occur both in the physician's office and at the insurance company. The charts are reviewed for accuracy and appropriateness of codes used for claims.
- Efficient, accurate processing of health insurance claims.

Coding and Insurance

All codes you use for patient billing must be complete and correct. The CPT codes reported on a patient's insurance claim form determine the amount insurance will pay for the service rendered. ICD codes help determine **medical necessity**. This means the procedure or service billed was reasonable for the patient's medical condition.

For example, an insurance company wouldn't consider a chest x-ray medically necessary if the ICD code was for an ear infection, but if the diagnostic code was acute bronchitis, the insurance company probably would pay. The diagnosis code justifies the procedure code. On the other hand, inaccurate coding can lead to:

- Delayed payment
- Reduced payment
- Denied payment

Of course, there must be documentation in the patient's chart to support the diagnoses and procedures used. Upcoding is assigning a code for services greater than the service provided to the patient. Upcoding is an unethical and illegal practice. **Downcoding**, would be the opposite, it represents coding for less than the actual service provided. This practice would then result in underpayment to the physician. Proper coding is critical to your office reimbursement.

Diagnostic Coding

The ICD is a system of classifying diseases developed by the World Health Organization (**WHO**) in the 1930s and 1940s. In 1948, the first ICD book was published. Since then, the list has been revised ten times. The latest revision, the ICD-10, has recently been adapted for use

in United States. The ICD-10-CM was published in the United States in 2015. It is updated each year with codes added, changed, and sometimes removed. The National Center for Health Statistics (**NCHS**), a US government agency, keeps the list of diagnoses current. The WHO approves all changes before they are published. Changes generally are published each October. Most health plans that require claims to be submitted after January 1 use the latest version of the codes.

ICD-10-CM code books are available from several publishers. Each publisher's book presents the information a little differently but the content is the same. Publishers also sell the annual updates to the ICD-10-CM. Your office should use the updates from the same publisher as your coding book.

ICD-10-CM Code Book

The ICD-10-CM is issued in two separate books, ICD-10-CM and ICD-10-PCS. The ICD-10-CM is divided into two volumes:

- *Volume 1: Tabular List of Diseases*—This section provides a numeric listing of codes. This section contains greater detail and is used second to the alphabetic index to insure the proper code is being assigned.
- *Volume 2: Alphabetic Index of Diseases*—As the name suggests, codes are listed alphabetically. This section is used first to obtain the numeric code and then is verified as the best code using Volume 1.

The ICD-10-PCS contains only *Volume 3: Tabular List and Alphabetic Index of Procedures*. This book includes codes for hospital procedures.

Symbols and Conventions

Prior to using the ICD-10 books, it is important to become familiar with the symbols and conventions used within each book. This information is found in the forward section of the book, the section immediately following the index. Some of the more commonly used symbols are also listed at the bottom of each coding page in Volume 2. A summary of all the symbols are located at the bottom of each page in Volume 1. For example, a red dot acts like a stop sign to alert you that the code requires additional digits. This is of significant importance as the more detailed the diagnose code is, the more accurately the claim can be processed. If digits are omitted from the claim, it will likely be rejected, resulting in a delay of payment. Pay special attention to the instructional notations at the beginning of each chapter. These notations will provide you with information regarding inclusions and exclusions within the chapter along with guidelines for seventh character placement. Table 12-1 provides a few examples of the coding conventions found in the ICD-10-CM.

Table 12-1	ICD-10-CM Coding Conventions
code first	Instructions indicating the underlying condition that should be coded first
use additional	Indicates another code may be required
Code also	Instructs that two codes are likely needed to fully explain the condition
N	Newborn

Organization of Codes

Volume 1 organizes diseases and other conditions into 21 chapters, according to **etiology**, the cause of the disease, or body system. The diseases are alphanumerically listed in sequence within each chapter and throughout the book beginning with A and ending with Z, excluding the letter U.

Special Codes

The V through Y codes are used to code conditions related to external causes. For example, if a person is injured due to a fall from non-in-line roller skates, the initial code would be V00.121. This code requires an additional character to indicate if this was the **initial encounter**, the first time seeing the patient. If it is a **subsequent encounter** or **sequela**, this indicates follow-up encounters. For example, if it is the initial encounter, the code used would be V00.121A. The A represents the initial encounter. Table 12-2 represents examples of codes used in External Causes. Take some time to explore the External Causes section of the ICD-10-CM coding manual to become familiar with the diagnoses covered in the section. Remember, these codes are in addition to the descriptive injury code.

The Z codes are used when a patient seeks care but is not ill or injured. These codes are used when a patient is not currently ill but is seeking care. A few types of care that the Z codes are used for include physicals, well examinations, and normal pregnancy.

Table 12-2	Examples of External Causes from ICD-10-CM

X ● W27.1 Contact with a garden tool
  Contact with: hoe, non powered lawnmower, pitchfork, or rake

X ● W32 Accidental handgun discharge

X ● indicates the need for a place holder (X) and additional characters

Recall from the case study that Jessica McNeil came to the office for her prekindergarten physical and immunizations. The diagnosis codes for her visit will be Z codes; annual physical examination of a child age 5 and vaccination against DPV and IPV. Using the ICD-10-CM coding manual, what are the correct diagnosis codes for her visit?

Coding Diagnoses

Diagnostic codes can range from three to seven characters in length. The more characters used within the code, the more detail is translated in the code. The ICD-10-CM coding manual is organized by chapters, according to the etiology (cause of the disease) or body system. Each section, within the chapter, has a three-character code that identifies the category. Additional characters are used to provide more detail about the condition, up to a total of seven characters. There will be times when you need a seventh digit but not a sixth. In these cases, you will use an X as a placeholder. This is extremely important as a change in the position of a number within a code changes its meaning. You should pay close attention to the symbols that indicate if additional characters are required. In cases where additional characters are required, there will be a box at the beginning of the section that contains the additional characters. You need to verify your code fails within those listed for the additional character box you are using. Some chapters have multiple boxes so you should use care to insure you are in the correct area.

Alphabetic Index to Diseases and Injuries

You should always begin the coding of a diagnosis in this section. This section allows you to look up the diagnosis alphabetically. Once you have selected a code from this section you will then use that code to look in the tabular list of diseases and injuries. As previously mentioned, this section provides more detail for the chosen codes. At times, you will find that the code you found in the alphabetic index may not be the best code for the diagnosis. Utilizing this practice every time you code will insure that you're coding to the greatest possible level of detail.

Table of Neoplasms

This section of the ICD-10 lists codes for neoplasms by anatomical site. You will need to know if the neoplasm is malignant, benign, or uncertain behavior. When dealing with malignant neoplasms, you need to know if it is primary, secondary, or in situ. This information will come from the physician. If the determination of benign or malignant has not been made, you will need the physician to specify whether it is a neoplasm with uncertain behavior or unspecified behavior.

Table of Drugs and Chemicals

This table contains a long list of medicines, drugs, and other substances. It shows the code to assign when a patient is harmed by a drug, or other substance, in each of these circumstances:

- *Accidental poisoning*—The patient received an accidental overdose of the drug or was given or took the drug by mistake.
- *Therapeutic use*—The patient took or received the drug in the right dose to treat or prevent a disease.
- *Suicide attempt*—The patient took the drug in an effort to poison or injure himself.
- *Assault*—Someone gave the patient the drug in a deliberate attempt to harm him.
- *Undetermined*—It's not known whether the poisoning or injury from the drug was intended or accidental.

The Main Term Rule

The first step in coding a diagnosis is to locate the main term in the diagnosis statement. This will usually appear on the progress notes in the patient's medical chart. The diagnosis usually will be listed there as the impression. The main term rule means that you look for the main term in the diagnosis or description. As you are coding, you need to look for the key words within the diagnosis.

Applying the Main Term Rule

For example, the main term for the diagnosis of malignant hypertension is hypertension, because it represents the actual condition. Hypertension is the term you look up in the alphabetic index. Under hypertension, you find all the different types of hypertension listed. Malignant will be one of the types.

Exceptions to the Main Term Rule

Keep these exceptions to the main term rule in mind when you use the alphabetic index:

1. Obstetric conditions may be found under these main terms:
   - Delivery
   - Pregnancy
   - Puerperal
2. Complications of medical or surgical procedures are listed under complication.

3. Z codes are found under main entries such as:
   - Admissions
   - Examination
   - History of observation
   - Problem (with)
   - Status
   - Vaccination
   - Encounter for

Study Skill

Proper coding takes time and practice, a lot of practice. Utilize every opportunity you have to explore the codes with the ICD-10-CM, CPT, and HCPCS. Look up diagnoses and procedures that interest you. Think through the process of patient care and then code accordingly. Use the tips throughout this chapter to help you become comfortable and efficient in your coding.

Primary Codes

A patient will have a **primary diagnosis** on each visit to the office. This is simply the patient's chief complaint or the reason he sought medical attention that day. The code for that diagnosis, complaint, or reason is the primary code for the visit. The primary diagnosis code is always listed first. In some cases, the primary diagnosis may not be the only reason for the visit. In cases of **comorbidity**, more than one disease or condition occurring at the same time, the reason for the patient's visit is complicated by a secondary diagnosis or diagnoses. These codes need to be listed to give an accurate picture of the patient's overall health. For example, a patient who has insulin-dependent diabetes mellitus comes in for the flu. Since the interaction between her diabetes and the flu will affect treatment and prognosis, list both diagnoses. Since her diabetes can complicate the treatment and progression of the flu, list it as a secondary code.

Therefore, you would code the diagnosis of type I diabetes mellitus below the primary code of the flu.

Late Effects

Late effects are conditions that result from a past injury or illness. They are present long after treatment for the injury or illness has ended. For example, patients who have suffered a stroke, known as a cerebrovascular accident (CVA) in the past, may have effects that linger after their recovery.

For instance, a patient may have a diagnosis of left hemiparesis (paralysis) resulting from a stroke 3 years earlier. For this patient's visit, you would code the current condition, left hemiparesis, first, as the primary diagnosis. The code number identifying the cause, the stroke, which is the original illness or injury, comes second.

Table 12-3 Late Effects Codes

Seventh character to be added to each S23 code

A   Initial encounter

D   Subsequent encounter

S   Sequela

Example of Late Effects Coding

S23.10   Subluxation and dislocation of unspecified thoracic vertebra

    S23.100   Subluxation of T1/T2 thoracic vertebra

    S23.101   Dislocation of T1/T2 thoracic vertebra

Note:

For an initial encounter with a diagnosis of subluxation and dislocation of unspecified thoracic vertebra = S23.10XA

X is used as a placeholder for digits that are not used.

A diagnosis of Initial Subluxation of T1/T2 thoracic vertebra = S23.100A

Table 12-3 is an example of the page showing the late effects codes that are always coded first, followed by the code identifying the cause. An example of this type of coding is also shown in the table.

Coding Suspected Conditions

In hospitals, medical coders don't list patients' diagnoses until testing is complete. In other words, they code from complete information. In a medical office, you have to report the reason for the patient's visit when it occurs. You'll be limited by the information available at the time. Often, this will be only the patient's complaint and the physician's best guess about what is causing it. The physician may write probable or rule out along with his suspected diagnosis. However, you cannot code this diagnosis as the reason for the visit until it's confirmed. You don't want to put in the patient's record that he has a condition he may not really have. Instead, you should code the reason the patient came in. That reason could be a test result that was abnormal, a sign or a symptom.

Here's an example: A patient makes an appointment because he's been having severe headaches. The physician suspects a brain tumor and schedules the patient for an MRI (magnetic resonance imaging) of his head. The physician writes rule out brain tumor in the patient's chart. But you can't code the diagnosis as brain tumor until the MRI test confirms it. You don't have that information on this visit. Therefore, you will code the symptom of severe headaches.

CPT-4 CODING MANUAL

The CPT-4 is the fourth edition of *Current Procedural Terminology*. The book lists codes for common medical procedures and services. It was first published by the American Medical Association (AMA) in 1966. The fourth edition was published in 1977. That was the last major revision of the book but it is updated every year.

A CPT code is a five-digit numeric code for a specific medical procedure or service that a physician provides to a patient. The main code for a procedure is listed first followed by other codes that offer additional services or details that are indented below it. CPT codes can also have modifiers, which offer additional special information. You'll read more about modifiers later in this chapter.

Patient Education

When a physician orders certain tests or procedures, they may require preauthorization the insurance company. Sometimes, this can be difficult to explain to the patient. It is important that the patient understands that even though the physician ordered the test or procedure we must follow the insurance companies guidelines. Be sure they understand that failure to obtain a preauthorization can result in the insurance company not paying for the test or procedure. MRI is one example of a test that must be preauthorized. The patient is responsible to pay for the cost of the test if the insurance company does not cover it.

CPT Coding

The CPT codes are divided into six sections. The codes in each section of the CPT-4 are listed by number and are organized by the type of service. The six sections of the CPT-4 are:

- *Evaluation and management*—These are the codes used to charge for office visits. All codes in this section begin with the number 9.
- *Anesthesia*—These codes are organized according to body site (head, thorax, hip, etc.). Then, under each body site, the specific procedure code is listed. These codes all begin with 0.
- *Surgery*—Surgery codes begin with numbers 1 through 6. Like the anesthesia codes, they are organized according to which part of the body is involved.
- *Radiology*—All radiology codes begin with the number 7.
- *Pathology and laboratory*—This section includes every lab test that can be ordered. These codes all begin with 8.
- *Medicine*—These codes cover nonsurgical treatments and services that ordinarily take place in a doctor's office such as injections and **global surgical follow-up**, an inclusive package of all the procedures and visits surrounding a surgical procedure. They all begin with a 9, just like the evaluation and management (E/M) codes.

Table 12-4 Examples of E/M Codes

99201—New Patient Visit:
 Problem-focused history and exam
 Straightforward decision making
 Face-to-face time 10 minutes

99202—New Patient Visit
 Expand Problem-focused
 Low complexity decision making
 Face to face time 20 minutes

Table 12-4 provides examples of E/M codes found in the CPT book.

Section Guidelines

Each section begins with a set of guidelines for coding the kinds of procedures listed in that particular section. Pay close attention to these guidelines as they contain useful information, such as:

- Definitions and explanations to assist the coder
- A list of procedures new to the section
- Modifiers that can be used with the section's codes
- Codes to use when an unlisted procedure is performed
- Directions on how to file a special report

Appendices

There are several appendices listed in the book of the CPT book immediately following the coding sections. The appendix you will use most frequently is Appendix A as it provides a complete listing of all modifiers. Additionally, Appendix C can be helpful if you are having difficulty determining an E/M code. Below is a guide to the appendices:

- Appendix A—all modifiers that are used to alter or modify codes
- Appendix B—complete list of additions to/deletions from and revisions of CPT manual
- Appendix C—clinical examples of many of the evaluation and management codes (E/M)
- Appendix D—lists all add-on codes (+)
- Appendix F—summary of CPT codes modifier –63 exempt –63 identifies procedures that are performed on infants <4 kg or 8.8 pounds and represents a significant increase in physician's work and complexity of service/procedure; may be reviewed for increase in reimbursement
- Appendix G—summary of moderate (conscious) sedation codes (bull's-eye)
- Appendix L—vascular families
- Appendix M—Summary of cross-walked deleted CPT codes, lists current-year code to replace a deleted code.

- Appendix N—Summary of resequenced CPT codes (re sequencing # symbol)
- Appendix O—multianalyte assays with algorithmic analyses

Symbols in the CPT-4

There are symbols used in the CPT coding book that require special attention. These symbols are listed at the bottom of each page and many of them correlate to a particular Appendix. Here are some of the symbols you will need to become familiar with:

- ● New code (Appendix B)
- ▲ Revised code-changed definition or terms (Appendix B)
- ; Separates "base definition" from "indented" code definitions
- ►◄ New or revised text
- + Add-on codes (Appendix D)
- | Modifier "–51" exempt (Appendix E)
- # Resequenced codes (Appendix N)
- ○ Recycled or reinstated code

The Index

The final part of the CPT-4 is an index that lists every procedure alphabetically. You use this index similar to the way you use the alphabetic index in the ICD-10-CM. That is, you look up the procedure in the CPT index first and then find the number it gives in the lists of codes.

Never use codes from the index without cross-referencing them. Additional information about each code is found in the numeric section. Sometimes, this additional information will change the initial code you selected.

HCPCS

The Healthcare Common Procedure Coding System (HCPCS) lists codes not included in the CPT. HCPCS codes are used for services and supplies provided to patients and covered by Medicare and Medicaid (as well as other insurances). These services include the following:

- Ambulance service
- Wheelchairs
- Orthotics (devices to assist a weakened limb)
- Hearing and vision services
- Medications (administered medications and chemotherapy drug, other than oral)
- Bandaging supplies
- Durable medical equipment

Outpatient surgery centers must use these codes when reporting charges for any patient who receives health benefits sponsored by the federal government. This requirement also applies to hospitals that perform outpatient surgery.

There are two levels of HCPCS codes:

- Level 1 codes are included in the CPT-4 lists. They are used with level 2 codes to provide greater detail about services and supplies.
- Level 2 codes are five-digit codes that begin with the letter A to V, followed by a four-digit number. For example, L8100 is the code for an elastic support stocking, ending below the knee and of medium weight.

CODING SERVICES AND PROCEDURES

It's helpful to know the basics about each type of codes, even if you never work in that kind of office. Here are some tips and examples for using each type.

Evaluation and Management Codes

The evaluation and management (E/M) codes are used to charge for the patient's visit with the physician. That visit can take place in any number of places. Here are just some of the possible settings for a patient visit.

- Office
- Hospital room
- Hospital emergency room
- Patient's home
- Nursing home
- Rehabilitation facility

Basically, each E/M code measures the physician's level of involvement with the patient. This can range from a short visit that deals with a single, simple problem to a longer visit in which the physician deals with several problems that are difficult or severe.

Selecting an E/M Code

It's always the physician's job to decide which E/M code to assign to a visit. However, you should know what each requires that supports the assigning of that code. That way, you can be sure the chart information supports the code and the billing will be correct. There may be times when you will have to discuss code assignments with the physician to insure the code assigned.

All E/M codes are based on these seven factors:

1. History
2. Physical examination
3. Medical decision making
4. Nature of the presenting problem
5. Counseling the patient or a family member
6. Time—the length of the visit
7. Coordination of care with other providers

The first three factors are **key components**—history, physical examination, and medical decision making. The rest are contributing factors in determining the level of the visit.

All three key components must be present to assign an E/M code to a new patient visit. For current or "established" patients, two key components are required.

Case Question

Remember from our case study that Jessica McNeil came to the office for a prekindergarten physical and immunizations. Her visit is coded as an E/M service. Do you think we should code this as a routine office visit or a physical examination visit? It's important to recognize when a patient is being seen for an annual well visit. Such visits must be coded as a physical examination with the proper CPT and ICD codes. Many insurance plans allow one annual physical per year payable at 100%.

Coding Consultations

There are four categories of consultations that include office, initial inpatient, follow-up inpatient, and confirmatory. Each category has its own reporting instructions. When a physician asks another provider for advice about a specific problem, the second provider becomes a consultant. The initial encounter is coded as a consultation. The documentation must support this.

- A letter must accompany the patient seeing the consultant.
- The consultant must send a letter back to the first physician outlining the findings.

If the consultant takes over part or all of the patient's care, follow-ups are coded as regular visits. A confirmatory consultation is considered a second opinion.

- The consultant offers only an opinion and advice.
- A confirmatory consultant does not take over treatment of the patient.

Anesthesia and Surgery Codes

The anesthesia codes and the surgery codes are closely related in these ways:

- Both are organized by the place on the body being treated.
- Both are then subdivided by the procedure being performed on that part of the body.
- Both are coded by medical office staff even if the procedure takes place in a hospital.

The anesthesia section of the CPT-4 uses two types of modifiers. These are letters, or numbers, added to a code to provide more detail. One anesthesia modifier is a standard type found in all sections of the CPT. The other type is a special **physical status modifier**. It is a two-digit code that begins with the letter P and ends in a number from 1 to 6. The physical status modifier tells the patient's condition, at the time of anesthesia administration. It helps determine the difficulty of the service the anesthesiologist performed. For example, a P1 modifier shows the anesthesia was given to a normal, healthy patient. A P5 modifier indicates a patient who was not expected to survive without the procedure.

Surgical Procedures

Many surgical procedures are coded as a surgical package. Included in the package CPT code are as follows:

- After the surgery has been decided, there can be one related E/M meeting immediately before or on the day of the surgery to gather history and other information.
- Administration of local anesthesia.
- The operation itself.
- Normal follow-up care after the operation.

These different components are bundled together and included in a single code. As long as the surgery goes as planned, there is no need for additional codes. Any procedures to deal with these complications are coded separately.

Each surgical code has a set number of follow-up days for care after surgery. Be sure that you know these limits are so that you can bill for any extra hospital, office, or other outpatient visits. Also, the surgical package only includes follow-up care directly related to the recovery from the procedure itself; not related conditions or complications.

Coding Inpatient Services

Most of the coding in a medical office is for outpatients; however, you may do inpatient coding too. This is because hospitals only bill for services they provide. For example, if a patient is hospitalized for surgery, the hospital will bill for the patient's room and meals, nursing care, the use of the operating room and recovery room, and so on. That bill does not include the surgeon or anesthesiologist services. Medical office coders are concerned only with the physician's services, no matter where they are performed. So if a physician from your office examines or treats a patient in the hospital, you'll code these services and submit the charges for them. Basically, billing is determined by who provides the service, not by where it's performed.

That's why you may be coding services that take place outside your medical office.

Other Surgical Coding Tips

Here are some other things you should know about using the surgical codes in the CPT-4:

- *The integumentary system*—This section of surgical codes has codes for which a measurement is needed. The size of the defect and the size of the specimen both must be measured before they are sent to the lab for testing. All codes listed in this section include simple closure.
- *Repairs*—The CPT-4 defines three types of repairs— simple, intermediate, and complex. Repairs should be measured in centimeters so they can be coded properly.
- *Cast reapplication*—You can't assign the same code to replacing a cast as you did to the original cast application. That's because the original code includes treatment of the fracture; replacing the cast does not. Therefore, the replacement code carries a lower payment rate.
- *Multiple procedures on the same day*—Code these procedures separately unless they are part of a package. They are coded in order, from major procedures to minor ones with the appropriate modifier(s).

Modifiers offer additional information that are added to a code. Table 12-5 shows a few of the more commonly used modifiers.

Radiology Codes

The radiology section of the CPT-4 is divided into four parts to match the four main types of radiology services:

- Diagnostic radiology (diagnostic imaging)
- Diagnostic ultrasound
- Radiation oncology (radiation therapy)
- Nuclear medicine

Table 12-5	**Common Modifiers**
25	Significant, Separately Identifiable Evaluation and Management Service by the Same Physician on the Same Day of the Procedure or Other Service
27	Multiple Outpatient Hospital E/M Encounters on the Same Date
22	Increased Procedural Services
50	Bilateral Procedure
51	Multiple Procedures
52	Reduced Services

Within each part, the codes generally are arranged by anatomic site—from the top of the body to the bottom. Many codes indicate the number of views in a particular test. That's because the more views there are, the greater the costs for film, developing, and the technician's time.

Some radiology tests require the use of a contrast medium, a liquid administered to the patient to enhance the image on the film. The codes for these tests indicate either with contrast or without contrast. Here is how to assign the correct code:

- If the contrast medium is given intravascularly (injected into the bloodstream), code the test *with contrast*.
- If the contrast medium is given orally or rectally, use the test code for *without contrast*.

If the same physician performs, supervises, and interprets the procedure, two codes are used. For example, the physician may inject the contrast medium, supervise the test, and interpret the results. The code for the procedure is found in the surgery, radiology, or medicine section. The code for supervision and interpretation is found in the radiology section. The physician must put a written report in the patient's medical record in order to bill this second code. If two physicians are involved in the procedure, for example, a surgeon and a radiologist, the radiology portion is billed by the radiologist.

Pathology and Laboratory Codes

These codes are divided into several sections that include the following:

- Drug testing
- Panels of tests
- Chemistry testing
- Antibody testing
- Urinalysis
- Consultations with pathologists

The pathology and laboratory section contains codes for just about every blood test and combination of tests a physician might order. The last part of the section includes services and procedures provided by a pathologist. These include the following:

- Gross (can be seen by the naked eye) examination of tissue removed during surgery
- Examination by microscope of tissue removed during surgery
- Postmortem examination or autopsy

Each tissue specimen is submitted under a different identifying code for diagnosis by the pathologist. The codes represent the level of the physician's work.

The CPT-4 also provides codes for reporting postmortem exams and autopsies.

Coding Automated Multichannel Tests

Some laboratory tests are ordered and performed in panels. This means a series of tests are performed together resulting in cost-savings. For this purpose, the codes from all the tests performed are **bundled** into one main code. It is important to remember that these panel codes cannot be **unbundled**, which means you cannot bill separately for the tests. They must be billed together under one code. For example, a Basic Metabolic Panel 80047 contains the following tests:

- Calcium, ionized (82330)
- Carbon dioxide (82374)
- Chloride (82435)
- Creatinine (82565)
- Glucose (82947)
- Potassium (84132)
- Sodium (84295)
- Urea nitrogen (BUN) (84520)

Using the Medicine Codes

Like the other five sections of the CPT-4 book, this section includes guidelines for proper coding. Pay special attention to the information about coding immunizations. Immunization injections are usually given when the patient comes to the office for a routine physical exam, or for some minor problem. When an immunization injection is given at such times, use two codes, one for the visit (E/M code) and the other for the injection. Another important tip to remember is that when you are coding for injections (other than immunizations), you will need two codes, the CPT code for the procedure of giving the injection along with a HCPCS code for the actual medication. Although you have two codes, there should only be one charge and should be listed with the medication.

CPT Tips

Here are some final tips for becoming a good medical coder:

- Always use the latest edition of the CPT code book.
- Refer to guidelines in each section regularly. Don't expect to know all the guidelines from memory. It can't be done!
- Make sure diagnosis codes clearly support CPT codes, but *never* change an ICD code just to accomplish this.
- Never hesitate to ask the physician to clarify a code, procedure, or chart documentation.
- Know the CPT modifiers and use them when appropriate.

Ethics

There are numerous cases in which physicians have lost their practice, and their freedom, due to Medicare and/or Medicaid fraud. Know what services were provided and code accordingly. If you have questions, ask. Never submit claims for procedures or services that were not provided. Protect your professional reputation. Always ask questions if you have any doubts before submitting a claim. If you witness fraud, be sure to report it to CMS, or OIG.

 CODING AND FRAUD

The **CMS** (Centers for Medicare and Medicaid Services) and the **OIG** (Office of Inspector General) define health-care fraud as:

To knowingly and willfully execute (or attempt to execute) a scheme to defraud any health care benefit program or to obtain money/property from a health care benefit program through false representations.

It's important to note that the mere act of filing a false claim is fraud, whether payment is made or not.

To combat fraud, CMS hires outside organizations to randomly review Medicare claims and compare them to the medical records of those patients. Many private insurance companies and state insurance departments also have units to combat fraud.

In medical coding, the most common examples of fraud are upcoding and unbundling.

- **Upcoding** is submitting a code for a service the physician hasn't performed. This often involves coding a service related to but more complex (and thus more expensive) than what was actually provided.
- **Unbundling** is submitting a code for each piece of a service package, instead of the single code for the entire package. Its goal is to gain greater payment by charging for each service separately.

Medicare has the same authority as the Internal Revenue Service (IRS) to audit your office's financial records. This means the claims you code and submit could be audited months or years after payment has been received. Remember if you find that you have made in error on any claim, it is vitally important that you inform the physician and/or office manager. Then notify the insurance company and make any necessary corrections.

The bottom line on fraud is don't do it! Not only is it illegal and the penalties severe, but submitting a false claim is a violation of your professional ethics as a medical assistant.

Procedure 12-1   Coding a Diagnosis or Diagnoses

Purpose: To accurately code the diagnosis or diagnoses for medical services and procedures provided to insure proper reimbursement from third-party payers.

Equipment: Patient records of diagnosis/diagnoses and treatment, current ICD coding book.

Step 1: Using the primary diagnosis, locate the main term (or cause) within the diagnosis. For example, if the diagnosis is CHF (congestive heart failure), the main term is failure.

Step 2: Locate the main term in the alphabetic section of the ICD coding book. Following our example, locate "failure."

Step 3: Refer to the additional descriptive terms or information within the diagnosis. For CHF, our next identifier would be "heart" as it describes the location

of the failure. Notice "heart" is indented under the main term "failure." Continue searching until all terms within the diagnosis have been located.

Step 4: Follow any special instructions given within the coding book. For example, "see also ...." If the section ever states "see condition," you will need to revisit your diagnosis and select a different main term. It does not mean go to the section "condition."

Step 5: Cross-reference the selected code with the numeric section of the ICD coding book. Read through the descriptive of the code selected. Look for any additional digit requirements to insure your code fully describes the diagnosis.

Step 6: Assign the code.

Procedure 12-2 Assigning a Procedural Code

Purpose: To determine and assign the most accurate code for services and procedures performed by the provider to insure full and proper reimbursement.

Equipment: Patient records of services and procedures performed, current CPT coding book.

Step 1: Identify the exact service or procedure performed.

Step 2: Using the index in the book of the CPT book, locate the procedure. Utilize the code or code range to cross-reference to the front of the book. *Important note: Even if only one code is listed for a particular service, it must be cross-referenced to insure that it is the correct code.*

Step 3: Locate the code or code range and read through the primary procedure(s) listed. Select the primary procedure that describes the service or procedure performed.

Step 4: Read through the indented description below the code you selected. Locate the code that matches the procedure in as much detail as possible.

Step 5: Be sure to read through the "Special Guidelines" section located at the front of the coding section to insure that all guidelines are followed.

Step 6: Determine if a modifier is needed. Remember, any unusual or special circumstance will require a modifier. A modifier allows for additional information to be provided.

Step 7: If a modifier is need, or if you are uncertain, review the modifier summaries on the front cover to locate possible modifiers. Then, cross-reference selected modifiers to the Modifier Appendix. Review the details of each modifier to select the correct one.

Step 8: Assign the selected code with modifier(s), if required.

Preparing for Externship

It is critical that a medical assistant know and understand their scope of practice. You are not allowed to practice medicine. So what does that mean? It means that you cannot diagnose a patient's problem nor can you make medical suggestions to a patient. For example, a patient may ask your opinion about something the physician has prescribed or recommended.

If you offer even an opinion, it can be interpreted as practicing medicine. So on your externship or when you are on the job, how do you deal with this type of situation? Always refer the patient's concerns or questions back to the physician. Support the physician's treatment plan for the patient. You can have an opinion but keep those opinions to yourself.

Chapter Recap

- Diagnostic coding involves using alphanumeric characters to describe diseases, injuries, and other reasons for seeking medical care.
- Diagnostic coding is linked to reimbursement because it assures that the services and procedures provided by physicians are medically necessary.
- ICD-10-CM is used for diagnostic coding.
- Procedural coding involves using numbers to describe procedures and other services physicians provide to patients.
- Complete and accurate coding is necessary to ensure proper reimbursement.
- The CPT-4 is used for procedural coding. It is organized by the type of service provided.

- Using the CPT-4 is similar to using the ICD-9-CM because the index in each book is consulted first.
- To ensure accuracy in diagnostic and procedural coding, the most recent version of each book must be used.
  - Modifiers are used to provide additional information about a procedure.
  - There can be up to seven characters in an ICD-10 code
  - HCPCS is used to code procedures and services not in the CPT book such as medications.
  - Z codes are used when a patient is not currently ill but is seeking medical care, such as annual physicals and pregnancy.

Online Resources for Students

Student Resources available on the text's online site include:

- Audio Glossaries
- Animations
- Competency Evaluation Forms

- Videos
- Anatomy & Physiology Module with Heart and Lung Sounds
- Weblinks
- Worksheets

Exercises and Activities

Certification Preparation Questions

1. When coding the patient's diagnosis you would use:
   a. CPT-4.
   b. HCPCS.
   c. ICD-10-CM.
   d. ICD-10-PCS.
   e. CPT-4-CM.

2. E/M codes can be found in:
   a. CPT-4.
   b. HCPCS.
   c. ICD-10-CM.
   d. ICD-10-HCP.
   e. CPT-4-CM.

3. Two-digit codes used to give additional information regarding procedures are referred to as:
   a. upcoding.
   b. modifiers.
   c. downcoding.
   d. bundling.
   e. unbundling.

4. ICD-10 codes can contain up to (maximum):
   a. five characters.
   b. four characters.
   c. six characters.
   d. three characters.
   e. seven characters.

5. Codes used when a patient is not currently ill but seeks medical advice are:
   a. V codes.
   b. Z codes.
   c. W codes.
   d. Y codes.
   e. U codes.

6. Submitting a code for services the physician did not perform or greater than those performed is called:
   a. downcoding.
   b. bundling.
   c. upcoding.
   d. unbundling.
   e. upbundling.

7. When a code contains more than one test it is called:
   a. downcoding.
   b. bundling.
   c. upcoding.
   d. unbundling.
   e. upbundling.

8. Sally is seen in the office for evaluation of a sprained ankle. Which coding book would you use to code her office visit?
   a. CPT-4
   b. HCPCS
   c. ICD-10-CM
   d. ICD-10-PCS
   e. CPT-4-CM

9. Sally had to have her ankle wrapped with a 3″ elastic bandage. Which book would you use to code for the bandage?
   a. CPT-4
   b. HCPCS
   c. ICD-10-CM
   d. ICD-10-PCS
   e. CPT-4-CM

10. After reviewing x-rays, the doctor diagnosed Sally with a third-degree sprain of her right ankle. Which book would you use to code her diagnosis?
    a. CPT-4
    b. HCPCS
    c. ICD-10-CM
    d. ICD-10-PCS
    e. CPT-4-CM

 Internet Resources

Access these Web sites for additional information on insurance coding and insurance fraud:

Center for Medicare and Medicaid Services: www. cms.gov

Office of Inspector General: www.oig.hhs.gov

13 Managing Medical Office Finances

Chapter Objectives

- Explain fee schedules and describe the main forms of payment.
- Summarize the process of identifying and collecting unpaid bills.
- Perform billing and collection procedures.
- Charge and payment entry.
- Perform accounts receivable procedures.
- Post adjustments.
- Process credit balance.
- Post NSF checks.
- Post collection agency payments.
- Process refunds.
- Describe how medical offices use bank services.
- Prepare a bank deposit.
- Identify accounts payable functions and relate how they are handled.

CAAHEP & ABHES Competencies

CAAHEP

- Define common bookkeeping terms.
- Describe banking procedures commonly used in the medical office.
- Identify precautions for accepting common types of payments.
- Describe types of adjustments made to patient accounts.
- Identify types of information required for patient billing.
- Explain patient financial obligations for office services.
- Perform accounts receivable procedures (posting of charges, payments, and adjustments).
- Prepare a bank deposit.
- Obtain accurate patient billing information.
- Demonstrate professionalism when discussing patient's financial obligations.

ABHES

- Demonstrate proper medical office billing and collection procedures.
- Explain accounts payable and accounts receivable.
- Demonstrate ability to post charges, payments, and adjustments.
- Explain payment procedures for credit balance, nonsufficient funds, and refunds.

Chapter Terms

Accounting	Charges	Cycle billing	Invoice
Accounts payable	Coinsurance	Debit	Nonsufficient funds check
Accounts receivable	Collections	Deductible	Packing slip
Adjustments	Copayment	Dunning	Posting
Aging schedule	Credit	Extension of credit	Restrictive endorsement
Bookkeeping	Credit balance	Fee schedule	

Abbreviations

EOB	FUTA	RBRVS	W-4
FICA	IRS	RVU	
FIT	NSF	UCR	

Case Study

Susan McNeil presented to the office for her visit. She failed to inform Bella, the medical assistant, that she had recently moved and had new insurance. The office sent a bill to the insurance company on file in Susan's patient record for an office procedure charge of $428. A week later, the insurance company informed the office that Susan was no longer covered under this plan. The office then mails a bill to the patient, only to have it returned a week later. Since Bella failed to check if the information in the system was correct, the office did not receive any payments and the account is already 2 weeks old.

A medical office is a business with two main goals. One is to provide patients the best possible medical care. The other is to make money. These two goals go hand in hand. A medical office must make money to keep its door open. As a medical assistant, you will aid in the financial success of the office by insuring patient accounts are current and correct. Therefore, you will be responsible for maintaining patients' accounts, collecting copayments and fees. Additionally, you may be in charge of accounts payable, which includes office expenses and payroll.

In this chapter, basic terminology and tasks to help you understand how to manage your medical office finances are presented.

SETTING AND COLLECTING FEES

When an office sets the fees that patients are charged, several factors are considered. One of these factors is the cost of running the office. A few office expenses to consider include the following:

- Office or building rent
- Utilities (heat, light, water, phone, etc.)
- Employees' wages
- Equipment and supplies
- Insurance, especially malpractice insurance

Additionally, the principles of RBRVS and UCR guide how an office structures its fees. **RBRVS** stands for "resource-based relative value scale." This guideline, used by Medicare to set its physician fee schedule, measures the relative value of a service in units (**RVU**). It does so by comparing a service to other services, considering their level of difficulty and the time required.

UCR stands for "usual, customary, and reasonable." The following items assist in determining the UCR fees:

Case Question

What should the medical assistant or receptionist done initially when the patient checked in for her appointment and procedure?

- Usual—the average fee the physician has charged for the service over a period of time.
- Customary—the average fee that other physicians in the same geographic area charge for the service.
- Reasonable—the fee that meets the criteria of the usual and customary fees.
- Insurance companies utilize RBRVS and UCR to determine what they will pay for each service.

Fee Schedules

A **fee schedule** is a list of charges for specific medical procedures. Each practice should have a fee schedule; this is important to insure that the charges are the same amount for the same procedure for all individuals. Remember that UCR uses the physician's usual fee for a service to determine payments. Suspicion of insurance fraud is likely if you charge different amounts for the same service, for example, more for patients with insurance and less for those without. In general, the best practice is to utilize one fee schedule and make adjustments as required by insurance allowable fees or patient's financial ability to pay.

Ethics

When creating the office fee schedule, it is of extreme importance that everyone understands that the fees are based on service level codes. Service levels are determined by three key factors (you will discuss these in more detail in another chapter), and all elements of these factors must be met to charge that level. Charging for higher levels of service or procedures than performed is illegal and unethical. Use care when entering information into the patient account. Never enter charges for procedures until they are completed.

Discussing Fees in Advance

It's a good idea to discuss fees before treatment begins. Patients need to know in advance whether the office is a preferred provider or participating provider with their health plan.

When scheduling appointments, it is important to inform patients of your office's payment policy as well as whether your office is a participating provider in their health care plan. Setting clear exceptions from the beginning will aid in the collection process. The first step of successful collections is to collect the payment at the time of service. **Collections** refer to the process of collecting money to pay on an account. Many insurance companies allow the office to view, online, a patient's policy including current out of pocket requirements. This information is used to determine the patient's portion of the bill prior to them leaving the office. The second step in successful collections is to have complete and correct billing information. Be sure to scan the patient's insurance card and check it at every visit to insure there are no changes. Patients sometimes change insurance and forget to inform the office. Additionally, you should scan the patient or responsible party driver's license and/or take a photo for your files to insure that you are billing for the correct patient.

Case Question

Thinking back to the case study, what steps could Bella have taken that would have improved collections in this case. Consider the difference it would have made if the following information had been obtained:

- A copy of the patient's insurance card (front and back)
- Confirmed and updated patient demographic information
- Collection of the patient's **copayment** at the time of service. The copayment is the amount the patient is responsible to pay with each medical service.

Forms of Payment

A patient usually can pay for services in a medical office in one of three ways:

- Cash—Many patients will request a receipt to keep for their own records.
- Personal/Electronic check—If a new patient pays by check (nonelectronic), get two forms of identification.
- Credit/Debit card—This is the best way to be paid, even though the credit card company charges the office a fee.

Although banks and credit card companies charge a fee (can be a percentage of the payment or flat fee based on type) for electronic checks, debit, and credit payments, the benefits normally outweigh this expense.

The insurance company payments make up the largest amount of money for services. For this reason, it's critical that you keep patients' insurance information up-to-date. Many offices ask for a patient's health insurance card at each visit. That way, any changes in insurance coverage are noted and recorded in the patient's account.

Adjusting Fees

Sometimes, you'll have to make **adjustments** (subtraction from the amount owed with no monetary exchange) to a patient's account. One type of adjustment is an insurance allowable fee adjustment. This occurs when your office contracts with an insurance company as a participating provider. The insurance company will outline the allowed amount and the difference will need to be adjusted. Adjustments are subtracted from the balance, similar to a payment, without the exchange of money or funds.

You will bill out the normal fee to the insurance company, even if the office is required by the contract to charge a lower fee. When the insurance payment is received, it will include an explanation of benefits (**EOB**). Once the EOB is received, you'll know how much the insurance company allows for the services rendered. You must then credit the patient's account for the difference between what the office charged and what the insurance company allowed. Once the credit adjustment is made, you can bill the patient if any unpaid balance remains due. Additionally, the EOB will tell you how much you can collect for the service, identified as **coinsurance** (contracted percentage owed by the insured/patient), **deductible** (annual amount owed by the insured prior to insurance payment), and **copayment** (amount owed by the insured/patient at time of service).

Case Study

Bella was able to get the correct information from Susan McNeil and filed her insurance. The insurance payment and explanation of benefits (EOB) was received today. Susan was charged $428.00, and the EOB shows $212.00 as the allowable fees. This means that $216.00 must be adjusted off as nonallowable fees per the contract with the insurance company (Charge $428.00 – Allowable $212.00 = $216.00 Nonallowable). The insurance paid 80% of the $212.00. Susan will owe the remaining amount as her coinsurance. The insurance payment 80% of $212.00 = $169.60. Susan will owe the difference of $42.40 ($212 – $169.60 = $42.40). The entry on her account will look like this:

Previous Balance $428.00 – Insurance Payment $169.60 – Insurance Adjustment $216.00 = Balance Due $42.40.

Case Question

How much will the office bill Susan?

Patient Credit

Depending on the treatment provided, health care costs can be very high. It's not always easy for patients to pay their bill—even a balance remaining after insurance has paid. Some offices extend patients' **credit**, or permission to pay later. Of course, this method results in additional costs to the office along with the risk of payments not being made. The following expenses are involved:

- Office supplies, including envelopes, the paper on which the bills are printed, and printer ink
- Employees' wages for the time it takes to prepare and mail monthly statements
- Postage costs

Because of these expenses, some offices charge patients interest on their monthly accounts. Another popular option is for the office to work with a credit company that would issue credit to the patient. Thus, allowing them to pay your bill and make payments (with interest) to an outside company. They allow patients to pay the amount due over time on a monthly payment plan.

Monthly Billing

You should send all patients who have an unpaid balance a bill each month. This applies to those whose insurance plan didn't cover all their charges, as well as to patients who have made credit arrangements to pay over time.

Each patient's bill should show all changes in the account since the last bill. These changes might include the following:

- Charges for any new visits and treatments
- Payments received from insurance plans
- Payments received from the patient
- Insurance discounts or other adjustments to the account

Extending Credit

Extension of credit is the practice of allowing a patient to pay on their account balance based on an established contractual agreement. State and federal laws control the extension of credit. Here are some points to keep in mind:

- Credit can't be denied because of some one's gender, race or nationality, age, marital status, religion, or source of income. In general, this means that if you give one patient credit, you can't refuse another patient the same terms.

- If your office charges interest on monthly accounts, the law requires that patients be given a truth-in-lending statement. This notice tells patients the interest rate and any other costs they incur if they pay their bill over time.
- Different states have different laws about extending credit. Some states have laws limiting the amount of interest that can be charged.

If the patient has received credit and is making monthly payments, the bill should show any interest charged. It should show the amount of the next scheduled payment as well.

All bills should clearly show the total unpaid balance that remains due. This allows the patient to pay more than her scheduled monthly payment, if desired, or even to pay off the balance in full.

When patient enters into a financial agreement with the office, it's important that the details of that agreement be put in writing. Figure 13-1 is an example of a contractual agreement for an extension of credit for a patient.

The patient's signature of the agreement demonstrates their understanding of the commitment.

Patient Education

Discussing finances can be uncomfortable for both the medical assistant and the patient. First, provide the patient with estimation of their cost (amount remaining after insurance pays) for the procedure or service. Then, review the payment options the office offers. Give a brief description of each option initially, detailed information can be given when the patient narrows the options down to suit their needs. Informing your patients of costs and options before procedures or services are delivered allows the patient to weigh their options prior to owing a large balance.

Bruce C. Collin, M.D. _____   305 Madison Avenue
                                               Anderson, Indiana 46027

I agree to pay $_____ per week/month on my account balance of $_____.

Payments are due by the _____ of each _____ and will begin _____.
                                    (week/month)   (date)

Interest will/will not be charged on the outstanding balance (see Truth-in-Lending form below for rate of interest).

I agree that if payments are not made in the full amount stated above or if payments are not received on time, the entire account balance will be considered delinquent and will be due and payable immediately.

I agree to be responsible for any reasonable collection costs or attorney fees incurred in collecting a delinquent account.

Date _____   Signature _____

This disclosure is in compliance with the Truth-in-Lending Act.

Patient's Name _____   Address _____

Responsible Party (if other than patient) _____   City, State, Zip Code _____

1.	Cash Price (Medical and/or Surgical Fee)	$
	Less Cash Down Payment (Advance)	$
2.	Unpaid Balance of Cash Price	$
3.	Amount Financed	$
4.	FINANCE CHARGE	$
5.	Total of Payments (3 + 4)	$
6.	Deferred Payment Price (1 + 4)	$
7.	ANNUAL PERCENTAGE RATE	%

The "Total of Payments" shown above is payable to Bruce Collin, M.D. at the address shown above in _____ weekly/monthly installments of $_____, the first installment being payable on this date _____, and all subsequent installments are due on the same day of each consecutive week/month until paid in full.

Date _____   Signature _____

Figure 13-1 Patient installment agreement form. (Reprinted from Kronenberger J, Ledbetter J. *Jones & Bartlett Learning's Comprehensive Medical Assisting.* 5th ed. Burlington, MA: Jones & Bartlett Learning, LLC; 2016.)

Cycle Billing

Larger offices have many bills they need to send each month. So, they utilize a system known as **cycle billing**. This system divides accounts alphabetically and bills them at separate intervals during the month. Here's an example of a typical billing cycle for a large office:

- Patients whose last names begin with *A* to *G* billed on the 1st of the month.
- Those with last names beginning with *H* to *N* billed on the 8th of the month.
- Patients whose last names begin with *O* to *S* billed on the 15th of the month.
- Those with last names beginning with *T* to *Z* billed on the 22nd of the month.

Some offices might create their billing cycle by type of insurance. Here's an example of that type of billing cycle:

- Medicare and Medicaid patients—Billed on the 1st of the month.
- Those with Blue Cross—Billed on the 8th of the month.
- Patients with all other PPOs and HMOs—Billed on the 15th of the month.
- All self-pay patients—Billed on the 22nd of the month.

Regardless of the type of billing system your office uses, it is important to maintain your office-billing schedule. The mailing of statements should not fluctuate by more than 10 to 14 days to insure timely payments.

Managing Overdue Accounts

If a patient does not pay his balance or make monthly payments as agreed, additional efforts are required to collect the balance owed. This process can be costly and time consuming. There are a number of federal laws that regulate bill collection practices. These laws must be followed when collecting any overdue bills.

Aging Accounts

One of your duties as a medical assistant will be to track patients' accounts. You must monitor unpaid accounts to limit the length of time they remain unpaid. This process is known as "aging" the accounts. The "age" of an account is determined by the date of the first bill, not by the date the service was provided. Here's an example: If a patient's office visit occurs on January 5th and the first bill is sent on February 1, the account will not become past due until the next bill is sent on March 1. Your computer software will keep track of the **aging schedule**. The aging schedule contains information that's very important to the financial health of the office. Accounts typically aged by 30, 60, 90, and 120 or more days past due. Generally, an account's "age" determines how you handle the account in the collection process.

Figure 13-2 demonstrates the number of accounts outstanding at the 60- and 90-day mark. The balance should be small and easy to manage.

Collecting Unpaid Bills

The "age" of your office's accounts receivable is utilized to measure its collection rate. This information should be reviewed at least quarterly to track your office collection percentage. Many offices utilize Web sites of insurance companies to calculate patients' copayments, deductibles, and coinsurance allowing them to collect fees at the time of service. Recall, the first step in the collection process is to collect at the time of service, thus reducing the risk of aged accounts. When tracking your office's collection ratio, be sure to use this information to develop and improve your collection practices.

The three most common methods for collecting past due accounts are as follows:

- Sending the patient an overdue notice
- Phoning to remind the patient the account is overdue
- Inquiring at the patient's next office visit

Additionally, your office computer system will likely have a **dunning** option. The dunning option allows you to set parameters with messages to be added onto statements when printing. For example, you could set a dunning message to post on accounts aged 45 to 60 days with the message: "*Your account with our office is currently past due and requires your immediate action. Please pay your balance as soon as possible to avoid further collection activity.*" Another method is to generate collection form letters to remind patients' that their account is past due. Whatever you send, it's a good idea to have a statement like this one printed somewhere on it:

> If you recently have sent your payment, please disregard this notice. Please contact us at the phone number above if you have any questions or concerns.

This message will help prevent patients from becoming concerned or upset if they have just made their payment. If a patient fails to respond to written overdue notices, you may have to phone the patient about his account. Always ask the patient when the office can expect to receive payment. Record the patient's response in his account file. If you don't receive the payment as promised, call the patient again.

Aging of Accounts Receivable Report: April 30, 2016

Patient Name	Account Number	Due Date	Amount
Accounts 30 Days Past Due:			
Doe, John C.	000-00-0000	3/6/16	625.00
Graham, Paula R.	000-00-0000	3/29/16	450.00
O'Toole, William Q.	000-00-0000	3/13/16	25.00
Parker, Mary W.	000-00-0000	3/25/16	299.00
Reeves, Chris A.	000-00-0000	3/11/16	58.00
South, Cheryl C.	000-00-0000	3/8/16	385.00
Yarkony, Ralph M.	000-00-0000	3/11/16	108.00
Accounts 60 Days Past Due:			
Forest, Patricia L.	000-00-0000	2/19/16	476.00
Heany, Beverly O.	000-00-0000	2/13/16	57.00
Thomas, Walter T.	000-00-0000	2/27/16	185.00
Accounts 90 Days Past Due:			
Glick, Rhonda K	000-00-0000	1/4/16	28.00
Payne, Robert A.	000-00-0000	1/25/16	456.00
Accounts 120 Days or More Past Due:			
Baird, Jane C.	000-00-0000	10/3/15	45.00
Wallace, Michael S.	000-00-0000	12/15/15	349.00
Total Overdue Accounts Receivable			**$3,546.00**

Figure 13-2   Aging accounts. (Reprinted from Kronenberger J, Ledbetter J. *Jones & Bartlett Learning's Comprehensive Medical Assisting.* 5th ed. Burlington, MA: Jones & Bartlett Learning, LLC; 2016.)

Rules for Collecting Accounts by Phone

The Fair Debt Collection Practices Act is a federal law that sets rules for collecting debts. Some general guidelines to follow when calling a patient about a past due account include the following:

- Not calling a patient at work.
- Never discuss details of the call with anyone but the responsible party. This includes saying that you are calling regarding a payment.
- Do not place calls before 8:00 A.M. or after 9:00 P.M.
- Do not contact the patient at all if he has filed for bankruptcy.
- Do not give the patient false or misleading information or make threats about further action unless the office intends to take it.
- If the patient asks in writing that such calls stop, you must do so. But you still can take legal action to collect the debt.

The failure to follow these rules could result in legal action. Despite the fact the patient owes money to the office if these rules are not followed he/she can file suit against the office.

Collecting from a Patient's Estate

Collecting a bill for treating a patient who later died is a sensitive situation. It requires special skills and approaches. Here are some guidelines to follow:

- Don't immediately contact the patient's family about the debt. They need time to grieve and accept the death. Most offices wait until at least a week after the funeral.
- At the proper time, call the next of kin listed in the patient's chart. Offer your sympathy. Then ask for the name of the patient's executor—the person who is handling the patient's affairs after death. This will likely be a relative, a friend, or an attorney.
- Contact the executor, introduce yourself, and explain the reason for your call. Get the executor's address and send the executor the final bill.

- It's important that the bill be sent promptly. If the patient's estate doesn't have enough funds to cover the patient's debts, the court will decide the order in which the debts will be paid.

Debt Collection Alternatives

Collecting unpaid debts is costly and time consuming to any business. Many medical offices find it easier and more effective to refer overdue accounts to collection agencies. These are companies specializing in collecting debts. The physician or office manager will set the guidelines to follow for sending an agent to a collection agency. For either a set fee or a percentage of the debt, a collection agency tries to collect the past-due amount. Since the collection agencies report accounts in their possession to the credit bureau, they may have more success than medical office employees. Another option that offices and collection agencies can use is small claims court. It's important to understand that even if your office or collection agency wins the case, the burden of collection still remains. Because of all the time, trouble, and expense involved, some medical offices don't seriously pursue collection of small debts from patients. If the office gives up trying to collect the money, it is referred to as "writing off" the debt. You will learn how to make this adjustment to the patient's account later in this chapter. The physician may wish to terminate the physician–patient relationship if the office is forced to write off the debt. Medical offices have the ability to report poor payment histories to credit bureaus as well.

ACCOUNTING AND BOOKKEEPING

Accounting is an organized system for keeping track of a business's finances. One accounting activity is **bookkeeping.** This involves keeping an organized record of a business' financial activities. Accounting and bookkeeping are both very important parts of a medical office's operations. In a large health care facility, a special department may do the accounting and billing. Other offices might hire an outside firm to perform these tasks. Many offices handle the daily bookkeeping themselves. For this reason, we'll focus on bookkeeping practices in this discussion.

Bookkeeping involves maintaining three primary financial accounts:

- **Accounts receivable**—Money owed to the office from patient accounts.
- **Accounts payable**—Money the office owes for operating expenses.

The daily financial operations of your medical office will be centered on patient accounts. These records change each day based on new charges, payments, and adjustments. Any time a patient receives service, a charge is entered onto the account. **Charges** refer to an increase on the accounts' receivable balance. Payments, made by the patient or insurance, along with adjustments, decrease the accounts' receivable balance. Remember that although adjustments are deducted from account balance, no monetary value is gained. Accounting is easier to understand if you remember that a **debit** is an addition to what is owed, and a **credit** is a reduction to what is owed.

Entering Charges, Payments, and Adjustments

The basic bookkeeping formula is Previous Balance + Charges – Payments – Debits = Current Balance. Although your medical bookkeeping software will calculate this automatically, understanding the fundamental formula insures you know accounting basics. Care is taken when entering charges into the system. Take time to insure that you enter all services rendered. Offices can enter charges through entries into the EHR program or independently at the end of the visit using a charge slip. At the time of service, copayments, coinsurance, and deductibles are collected and recorded. Many offices will collect copayments and deductibles prior to the patient seeing the physician. Any payment made should be entered immediately to avoid error and confusion. Additional payments received from insurance companies or mailed in payments should also be entered immediately. When posting insurance payments, be sure that you record any necessary adjustments at the same time. Your system automatically updates your patient accounts each time an entry is entered. At the end of the day, you can verify that all patients seen have been assessed a charge. The amount entered for payments must equal the amount of your deposit for that day. After you have verified charge entries and payments, this is called rectifying accounts, you will need to save and post the day's activity. **Posting** daily activities means the program saves activity for that day in the system for that month and resets the daily balance for your next day. If you fail to post the day's activities, your balances for the next day will be completely off as they will equal 2 days of activity. Most systems will not reset the date if the system information has not been posted.

Figure 13-3 demonstrates how the electronic entry of charges, payments, and adjustments are entered into the system at the time of service or receipt of payment.

Overpayments and Refunds

Overpayment of an account is more common than you might think. It can happen easily when you are collecting some money from the patient as well as billing one

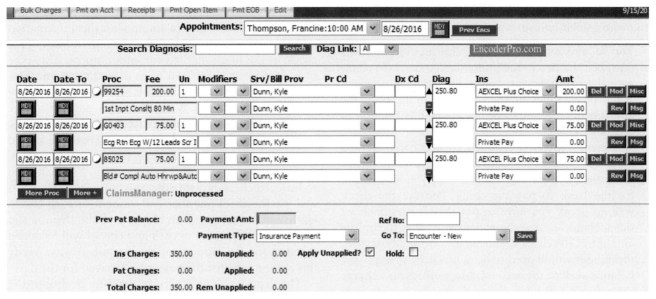

Figure 13-3 Computerized billing screen. (Courtesy of Harris CareTracker™.)

or more insurance companies for the patient's charges. Sometimes, payments from the patient and his insurance total more than the charge for the visit. This will show on the patient's ledger card as a **credit balance**. A credit balance is different from a balance due. A balance due is what is owed on the account. A credit balance is an overpayment. A credit balance is demonstrated by the presence of brackets around the amount in the balance column—for example, [*$125.64*]. Brackets are used in accounting to show the opposite of a column's normal meaning. In this case, it means that the amount in the balance due column is not what the patient owes, but what the office owes the patient or insurance company instead.

The office is legally and ethically required to return insurance overpayments to the insurance company. Overpayments, by a patient, are handled by mailing a check back to the patient, typically within 30 days.

Credit Adjustments

The adjustments column on the ledger card and day sheet is used to make adjustments to the patient's account that don't involve charges or payments. There are two basic types of adjustments—credit adjustments and debit adjustments.

The most common reason for making a credit adjustment to an account involves insurance. Most medical offices are providers for one or more insurance plans. This means the provider agrees to accept lower fees set by the insurance company instead of the office's normal fees.

Recall that you must charge every patient the same fee for the same service based on the office fee schedule. As previously discussed, this will result in the need for an adjustment as the contract fee will most likely be less than billed amount.

You'll post the insurance payment then you must write off the difference between the contracted fee and the amount you charged. You do this by making a credit adjustment for the difference.

Suppose, for example, your office charges $40 for an office visit; however, the contracted insurance amount is $35. You would post $40 in the charges column. Then, when the insurance payment is received, you would enter the payment and a $5 in the adjustment to arrive at the agreed-on amount for this service (any remaining balance would be billed to the patient).

Another time you would use a credit adjustment would be if an account is being sent to collections. In this situation, the entire account balance would need to be adjusted, for example, if a patient's account is delinquent $1,200 and is turned over to a collection agency, you would enter a collection adjustment in the amount of $1,200. This will bring the balance of the account to zero.

Debit Adjustments

Unlike credit adjustments, debit adjustments add to or increase the patient's balance.

Let's go back to the last example of a credit adjustment. Suppose the collection agency collects the $1,200 from the patient and sends in a check for that amount. Remember that the patient's balance has been adjusted to 0. You must charge money to the account in order to post the collection agency's payment. Otherwise, the account will have a credit balance of $1,200. Since these are not new charges, you would not add the $1,200 in the charges column. Instead, you will make a $1,200 debit adjustment in the adjustments column. Then, when you post the collection agency's check, the patient's balance will be zero (0) again.

Here are two other examples of when you will need to make a debit adjustment to a patient's account:

- You've already read that insurance overpayments must be refunded to the insurance company. To eliminate the overpayment, you must debit the account. Write the amount of the refund in brackets in the adjustments column. Code this amount as a refund to insurance carrier.
- A patient's check is returned by the bank marked **NSF**. This stands for **nonsufficient funds**. It means the patient doesn't have enough money in his account for the bank to pay the check. Because the check was no good, you have to put the charges back on the account because the patient still owes them. The amount of the check is entered as a debit adjustment, meaning it would need to be in brackets, to apply the balance back to the account. Most offices also charge the patient a fee for returned checks; this amount is entered as a charge (as it will be a new charge, over and above the amount of the original fee). You would contact the patient to make them aware of the returned check and fees owed to your office. Most offices would require that this amount be paid with cash, credit, or debit card. NSF checks not cleared by the patient within a reasonable time (usually 14 days) are sent to collections or the prosecuting attorney's office, unless special arrangements have been made.

 BANKING

Several things are important in choosing a bank for the office's business account.

- Bank location—A nearby bank would be the most convenient since deposits are made daily.
- Monthly service fees—Some banks charge a monthly; others, however, don't charge any monthly fee if the account's balance doesn't fall below a specific dollar amount.
- Returned check fees—Make sure you consider the amount charged for NSF paid to your office.
- Overdraft protection—This service guarantees that the bank will pay the checks you write even if not enough money is in the office's account. Review the terms and charges, including interest, that are associated with this type of protection.
- Special services—Includes paying interest on checking account.

Deposit

The first thing you should do when a check comes into the office is check to be sure it is made out to your office and filled in correctly. Next, you must endorse the check. This involves writing the name of the physician or medical office and account number on the back of the check. Most offices have a stamp with this information already on it. All you have to do is stamp the back of the check in the place marked for endorsement. This type of endorsement is referred to as a **restrictive endorsement**, as it restricts the depositing of this check only to the account listed. When the day's payments have been received, posted, and processed, add all the checks, credit card receipts, and cash received. This total should match the total of the payments for the day. If it does, you're ready to prepare the deposit slip. You will need to list each check individually on your deposit slip. You will list the check number and amount of each check. Cash will be recorded on the top of the deposit slip and totaled. The total of cash and checks will be added together for the amount of the deposit. Always verify this amount against the payments received for the day.

The deposit can be mailed to the bank or dropped in the bank's secure night deposit box. But if the deposit includes any cash, you should take it directly to a bank teller. Always get a receipt from the teller for any deposits that contain cash.

All checks should be endorsed with a restrictive endorsement. This endorsement clearly defines how the check can be processed. Figure 13-4 is an example of an endorsement on the back of a check.

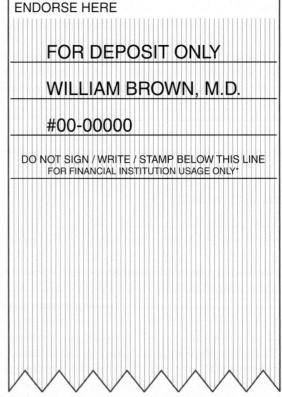

Figure 13-4   Check endorsement. (Reprinted from Kronenberger J, Ledbetter J. *Jones & Bartlett Learning's Comprehensive Medical Assisting.* 5th ed. Burlington, MA: Jones & Bartlett Learning, LLC; 2016.)

Types of Checks

Certain kinds of checks are more "secure" than the personal checks patients may write to pay on their accounts. Examples include the following:

- Certified checks are written from the patient's account and stamped by the bank. The bank guarantees that it's holding enough money in the patient's account to pay the check.
- Cashier's checks are written by the bank and sold to the customer for the amount of the check plus an additional fee. This process gives the receiver of the check confidence that it is good.
- Money orders are not true checks, but they do guarantee payment just like cashier's checks. Banks, the U.S. Postal Service, stores and businesses sell these to customers.

Writing Checks

Another of your administrative duties may be handling accounts payable—that is, paying the office's bills. Accounts payable usually include such things as follows:

- Rent and utilities
- Refunds to patients and insurance companies
- Payment for supplies and services
- Repayment to the office's petty cash fund
- Employees' salaries
- Taxes

Accounts payable can be paid by check or electronic transfer. You may produce these checks on the computer or write them by hand. In either case, you probably won't be signing the checks, and if you will be signing checks your signature must be listed at the bank as an authorized agent. In most offices, the office manager, business manager, or physician signs the accounts payable checks. Some offices require two signatures on checks, especially if they're over a certain amount.

Here are some points to remember when you prepare accounts payable checks.

- Be sure you make the check payable to the correct name of the person or business.
- Place the current date on the check.
- Enter the payment amount in both words and numbers.
- Put the reason for the check on its memo line for reference.
- Record the date, check number, amount of the check, and who it's payable to in the checking account register.
- Subtract the check's amount from the register balance.

- Post the payment to the appropriate category or account in the office's financial records.

If you are preparing checks by hand, be sure your handwriting is clear.

In addition to the checkbook register, the office should keep a logbook of all checks written. Along with the date, number, and amount of the check, the log should include why the check was written—for example, office supplies, payroll taxes, monthly credit card bill, and so on.

Bank Statements

Banks mail a monthly statement to account holders. This statement shows all account activity since the previous statement. It lists the following information:

- All checks written and their amounts
- All deposits made and their amounts
- All electronic transactions
- Any service charges

You must reconcile each monthly statement. This means you must compare it with your office records for the account. The main office record you'll use is the checkbook register. You would follow these steps:

1. Compare the amounts of all checks and deposits listed on the statement with their listing in the register. Verify that the information is identical.
2. Make a check mark in the register for each check the statement shows has been paid by the bank.
3. Make a check mark in the register for each deposit the statement shows was received by the bank.
4. Total all deposits that have no check marks in the register. Add that total to the ending balance shown on the statement. This is the revised ending balance.
5. Total all the checks that have no check marks in the register. Subtract that total from the revised ending balance you calculated in step 4.
6. Subtract from the register balance any fees and charges shown on the statement that are not recorded in the register. (Enter these fees and charges in the register so the register is balanced.)
7. The balance you reach in step 6 should equal the balance you reached in step 5. If it does not, there is a problem. Check your math and make sure the numbers are all correct. If no errors in the math are found, there could be a problem with your checking account.

Figure 13-5 is a sample of a reconciliation sheet used to check the account balance for accuracy.

Reconciliation of the office banking account is an important monthly task.

1. Subtract any fees or charges that appear on this statement from your checkbook balance.
2. Add any interest paid on your checking account to your checkbook balance.
3. List the checks you have written that have not been paid (these checks did not yet appear on your bank statement). You can also include in this list any withdrawals you have made since the ending date of the banking statement that do not appear on the statement.

Check Number	Amount
6217	32.94
6218	50.00
6219	119.24
Total	202.18

4. If you have entered deposits or other additions to your checkbook that do not appear on the statement, list them here:

Date	Amount
12-8-15	592.00
Total	592.00

5. Enter the ending balance from your statement here: 9542.91
   Add the total deposits from Step 4:   +   592.00
   Subtract the total from Step 3:   −   202.18
   Total (this should equal your checkbook balance):   9932.73

If these balances do not equal your checkbook balance:
• Check the addition and subtraction in your checkbook
• Check the amount of each transaction in your checkbook with the amount shown on your statement
• Check to see that all transactions from your previous statement have been accounted for
• Call your bank manager for assistance

Figure 13-5 Checking account reconciliation. (Reprinted from Kronenberger J, Ledbetter J. *Jones & Bartlett Learning's Comprehensive Medical Assisting.* 5th ed. Burlington, MA: Jones & Bartlett Learning, LLC; 2016.)

ORDERING SUPPLIES

Like all businesses, one of your office's goals is financial success. You've already read how billing, collections, and bookkeeping practices contribute to this goal. Keeping the office's expenses well managed is also required to help the practice finances.

There are many ways to save money when buying office supplies. Here are just a few of them.

• A purchasing cooperative (co-op) allows the office to join with others in buying supplies. The co-op's members benefit from the lower prices that go with large orders.
• Some suppliers offer price discounts for prompt payment.
• Large warehouse-type sellers and companies with discount catalogs also offer low prices.

Finding the best deals can take time. But the savings can be worth the effort, especially for items you use a lot.

There are things other than cost to consider in deciding what and where to buy. Consider the following:

• All supplies should be high quality, not just inexpensive. Many offices use several suppliers to get this mix of good quality and good price.
• Office supply companies often deliver for free. Office warehouse chains may charge a delivery fee or require a minimum order for free delivery.

Receiving and Paying for Supplies

Arriving supplies should always have a **packing slip** that lists the items the delivery contains. Always compare the packing slip to the actual contents received. This is a check to make sure the order is accurate and complete. If all items were received, initial the slip. Place all packing slips in a bills-pending file so they can be compared to the invoice, or bill, when it arrives. If the supplies were paid for in advance, place the packing slip in the appropriate accounts-paid file. If any items were missing, mark them on the packing slip, and contact the company. Invoices for supplies and other bills the office has not yet paid should be kept in a bills-pending file. This will help prevent them from being lost or misplaced. Bills may be paid daily, weekly, bimonthly, or monthly. Generally, office policy will determine how often accounts payable checks are written. Figure 13-6 is a medical assistant checking in supplies received in the office.

Verify receipt of all items shipped by comparing the packing slip to the contents received. Check each item as received and circle any items not received. Follow up immediately on items that are listed as shipped yet not received. Make note of any items listed as on back order and be sure to watch for their arrival. Packing slips should be stored safely to be used to compare against the billing statement.

Petty Cash

Most offices keep a petty cash fund to make small purchases. For example, suppose you run out of file folders

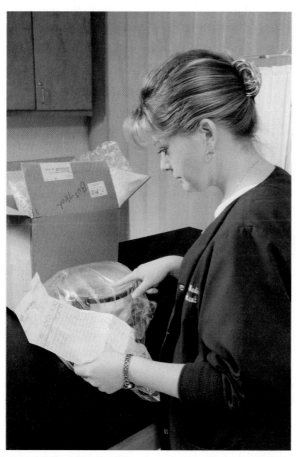

Figure 13-6 MA checking in supply order. (Reprinted from Kronenberger J, Ledbetter J. *Jones & Bartlett Learning's Comprehensive Medical Assisting.* 5th ed. Burlington, MA: Jones & Bartlett Learning, LLC; 2016.)

and need more right away. Since it will take time to get more from your office supplier, you could buy a box at a local store to use until the new supply arrives. You would take money from petty cash to pay for this small purchase.

The value of a petty cash always remains the same. This means that when you take money out, you replace it with the receipt for money spent. The cash remaining in the fund and the total of the receipts should always equal the set value of the fund.

The petty cash fund usually is renewed once a month. This is done by writing and cashing an accounts payable check for an amount that equals the total of the receipts in the fund. The receipts are removed and filed, and the money from the cashed check is put in the fund.

PAYROLL

Many medical offices hire an outside service to maintain and process payroll records and issue pay checks to the staff. But in some offices, these checks will be written by a medical assistant or office manager.

Generally, paychecks are issued on one of the following schedules:

- Weekly (52 pay periods per year)
- Biweekly (26 pay periods per year)
- Monthly (12 pay periods per year)

Your employer decides the pay period in your office. Usually, all the employees are paid on the same schedule.

Deductions and Withholdings

Writing payroll checks requires more than just knowing each employee's pay rate. A number of amounts are deducted from employees' pay. Here are the common payroll deductions.

- Health, life, or disability insurance premiums
- Employee contributions to the company-sponsored retirement plan
- Court-ordered withholdings to pay a debt the employee owes
- Federal taxes

In most states, state income tax must be withheld, too. Many cities and towns also tax the earnings of people who live or work there.

Federal Taxes

The federal taxes you must withhold from employees' paychecks are as follows:

- Federal income tax (**FIT**)
- Social Security (also known as **FICA**)
- Medicare

All three of these withholdings are based on the amount of the employee's earnings. In general, the greater the employee's pay, the larger the amount that is withheld. FICA tax is based solely on the amount earned without regard to their marital status or number of dependents.

The size of the FIT withholding is affected by the employee's marital status and by the number of exemptions the employee claims. This information is contained on the employee's W-4 form. If an employee does not have a W-4 form on file, you must withhold FIT at the highest rate, that is, the tax rate for a single person with no dependents. It is extremely important that all employees have a W-4 on file.

Each employee must complete a federal W-4 form on the first day of hire. The **W-4** form contains the employee's name, address, Social Security number, marital status, and number of exemptions she claims. In general, employees can claim one exemption for each person who depends on their income. An employee's dependents usually are her spouse or minor children.

Employee Records

No matter who does your office payroll, the office should have a personnel file on each employee. The file should contain the following items and information:

- Employee's original job application or resume
- Job references
- Salary or hourly rate at time of hire
- Dates and amounts of pay raises
- Performance reviews and evaluations
- All employee withholding authorization forms, such as W-4 forms
- Pension plan, health, and life insurance paperwork
- Vital facts such as employee's date of birth, name of spouse, address and phone number, and name and daytime phone number of an emergency contact person

Calculating Federal Withholdings

You can easily find out how much of federal taxes to withhold from each employee's check by using tax tables provided by the U.S. Internal Revenue Service (**IRS**). Combined tax tables found in IRS publications for businesses calculate the withholding for FIT, Social Security, and Medicare for you.

The tables tell how much to withhold for weekly, biweekly, monthly, and other payroll periods. Your office's payroll period and the marital status of the employee will determine which table to use. If an employee's wages are greater than the highest bracket on the table, you will have to use one of the other methods described in the publication to calculate the withholding.

Employer Taxes

An employer must match the amount withheld from each employee's check for Social Security and Medicare. Suppose, for example, that you withhold $150 from an employee's check for these taxes. The office must pay $300 to the IRS—$150 for the employee's withholding and $150 for the employer's match.

Each pay period, or at least once a month, you will write an accounts payable check to the IRS for the federal taxes you have withheld from employees' pay checks. This check will be for the total of the following amounts:

- Federal income tax withheld from employees' pay
- Medicare tax withheld from employees' pay plus the employer's matching contribution
- Social Security tax withheld plus the employer's matching contribution

The medical office's accountant will give you the federal deposit forms you will need to include with the check.

The office's accountant will calculate how much federal unemployment tax (**FUTA**) your employer must pay. This tax is paid either quarterly (every 3 months) or once a year. Most states also require employers to pay a state unemployment tax. The accountant also will calculate how much this state tax will be.

Study Skill

This chapter has many new terms related to finances and money that may be new to you. This would be a great time to make some flash cards to study these terms so you are clear on the difference between them. Students frequently get confused about accounts receivable and accounts payable as well as credits and debits. If you understand these terms, you will be a great asset to the medical office on your externship and into employment.

Procedure 13-1 Posting Charges, Payments, and Adjustments

Purpose: To maintain proper accounting of all charges, payments, and adjustments within the practice for management of the practice A/R (accounts receivable).

Equipment: Computer system equipped with medical practice accounting software, current fee schedule, completed encounter forms, and current coding books (ICD, CPT, and HCPCS).

1. Log into the practice accounting software and insure that the current date appears on charge entry screen.

2. As patients checkout, verify that all billing and insurance information was updated at check in.

3. Enter each procedure, using the appropriate code for service, and charge (charges may automatically appear if they have been loaded into the software by procedure code).

4. Calculate patient's responsibility and collect this amount (or if collected at check in, insure that it is applied to current charges).

5. Enter the payment type and payment amount using appropriate payment codes. For example, a patient paying cash for their copay might be entered at PPC or patient payment cash. Each office will determine the payment types and codes they will use.

6. Save the changes made to the patient's account.

7. Offer the patient a receipt, print the receipt and explain that the remaining balance will be sent to insurance for processing. Be sure they understand any remaining balance following insurance payment will be their responsibility.

8. Once payment is received from insurance, post the payment (using the appropriate payment code) using the EOB as your guide. Sometimes it's helpful to highlight the final payment amount for each account in one color and the allowable fee or adjustment (if already calculated for you) in a different color.

9. Calculate the amount of the adjustment (amount charge – allowable fee). Enter this amount as an adjustment to the account.

10. Bill for any remaining balance.

Procedure 13-2 Managing Accounts in Collection

Purpose: To ensure proper handling of accounts sent to collections. Accounts should be adjusted when sent to collections. Credit adjustments will need to be made as payments are received from the collection agency.

Equipment: Computer with medical practice accounting software, collection agency data sheets and listing of delinquent accounts.

1. Determine which accounts will be sent to the collection agency.

2. Adjust each account individually. Each account will have an adjustment equal to the total balance being sent to collection. Tag the account as Collections so no new charges will be allowed.

3. Gather all necessary information from each account, to include all billing information and the amount of each account. Submit this information to the collection agency.

4. As payments are received on a collection account, a reverse or credit adjustment will need to be made. The adjustment should only be for the amount of the payment.

5. Once the reverse adjustment has been made and the account shows a balance equal to the amount of the payment. Post the payment as a collections payment.

Procedure 13-3 | Processing an NSF (Nonsufficient Funds) Check

Purpose: To document and charge the account of the nonsufficient fund payment along with fees to insure proper restitution of the account.

Equipment: Computer with medical practice accounting software, NSF check, and posted signage of fees charged for returned checks.

1. Upon receipt of the NSF check first post the amount of the check back to the appropriate account using a reverse or credit adjustment.

2. Enter a charge for the returned check fee. This is entered as a charge as it is a new fee to this account.

3. Contact the patient by phone notifying them of the returned check and fees charged. Make arrangements for payment in full. Set a clear deadline.

4. If unable to reach the patient by phone, send them a certified letter with return receipt explaining the situation. Give a clear deadline as to when the payment is due in the office to avoid further action.

5. When payment is received (cash, debit, or credit card only), post to the account as a payment. Note that the payment is for NSF plus fees.

6. If payment is not received timely, the check can be sent to the prosecuting attorney's office in your area for collection or your office can send the account to a collection agency.

Procedure 13-4 | Reconciling the Office Bank Statement

Purpose: To maintain the financial well-being of the office practice through proper management of the practice banking account.

Equipments: Bank statement, reconciliation worksheet, checkbook ledger, ending balance of previous bank statement, calculator, and pen.

1. Compare the opening balance on current bank statement with the closing balance of the previous bank statement.

2. Check the bank statement for service fees, withdraws, and automatic payments. Insure these all appear on the ledger. If any are missing from the ledger, make an entry noting the date and amount then subtract from the ledger balance (this will be your current balance). Enter the current balance of the account, from the checkbook ledger, on the reconciliation form.

3. Compare check entries on the bank statement with the ledger. Please put a check mark by each cleared check, and be sure to verify that check amounts are the same.

4. Record any checks not cleared by the bank that appear on the ledger (those without check marks).

5. Add the amount of all outstanding checks, and record the total on the reconciliation form.

6. Compare all deposits listed on the bank statement with those on the ledge. Please put a check mark by each deposit that appears on both.

7. Record any outstanding deposits that are listed on the ledger, however, are not listed on the bank statements on the reconciliation form.

8. Total the outstanding deposits.

9. Add the total of outstanding checks to the starting balance.

10. Subtract the total of any outstanding deposits from the balance.

11. The balance on the reconciliation sheet should match the balance on the bank statement.

12. If the balance do not match, double check your math first. Then, repeat the process to insure that you haven't missed any fees, checks, or deposits.

Preparing for Externship

While performing your externship, you need to overcome any personal challenges that may get in the way of your success. Some students allow personal issues to obstruct their path to completion of the externship. Issues that may be the cause include not arranging backup plans for transportation or child care. Prior to starting your externship, decide the transportation required to get to the site and then think about a backup plan if that transportation fails. For example, if you drive a vehicle and have a flat tire or dead battery, what will you do that day to get to the site? Ask family members for assistance if possible. What if you have small children and the babysitter calls you in the morning sick and unable to watch the children? What do you do? Hopefully you have a backup plan for that problem too. If you are unable to secure an alternate plan for the problem, make sure you notify the site right away and then call your school. Don't give up for the entire day. You may be able to find a solution to your problem in an hour or so and be able to get to the site to complete the day. This solution will prove to the site how serious you are about your externship.

Chapter Recap

- The financial health of a medical office is based on its ability to collect the fees it charges.
- Credit arrangements, monthly billing, and attention to the collection of aging accounts help keep office finances running smoothly and efficiently.
- Accurate posting of charges, payments, and adjustments to patients' accounts require attention to detail.
- Checks should be immediately endorsed for deposit into the office account.
- Patients should be informed of the approximate cost of procedures prior to performing them.
- Always verify billing and insurance information prior to each visit.
- W-4 forms should be obtained yearly for each employee to insure proper taxes are withheld from their earnings.
- Payments must be made to the IRS for employment taxes at least monthly.
- Unemployment taxes must be paid quarterly or yearly.

Online Resources for Students

Student Resources available on the text's online site include:

- Audio Glossaries
- Animations
- Competency Evaluation Forms
- Videos
- Anatomy & Physiology Module with Heart and Lung Sounds
- Weblinks
- Worksheets

Exercises and Activities

Certification Preparation Questions

1. The term debit in accounting means to:
   a. add to an account balance.
   b. subtract from an account balance.
   c. adjust an account balance.
   d. write off an account balance.
   e. move the current balance forward.

2. The term credit in accounting means to:
   a. add to an account balance.
   b. subtract from an account balance.
   c. adjust an account balance.
   d. write off an account balance.
   e. move the current balance forward.

3. The bookkeeping formula is:
   a. previous balance + charges – payments = balance due.
   b. charges + payments – adjustments = balance due.
   c. current balance + charges – payments – adjustments = previous balance.
   d. previous balance – payments – adjustments = balance due.
   e. previous balance + charges – payments – adjustments = balance due.

4. Cycle billing means to:
   a. divide active accounts into sections and bill each section at different times throughout the month.
   b. bill all accounts on the 5th of each month.
   c. rotate accounts each month so that accounts are never billed on the same date.
   d. divide active accounts and bill sections on different days throughout the same week.
   e. divide accounts by balance due and bill those with the highest balance first.

5. The proper steps to take when handling a check that has been returned for nonsufficient funds:
   a. wait for the patient to return to the office and then discuss it.
   b. notify the patient, post the amount of the returned check as an adjustment in brackets, and post the service fee as a charge on the patient's account.
   c. notify the patient, post the amount of the returned check and fees as a charge on the patient's account.
   d. post the amount of the returned check as an adjustment and post the service fee as a charge.
   e. post the amount of the returned check and service fee as an adjustment with brackets.

6. Accounts payable refers to money that is owed:
   a. to the office from patient accounts.
   b. by the office to patients only.
   c. to the office from other businesses.
   d. by the office to all creditors.
   e. by the office to their employees only.

7. Accounts receivable refers to funds that are payable:
   a. by the office for services received.
   b. to the office from patient accounts.
   c. from employee payroll for taxes.
   d. by the office to patients.
   e. to the office from the IRS.

8. Employees should complete this form at the beginning of each year or when a change that will affect the amount they want withheld for taxes changes:
   a. W-2 form
   b. 1099 form
   c. W-4 form
   d. 1040 form
   e. I-9 form

9. Which of these are the withholding taxes that employers are required to withhold from employees' earnings?
   a. FIT, FICA, and Medicare
   b. FICA, Medicare, and unemployment
   c. Medicare, FIT, and unemployment
   d. FIT, FICA, and unemployment
   e. FIT and FICA

10. An adjustment made on an account reflects a:
    a. decrease in the balance from a payment.
    b. increase in the balance due to an error.
    c. decrease in the balance without a payment.
    d. increase in the balance due to a charge.
    e. increase in the balance due to interest.

 CareTracker Connection

Managing the Finances of a Medical Practice

 HARRIS CareTracker   CareTracker Activities Related to This Chapter

- Case Study 10: Entering Coding, Billing, and Payment Information

Perhaps no service is more expensive or has a more complicated payment process than health care. The complexity of most health insurance plans and the sheer volume of transactions that take place in most medical offices make it a challenge to determine who owes what, who has paid and who hasn't, and what the current balance is for any given patient. This is another area in which integrated practice management and electronic health record systems, such as CareTracker, can make a medical assistant's life much easier. Because of this integration, diagnosis and procedure codes that are entered into a patient's health record can be automatically imported into the practice's financial applications, making accurate and timely billing much more feasible.

Tasks discussed in this chapter that can be performed in CareTracker include the following:

- Establishing and maintaining a fee schedule
- Entering patient charges, manually and in bulk
- Generating claims
- Performing billing and collection procedures
- Entering payments from patients and third parties
- Posting adjustments
- Processing credit balances
- Reversing charges
- Processing refunds
- Managing overdue accounts
- Performing accounts payable functions

A task we'll consider here is entering bulk charges for patients.

Throughout the day in a medical office, medical assistants capture patient visit information, including diagnosis and procedure codes and their associated fees, when they enter these data into CareTracker. Typically, all visits on a given day are grouped together in a "batch," so that visits and charges may be processed in bulk rather than individually. To generate claims for payment, all visits in a given batch must be entered as charges in the system. One way to access these visits is via the Practice tab of the Dashboard application found in the Home module in CareTracker, as shown below.

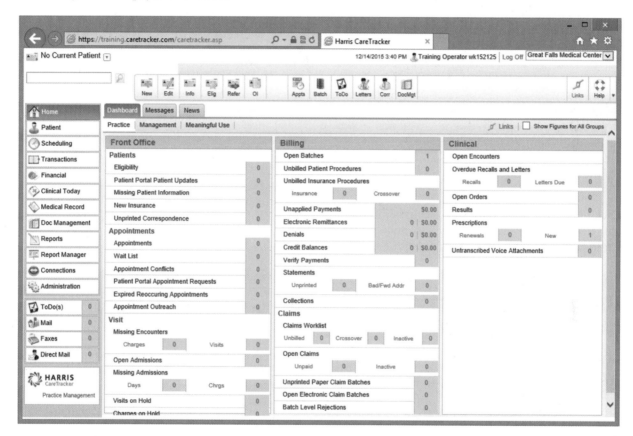

Under Visit in the Front Office column of the Practice tab of the Dashboard, find the Missing Encounters section.

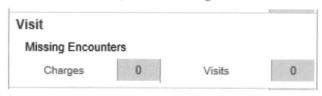

Clicking on the word "Charges" will cause the Missing Encounters screen to display. By entering today's date and clicking on Go, all of the visits that have been captured that still have charges waiting to be entered will appear.

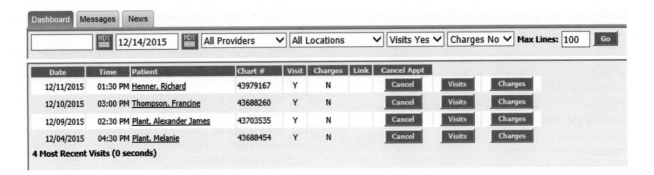

Bulk charges are entered for all patient visits recorded on the same day. In the example above, each of these four visits is on a different date, so each will be entered separately by clicking on the Charges button to the right of the visit. Clicking on the Charges button causes the screen below to appear.

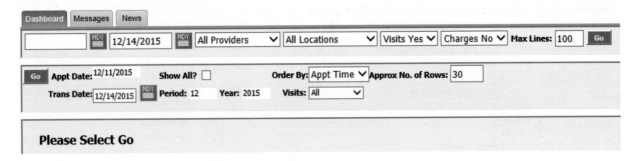

Clicking on the Go button on the left side of the screen, next to Appt Date, causes the Bulk Charges screen for this date to appear.

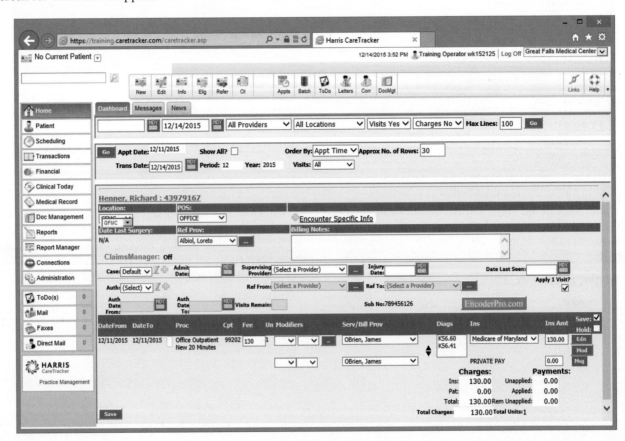

Note that all of the details pertaining to the visit(s) appear at the bottom of the screen, including the procedures, diagnoses, insurance information, and charges. Clicking on Save causes the charges associated with the visit(s) to be entered into Care-Tracker.

This process is repeated for each separate day listed, until all charges have been saved.

14 Health Insurance and Processing Claims

Chapter Objectives

- Describe the differences between group, individual, and government-sponsored health benefit plans.
- Explain the difference between Medicare and Medicaid.
- Explain how managed care programs work.
- Point out similarities and differences between HMOs and PPOs.

- Apply third-party guidelines.
- Apply managed care policies and procedures.
- Summarize how to file claims with Medicare, Medicaid, workers' compensation, and private insurance.
- Complete insurance claim forms.

CAAHEP & ABHES Competencies

CAAHEP

- Identify types of third-party plans.
- Demonstrate understanding of information required to file a third-party claim.
- Identify the steps for filing a third-party claim.
- Outline managed care requirements for patient referral.
- Describe processes for verification of eligibility for services.
- Describe processes for precertification and preauthorization.

- Define a patient-centered medical home (PCMH).
- Differentiate between fraud and abuse.
- Interpret information on an insurance card.

ABHES

- Process insurance claims.
- Differentiate between procedures of private, federal, and state payers.
- Understand the difference of HMO, PPO, and IPA managed care programs.
- Explain the process for obtaining referrals and precertification.

Chapter Terms

Assignments of benefits	Crossover claim	Participating provider	Third-party payments
Balance billing	Deductible	Preauthorization	TRICARE
Birthday rule	Dependents	Precertification	Utilization management
Clearinghouse	Gatekeeper	Preexisting conditions	Utilization review
Coinsurance	Medicaid	Referrals	
Coordination of benefits	Medicare	Third-party administrator	
Copayment	Medigap	Third-party payer	

Abbreviations

CHAMPVA	HDHP	POS	UR
EOB	HMO	PPO	
EPO	PCP	UM	

Case Study

Sally, an 85-year-old patient, called the office to schedule an appointment. She recently changed her insurance from Medicare to Coventry. Sally asked the medical assistant if the office participated in Coventry. The medical assistant assured her that the physician was a participating provider in the Coventry system. An appointment was scheduled. When Sally arrived for her appointment, the medical assistant noticed that her insurance was with Coventry One. Although Coventry One is a plan offered by Coventry, it was not a plan that the physician participated with. The medical assistant explained to Sally that the physician did not take her particular plan. Sally was very upset, as she had asked when she made the appointment if the doctor took her plan. She waited 2 weeks to see the doctor and now will not be seen due to a serious misunderstanding of insurance. The medical assistant was very apologetic and offered to help Sally find a provider within her plan.

Health insurance, third-party payment, is constantly changing. There are numerous types of plans offered by a vast number of companies. The increase in options, at times, causes confusion for patients, thus making things more complicated for you. This chapter will present information about different types of plans and the procedures necessary to insure proper payment.

HEALTH BENEFIT PLANS

Health care insurance is categorized into three general groups:

- Group health plans
- Individual health policies
- Government-sponsored benefits

Group plans are offered through employers or other groups. These plans usually provide a lower cost for benefits for its' participants and their families. Individual policies can be purchased through an insurance broker or from a state Marketplace. Government-sponsored benefit plans include Medicare, Medicaid, and Children's Health Insurance Program (CHIP). The federal government sponsors TRICARE and CHAMPVA are benefit plans for military members, retirees, and their families.

Case Question

How would you interact with this patient if you are the medical assistant who made the appointment?

In addition, group plans and individual policies offer four common types of plans:

- Health maintenance organizations (**HMO**)
- Preferred provider organizations (**PPO**) or exclusive provider organizations (EPO)
- Point of service (**POS**)
- High-deductible health plans (**HDHP**)

Handling insurance matters effectively is of great importance in operation of the practice, as well as to the patients your office serves. There are many differences between plans and knowing where to find individual requirements will aid in efficiency. Most insurance companies offer provider access to Web sites where you will be able to view the insurance accounts of your patients. These sites provide information regarding patient deductible (including amounts met), coinsurance, or copayment amounts, along with requirements for referral or preauthorization. Due to the vast number of plans and policies available, sometimes it is necessary to use the insurance payer identification number when assigning insurance to a patient's account. The payer identification number is listed on the patient's identification card. Figure 14-1 shows a typical patient insurance card that is scanned on both sides when the patient checks in the office. This ensures that all the necessary information will be accessible.

Group Health Plans

A group health plan is sponsored by an organization. Any person who is a member of the organization is eligible to be covered by the plan. If they choose to have this health coverage, they become part of the group. Members can usually add their dependents to the group too. **Dependents** generally include the member's spouse and minor children.

Associations and labor unions are among the kinds of organizations that offer these plans. Employers sponsor most group health plans. Employers offer insurance as a benefit to their employee.

Third-Party Payer

A payment from any source other than the patient is referred to as a **third-party payer**. Therefore, payments received from health insurance policies are considered **third-party payments**. Other examples of third-party payers include liability cases, in which another individual's liability insurance covers expenses, or legal cases where payments are received directly from the attorney. Time should be spent learning your office policy regarding liability cases and how the office wants them handled. Remember, the physician is not required to accept payment from all third-party payers (especially in liability cases); she can elect to require payment directly from the patient or the patient's health insurance.

Insurance companies charge a fee for benefits. The employer, employee, or both pay this monthly premium.

Self-Funded Plans

With self-funded plans, the employer itself is the insurer. It hires an insurance company or other company to review claims and make payment from the employer's funds. In this case, the company is only the agent for the plan. Therefore, it's a **third-party administrator** (TPA), not a third-party payer.

Marketplace Health Insurance

Varieties of insurance plans are available to individuals without other insurance options. Just as with other plans, it is important for to you verify a patient's insurance prior to the appointment. If a patient has a policy that the office doesn't participate in, there will be additional (unanticipated) costs to the patient.

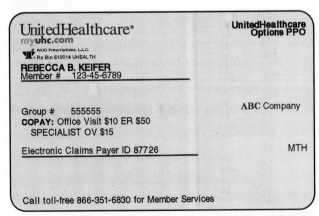

Figure 14-1 Patient identification card. (Reprinted from Kronenberger J, Ledbetter J. *Jones & Bartlett Learning's Comprehensive Medical Assisting.* 5th ed. Burlington, MA: Jones & Bartlett Learning, LLC; 2016.)

Determining Eligibility

Group insurance policies often have requirements that must be met prior to participant enrollment in the plan. Eligibility requirements are defined in the policy or plan document. They often include the following:

- Work requirement—The employee must work a minimum number of hours per week.
- Waiting period—A stated length of time must pass from the date of employment before health benefits take effect.

The employee also must have enrolled in the group. This usually means completing required forms during an enrollment period. Not all employees will necessarily be members of the group health plan. Group membership is not automatic with employment. Employees must choose coverage by their employer's health benefits.

The eligibility of a dependent is based on the employee's eligibility. Children of the insured can be covered until the age of 27. Spouses and domestic partners can also be included in coverage. Additional premiums will apply to spouses and children based on rates set by the group policy contract.

Individual Health Plans

People buy individual health policies from an insurance company. They pay their premiums directly to the insurance company. The insurance company may:

- Pay the doctor or hospital directly
- Reimburse the person for eligible medical expenses

The process and requirements for filing claims under individual health plans are the same as those for group health plans. Individual policies, however, often offer less coverage than group plans do. For example, the **deductible** for an individual policy may be higher. The patient must pay this amount before insurance starts paying.

Case Questions

 When the patient in the case study called the office, she was informed her insurance was accepted by the office. Why should the medical assistant ask about the patient's insurance payer identification number on the patient's insurance card? Do you think patients should know this information to avoid issues or problems?

 # HEALTH INSURANCE AND HIPAA

The Health Insurance Portability and Accountability Act of 1996 (HIPAA) brought major changes to the health care and health insurance industries. Some ways HIPAA has affected health insurance include the following:

- Limited exclusions for preexisting conditions in employer-sponsored health plans
- Banned the use of genetic testing information to deny health coverage
- Eased confidentiality requirements for providing patient information to insurance companies
- Required standards for the electronic transmission of insurance claims
- Required standards for attachments to insurance claims
- Required diagnostic and procedural coding to be standardized
- Strengthened protections against fraud and abuse in insurance billing

An individual policy also may have a provision that denies or limits benefits for certain **preexisting conditions**. These are injuries or illnesses the patient had before the policy took effect. Sometimes, these conditions are not covered by the policy even if the patient was not being treated for them at the time. Preexisting conditions generally won't apply to most patients covered by group health plans. That's because the Health Insurance Portability and Accountability Act of 1996 (HIPAA) severely limited this exclusion in employer-sponsored plans.

Government Health Plans

Government-sponsored health benefit programs are funded and operated by the federal government and the individual states. These programs are designed to provide health benefits for the elderly, the poor, and others who might not be able to get benefits on their own. Also included in government health plans are those offered to military members, retirees, veterans, and their families. These programs include the following:

- Medicare
- Medicaid
- TRICARE
- CHAMPVA

Medicare

Congress created **Medicare** in the 1960s as a health benefit plan for persons age 65 and over. At the time, only about half of elderly Americans had health insurance coverage.

All persons who are entitled to receive Social Security retirement benefits become eligible for Medicare when they reach age 65. This is true even if they don't retire. As long as they are covered by an employer's group health plan, that plan is the primary coverage and Medicare is secondary.

In the 1970s, Congress expanded the Medicare program to cover other groups who had difficulty obtaining health insurance. These groups include the following:

- Disabled persons who cannot work and are receiving Social Security disability benefits; they must receive these benefits for 24 months before they are eligible for Medicare.
- Persons suffering from end-stage renal disease; these are persons whose kidneys have failed permanently and who are receiving dialysis.

In recent years, Congress changed Medicare again, to create more choices for coverage. The early Medicare program (now called Original Medicare) consisted of two parts:

- Medicare Part A—Covers hospital expenses
- Medicare Part B—Covers outpatient services (including physician services)

Eligible persons still may enroll in Original Medicare, or they may choose to elect coverage through one of the Medicare Advantage plans.

Medicare Part A

Everyone enrolled in Original Medicare is covered by Part A. There's no monthly charge for this coverage, although the plan has deductibles and coinsurance. **Coinsurance** is money a patient must pay as his share of the cost of treatment. Part A covers hospital expenses (inpatient).

Medicare Part B

Medicare Part B is optional. All Part B charges are subject to deductibles and coinsurance.

Patients who have this coverage pay a monthly fee for this benefit. Part B pays physicians' fees for both inpatient and outpatient care and outpatient services. These services include the following:

- Diagnostic testing
- Certain immunizations such as influenza and pneumonia
- Specific screening tests such as PSA, mammograms, Pap smears, bone density testing, and colorectal screening
- Medical equipment such as canes, crutches, walkers, commodes, and chairs

Medicare Advantage

Medicare Advantage offers a variety of managed care and traditional insurance plans through private insurance companies. Patients who qualify for Medicare may choose between traditional Medicare and any of the advantage plans. These plans operate much like other managed care and traditional insurance plans.

Medicare Part D

Part D is a prescription plan that Medicare beneficiaries can elect to purchase to help offset the costs of medications. Similar to other pharmaceutical plans, patients will pay a copayment based on the tier level of the medication. People enrolled in Medicare Advantage plans may already have drug benefits within their selected plan. Medicare Part D plans are offered through private companies.

Medigap

Medigap is the name given to policies that private companies sell to fill the gaps in original Medicare. These policies are voluntary and cost the patient an additional monthly fee. They pay for things Medicare Parts A and B do not. For example, a Medigap policy may pay the following gaps in Part B coverage:

- The annual deductible
- Coinsurance for physicians' services
- An annual physical examination
- Other services, treatments, and supplies not covered by Medicare

Electronic Medicare claims can automatically crossover to Medigap or other secondary plans. When claims crossover information from Medicare, including contracted amounts, nonallowable fees, coinsurance, and deductible amounts are electronically forwarded to secondary insurances. Figure 14-2 is a copy of a printed CMS-1500 form. All insurance claims are formatted using the CMS-1500 standard.

Patient Education

Insurance can be very complex and confusing, especially to patients. When patient requires special testing, imaging or certain medications that require preauthorization take time to explain this procedure to the patient. Sometimes, the patient can assist in the authorization process by calling the insurance company directly and discussing their symptoms and past treatments. Prior to suggesting any patient, call their insurance company check with the physician and insure that the patient is comfortable speaking with them.

PLEASE
DO NOT
STAPLE
IN THIS
AREA

CARRIER →

HEALTH INSURANCE CLAIM FORM

| □□ PICA | | | | | | | | PICA □□ |

1. MEDICARE	MEDICAID	CHAMPUS	CHAMPVA	GROUP HEALTH PLAN	FECA BLK LUNG	OTHER	1a. INSURED'S I.D. NUMBER	(FOR PROGRAM IN ITEM 1)
X (Medicare #)	□ (Medicaid #)	□ (Sponsor's SSN)	□ (VA File #)	□ (SSN or ID)	□ (SSN)	□ (ID)	000-00-0000A	

2. PATIENT'S NAME (Last Name, First Name, Middle Initial)
Naomi A Dishman

3. PATIENT'S BIRTH DATE MM 04 DD 14 YY 24   SEX M □ F X

4. INSURED'S NAME (Last Name, First Name, Middle Initial)
Same

5. PATIENT'S ADDRESS (No., Street)
405 Carolina Ave

6. PATIENT RELATIONSHIP TO INSURED Self □ Spouse □ Child □ Other □

7. INSURED'S ADDRESS (No., Street)

CITY Danville   STATE VA

8. PATIENT STATUS Single □ Married X Other □

CITY   STATE

ZIP CODE 24540   TELEPHONE (Include Area Code) (434) 555-5555

Employed □ Full-Time Student □ Part-Time Student □

ZIP CODE   TELEPHONE (INCLUDE AREA CODE) (   )

9. OTHER INSURED'S NAME (Last Name, First Name, Middle Initial)
NONE

10. IS PATIENT'S CONDITION RELATED TO:

11. INSURED'S POLICY GROUP OR FECA NUMBER

a. OTHER INSURED'S POLICY OR GROUP NUMBER

a. EMPLOYMENT? (CURRENT OR PREVIOUS) □ YES X NO

a. INSURED'S DATE OF BIRTH MM DD YY   SEX M □ F □

b. OTHER INSURED'S DATE OF BIRTH MM DD YY   SEX M □ F □

b. AUTO ACCIDENT? □ YES X NO PLACE (State)

b. EMPLOYER'S NAME OR SCHOOL NAME

c. EMPLOYER'S NAME OR SCHOOL NAME

c. OTHER ACCIDENT? X YES □ NO

c. INSURANCE PLAN NAME OR PROGRAM NAME

d. INSURANCE PLAN NAME OR PROGRAM NAME

10d. RESERVED FOR LOCAL USE

d. IS THERE ANOTHER HEALTH BENEFIT PLAN? □ YES □ NO *If yes*, return to and complete item 9 a-d.

READ BACK OF FORM BEFORE COMPLETING & SIGNING THIS FORM.
12. PATIENT'S OR AUTHORIZED PERSON'S SIGNATURE I authorize the release of any medical or other information necessary to process this claim. I also request payment of government benefits either to myself or to the party who accepts assignment below.

SIGNED Signature on File   DATE 010516

13. INSURED'S OR AUTHORIZED PERSON'S SIGNATURE I authorize payment of medical benefits to the undersigned physician or supplier for services described below.

SIGNED

14. DATE OF CURRENT: MM 05 DD 28 YY 16 ILLNESS (First symptom) OR INJURY (Accident) OR PREGNANCY(LMP)

15. IF PATIENT HAS HAD SAME OR SIMILAR ILLNESS. GIVE FIRST DATE MM DD YY

16. DATES PATIENT UNABLE TO WORK IN CURRENT OCCUPATION FROM MM DD YY TO MM DD YY

17. NAME OF REFERRING PHYSICIAN OR OTHER SOURCE

17a. I.D. NUMBER OF REFERRING PHYSICIAN

18. HOSPITALIZATION DATES RELATED TO CURRENT SERVICES FROM MM DD YY TO MM DD YY

19. RESERVED FOR LOCAL USE

20. OUTSIDE LAB? □ YES □ NO $ CHARGES

21. DIAGNOSIS OR NATURE OF ILLNESS OR INJURY. (RELATE ITEMS 1,2,3 OR 4 TO ITEM 24E BY LINE)
1. L845.03
2. L250.00
3. L___.___
4. L___.___

22. MEDICAID RESUBMISSION CODE   ORIGINAL REF. NO.

23. PRIOR AUTHORIZATION NUMBER

24. A DATE(S) OF SERVICE						B Place of Service	C Type of Service	D PROCEDURES, SERVICES, OR SUPPLIES (Explain Unusual Circumstances) CPT/HCPCS MODIFIER	E DIAGNOSIS CODE	F $ CHARGES	G DAYS OR UNITS	H EPSDT Family Plan	I EMG	J COB	K RESERVED FOR LOCAL USE
From MM	DD	YY	To MM	DD	YY										
1	05	28	16	05	28	16	11		99213	1	100 00	1				
2	05	28	16	05	28	16	11		82947	2	25 00	1				
3																
4																
5																
6																

25. FEDERAL TAX I.D. NUMBER 54-0000000 SSN □ EIN □

26. PATIENT'S ACCOUNT NO. 1234

27. ACCEPT ASSIGNMENT? (For govt. claims, see back) X YES □ NO

28. TOTAL CHARGE $ 125 00

29. AMOUNT PAID $

30. BALANCE DUE $ 125 00

31. SIGNATURE OF PHYSICIAN OR SUPPLIER INCLUDING DEGREES OR CREDENTIALS (I certify that the statements on the reverse apply to this bill and are made a part thereof.)

SIGNED   DATE

32. NAME AND ADDRESS OF FACILITY WHERE SERVICES WERE RENDERED (If other than home or office)

33. PHYSICIAN'S, SUPPLIER'S BILLING NAME, ADDRESS, ZIP CODE & PHONE #
JOSEPH G NORTH, MD
1111 GRAYSON STREET
DANVILLE VA
PIN#   GRP#

PATIENT AND INSURED INFORMATION →
PHYSICIAN OR SUPPLIER INFORMATION →

(APPROVED BY AMA COUNCIL ON MEDICAL SERVICE 8/88) **PLEASE PRINT OR TYPE**
APPROVED OMB-0938-0008 FORM CMS-1500 (12-90), FORM RRB-1500,
APPROVED OMB-1215-0055 FORM OWCP-1500, APPROVED OMB-0720-0001 (CHAMPUS)

Figure 14-2 Sample CMS-1500 claim form indicating proper sequencing. (Reprinted from Kronenberger J, Ledbetter J. *Jones & Bartlett Learning's Comprehensive Medical Assisting.* 4th ed. Burlington, MA: Jones & Bartlett Learning, LLC; 2013.)

Medicaid

Medicaid is a health assistance program funded by both federal and state governments. The federal government sets general guidelines that must be followed. Each state government can set additional eligibility standards and benefits. Federal guidelines require that every state offer a Medicaid program. Some states offer several options for coverage with policies available through various independent insurance companies. You will need to learn the various plans available in your area and the specific plans your office participates in.

The federal government sets Medicaid's minimum coverage. However, states can provide coverage beyond the minimum. Therefore, like eligibility for Medicaid, benefits vary from state to state. All states provide at least these areas of coverage:

- Inpatient hospital care
- Outpatient treatment and services
- Diagnostic services
- Family planning
- Skilled nursing facilities
- Diagnostic screenings for children

Cultural Connection

Bias can affect not only your feelings about a group of individuals but also the manner in which you treat them. Frequently, bias is based on thought or opinion with limited factual information. Many people, including those in health care, have biased opinions of individuals covered under the Medicaid program. Regardless of the reasoning behind this bias, there is no place for it in a professional environment. Every patient regardless of economic background or insurance should be treated with respect and receive the best care possible.

TRICARE and CHAMPVA

TRICARE formerly known as CHAMPUS is a government program sponsored by the U.S. Department of Defense. It provides health benefits for:

- Dependents of active duty military personnel
- Dependents of military personnel who died while on active duty
- Retired military personnel and their dependents

The TRICARE system provides health care through civilian hospitals and clinics. **CHAMPVA** stands for the Civilian Health and Medical Program of the Veterans Administration. It covers dependents of two types of military veterans. These are:

- Dependents of veterans who have total and permanent service-connected disabilities
- Dependents of veterans who died from service-connected disabilities

CHAMPVA patients can choose their own civilian physician. This allows them the same benefits as a traditional insurance program.

The provider also may bill the patient for any other amounts not paid by insurance. For example, the insurance company's maximum allowable payment for a service may be less than the provider's fee. In some cases, the provider can require the patient to pay the difference. Also, an insurance plan may not cover certain equipment or supplies.

 ## TYPES OF INSURANCE COVERAGE

There are various types of insurance coverage. Let's take some time to review the various types of coverage:

- Basic medical benefits pay all or part of a physician's charges for nonsurgical services. These include office, hospital, and home visits as well as most lab tests and x-rays.
- Hospitalization coverage pays all or part of the costs for a patient's hospital room, food, and health care services that don't involve a physician. It also pays for use of hospital facilities, such as an operating room.
- Surgical coverage pays all or part of a surgeon's fees. The surgery can take place in the hospital or the physician's office. If the procedure requires anesthesia, this is paid by the surgical benefits as well.
- Major medical coverage pays for very large bills that can result from a long or extremely serious illness. This coverage usually takes effect when benefits under the plan's other coverage have been exhausted. Deductibles and coinsurance usually apply to most of the coverage. If major medical coverage is in effect, however, the patient may have already paid his maximum required amount.

 ## COST MANAGEMENT

Health care plans control costs in several ways including:

- **Precertification (preauthorization)**—Most insurance plans require that certain procedures are precertified or preauthorized before the patient can receive the treatment. These usually include hospitalization and other procedures except in emergencies. The goal is to provide services in the most cost-effective way. For example, surgeries for which patients were once hospitalized are now performed in outpatient settings. Precertification is sometimes called **utilization management (UM)** or **utilization review (UR)**.

- **Referrals**—Many health care plans will not pay for treatment by specialists, unless the patient is referred by his Primary Care Physician (**PCP**). Some plans require preapproval by the plan administrator as well. The goal is to ensure that a specialist's services are medically necessary. Insurance-required referrals are assigned a referral number, outline the number of treatments (frequently including CPT codes), and the time frame for completion of these treatments.

Health Maintenance Organizations (HMO)

Health Maintenance Organizations contract with providers at a contracted rate to provide services to those covered under the plan. Patients select a Primary Care Physician (PCP), or **gatekeeper**, who coordinates the patients' care. The PCP would be responsible for any referral to specialists as needed. Such referrals must be completed prior to the patient being seen by the specialist and the referral authorization number should be recorded on the claim form. Patients usually pay a set **copayment** for services. Copayments can vary based on service provider, for example, the PCP copayment might be $20 with a specialist copayment of $50. Deductibles and coinsurance generally do not apply to such services.

Preferred Provider Organizations

A preferred provider organization (PPO) is a network of physicians, hospitals, and other providers that contract with one or more health plans. The PPO's provider members agree to accept less than their normal charges and to follow the plan's requirements for providing services. Unlike an HMO, patients in a health plan with a PPO can go to any provider they wish. The plan generally offers two levels of service, called *in-network* and *out-of-network*.

If the provider is in-network, referred to as a **participating provider**, the plan's benefits are greater. Providers that are out-of-network (called a nonparticipating provider) will cost the patient more. Although the PPO system gives patients free choice, they have a strong financial incentive to see in-network providers. Table 14-1 lists the basic PPO guidelines.

Exclusive Provider Organizations (EPO)

EPO, exclusive provider organization, is similar to the PPO in that a PCP is not required. The patient can choose to see any provider they would like as like as the

Table 14-1	PPO Guidelines	
Benefit	**In-Network**	**Out-of-Network**
Yearly patient deductible	$100	$300
Patient coinsurance	10%	30%
Routine care benefit	$200 per year	0
Mental health benefit	80% of charges	50% of charges
Office visit—patient share	$10 copay; no deductible	70% of charges

provider in the EPO network. No benefits are paid if the patient uses a provider outside of the network.

Point of Service (POS)

POS, point of service, is similar in nature to the HMO in the PCP are required. The patient was limited to providers within the plan. Additionally, referrals are required for the patient to see a specialist.

High-Deductible Health Plan (HDHP)

HDHP plans have lower monthly premiums, however, come with high deductible. Since the deductibles are very high, the patient will pay for most routine care out of pocket. As with all plans, the policy will not pay until the deductible liability has been paid.

Ethics

Most insurance companies require preauthorization prior to the performance of expense testing, including MRI. Often insurance companies will require specific information in regard to the patient's symptoms, diagnosis, and treatments. This information must be true and documented in the patient EHR. Always verify symptoms, diagnosis, and treatment. Do not exaggerate any of the information. For example, if eight physical therapy sessions are ordered but the patient has only attended one session, you could not state the patient has had eight physical therapy sessions. All information should be accurate and well documented in the EHR. Remember, if it's not documented, it didn't happen.

FILING CLAIMS

Many pieces of information are necessary to process insurance claims. It's of extreme importance that this information be entered into the electronic health record accurately and completely. The patient's ID card is your basic resource for processing insurance. This card contains information that's essential to the accurate filing of claims including:

- The name of the plan that provides the patient's coverage
- The patient's plan ID number and group number if it's group coverage
- Phone numbers for questions about benefits, coverage, and approval requirements
- Directions on where to file claims

Keep a copy of the patient's ID card in the patient's file. Update it at least yearly. Also, verify the information at each visit, since the patient's employment and eligibility may change.

Coordination of Benefits

It's not uncommon for a patient to be eligible for benefits from more than one health plan. For example, a patient may be covered under her employer's plan and also as a dependent on her spouse's group plan. The plan that pays first—the primary plan—is the plan provided by the patient's employer. The spouse's group plan is secondary. It will consider any amounts up to the allowable limit for the policy not paid by the primary insurance. This is called **coordination of benefits.**

Study Skill

Create key points that break down the information you are trying to learn. By dividing large or complicated information into small simpler pieces of information, it will be easier to learn.

The Birthday Rule

Dependent children may be covered under the insurance plans of both parents. When this happens, the primary plan is usually the plan of the parent whose birthday occurs first during the year, not necessarily the older parent. This is known as the **birthday rule.**

Consider this example of a married couple:

- Brad's birthday is December 20, 1963.
- Maria's birthday is October 11, 1965.

Whose insurance would be primary? It would be Maria because the month and day of her birthday come before Brad's birthday. It doesn't matter that Brad is the older of the two.

If the parents are divorced or legally separated, the primary plan is usually the plan of the parent who has custody. In some instances, however, a court order or the divorce decree may make the other parent's plan primary.

Electronic Claims Submission

The size of the office you are working in will dictate how frequently you will submit claims. Claims can be submitted anywhere from daily to weekly. Files will electronically be prepared for submission. This process takes the information entered during charge entry and converts it into the standard format, referred to as CMS-1500. The CMS-1500 is the industry standard for claim submission. HIPAA requires that all claims are electronically filed by computer. Several regional and national clearinghouses receive these claims and electronically direct them to the proper claims administrators. A **clearinghouse** is a company that simplifies the medical insurance claims process by providing electronic submission and translation services between doctor offices and insurance companies. This system allows you to send all claims to one place instead of filing each one separately with many different claims administrators.

The clearinghouse system reviews all claims upon receipt. Any claim that is missing information or does not meet the requirements of the patient's health plan will be rejected. When this occurs, the claim is returned electronically to the sender for correction. Figure 14-3 is a sample of an electronically submitted claim that can be previewed prior to submission.

Assignment of Benefits

Assignment of benefits means that the patient allows the insurance company to send payments directly to the physician. Additionally, accepting the assignment of benefit also commits the provider to accepting the allowable fee as payment in full. Meaning, if the physician charged $425.00 and the insurance's allowable fee is

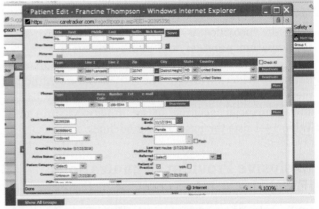

Figure 14-3 Screenshot of insurance information "form" in an electronic version. (Courtesy of Harris CareTracker™.)

$250.00, the provider will need to adjust the difference of $175.00. If the physician elects not to accept the assignment of benefits, the payment will go directly to the patient and the full charge can be collected.

HANDLING DENIED CLAIMS

Denied claims can lead to lengthy delays in payment to the physician. Here are the most frequent reasons for denial of a claim and actions you should take to address them:

- The patient cannot be identified as a covered person. Confirm that the coverage information on file is correct, including the health plan's name, policy or group number, and the patient's Social Security number.
- Coding is not appropriate for the services provided. Review provided services and recode as necessary.
- The patient is no longer covered by the plan. Bill the patient for the charges. The patient may produce evidence of new coverage. Verify coverage prior to every visit.
- The data are incomplete. Complete the required data and resubmit the claim.
- The services are not covered by the plan. Bill the patient for the services unless there's a basis for an appeal. Always verify benefits prior to the patient's visit.

Most managed care plans require participating providers to accept assignment of benefits. Here's what you'll need to do:

- Obtain the patient's electronic signature assigning insurance benefits to the office.
- If you are unable to obtain an electronic signature, have the patient sign a hard copy and scan it into their record.
- Finally, enter *signature on file* on the patient's signature line when you file the claim.

Balance billing is the practice of billing the patient for the difference between the physician's usual charge and the health plan's allowable charge. The patient is responsible for payment of this amount.

Explanation of Benefits

When a claims administrator settles a claim, it sends an explanation of benefits (**EOB**) to both the patient and the provider. The EOB tells about the payment (if any) the plan made. It also includes information about deductible amounts and coinsurance as they apply to the claim. The EOB may include information for several claims for several patients the plan has processed during a stated period. You may be responsible for checking the EOB to make sure all payments are for the correct procedures and amounts. These payments are credited to the patients' accounts and any deductibles and coinsurance billed to the patient.

Figure 14-4 shows an explanation of benefits listing the insurance allowable, amount applied to the deductible, and the coinsurance or copayment amounts.

Worker's Compensation Claims

In every state, a workers' compensation program covers employees. This program is operated by the state or by a TPA, the state hires to run the plan. The plan's benefits cover medical expenses resulting from work-related illnesses or injuries.

If you bill the patient's health plan for services related to a work-related condition, the plan will return your claim with instructions to file it with the workers' compensation claims administrator.

When your office treats patients for injuries, always inquire if the injury is work related. Also, be aware that some illnesses can be work related too. It's important to know this before services are provided so you can account and file for the charges correctly. In Worker's Compensation claims, it is important to submit the First Report of Injury within 48 hours of the patient's visit. Delay in filing of this claim and paperwork will delay the patient's benefits and could affect his care.

Medicare Claims

Whether or not your office participates in the Medicare program, you must file all Medicare claims. Physicians who participate in the Medicare program are required to accept assignment of benefits. Most physicians are participating providers (PAR providers) with Medicare. A PAR provider must agree to Medicare's fee schedule. They submit the bill to Medicare and get payment in return. The payment will be for 80% of the Medicare-approved amount for the service. The remaining 20% is patient coinsurance.

PAR providers can bill a Medicare patient for the coinsurance and any deductible amount. PAR providers are not allowed to do balance billing. This makes PAR providers much like members of a PPO. They must accept the insurer's approved fee as payment in full.

Physicians who aren't PAR providers also must file the patient's claim. Medicare will send the payment to the patient instead of the provider. This means non-PAR providers must collect both Medicare's share and the coinsurance from the patient. However, non-PAR providers are permitted to balance bill patients for charges that exceed what Medicare allows.

Some non-PAR providers ask patients to make part or full payment at the time of the service. This can be a financial hardship for the patient, especially until Medicare reimburses the patient.

Crossover Claims

Medicare patients whose financial hardship is great may be excused from paying the 20% coinsurance. In some

Explanation of Benefits

Employee Name: Joe Doe

SSN: 555-55-5555 **1**

Group No. 55555

Patient Name: Joe Doe

Date of Service: 6-15-2016

Provider: Dr. Jones

Provider TIN: 35-5555555

Date of Service **2**	Comment Code **3**	Amount of Charge **4**	Amount Allowed **5**	At **6**	Amount Paid **7**
6-15-2009	57	87.00	82.00	80%	65.60
			Total **8**		65.60
			Less Deductible **9**		25.00
			Amount Paid **10**		40.60

Payable to: Dr. Jones
Address

Comment Code:
57 - The amount charged exceeds Usual and Customary

Reading the EOB (Explanation of Benefits)

After the claim has been processed, an EOB will be issued. Although each payer has his or her own EOB format, this sample EOB illustrates the key points included in an EOB. The terms used may differ, and the formats differ widely.

1 The top section typically includes the name of the employee and the Social Security number (SSN) or other identifying number, as well as the name of the patient, the group number, the date of service and provider name, and employer identification number (EIN) (Federal identification number assigned to the physician).

2 The date of service is included and is shown as the date the service is actually rendered, not the date that was posted or billed.

3 The Comment Code is a tool used on many EOBs to indicate a coded comment that is on the bottom as exceeding "Usual and Customary." In this situation, the claim will be processed on the Usual and Customary amount. The difference between the amount charged ($87.00) and the amount allowed ($82.00) is $5.00. Unless the physician is contractually bound by an agreement with a managed care plan that forbids the practice of balance billing, that difference of $5.00 may be billed to the patient.

4 Amount of Charge shows the amount that the physician's office billed for the service.

5 Amount Allowed shows the amount of charge upon which the claim processing will be based (in this example, it is the amount of Usual and Customary).

6 This indicates the percentage of co-insurance payable by the plan.

7 Amount Paid shows the amount payable by the plan after co-insurance has been applied, but is not necessarily the amount that is actually paid (see #10).

8 The Total shows the total submitted and payable after the claim has been processed.

9 After all processing on the claim has been completed, any deductible is applied. In this example, Joe still had $25.00 to be applied to his annual deductible. Therefore, $25.00 is deducted from the amount paid and the actual reimbursement to the physician is $40.60. The amount applied to the deductible should be billed to the patient.

10 The amount actually reimbursed.

Figure 14-4 Explanation of benefits. (Reprinted from Kronenberger J, Ledbetter J. *Jones & Bartlett Learning's Comprehensive Medical Assisting.* 5th ed. Burlington, MA: Jones & Bartlett Learning, LLC; 2016.)

cases, such patients also may be eligible for Medicaid. This is referred to as a **crossover claim** because the unpaid amount of the Medicare claim crosses over automatically to Medicaid.

When both Medicare and Medicaid cover a patient, Medicare is billed first. Medicare is always primary and Medicaid is secondary. Always ask Medicare patients if they have any other coverage. Many who are not eligible for Medicaid may have Medigap insurance.

Procedure 14-1 | Obtaining Preauthorization for Services

Purpose: To obtain approval prior to certain services to insure the procedure is covered by the patient's insurance.

Equipment: Computer with access to the patient's EHR, telephone or secure Internet, CPT for procedure to be performed, date of service, location of service, physician's name, and tax identification number.

1. Locate the appropriate phone number or Web site to begin the preauthorization request. Call or access the Web site.

2. Provide complete details of the procedure or service to be performed including date, time, physician information, CPT code with detailed information about the procedure, and information regarding past treatments the patient has received.

3. After providing all necessary information, either by phone or computer, wait for the approval authorization or denial. If denied, obtain information regarding the appeals process.

4. If approved, notify the patient proceed with the procedure or service. If declined, notify patient and cancel the procedure or service. Inform the physician to see if he/she wants to move forward with an appeal.

Externship

Demonstrate your strong work ethic and quality skills every day while at extern to insure a great reference or possibly even a position. Oftentimes, cell phones become a distraction and block the ability to focus. Keep your cell phone on silent or off and stored out of sight. This will protect you from the urge to send that one quick text or e-mail. Your focus should be 100% dedicated to your patients and work. Only check your cell phone during your lunch break or after work hours.

Chapter Recap

- Medicare Part A benefits cover hospitalization and are provided at no charge to those who qualify for coverage.
- Scan insurance cards, front and back, into the patient record.
- Worker's Compensation claims require that the First Report of Injury be submitted within 48 hours of the initial visit.
- Payments from health plans provide the majority of most offices' income.
- Types of health plans include group, individual, and government-sponsored plans.
- Many physicians have contracts with managed care plans such as HMOs and PPOs.
- Each plan and type of plan has certain requirements about eligibility for payment of services.
- Your primary duty in filing claims is to do so in a timely and correct manner that will ensure maximum reimbursement for the office.

Online Resources for Students

Student Resources available on the text's online site include:
- Audio Glossaries
- Animations
- Competency Evaluation Forms
- Videos
- Anatomy & Physiology Module with Heart and Lung Sounds
- Weblinks
- Worksheets

Exercises and Activities

Certification Preparation Questions

1. An insurance plan with lower monthly premiums due to high deductible is:

   a. HMO.
   b. PPO.
   c. HDHP.
   d. HPHD.
   e. EPO.

2. The insurance plan that covers retired individuals aged 65 or older:

   a. Medicare
   b. Medigap
   c. Medicaid
   d. TRICARE
   e. CHAMPVA

3. A health care assistance program funded by both federal and state governments:

   a. Medicare
   b. Medigap
   c. Medicaid
   d. TRICARE
   e. CHAMPVA

4. The percentage owed by the patient after the insurance has paid:

   a. copayment.
   b. coinsurance.
   c. deductible.
   d. third-party payer.
   e. third-party administrator.

5. Sue Smith has two insurances, one through her employer and one through her husband. Sue's insurance company processed and paid their potion of the bill. Which of the following clauses would come into play when collecting from her husband's insurance?

   a. Birthday rule
   b. Coordination of benefits
   c. Third-party administrator
   d. Assignments of benefits
   e. Crossover claim

6. If a patient is covered by Medicare and Medicaid, which of the following would describe how the claim is transferred from one insurance to the other?

   a. Balance billing
   b. Coordination of benefits
   c. Crossover claim
   d. Assignment of benefits
   e. Third-party payments

7. When a child is insured by both parents, which of the following is used to determine which insurance is billed as primary?

   a. Crossover claim
   b. Coordination of benefits
   c. Birthday rule
   d. Balance billing
   e. Assignment of benefits

8. Prior to a patient having expense testing or an MRI, you must first acquire:

   a. precertification.
   b. utilization review.
   c. utilization management.
   d. assignment of benefits.
   e. coordination of benefits.

9. When electronically submitting claims instead of sending each claim separately to their insurance provider, which of the following can be used?

   a. Utilization management
   b. Participating provider
   c. Clearinghouse
   d. Third-party administrator
   e. Gatekeeper

10. The physician who coordinates care for patients with an HMO is referred to as:

    a. participating provider.
    b. nonparticipating provider.
    c. third-party payer.
    d. gatekeeper.
    e. dependent.

CareTracker Connection

Generating, Filing, and Managing Insurance Claims

> **HARRIS** CareTracker Activities Related to
> CareTracker This Chapter
> • Case Study 14: Submitting an Electronic Claim
> • Case Study 15: Generate and Print Paper Claims

NOTE: Case Studies 14 and 15 have prerequisite cases (in addition to Cases 1–13), which must be completed first.

Health care services can be extraordinarily expensive. Because of this, most people in the United States rely on health insurance—whether public or private—to cover their health care expenses. With the passage of the Patient Protection and Affordable Care Act in 2010, Americans are required to have health insurance of some type. Therefore, properly generating, submitting, and following up on insurance claims are critical skills for the medical assistant to possess. Practice management and electronic health record systems, such as CareTracker, simplify this process by integrating health insurance plan parameters and data into the financial system of the practice and allowing automatic electronic claim submission and payment.

Tasks discussed in this chapter that can be performed in CareTracker include the following:

- Generating electronic and paper claims
- Filing claims with Medicare, Medicaid, workers' compensation, and private insurance
- Handling denied claims
- Performing balance billing and collection procedures
- Entering payments from third-party payers

Many of these tasks are discussed in CareTracker Connection features in other chapters. A task we'll consider here is making payments on open items.

Once a patient's office visit is completed and has been captured in the system, charges related to the visit have been entered (as discussed in the CareTracker Connection feature in Managing Medical Office Finances), claims to the patient's insurance company have been submitted, and payments from the insurance company have been received, then the medical assistant may enter these payments into CareTracker. Payments may be entered in the Charge application of the Transactions module when a patient is in context.

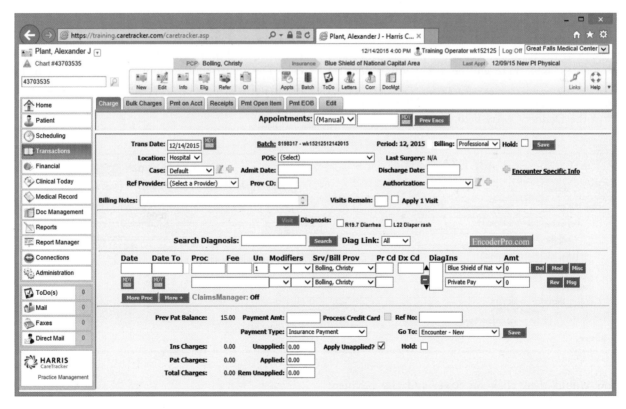

Clicking on the Pmt Open Item tab in this application will cause a list of procedures and their associated charges for the patient in context to display. Note that the charges are divided between private pay (what the patient is required to pay out of pocket) and the patient's insurance company or companies.

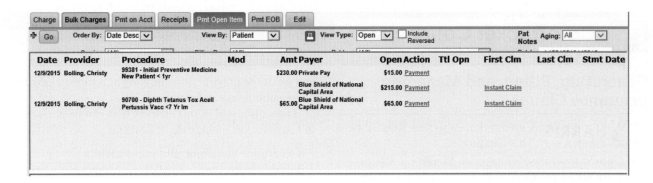

To enter a payment by an insurance company, you simply click on the Payment link next to insurance company's name (such as "Blue Shield of National Capital Area" above) and the associated charge (such as "$215.00" above), and a new window will appear.

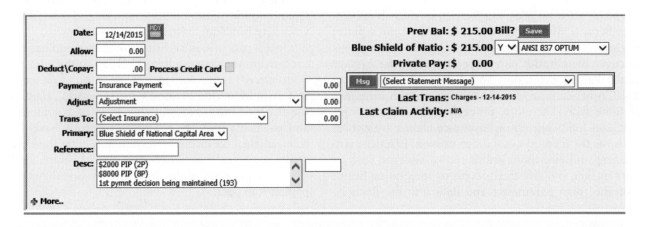

In this case, the insurance company has found that only $215 of the total $230 charged for this procedure is allowable. Thus, there will be a $15 adjustment on this account.

You would enter "215" in the Allow field and "15" in the Deduct\Copay field, as this is the patient's copayment. Once entered, "200.00" appears in the Payment field and "15.00" appears in the Adjustment field. The adjustment amount will later have to be billed to the patient or assumed as a loss by the practice.

You would then click on Save, and the payment would be made.

You'll get a chance to practice this task in Case Studies 14 (Submitting an Electronic Claim) and 15 (Generate and Print Paper Claims).

Section IV

Clinical Medical Assistant Skills

15 Medical Asepsis and Infection Control

Chapter Objectives

- Describe the conditions that help microorganisms live and grow.
- Explain the chain of infection process.
- List different ways that microorganisms are transmitted.
- Describe how the immune system works to fight infection by microorganisms.
- Compare the three levels of infection control and their effectiveness.
- Explain the concept of medical asepsis.
- Perform hand washing.
- Demonstrate knowledge of OSHA guidelines for risk management in the medical office.

- List the components of an exposure control plan.
- Practice standard precautions.
- Identify situations when personal protective equipment should be worn.
- Demonstrate how to use and remove personal protective equipment.
- Prepare and maintain examination and treatment areas.
- Dispose of biohazardous materials.
- Explain the facts about the transmission and prevention of HBV and HIV in the medical office.
- Describe how to avoid becoming infected with HBV and HIV.

CAAHEP & ABHES Competencies

CAAHEP

- Participate in training on standard precautions.
- Practice standard precautions.
- Select appropriate barrier/personal protective equipment (PPE) for potentially infectious situations.
- Perform hand washing.
- Describe the infection cycle, including the infectious agent, reservoir, susceptible host, means of transmission, portals of entry, and portals of exit.
- Define asepsis.
- Identify personal safety precautions as established by OSHA.

- List major types of infectious agents.
- Compare different methods of controlling the growth of microorganisms.
- Match types and uses of personal protective equipment (PPE).
- Discuss the application of standard precautions with regard to all body fluids, secretions, and excretions, blood, nonintact skin, and mucous membranes.

ABHES

- Infection control
- Biohazards

Chapter Terms

Aerobe	Contaminated	Pathogen	Vector
Anaerobe	Disinfection	Protozoa	Viable
Antibody	Fungi	Resident flora	Virus
Asepsis	Immunity	Resistance	
Bacteria	Microorganisms	Sanitization	
Contagious	Normal flora	Sterilization	

Abbreviations

CDC	HIV	PPE	TB
EPA	OPIM	SDS	
HBV	OSHA		

Case Study

Lucille Hawkins, an elderly patient, arrives at your clinic with her hand wrapped in a large handkerchief. As Judy Simmons, the medical assistant, escorts her to an exam room, she removes the bandage from her hand to reveal that she has an open wound on the palm of her hand. When the medical assistant questions her about the wound, the patient states that her cat scratched her over 2 weeks ago. She added that she has been taking care of it at home but it doesn't seem to be getting better.

Patients have different reasons for visiting a medical office. You are probably familiar with many of them. Some patients need physical examinations for their jobs. Others require follow-up care after surgery or care for an ongoing condition. Many patients visit the medical office because they have an illness.

When patients are ill, they can carry disease. **Contagious** diseases are those that can spread easily from one person to another. The words contagious, communicable, and infectious are all used to refer to diseases that can be transmitted from one person to another. As a medical assistant, part of your job will be to prevent the spread of disease. You need to protect patients as well as yourself from contracting contagious diseases.

DISEASE AND THE BODY

Many diseases spread through **microorganisms**—tiny living things that are too small to see without a microscope. Some people call them microbes. Many microbes are a normal part of the environment, but others can cause disease.

Stop Disease from Spreading

Medical assistants help prevent disease from spreading in two ways:

- Practice medical asepsis. **Asepsis** is a condition in which there are no living pathogens, a state of sterility. Medical asepsis is a set of procedures for preventing the spread of disease. As a medical assistant, you'll use specific procedures to control the spread of disease in the medical office. Proper hand washing is one example of a medical aseptic procedure.
- Teach others. Medical assistants show patients and their families how to prevent the spread of disease at home. Reminding a patient to cover his nose and mouth when coughing and sneezing is just one example of a teaching point.

Case Questions

What should Judy, the medical assistant, do to avoid contact with the wound on Lucille's hand? Where should the medical assistant discard the bandage that Lucille had on her hand?

Bugs and Germs

You may have heard people say, "I've caught a flu bug" or "Sneezing spreads germs." When people say these things, they are really talking about microbes that cause disease. In health care, such microbes are called **pathogens**—capable of causing disease. Most pathogens belong to one of four main groups—bacteria, viruses, fungi, or protozoa.

Bacteria

Bacteria are tiny one-celled creatures found in soil or water or on other organisms. Thousands of different types of bacteria exist on earth. Many are harmless, and some are even helpful to humans. But some bacteria cause disease. For example, strep throat is caused by a type of bacteria called streptococcus group A.

Bacteria are capable of forming spores. Spores are protective protein capsules that some bacteria form around them. It is like they form a coat of armor around them. The bacteria rest in this state until the conditions are right for growing.

Viruses

Viruses are tiny bits of protein-coated nucleic acid that invade and take over cells in other living organisms. They need living cells to reproduce. Most viruses cause disease. Influenza, commonly known as "the flu," is caused by a virus. So is the common cold.

Fungi

Fungi are a type of plant. They may be familiar to you as mushrooms or mold. Fungi live in the air, in the soil, on plants, and in water. Some tiny fungi also live in the human body. Only some of these fungi cause disease. An example of a disease caused by a fungus is ringworm, a disease of the skin.

Protozoa

Protozoa are tiny parasites—animals that live in or on another organism. They prefer to live in moist environments. In humans, protozoa often cause disease. One disease caused by protozoa is malaria, a disease with symptoms of high fever and chills.

Good Bugs Gone Bad

Most microbes are not pathogens. In fact, some microbes are necessary to stay healthy. These include some kinds of bacteria, fungi, and protozoa. They are referred to as **normal flora** or **resident flora** because they normally live in your body. Here are some places where normal flora are normally found:

* On your skin
* In your respiratory system
* In your gastrointestinal system
* In your genitourinary system

Normal flora is usually not disease causing. But they can sometimes become pathogens. This may happen if:

* They multiply until there are too many
* They move to a part of the body where they are not normally found

When microbes begin living in a part of the body where they usually are not found, they are called transient flora. A key factor that affects whether transient flora will become pathogenic is the body's level of resistance. **Resistance** refers to how well the human body fights disease. If a person's resistance is low, transient flora may become pathogens.

Body Protection

The human body has several ways to protect itself from disease. Natural defenses help to keep pathogens out of body organs.

* *Skin.* Clean, unbroken skin acts as a barrier. It stops pathogens from getting into the body.
* *Eyes.* Eyelashes trap many microbes before they reach the eye. Some are destroyed by tears. Tears contain lysozyme, a substance found in the body that kills some kinds of bacteria.
* *Mouth.* More kinds of microbes are found in the mouth than anywhere else in the body. Luckily, saliva is slightly bactericidal. This means that it can destroy bacteria. Good oral hygiene can stop the growth of many pathogens in the mouth.
* *Gastrointestinal (GI) tract.* The stomach stops many microbes that enter the GI tract. Hydrochloric acid, an acid usually found in the stomach, destroys many pathogens.
* *Respiratory tract.* Hairs and cilia (fine hair-like structures) on membranes inside the nostrils stop microbes in the air from entering the nose. If these structures are unable to keep pathogens out, there's a second line of defense. Mucus membranes in the respiratory tract trap microorganisms. They help remove them from the body through sneezing, swallowing, or coughing.
* *Genitourinary tract.* Most microbes don't last long in the reproductive or the urinary systems because the environment is slightly acidic.

These protective systems often prevent pathogens from taking over in the human body. But the systems sometimes fail when they must deal with a virulent organism. A virulent organism is one that can overpower the body's defenses.

How Microorganisms Survive

Like other living things, microbes need certain things to live and grow.

- *Moisture.* Most microbes need water or moisture to live. Bacterial spores will not be active until they are moistened.
- *Nutrients.* All living things take in nutrients or substances that help them grow and live. Humans get nutrients from food. Microbes find nutrients in the environment around them.
- *Temperature.* Some microbes grow best at the normal body temperature for humans (98.6°F). These are the ones most likely to become pathogens. Some microbes can survive even in freezing or boiling temperatures.
- *Darkness.* Many pathogenic bacteria cannot survive in bright light, such as sunlight.
- *Neutral pH.* pH measures the acid–base balance of a solution on a scale from 1 to 14, where 7 is neutral. Many microbes that invade the body prefer pH levels like those in human blood (7.35 to 7.45).
- *Oxygen.* Microbes that need oxygen to survive are called **aerobes**. But a few types of microbes do not need oxygen to survive. They are called **anaerobes**.

The Process of Infection

Many pathogens live in the environment, but they do not always cause disease. Infection occurs when pathogens invade the body and start growing. As a medical assistant, you must understand the process of infection. This process can damage body organs and tissues and can lead to disease.

Think of the process of infection as a chain. Breaking any link in the infection chain can stop pathogens from spreading. There are five links in the chain of infection. See Figure 15-1.

Link #1 Reservoir

The first link in the chain is the place where a microorganism lives and grows. A person or animal infected with a microorganism is a reservoir host. The host's body is a source of nutrients for the microbe. The reservoir host may or may not show signs of infection. But the reservoir host is a carrier of the pathogen with the potential to spread it to others.

Link #2 Exit from the Reservoir

The reservoir host transmits disease if there is an escape route from the host's body. Some ways in which the microbe may exit the reservoir host are the mucous membranes of the nose and mouth, openings of the gastrointestinal system (mouth and rectum), or an open wound.

Link #3 Vehicle of Transmission

The vehicle of transmission is the way the microbe is carried through the environment. For example, mucus or air droplets from the nose or mouth can be a vehicle of transmission. Coughing or sneezing can send microbes into the environment. Touching another person or object with an unclean hand also can transmit microbes.

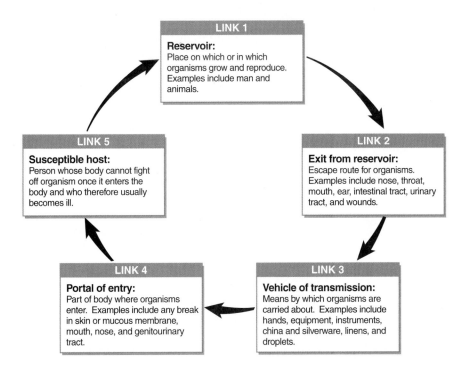

LINK 1
Reservoir: Place on which or in which organisms grow and reproduce. Examples include man and animals.

LINK 2
Exit from reservoir: Escape route for organisms. Examples include nose, throat, mouth, ear, intestinal tract, urinary tract, and wounds.

LINK 3
Vehicle of transmission: Means by which organisms are carried about. Examples include hands, equipment, instruments, china and silverware, linens, and droplets.

LINK 4
Portal of entry: Part of body where organisms enter. Examples include any break in skin or mucous membrane, mouth, nose, and genitourinary tract.

LINK 5
Susceptible host: Person whose body cannot fight off organism once it enters the body and who therefore usually becomes ill.

Figure 15-1   The infectious process cycle. Infections and infectious diseases are spread by starting from the reservoir (Link #1) and moving in a circle to the susceptible host (Link #5). Microorganisms can be controlled by interfering at any link in the cycle. (Reprinted from Kronenberger J, Ledbetter J. *Jones & Bartlett Learning's Comprehensive Medical Assisting.* 5th ed. Burlington, MA: Jones & Bartlett Learning, LLC; 2016.)

Link #4 Portal of Entry

Microbes in the environment need nutrients to survive. They can find these nutrients in a new host. The portal of entry is a place where microorganisms can enter the next host's body. Microbes in air droplets can enter through the nose and respiratory system. For microbes in food or drink, the portal of entry is the gastrointestinal system. For some microbes, a portal of entry can be a cut in the skin.

Link #5 Susceptible Host

Once a pathogen has entered a new host's body, that person is at risk for developing a disease. A susceptible host is a person who cannot fight the pathogen once it enters the body. It is the last link in the infection chain. If the body of the susceptible host provides the right conditions and nutrients, the microbes will grow and multiply. The susceptible host then becomes a carrier, or reservoir host, starting the infection chain again.

FIGHTING INFECTION AND DISEASE

Skin, cough reflexes, tears, and stomach acid are some of the body's natural barriers to stop microbes from entering. But natural barriers do not always work. If pathogens get past the body's natural barriers, they can enter the body and start the process of infection. Then the body must fight back.

Inside the body, the immune system is a complex system of organs, tissues, and cells that work together to protect the body from infection and disease. The immune system works to:

- Find invading pathogens
- Attack pathogens before they start to reproduce
- Minimize the damage caused by pathogens
- Provide future protection from pathogens

The Body's Response

Inflammation is the first way the body responds to any outside attack. It is called a nonspecific response, because it occurs regardless of the kind of threat there is to the body. Some of these threats include the following:

- A foreign object, such as a splinter in the finger or a particle in the eye
- Extreme temperatures
- Trauma or injury
- Pathogens entering the body

There are four main signs of inflammation:

- Redness
- Swelling
- Heat
- Pain

These signs are part of the body's natural response to infection or injury. Inflammation does not always mean the body is fighting infection caused by pathogens. But when infection occurs, inflammation will be part of the body's response.

The signs of inflammation occur when the body sends fluid into the damaged tissue. Swelling helps to keep invading pathogens away from other tissues. The fluid also contains cells from the immune system. They move into the damaged tissue to fight infection.

Case Question

When Lucille arrived at the office, she stated that she tried to take care of her wound for 2 weeks and it was not getting better. What signs or symptoms were most likely present that indicated to her that it was not healing?

The Direct Attack

The immune system produces several kinds of cells to fight infection. Some are white blood cells that attack and destroy any pathogens. In some cases, the immune system will create an **antibody**—a structure that are designed to attack specific pathogens. Antibodies also can protect the body against future attacks by that type of pathogen.

The Immune System Remembers

A host's susceptibility to disease is related to the body's immunity to the disease. **Immunity** refers to the body's ability to fight specific pathogens. The immune system already may be able to produce antibodies for a specific pathogen. Immunity can result from:

- Previous infection by a specific pathogen
- Immunization with a vaccine

Immunization is a way to protect the body from a specific pathogen. It involves the injection of a vaccine—a substance that signals the immune system to produce antibodies for the disease. Vaccination can provide permanent immunity from the disease caused by that pathogen.

Types of Immunity

There are different types of immunity. Some individuals are born with natural immunity to certain diseases. This type of immunity does not involve antibodies. It is already programmed into the person's DNA.

Another important type of immunity is called acquired immunity. Acquired immunity does involve antibodies. This type of immunity may be acquired either passively or actively. There are four different kinds of acquired immunity.

- Passive acquired natural immunity. Passive acquired natural immunity comes from another source, such as from the mother to the fetus across the placenta. It also can be passed from a nursing mother to her baby through breast milk.
- Passive acquired artificial immunity. Passive acquired artificial immunity is produced by injections of a special type of antibodies after possible exposure to an infectious pathogen. These antibodies are not a vaccine and only provide temporary protection. For example, a patient with no tetanus immunization can have an injection to prevent tetanus after stepping on a rusty nail.
- Active acquired natural immunity. Active acquired natural immunity develops in a person who contracts a specific disease. It causes the body to produce antibodies and memory cells. For example, a person who gets chicken pox develops an active acquired natural immunity to the disease that should prevent him from getting chicken pox again in the future.
- Active acquired artificial immunity. Active acquired artificial immunity results from a vaccine. The vaccine stimulates the production of antibodies and memory cells to prevent specific diseases by killing the pathogen if it enters the body. Vaccines are available to prevent diseases such as measles, mumps, and rubella to name just a few.

When the Immune System Fails

Sometimes, the immune system cannot control an infection. It may not stop pathogens from growing for one or both of two reasons:

- A virulent pathogen may be too powerful for the immune system to fight.
- The immune system may be depleted. That means it does not have the resources it normally possesses to fight infection or disease.

For example, in a person who is ill, the immune system may have already used up many cells fighting one illness. There may not be enough cells available to fight infection by another pathogen. This is why a person with a depleted immune system is more susceptible to infection and disease.

From Infection to Disease

Infection occurs when pathogens enter a host and begin to multiply. Infection may or may not cause disease. Infection leads to disease if the immune system is not able to stop the pathogen from damaging cells or tissues. Diseases that result from infections are called infectious diseases.

Symptoms are physical signs that the patient has a disease. There are many physical signs of infectious disease. Common symptoms include fever, weakness, fatigue, pain, and loss of appetite.

Spotting a Susceptible Host

There are many reasons why a susceptible host cannot fight off pathogens. Some of these include the following:

- Age. Body defenses against disease become less effective as you age. Elderly people may have weaker immune systems. At the other end of the spectrum, infants may not have fully developed immune systems. They are less able to fight pathogens.
- Existing disease. A person who already has an illness may have more trouble fighting off a pathogen. An ill person may have a depleted immune system.
- Poor nutrition. A diet lacking in nutrients (proteins, fats, carbohydrates, vitamins, and minerals) can harm the body's cells, making it difficult for the body to repair damage.
- Poor hygiene. Keeping the body clean will keep down the number of microorganisms on the skin. That means there are fewer microorganisms to spread disease.

Types of Infections

Some pathogens make you very sick for a short period of time. Others can leave you ill for a long time. There are three main types of infections—acute infections, chronic infections, and latent infections.

Acute Infections
Acute infections develop quickly and last only a short time. Influenza, or the flu, is an example of an acute infection. The immune system destroys the virus that causes the flu within 2 or 3 weeks and symptoms disappear.

Chronic Infections
Chronic infections last for long periods of time, possibly even a lifetime. Their symptoms may not always be noticeable. For example, hepatitis B is a chronic infection of the liver that is caused by a virus. People with hepatitis B may not show symptoms, but the virus can be detected in their blood.

Latent Infections
Latent infections have periods when the pathogen is dormant, or not active, for months or even years. Viruses often cause these kinds of infections. When the conditions are right for the virus to grow, the infection

often reappears. During this active phase, the virus can be transmitted to other people. Cold sores and genital herpes are latent infections caused by viruses.

Stages of Infectious Disease

Different pathogens lead to different kinds of infectious disease. But many of these diseases develop in a similar way. There are five identifiable stages of infection.

Stage One: Incubation Stage

After a person is exposed to a pathogen, some time passes before any symptoms appear. During this incubation stage, the pathogen grows and establishes itself in the body. For some diseases, the incubation stage lasts only a day or two before the first symptoms appear. For other diseases, it may take years before the person notices any symptoms.

Stage Two: Prodromal Stage

At the prodromal stage, the person may have only a general feeling of illness or fatigue. These general symptoms may suggest that an infectious disease might be developing.

Stage Three: Acute Stage

In the acute stage, specific symptoms become obvious. The infectious disease reaches its most severe point. The body's inflammatory process is at work. Medical treatments may be given to reduce pain or discomfort. Other treatments, such as antibiotics, may be prescribed to promote healing. Antibiotics fight infections caused by bacteria and other microorganisms.

Stage Four: Declining Stage

During the declining stage, symptoms start to fade. However, the disease is still present. Because patients are feeling better, they sometimes stop taking their medications at this stage. They should be educated not to do this.

Stage Five: Convalescent Stage

At last, the disease is defeated! During the convalescent stage, the patient is recovering. The patient's body is working to return to its previous state of good health.

 HOW GERMS ARE SPREAD

Some patients in a medical office might be in one of the stages of infectious disease. This can expose you, other staff, and other patients to potential pathogens. By understanding their vehicles, or modes of transmission, you can break this link in the infection chain and prevent disease from spreading. It is important to cover your nose and mouth when you cough or sneeze. It is recommended that you cough or sneeze into the sleeve of your arm so you do not get the germs on your hands. Also remember to wash your hands frequently especially after coughing or sneezing.

Direct Transmission

Direct transmission occurs when there is direct contact between the reservoir host and the susceptible host. Examples include the following:

- Shaking hands
- Touching the blood or body fluids of the reservoir host
- Inhaling infected air droplets of the reservoir host
- Intimate contact such as kissing or sexual intercourse

Indirect Transmission

Not all pathogens are spread through direct contact with an infected person. Indirect transmission occurs through a vector. A **vector** is an object that contains pathogens. Examples of indirect transmission include the following:

- Eating food that is contaminated (Something that is **contaminated** has been touched by a source of pathogens.)
- Drinking from an infected person's glass
- Getting bitten by a disease-carrying insect
- Using an improperly disinfected medical instrument
- Touching a contaminated surface, such as a doorknob

Sources of indirect transmission often are not easy to see. Many microbes can stay **viable**, or alive—capable of living, for long periods of time outside the human body. For example, a surface that once was in contact with saliva, blood, or pus from an infected wound can be full of pathogens even if it does not look contaminated.

Who Transmits Pathogens?

Most reservoir hosts are humans, animals, or insects.

Human Hosts

The most common source of pathogens that cause infectious disease in humans is humans themselves. Human hosts are typically:

- People who are obviously ill with an infectious disease
- People who show no symptoms but are incubating an infectious disease
- People who are carriers of an infectious disease

Animals

Many people worry about animals spreading disease. In fact, animals are not a common vehicle for diseases that affect humans. However, those that can be a source of pathogens include the following:

- Dogs
- Cats
- Birds
- Cattle
- Rodents
- Animals that live in the wild

Rabies and avian flu are examples of diseases that can be transmitted to humans by infected animals. Avian flu, or bird flu, is caused by a virus that birds can pass to one another. The virus usually doesn't affect humans, but when it does, it can be deadly.

Insects

Insects are another source of disease. Flies and cockroaches carry many kinds of pathogens. Some insects feed on the blood of the reservoir host. When they bite another person, they can pass on the pathogens. For instance, ticks can cause Lyme disease, a bacterial disease that can affect the skin, joints, and nervous system. Some mosquitoes carry the West Nile virus, which can lead to swelling in the brain and spinal cord. See Table 15-1, which lists some of the common infectious diseases and how they are spread.

 CONTROLLING INFECTIONS

An important part of your job as a medical assistant will be to help control and prevent infections in the medical office. One of the best ways to do this is to follow guidelines set by the Occupational Safety and Health Administration (**OSHA**) and the Centers for Disease Control (**CDC**).

Medical Asepsis

Medical asepsis is a set of practices to keep an object or area free from microbes. These practices are sometimes called clean techniques because they prevent the spread of microorganisms within the medical office.

Table 15-1	Common Infectious Diseases and How They Spread
Disease	**How It Spreads**
AIDS	Direct contact or contact with contaminated needles
Chicken pox	Direct contact or droplets
Hepatitis B	Direct contact with infectious body fluid
Influenza	Droplets in the air; direct contact with infected carriers or with contaminated articles such as used tissues
Measles	Infected droplets in the air; direct contact with infected carrier
Mononucleosis	Infected droplets in the air or contact with saliva
Pneumonia	Infected droplets in the air or direct contact with infected mucus
Rabies	Direct contact with saliva of infected animal, such as through an animal bite

Clean Hands

Hand washing is the simplest but the most important medical aseptic practice. This practice is the single best way to stop the spread of disease. Always wash your hands in these situations:

- Before and after patient contact
- After contact with any blood or body fluids
- After contact with contaminated material
- After handling specimens
- After coughing, sneezing, or blowing your nose
- After using the restroom
- Before and after going to lunch and taking breaks
- Before leaving for the day

Wear disposable gloves when handling specimens or if you think you might come into contact with contaminated material. Always assume blood and body fluids are contaminated. But even then, remember to wash your hands. To stop disease from spreading, you need to wash your hands before putting gloves on and after taking them off.

Clean Workplace

Medical asepsis also involves keeping the office clean. Areas to clean include examination and treatment rooms, waiting and reception areas, and clinical work areas.

- Take care to keep soiled linen, table paper, supplies, or instruments from touching your clothing. Always roll used table paper or linens inward so the unused side is facing out.
- Always think of the floor as contaminated. Anything dropped on the floor is no longer clean. It must be thrown away or cleaned to its former level of asepsis before being used.
- Clean tables, counters, and other surfaces often. If they become contaminated, they must be cleaned immediately. Microbes are less likely to live and grow on clean surfaces.
- Assume that body fluids and blood from any source are contaminated. Follow guidelines from OSHA and the CDC to stop the spread of disease. Protect yourself and your patients.

Levels of Infection Control

Medical instruments, equipment, and supplies need to be kept clean to prevent the transmission of disease. There are different levels of infection control for the various kinds of tools—sterilization, disinfection, and sanitization. Each level has a different result and procedures. Table 15-2 lists the levels of infection control.

Sanitization

The lowest level of infection control is **sanitization**—cleaning items using soap or detergent. Your goal is to reduce the number of microbes on objects or surfaces. Clean objects and surfaces thoroughly by rubbing and scrubbing using warm, soapy water. Any contaminants you can see should be removed. Sanitization must be done before disinfection or sterilization.

Disinfection

Disinfection refers to the destruction of pathogens by direct exposure to chemical or physical agents. It offers an intermediate level of infection control. Using germicides or disinfectants, you can destroy many pathogens and other microbes. Disinfection does not destroy all microorganism or bacterial spores. But high levels of disinfection are almost as effective as sterilization. Some disinfection methods work better than others. Levels of disinfection and procedures are listed in Table 15-3.

Various products used for disinfection are shown in Figure 15-2. Here are some factors to consider:

- *Prior cleaning.* Disinfection is more effective if items are sanitized first.
- *Type of microorganism.* Some microbes are more resistant to certain methods and disinfectants than others.
- *Strength of the disinfecting solution.* Concentrated germicides are most effective. Disinfectants that are diluted with water may not kill as many pathogens.
- *Length of exposure.* Leave the object in germicide or disinfectant for the length of time recommended by the manufacturer.
- *Complexity of the object.* Objects with corners, edges, or rough spots may be more difficult to disinfect.
- *Temperature.* Many disinfectants work best at room temperature.

Table 15-2   Levels of Infection Control

Level of Control	Type of Control	Effect	Procedures
Low	Sanitization	Removes contaminants	Cleaning with soaps and detergents
Medium	Disinfection	Destroys many pathogens	Using different chemical solutions
High	Sterilization	Destroys all microbes and spores	Several different methods including autoclaving

Table 15-3 Levels of Disinfection and Procedures

Level	Procedures	When to Use	Effect
Low	Commercial products without tuberculocidal properties	Routine cleaning; to clean objects or surfaces with no visible blood or body fluids	Destroys many bacteria and some viruses; does NOT destroy *M. tuberculosis* or bacterial spores
Intermediate	Commercial germicides that kill *M. tuberculosis*; solutions containing 1:10 dilution of household bleach (2 oz. of chlorine bleach per quart of tap water)	To clean instruments that have touched unbroken skin, such as blood pressure cuffs, stethoscopes, and splints	Destroys many viruses, fungi, and some bacteria, including *M. tuberculosis*; does NOT destroy bacterial spores
High	Immersion in approved disinfecting chemical for 45 min or according to guidelines on label; immersion in boiling water for 30 min (rarely used)	To clean reusable instruments that contact body cavities with mucous membranes, such as the vagina and rectum, that are not considered sterile	Destroys most microorganisms except certain bacterial spores

Sterilization

Sterilization offers the highest level of infection control. It destroys all forms of microorganisms, including bacterial spores. The four basic methods of sterilization are as follows:

- High pressure/steam heat from an autoclave
- Sterilization gases, such as ethylene oxide
- Dry heat ovens
- Immersion in approved chemical solutions

What Needs to be Sterilized?

Many of the instruments used in a medical office need to be sterilized. These types of equipment must be sterilized:

- Instruments that break, penetrate, or cut the skin
- Instruments that contact areas of the body considered sterile, such as the bladder
- Instruments that come in contact with surgical incisions
- Any instrument that becomes contaminated or soiled during a procedure

Medical equipment may come in sterile, ready-to-use packages (Fig. 15-3). Many medical offices use disposable sterile supplies. These supplies are used once and discarded immediately after use.

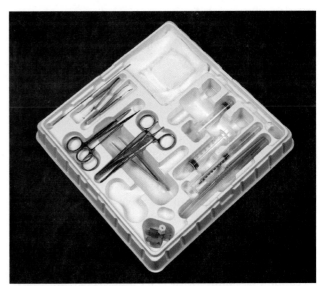

Figure 15-3 Equipment that must be sterile includes items that will penetrate the skin or come into contact with surgical incisions, such as surgical instruments. These items are disposable and meant for one-time use only. (Reprinted from Kronenberger J, Ledbetter J. *Jones & Bartlett Learning's Comprehensive Medical Assisting.* 5th ed. Burlington, MA: Jones & Bartlett Learning, LLC; 2016.)

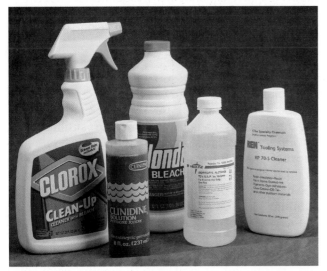

Figure 15-2 These products destroy many pathogenic microorganisms if used correctly. (Reprinted from Kronenberger J, Ledbetter J. *Jones & Bartlett Learning's Comprehensive Medical Assisting.* 5th ed. Burlington, MA: Jones & Bartlett Learning, LLC; 2016.)

GUIDELINES FOR THE MEDICAL OFFICE

The Occupational Safety and Health Administration is responsible for ensuring the safety of all workers. This federal agency makes and enforces safety rules for medical offices.

By law, a medical office must establish practices to keep employees healthy and safe. These practices must be written into a policy or procedure manual or put in a separate infection control manual. They should be kept in a place where employees and OSHA inspectors can find them easily.

The Infection Control Manual

The medical office must provide clear instructions to protect you from exposure to disease and biohazardous materials. Biohazardous means that the materials are capable of causing disease or infection. Biohazardous materials may be contaminated with pathogens. They present a risk to your health and the health of patients. It is important that the medical office has written instructions for the employees to follow when dealing with biohazards. Here are two key things the instructions should contain:

- Exposure risk factor. Written policy must include an exposure risk factor for each job description. This measures each employee's risk of being exposed to a communicable disease while performing the duties of their position.
- Exposure control plan. Every medical office with more than 10 employees also must have a written exposure control plan. It explains what to do if employees or visitors are exposed to biohazardous material in spite of precautions.

Medical Assistant Risks

Not all medical assistants will have the same exposure risk factor. Administrative medical assistants have a low exposure risk, for instance. They will be typically assigned to duties that do not involve hands on patient care or performance of invasive procedures. They require only minimal protection on the job. Clinical medical assistants have greater exposure to pathogens and therefore have a higher risk. Their duties typically involve invasive procedures increasing their possibility of coming in contact with body fluids. They must have access to personal protective equipment (**PPE**), such as gloves, gowns, goggles, and/or face shields. Figure 15-4 shows a medical assistant with appropriate goggles and gloves ready to perform procedures that may put her at risk of contact with body fluids.

The employer also must provide immunization against hepatitis B at no charge.

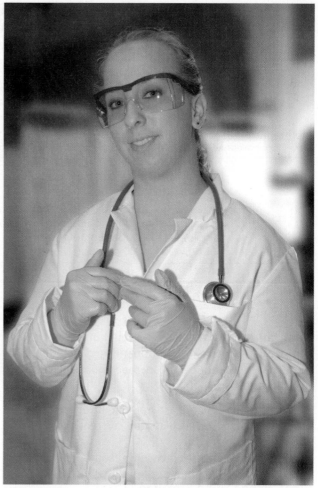

Figure 15-4 Personal protective equipment that must be provided for employees who may come into contact with contaminated materials includes gloves, goggles, face shields, and gowns or aprons to protect clothing. (Reprinted from Kronenberger J, Ledbetter J. *Jones & Bartlett Learning's Comprehensive Medical Assisting.* 5th ed. Burlington, MA: Jones & Bartlett Learning, LLC; 2016.)

Study Skill

Are you a procrastinator? Procrastination means to postpone things until later, sometimes much later. Procrastination causes students to submit late, incomplete assignments or wrong assignments because they did not plan ahead or take the time to do it correctly. Typically, students procrastinate because the assignment seems difficult or time consuming. They may have trouble getting started on the assignment or are just afraid of failing by not knowing how to correctly do the assignment. To avoid procrastination, get organized and break up the assignment or project into smaller segments. You should plan ahead and develop a schedule to keep you on track, toward completion of the assignment. After you complete each segment of the assignment, reward yourself.

The Exposure Control Plan

It is important to follow the guidelines in the exposure control plan for your medical office. If you think you or a patient has been exposed to a biohazard, apply first aid principles right away. Then, tell your supervisor, office manager, or office physician. Some kinds of exposures might require postexposure testing or procedures.

After exposure, you will need to complete a report called an incident report or exposure report. In the report, you will describe how the exposure occurred. The report can help your medical office change its policies to prevent this kind of exposure in the future. Your employer also must record the exposure on an OSHA 300 Log form (Fig. 15-5).

Exposure to Biohazards

Medical assistants need to understand what to do immediately when exposed to a biohazard. For example, even though you are very careful performing duties, one day, your glove tears and the patient's blood seeps into the glove and comes in contact with your skin. Now, you have an exposure situation that you need to tend to immediately. It is important to remain calm and follow safety procedures.

- If the blood gets in your mucous membranes (eyes, nose, or mouth), you need to flush the area right away with water or saline.
- If you're stuck by a needle, you must let the site bleed. Then, clean the site with soap and water.
- Next, you must report the exposure to your employer right away. Your employer will need to follow OSHA guidelines to manage the exposure.
- You will need to be evaluated to determine if you may have come in contact hepatitis B, hepatitis C, or HIV.
- Your office must check the patient's medical records to determine if they are infected with hepatitis B, hepatitis C, or HIV. If this information is not known, the patient should be asked to give consent to be tested. If the patient is infected with any of these blood-borne pathogens, you must be treated following OSHA standards to prevent illness.
- If the injury was caused by a needle, your employer must keep track of this type of exposure in a sharps injury log.

Reporting to OSHA

If one or more of the following criteria are met, exposures to biohazardous material must be reported to OSHA. Your employer normally takes care of this task. Reporting is required when any of these exposures have occurred.

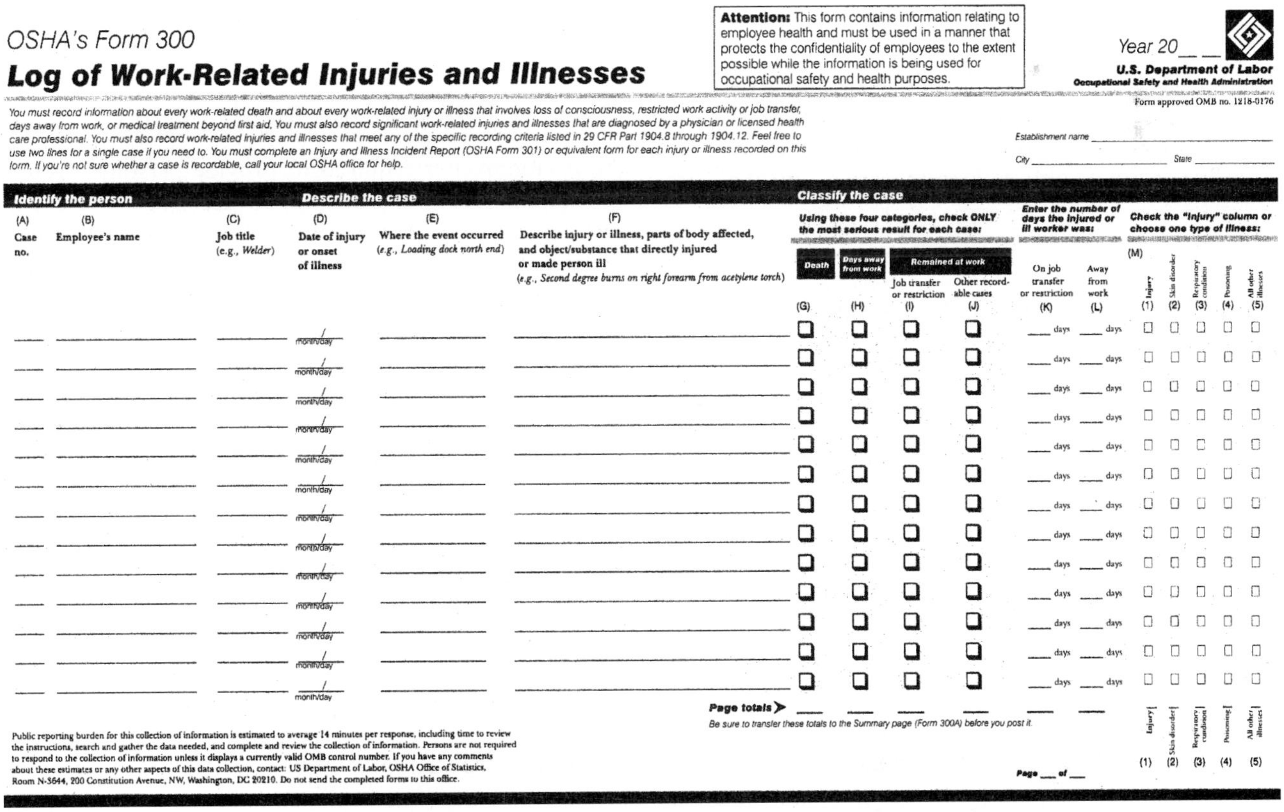

Figure 15-5   The OSHA 300 Log form. (Courtesy of the U.S. Department of Labor.)

- The exposure was work related and required medical treatment beyond first aid (such as medication or vaccination).
- The employee lost consciousness or had to be medically removed.
- The employee lost days at work or needed to transfer to another job.
- An accident involved an injury from a needle or a sharp object that was contaminated with another person's blood or another possibly infectious material.
- The exposure involved a known case of tuberculosis (**TB**) and resulted in a positive skin test for TB or a diagnosis of TB by a physician.
- A negative blood test for a contagious disease changed to a positive test after the exposure.

OSHA Blood-borne Pathogen Training Requirements

OSHA requires that newly hired medical office employees who will be exposed to blood have special training. The training must be repeated every year. It will include any new policies recommended by OSHA, the CDC, the Department of Health and Human Services, or the U.S. Public Health Service. The training should include these key points:

- Descriptions of blood-borne diseases, how they are transmitted, and related symptoms
- The kinds of personal protective equipment available and its location in the medical office
- Information about the risks of contracting hepatitis B and about the HBV vaccine
- The exposure control plan and postexposure procedures, along with follow-up care if an exposure occurs

Practicing Standard Precautions

Standard precautions are a set of procedures recognized by the CDC. The goal of the procedures is to reduce the transmission of microorganisms in any health care setting, including medical offices. For safety reasons, remember to always treat blood and all other body fluids as contaminated.

You need to use standard precautions whenever you will be touching blood, body fluids, damaged skin, or mucous membranes including these important procedures.

- Wash your hands with soap and water after touching blood, body fluids, secretions, or other contaminated objects—whether you have worn gloves or not.

- You can use alcohol-based hand rub to decontaminate your hands if your hands are not visibly dirty or contaminated.
- Wear clean, nonsterile examination gloves if you think you might come into contact with blood, body fluids, secretions, mucous membranes, damaged skin, or contaminated objects.
- If you have touched infective material, change your gloves between procedures, even if the procedures involve the same patient.
- Wear equipment to protect your eyes, nose, and mouth. Keep your clothing clean by wearing a disposable gown, especially for procedures that might splash or spray blood, body fluids, or secretions.
- Dispose of single-use items appropriately. Do not disinfect them, sterilize them, or reuse them.
- Take care to avoid injuries before, after, and during procedures that involve scalpels, needles, or other sharp instruments.
- Do not recap used needles or bend or break them. When giving injections or drawing blood, make sure you have a sharps container within reach to throw away used needles.
- Use safety lock devices when performing invasive procedures.
- Place used disposable syringes, needles, and other sharps in the closest puncture-resistant container (sharps container).
- Use barrier devices such as mouthpieces or resuscitation bags as alternatives to mouth-to-mouth resuscitation.

Personal Protective Equipment

Your employer is required to provide personal protective equipment (PPE) for you to use when you are at risk of coming in contact with blood-borne pathogens. If you might be exposed to biohazardous materials in your work, you must have access to PPE including disposable gowns, goggles, face shields, and gloves—either latex or vinyl.

Gowns, goggles, and face shields are worn in any areas where splashing or splattering of airborne particles may occur. You must wear gloves whenever you perform a procedure that involves a risk of exposure to blood or body fluids. For example, you must wear gloves to:

- Draw blood specimens
- Dispose of biohazardous waste
- Touch contaminated surfaces
- Handle contaminated equipment
- Give injections
- Clean biohazard spills

Gloves should fit comfortably. Be sure to choose the right size for your hands. They should not be too loose or too tight. If you or patients are sensitive to the latex in regular examination gloves, an alternative must be made available.

Applying and Removing PPE

There is a specific sequence used to apply and remove personal protective equipment. When applying PPE, put on the gown, then the mask or face shield or goggles, and then put on your gloves last. After completion of procedures, take off your gloves first and then the goggles, gown, and mask last. Once you have removed the personal protective equipment, including your gloves, always wash your hands.

Biohazard and Safety Equipment in the Medical Office

The medical office where you work must offer the following protections from biohazardous and other dangerous materials.

- SDS binder. Safety data sheets (**SDS**), formerly known as material safety data sheets (**MSDS**), are forms prepared by the manufacturers of all chemical substances and products used in a medical office. The binder in your office should contain sheets for all chemicals used in your workplace. Each sheet tells how to handle and dispose of the chemical and lists any protective gear you will need. It also gives you information about the health hazards and other possible dangers of the chemical, the safety precautions you need to take when using it, and how to fight any fires involving it. These sheets also outline first aid in the event that you do have harmful exposure to the chemical.
- Biohazard waste containers. These are special containers used only for waste contaminated with blood, body fluids, or other potentially infectious material (**OPIM**). Sharps containers are one type of biohazard waste container. They are used to dispose of items that puncture or cut the skin.
- Personal protective equipment. Gloves and other PPE must be available for use in areas where there is a risk of exposure to blood or body fluids. See Box 15-1 for information about latex allergy in the medical office.
- Eyewash station. The eyewash basin can remove contaminants or chemicals that accidentally get in your eyes. For chemical exposure, the eyes should be washed for the amount of time recommended on the SDS or for at least 15 minutes. OSHA

requires every laboratory to contain an eyewash station.
- Immunization. Employers are required by OSHA to provide immunization against blood-borne pathogens, such as hepatitis B, if vaccines are available. If the employee does not want the immunization, a document of declination or waiver must be signed for the employee's file.

Box 15-1 | **Latex Allergy and the Medical Assistant**

Many health care workers develop allergic reactions to latex. Latex is a product of the rubber tree. Proteins in latex can cause allergic reactions. Unfortunately, many products, including examination gloves, are made of latex.

Reactions to latex can range from mild to severe. Symptoms of a mild allergy are skin redness, rash, itching, or hives. A severe allergy can result in difficulty breathing, wheezing, or coughing.

You are most likely to see respiratory responses after gloves are removed. Powder inside the gloves goes into the air. It enters the respiratory system when you breathe. Protect yourself from latex allergy by following these guidelines. Patients may also be allergic to latex many practices use gloves made of nitrile or vinyl.

- Find out about other latex-free equipment, including blood pressure cuffs for taking a patient's blood pressure.
- Avoid using oil-based lotions or hand creams before putting on latex gloves. Oils can break down the latex and release the proteins that cause allergic reactions.
- Wash your hands thoroughly after removing any gloves.
- Know the symptoms of latex allergy so you can recognize them in yourself, your coworkers, or patients.

 ## HANDLING CONTAMINATION IN AND AROUND THE OFFICE

Some of your duties as a medical assistant may involve keeping equipment and surfaces in the office clean. You will need to follow proper procedures. To sanitize, clean off any soil you can see on surfaces and equipment using detergent or low-level disinfectant. Floors, examination tables, countertops, and cabinets all need to be cleaned routinely. They also must be cleaned when they have become soiled with blood or body fluids.

Biohazard Cleanup

Surfaces contaminated with biohazardous materials must be cleaned right away. You need to use an approved germicide or a diluted bleach solution to destroy microorganisms.

Some offices purchase commercial spill kits. These kits include all the materials you need to clean contaminated surfaces. Some kits may contain different materials depending on the manufacturer. If your office does not purchase kits, you must gather the materials from the office yourself. It is a good idea to store them together in case a biohazardous spill occurs—you will be ready for action. Here are items you will need:

- Clean examination gloves
- Disposable gowns
- Eye protection, such as goggles
- Face shields and masks
- Absorbent crystals, gel, or powder (such as sodium bicarbonate)
- A disposable scoop
- Paper towels
- At least one biohazard waste bag (usually called a "red bag")
- A chemical disinfectant
  - A sharps container or spill control barriers
  - Shoe covers (for large amount of contamination on the floor)

Waste Containers

In the medical office, there are separate containers for disposing of different kinds of waste. You need to make sure you put waste in the right place.

Regular Waste Container

The regular waste container is used only for waste that is not contaminated. Some examples include the following:

- Paper
- Plastic
- Disposable tray wrappers
- Packaging material

Liquids should be discarded in a sink or other washbasin, not in the plastic bag inside the regular waste container. This will keep you from having to clean up leaks and mess from the waste container.

When the plastic bag in the container is about two-thirds full, it should be removed from the waste can. Bring the top edges of the bag together and tie them, or use a twist tie. Follow your office policy and procedure for where to dispose of regular waste. Remember to put a fresh bag in the waste container.

Sharps Waste Container

The sharps waste container is used only for sharp objects that may puncture or injure someone. These include needles, microscope slides, used ampoules, scalpel blades, and razors. *Never* put any sharps in plastic bags. For safety reasons, they need to go in an approved, puncture-resistant container like the one shown in Figure 15-6.

Biohazard Waste Container

The biohazard waste container is used ONLY for waste contaminated with blood or body fluids. A red colored plastic bag is used to distinguish this container from a regular waste basket. The waste container shown in Figure 15-7 appears to be a typical waste can, but with a red colored plastic liner, it is designated as a biohazard waste container and not used for regular trash.

Some examples include the following:

- Soiled dressings and bandages
- Soiled examination gloves
- Soiled examination table paper
- Cotton balls and applicators that have been used on the body

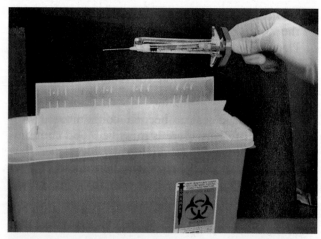

Figure 15-6 All sharps should be disposed of properly by placing them in a plastic puncture-resistant sharps container like the one shown here. Note the biohazard symbol on the sharps container. (Reprinted from Kronenberger J, Ledbetter J. *Jones & Bartlett Learning's Comprehensive Medical Assisting.* 5th ed. Burlington, MA: Jones & Bartlett Learning, LLC; 2016.)

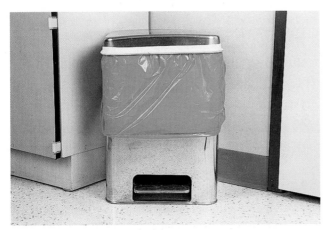

Figure 15-7 Biohazard waste disposal container with red plastic bag liner. Nonsharp items, visibly soiled with blood or body fluids, are discarded in this container. (Reprinted from Kronenberger J, Ledbetter J. *Jones & Bartlett Learning's Comprehensive Medical Assisting.* 5th ed. Burlington, MA: Jones & Bartlett Learning, LLC; 2016.)

Your Medical Office and Biohazard Waste

The Environmental Protection Agency (**EPA**) and OSHA set regulations and guidelines for disposing of hazardous materials. Individual states use these guidelines to determine their own policies.

Policies for disposing of infectious waste may be different in different states. You need to check your state and local regulations before making decisions about biohazardous waste.

Many medical offices, small waste generators, produce <50 pounds of waste each month. Hospitals and larger clinics that produce more than 50 pounds of waste each month are considered large generators. They must obtain a certificate of registration from the EPA. They also need to keep records of the quantity of waste and their disposal procedures.

Many facilities use a company that specializes in biohazard waste services. This ensures that they comply with state and federal laws and that biohazardous waste will be disposed of appropriately and safely.

Biohazard waste disposal services supply offices with appropriate waste containers. They pick up filled containers regularly. After they pick up filled containers, they dispose of waste according to EPA and OSHA guidelines.

The service keeps a tracking record. The record lists the type of waste, its weight in pounds, and its disposal destination. After the waste has been destroyed, the tracking record is sent to the medical office.

The tracking record must be kept in on file in the office for 3 years. It must be given to the EPA if an audit is performed to check whether the medical office is following regulations. States may have stiff penalties for violating disposal regulations, including fines and/or imprisonment.

Biohazard waste services determine their fees based on the type and amount of waste that is generated. Because of this, it is important to dispose of only biohazardous waste in these containers. You do not want your office to be charged for the removal of everyday trash.

CONCERNS ABOUT HEPATITIS B AND HIV

As a medical assistant, you may worry about transmission of the hepatitis B virus (**HBV**) and the human immunodeficiency virus (**HIV**). You may already be familiar with public concerns about HIV. HBV also has been a hazard for health care professionals for many years.

There are good reasons to be concerned about HBV. It is more viable than HIV. HBV can survive in a dried state on counter surfaces and clinical equipment at room temperature for more than a week. That means there is a chance it can be spread through the medical office by direct contact, such as through contaminated hands or gloves. HBV can be contained by proper use of standard precautions. It can be killed easily by cleaning with a diluted bleach solution.

Preventing Exposure

HIV and HBV are both transmitted through exposure to blood and body fluids. If you have direct contact with surfaces that are contaminated, there is a possibility the virus can enter your body.

The virus can enter the body through accidental punctures with sharp objects contaminated with blood, such as used needles. It also might be able to enter through broken skin. Broken skin can result from a cut or wound. Several skin disorders also involve breaks in the skin:

1. Dry, cracked skin
2. Dermatitis
3. Eczema
4. Psoriasis

If you have one of these skin disorders, you need to be sure you wear PPE, especially if you think you might come into contact with blood or body fluids.

There is no vaccine to prevent infection by HIV, but you can protect yourself from HBV with the HBV vaccine. The HBV vaccine is given in a series of three injections. These injections normally produce immunity to the disease.

To test for immunity, it is recommended that you have a blood sample taken and tested 6 months after the last injection. The blood test checks for the presence, or titer, of antibodies against hepatitis B. If the test finds that you are not immune, the vaccine series can be repeated. Immunity to HBV can last as long as 15 years; however, this is a topic that is still being researched and debated in the medical world.

Your Right to Protection

If your duties at work place you at risk for exposure to HBV, OSHA recommends that you be vaccinated to prevent infection. Your employer is required by law to offer to you and provide the vaccine at no cost.

If you choose not to receive the HBV vaccine, you must sign a waiver or release form declining the vaccination series. This form states that you are aware of the risks related to HBV. Individuals who contract hepatitis B may develop cirrhosis (damaged liver cells). They also may have a greater risk of developing liver cancer.

If You Have Been Exposed

If you have been exposed to blood or body fluids infected with HIV or HBV, the postexposure plan provides guidelines for what to do. The plan should include immediate blood testing. Your blood needs to be tested again at specific intervals, usually 6 weeks, 3 months, 6 months, 9 months, and 1 year.

If you have already been immunized against HBV, further treatment is not normally needed. But if you have not been immunized against HBV, you can receive hepatitis B immunoglobulin by injection to begin protecting your body right away. The series of immunizations for the HBV vaccine can be started to offer longer-term protection.

Patient Education:

Stopping the Spread of Disease at Home

As you work with patients, take time to teach them basic aseptic practices they can use at home.

1. *Hand washing.* Remind patients that they can stop the spread of disease by washing their hands. Patients should wash their hands before and after meals; after sneezing, coughing, or blowing the nose; after using the bathroom; before and after changing a dressing; and after changing diapers.
2. *Using tissues.* Encourage patients with respiratory symptoms (coughing and sneezing) to use tissues to cover their mouths and noses so they do not spread their illness through the air. Remind them to throw out used tissues right away and then wash their hands. Tissues are thin and it is easy for body fluids to soak through to a person's hands.
3. *Changing bandages.* Explain procedures to patients and family members who will need to change bandages. Take care to demonstrate how to apply sterile dressings and clean bandages. To check their understanding, ask the patients or family members to repeat what you showed them.
4. *Staying sanitary.* Talk to patients about how to dispose of waste from household members who have infectious diseases.
5. *Sharing glasses.* Explain to patients that each family member needs to use their own drinking glasses and eating utensils.

Procedure 15-1   Handwashing for Medical Asepsis

Equipment: Sink, paper towel, soap, and orangewood stick.

1. Take off your rings and your wristwatch. It is not a good idea to wear rings when working with material that could be infectious. Rings can provide a great environment for germs to hide.

2. Stand close to the sink, but avoid touching it. The sink is considered contaminated. If you stand too close, you might contaminate your clothing.

3. Using a paper towel, turn on the faucet. Adjust the temperature and then dispose of the paper towel.

Warm water is best. Water that is too hot or too cold can crack or chap the skin on your hands and break one of your natural body barriers against pathogens.

4. Wet your hands and wrists under warm running water. Use a clean towel to push the soap dispenser. Then, apply soap and lather up, rub your palms together, and rub the soap between your fingers at least 10 times. The rubbing action will loosen microorganisms between your fingers. You are removing transient flora and some resident flora, too.

Procedure 15-1 | Handwashing for Medical Asepsis (*continued*)

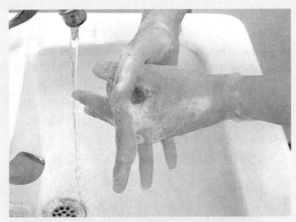

(Reprinted from Kronenberger J, Ledbetter J. *Jones & Bartlett Learning's Comprehensive Medical Assisting.* 5th ed. Burlington, MA: Jones & Bartlett Learning, LLC; 2016.)

5. Scrub the palm of one hand with the fingertips of the other using a circular motion. Then, switch hands to scrub the other palm. Friction helps remove microorganisms. You will also need to scrub your wrists.

6. Rinse hands and wrists well under running warm water. Hold your hands below your elbows and wrists—that way microbes can flow from your hands and fingers, rather than back up your arms. Take care not to touch the inside of the sink—remember, it is considered contaminated.

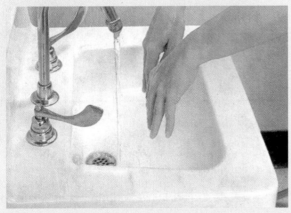

(Reprinted from Kronenberger J, Ledbetter J. *Jones & Bartlett Learning's Comprehensive Medical Assisting.* 5th ed. Burlington, MA: Jones & Bartlett Learning, LLC; 2016.)

7. Next clean your nails. Microbes can hide under your nails, too. Use an orangewood stick or nail brush to clean under each nail. Metal files or pointed tools might break the skin, creating an opening for microbes. You can clean your nails at the beginning of the day, before leaving for the day, or after touching potentially infectious material.

8. Use a clean paper towel to push the soap dispenser again. Use more liquid soap and warm, running water to wash your hands and wrists again. You need to wash away any microbes that might have been removed with the orangewood stick.

9. Rinse your hands thoroughly again. Be sure to hold your hands lower than your elbows.

10. Dry your hands gently with a paper towel. They need to be completely dry to prevent your skin from drying and cracking. Discard the paper towel and used orangewood stick when you are finished.

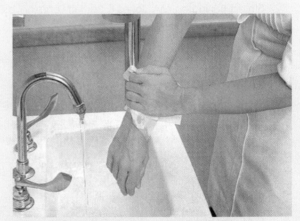

(Reprinted from Kronenberger J, Ledbetter J. *Jones & Bartlett Learning's Comprehensive Medical Assisting.* 5th ed. Burlington, MA: Jones & Bartlett Learning, LLC; 2016.)

11. Use a dry paper towel to turn off the faucets. Your clean hands should not touch the faucet handles—they are also considered contaminated. Discard the paper towel.

Procedure 15-2   Removing Contaminated Gloves

Equipment: Nonsterile gloves and biohazard waste bin.

1. To remove gloves, grasp the glove of your nondominant hand at the palm. (If you are right handed, grasp the glove on your left hand.) Avoid grasping the glove at the wrist—you might transfer contaminants from your glove to your wrist. Make sure hands are pointed down and away from the body, preferably directly over the biohazard container.

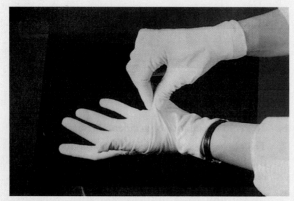

(Reprinted from Kronenberger J, Ledbetter J. *Jones & Bartlett Learning's Comprehensive Medical Assisting.* 5th ed. Burlington, MA: Jones & Bartlett Learning, LLC; 2016.)

2. Tug the glove toward the fingertips of your nondominant hand.

3. Slide your nondominant hand out of the glove by rolling the glove against the palm of your dominant hand. You must be careful not to touch either glove with your bare hand.

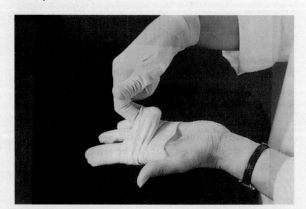

(Reprinted from Kronenberger J, Ledbetter J. *Jones & Bartlett Learning's Comprehensive Medical Assisting.* 5th ed. Burlington, MA: Jones & Bartlett Learning, LLC; 2016.)

4. Keep holding the soiled glove in the palm of your dominant hand. Slip your bare fingers under the cuff of the glove you are still wearing. Be careful not to touch the outside of the glove. Skin can touch skin, but never the soiled part of the glove.

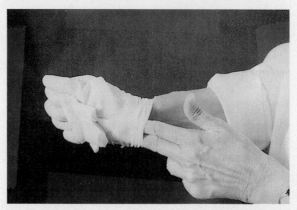

(Reprinted from Kronenberger J, Ledbetter J. *Jones & Bartlett Learning's Comprehensive Medical Assisting.* 5th ed. Burlington, MA: Jones & Bartlett Learning, LLC; 2016.)

5. Stretch the glove of the dominant hand up and away from your hand. At the same time, turn the glove inside out. The glove you removed first should be balled up inside. All the soiled surfaces of the gloves should be inside. The first glove should be inside the second glove, and the second glove should be inside out.

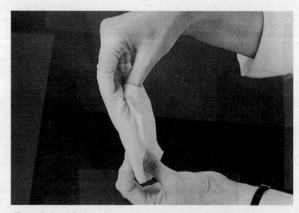

(Reprinted from Kronenberger J, Ledbetter J. *Jones & Bartlett Learning's Comprehensive Medical Assisting.* 5th ed. Burlington, MA: Jones & Bartlett Learning, LLC; 2016.)

6. Discard the gloves as they are (without taking them apart) in a biohazard waste bin or bag.

7. Wash your hands. Wearing gloves does not replace the need for good hand washing.

Procedure 15-3   Cleaning Examination Tables

Equipment: Clean gloves, biohazard waste bag, and germicide.

1. Put on clean gloves. If there is a possibility of contact with used dressings, body fluids, or other contaminated items on the table, further protect yourself with a gown or apron, protective eyewear, and shoe coverings.

2. Even though you are wearing gloves, try to handle the soiled table paper or linen as little as possible. Fold it carefully so the most soiled surface is turned inward. This will help stop contaminants from getting into the air or touching your clothes.

3. Dispose of soiled table paper in a biohazard waste bag. If your office uses cloth linens, place them in a biohazard laundry bag in the examination room. Do not carry unbagged dirty linen through the office for laundering.

4. Spray the table with a commercial germicide or diluted bleach solution. Then, wipe with disposable paper towels. Discard the towels in the biohazard waste bag. Remove gloves and wash hands.

5. Apply new examination table paper or linens.

6. Dirty linens may be sent to an outside company for laundering. If they are laundered at the office, use normal laundry cycles and follow office policy and procedure. Follow the manufacturers' recommendations for the washer, detergent, and fabric.

Procedure 15-4   Cleaning Biohazardous Spills

Equipment: Disposable gloves, gown or apron, protective eye wear, shoe covers, germicide.

1. Put on your gloves first. If you think there will be any splashing, protect yourself. A gown or an apron will protect your clothing from contaminants. Wear protective eyewear and shoe coverings.

2. Follow your office policy for cleaning up spills. Use chemical gels, crystals, or powders to absorb the spill. Clean up the spill with disposable paper towels or a scoop. Be careful not to splash.

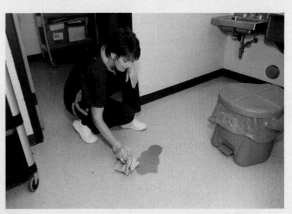

(Reprinted from Kronenberger J, Ledbetter J. *Jones & Bartlett Learning's Comprehensive Medical Assisting.* 5th ed. Burlington, MA: Jones & Bartlett Learning, LLC; 2016.)

Procedure 15-4 Cleaning Biohazardous Spills (*continued*)

3. Dispose of paper towels and absorbent material in a biohazard waste bag. The bag will alert anyone handling the waste that it contains biohazardous material.

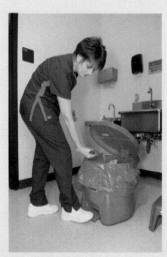

(Reprinted from Kronenberger J, Ledbetter J. *Jones & Bartlett Learning's Comprehensive Medical Assisting.* 5th ed. Burlington, MA: Jones & Bartlett Learning, LLC; 2016.)

4. Spray the area with a commercial germicide or diluted bleach solution. Then, wipe with disposable paper towels. Be sure to discard towels in the biohazard waste bag.

5. Keeping your gloves ON, remove any protective eyewear being careful not to touch your face. Discard the eyewear or disinfect it, depending on the policy in your office. Take off the gown or apron and shoe coverings. If they are disposable, put them in the biohazard waste bag. If they are reusable, put them in the biohazard laundry bag.

6. Place the biohazard waste bag in the biohazard waste bin for your office.

7. Take off your gloves and wash your hands thoroughly.

Procedure 15-5 Guidelines for Waste Disposal

Equipment: Sharps container, biohazard waste container, and gloves.

1. Use separate containers for each type of waste. Sharps containers are only for sharps. Paper towels used for routine hand washing do not go in a biohazard waste bag.

2. Use only approved biohazard waste containers.

3. Fill sharps containers two-thirds full before disposing of them. Look for a fill line on the container to show you how much goes in.

4. If you need to move a filled biohazard waste container, make sure the bag is secure. A closure should be provided with the container.

5. Take extra care when the biohazard waste container is contaminated on the outside and wear gloves. Put the container inside another approved biohazard waste container. And be sure to wash your hands thoroughly afterward.

6. Place biohazard waste for pick up by the service in a secure, designated area.

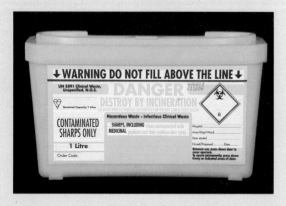

Preparing for Externship

your medical assistant program. This is especially true during your externship. You will be exposed to many patients who are ill with infections that are easily transmitted, such as colds and the flu. You need to be able to resist the bacteria and viruses that you may come in contact with. You need to get plenty of rest, eat good nutritious meals and perform frequent hand hygiene. Don't forget to wash your hands before and after working with each patient. You may want to use a hand sanitizer gel when you cannot get to the sink to wash with soap and water. Remember that friction, by rubbing your hands together, is the key to getting your hands scrubbed well.

Chapter Recap

- Medical assistants use specific procedures and practices to prevent the spread of microorganisms that carry disease.
- The human body has natural barriers to protect itself. These barriers can be overpowered by virulent pathogens, especially in a susceptible host.
- By understanding what microorganisms need to survive and how they are transmitted, the medical assistant can break the chain of infection.
- The medical assistant follows guidelines from OSHA and the CDC. These standard precautions will control and prevent infections in the medical office.
- Medical asepsis keeps office areas free of microorganisms. The medical assistant also teaches patients basic aseptic practices to prevent the spread of microorganisms in their homes. Hand washing is critical.
- Different objects and equipment require different levels of infection control. The highest level of infection control is sterilization. It destroys all microorganisms and spores.
- It is important for the medical assistant to know when and how to use different disinfection methods. There are three different levels of disinfection.
- Specific policies and regulations protect medical assistants from biohazardous materials and infectious disease. Written policies in the medical office outline the exposure risk factor for each employee. They also provide an exposure control plan.
- Medical assistants protect themselves and their patients by following strict procedures for cleaning biohazardous waste. Improper disposal of biohazardous waste can lead to fines or imprisonment.
- Many medical assistants worry about exposure to HIV and HBV. Knowing how these viruses are transmitted helps reduce the risks. Medical assistants have a legal right to a vaccine for HBV at no cost. Exposure to HIV or HBV requires follow-up testing.

Online Resources for Students

Student Resources available on the text's online site include:
- Audio Glossaries
- Animations
- Competency Evaluation Forms
- Videos
- Anatomy & Physiology Module with Heart and Lung Sounds
- Weblinks
- Worksheets

Exercises and Activities

Certification Preparation Questions

1. Which of the following represents an example of indirect transmission of disease?

   a. Shaking hands with an infected person
   b. Kissing a person who is infected
   c. Inhaling droplets from a reservoir host
   d. Touching a contaminated doorknob
   e. Touching blood from a reservoir host

2. Which stage of infectious disease will a person only have a general feeling of illness or fatigue?

   a. Incubation
   b. Prodromal
   c. Acute
   d. Declining
   e. Convalescent

3. When a person becomes infected with chicken pox and develops immunity, it is an example of:

   a. active acquired natural immunity.
   b. active acquired artificial immunity.
   c. natural artificial acquired immunity.
   d. passive acquired natural immunity.
   e. passive acquired artificial immunity.

4. Which of the following is NOT a main sign of inflammation?

   a. Redness
   b. Swelling
   c. Heat
   d. Pain
   e. Fatigue

5. The difference between an aerobe and anaerobe is that:

   a. an aerobe is pathogenic and an anaerobe is not.
   b. an anaerobe is pathogenic and an aerobe is not.
   c. aerobes are found where there is an absence of oxygen.
   d. anaerobes do not require oxygen to survive.
   e. aerobes cause disease and anaerobes do not.

6. Which of the following would be appropriate to discard in a biohazard waste container (red bag)?

   a. Disposable lancets
   b. Microscope slides
   c. Safety lock needle
   d. Soiled exam table paper
   e. Filter needle

7. Which of the following represents a microorganism that is a type of plant?

   a. Bacteria
   b. Virus
   c. Fungus
   d. Parasite
   e. Protozoa

8. Where can a medical assistant locate information regarding the safe use of chemical products in the medical office?

   a. EPA
   b. SDS
   c. OPIM
   d. CDC
   e. OSHA

9. Which of the following is a true statement regarding the HBV vaccine?

   a. HBV is a vaccine used to protect against chicken pox.
   b. All employees are required to receive the HBV vaccine in order to avoid being terminated from employment.
   c. An employee may sign a waiver to not receive the HBV vaccine.
   d. HBV is a vaccine intended to protect against all viral diseases.
   e. HBV vaccine is given in two doses and will protect an individual for 1 year.

10. An example of a disease caused by a protozoa is:

    a. malaria.
    b. chicken pox.
    c. strep throat.
    d. mononucleosis.
    e. hepatitis.

 Internet Activities

1. Access the Web site for OSHA, Occupational Safety and Health Administration. Locate the fact sheet for blood-borne pathogens standard. Review the specific requirements of the standard as they apply to employers at health care facilities.

2. Access the Web site for the World Health Organization and research statistical data regarding hepatitis B including number infected and deaths attributed to this disease.

Reference

Source: World Health Organization; http://www.who.int/about/en/

16 | Medical History and Patient Assessment

Chapter Objectives

- List the typical information included on a medical history form.
- Explain the use of different techniques used to collect information during a patient interview.
- Explain how to use open-ended and closed-ended questions during a patient interview to obtain information.
- Perform patient screening via telephone and face to face.
- Explain the difference between patient signs and symptoms.
- Explain the difference between a chief complaint and present illness.
- Summarize how to measure and record a patient's height and weight.

- Explain the differences in taking a patient's temperature using the oral, rectal, axillary, and tympanic methods.
- Explain how the body controls temperature and the factors that influence it.
- Describe how to assess and record a patient's respiration.
- Identify body sites used for palpating a pulse.
- Explain how to choose the correct blood pressure cuff size.
- Describe the five phases of Korotkoff sounds.
- Identify the factors that may affect blood pressure.
- Accurately obtain and record vital signs including blood pressure, pulse, temperature, respiration, and pulse oximetry.

CAAHEP & ABHES Competencies

CAAHEP

- Obtain vital signs.
- Apply critical thinking skills in performing patient assessment and care.
- Use language/verbal skills that enable patients' understanding.
- Demonstrate respect for diversity in approaching patients and families.
- Differentiate between subjective and objective information.

ABHES

- Gather and process documents.
- Obtain vital signs, obtain patient history, and formulate chief complaint.

Chapter Terms

Afebrile
Anthropometric
Assessment
Diagnosis

Familial disorder
Febrile
Hereditary disorders
Homeopathic

Hyperpyrexia
Metabolism
Paraphrasing
Pyrexia

Reflecting
Signs
Sphygmomanometer
Symptoms

Abbreviations

BP
CC
FH

Ht
P
PH

PI
R
ROS

T
Wt

Case Study

Robert Foster is a new patient recently seen by Dr. Kauffman in the emergency room for abdominal pain and now has arrived at the physician's office for a follow-up appointment. MaryAnn Hastings, Dr. Kauffman's medical assistant, provided a new patient history form for Mr. Foster to complete. He tries to complete the form but does not understand some of the terms used on the form. He is embarrassed to ask the medical assistant for help so he leaves those areas blank. When he gives the form to MaryAnn, she notices that he has not completed all the required fields on the form.

It is imperative that a physician knows a patient's past and current health information in order to diagnose and treat the patient's present illness. The physician will try to establish a **diagnosis**, the process of identifying a disease or illness. As a medical assistant, you play a large role in collecting the information the physician needs for a medical history and assessment.

The patient's medical history is information about the patient's past and present health status. It also includes information about the health of family members and information about the patient's social habits, such as smoking and alcohol use. The patient's family should include only those members who are biologically related to the patient.

Assessment is the process of gathering information in order to determine the patient's problem. It begins with asking standard questions and recording the patient's answers. The methods used will be outlined in the office policy and procedure manual.

 THE MEDICAL HISTORY

It is the medical assistant's responsibility to work initially with the patient to gather the medical history information. An example of a typical history form, front and back, is shown in Figure 16-1.

The following are the methods used by most offices to collect and record the patient's medical history.

- The patient completes a form upon arrival for their first visit, before seeing the physician.
- The patient returns a form that was mailed to them prior to their first appointment.
- The patient completes an electronic form online prior to their first visit.
- The medical assistant interviews the patient using a medical history form with a list of questions.
- The physician completes the medical history form during the patient's examination.

It is important for the medical assistant to know and understand all aspects of the medical history forms used in the medical practice. When the patient has completed their portion of the medical history form, the medical assistant should review the form to make sure the patient did not leave any areas blank and that the information provided by the patient is understandable.

Medical History Information

Medical history forms may be differently formatted, but the information required is typically the same for all of them. There may be additional questions asked

Professional Medical Associates – History Form

NAME: _____ DATE OF BIRTH: _____

What is the main reason for your visit to the doctor? _____

_____

Were you referred? _____ if so, by whom? _____

PAST MEDICAL HISTORY:

Are you allergic to any medication? _____

If so, list medications: _____

List current medications, dosage, and how many times a day you take them:

Medication	Dose	Times a Day

Alcohol Consumption: What type? _____ Amount _____ How Often? _____

History of Alcoholism? _____

When was your last TB or Tine test? _____

Have you ever had a positive test for tuberculosis? _____

When was your last Tetanus shot? _____

List all surgeries you have had in the past:

Date	Type of Surgery

List all past hospitalizations (not involving surgeries above):

Date	Reason for Hospital Stay

List all past problems with trauma (broken bones, lacerations, etc.):

_____

REVIEW OF SYSTEMS, PAST MEDICAL PROBLEMS:
If you have been told you have any of the problems listed below, or are having any of the problems listed below, please CIRCLE:

1. <u>GENERAL:</u> Weight loss, weight gain, fever, chills, night sweats, hot flashes, tire easily, problems with sleep, crying spells, history of cancer.

2. <u>SKIN:</u> Rash, sores that won't heal, moles that are new or changing, history of skin problems.

3. <u>HEENT:</u> Headache, eye problems, hearing problems, sinus problems, hay fever, dizziness, hoarseness, sores in your mouth that won't heal, dental problems.

   Do you chew tobacco or dip snuff? _____

4. <u>METABOLIC/ENDOCRINE:</u> Thyroid problems, diabetes or sugar problems, high cholesterol.

Figure 16-1   A sample medical history form, front and back. (Reprinted from Kronenberger J, Ledbetter J. *Jones & Bartlett Learning's Comprehensive Medical Assisting.* 5th ed. Burlington, MA: Jones & Bartlett Learning, LLC; 2016.)

5. <u>RESPIRATORY:</u> Cough, wheezing, breathing problems, history of asthma, history of lung problems.

   Do you smoke cigarettes or pipe? _____

   How much? _____ For how long? _____

6. <u>BREAST (WOMEN):</u> Breast lumps, changes in nipples, nipple discharge, breast problems, family history of breast cancer. When was your last mammogram? _____

7. <u>CARDIOVASCULAR:</u> Heart murmur, rheumatic fever, high blood pressure, angina, heart problems, heart attack, abnormal heart rhythm, chest pain, palpitations, leg swelling, history of phlebitis or blood clots.

8. <u>GI:</u> Problems with appetite, swallowing, heartburn, nausea, vomiting, pain in the abdomen, constipation, diarrhea, blood in stool, history of ulcers, liver problems, hepatitis, jaundice, pancreas problems, gallbladder problems, or colon problems.

9. <u>REPRODUCTIVE (WOMEN):</u> Problems with irregular menstrual cycles, abnormal vaginal bleeding or discharge, history of sexually transmitted diseases, sexual problems.

   AGE OF FIRST MENSES (PERIOD) _____ AGE OF MENOPAUSE _____

   LAST PAP SMEAR _____ METHOD OF CONTRACEPTION _____

   Obstetric History (Women)

   NUMBER OF PREGNANCIES _____ PLEASE LIST AS FOLLOWS:

   Delivery Date   Pregnancy Complications   Type Delivery   Baby's Weight

   _____

   _____

   <u>MEN:</u> Problems with genital discharge, history of venereal diseases, sexual problems, prostate problems.

   METHOD OF CONTRACEPTION _____

10. <u>UROLOGIC:</u> Problems with painful urination, urinary frequency, blood in urine, weak urinary stream, history of bladder or kidney infections, or kidney stones.

11. <u>MUSCULOSKELETAL:</u> Arthritis, back pain, cramps in legs.

12. <u>NEUROLOGIC:</u> Seizures, stroke, arm or leg weakness or numbness, black-out spells, memory or thinking problems, depression, anxiety, psychiatric problems.

13. <u>HEMATOLOGIC:</u> Anemia, bleeding problems, enlarged lymph nodes.

HAVE YOU EVER HAD A BLOOD TRANSFUSION? _____ DATE _____

FAMILY HISTORY:

List any medical problems that run in your family and which family members have these problems.

_____

_____

SOCIAL HISTORY:

MARITAL STATUS: _____

OCCUPATION: _____

EDUCATION: _____

HOBBIES: _____

WHAT DO YOU DO FOR ENJOYMENT? _____

Figure 16-1 (*continued*)

on medical history forms used in specialty practices. Common information included on standard medical history forms includes the following:

- Demographic data
- Past history (**PH**)
- Review of systems (**ROS**)
- Family history (**FH**)
- Social history

Demographic Data

Demographic data are the patient's identifying information. Most of this information is required for the practice's business operations. In addition to the patient's name, mailing address, and phone number, it also includes the following:

- The patient's emergency contact information
- The patient's gender, marital status, and race
- The patient's Social Security number
- The name, address, and phone number of the patient's employer
- The name, address, and phone number of the patient's insurance carrier
- The patient's health insurance policy number

Past History

The past history (PH) refers to any information about the patient's past health status. This helps the physician plan the patient's current care. The past history includes information about the patient's:

- Allergies
- Immunizations
- Childhood diseases
- Current and past prescribed medications
- Over-the-counter medications and herbal supplements
- Prior illnesses
- Prior surgeries
- Prior hospitalizations
- Prior accidents

Case Question

 When MaryAnn, the medical assistant, asks Mr. Foster about the blank areas of the medical form, Mr. Foster says he doesn't understand some of the medical terms used on the form and is unsure how he should answer. How can MaryAnn help him feel more comfortable and assist him in providing the necessary information to complete the form?

Review of Systems

The review of systems (ROS) section contains questions about overall health and specific symptoms or diseases of each body system. Information may be revealed that a patient may have forgotten to note in the PH section or thought was unimportant. The questions are usually in a sequence from head to toe.

Family History

This section of the medical history form asks for information about the health of the patient's biological relatives. Some diseases or disorders have familial or hereditary links. A **familial disorder** is a problem that is unusually common within a family. **Hereditary disorders** are passed from parents to their offspring. In the family history (FH) section, health information is gathered about the patient's parents, brothers, sisters, and grandparents. If any immediate family member is deceased, the cause of death should be noted in the patient's medical history.

Social History

The social history section covers the patient's lifestyle. It includes information about marital status, occupation, education, and hobbies. It may also include information about:

- Diet
- Tobacco use
- Alcohol use
- Sexual history
- Sleeping habits
- Exercise

The social history information helps the physician understand how the patient's illness and any treatment may affect the patient's lifestyle. It also helps the physician see how the patient's lifestyle and illness may be related.

This information also can be a guide to the need for patient education. The physician may want to address some patient behaviors in order to avoid future medical problems. For example, high tobacco use or a diet high in fat may lead to illness or disease.

Interviewing Patients

To complete the medical history, the medical assistant needs to interview the patient. Figure 16-2 shows a medical assistant with a patient she is interviewing. You can see the medical assistant is maintaining good eye contact with the patient.

The goal is to obtain accurate and relevant information. Throughout the interview process, the medical assistant is required to treat the information in a patient's medical history as confidential. The Health Insurance Portability and Accountability Act (HIPAA) is a federal law that protects the privacy of health information. To comply with HIPAA, patient records must be stored in a secure place. Electronic records need to be

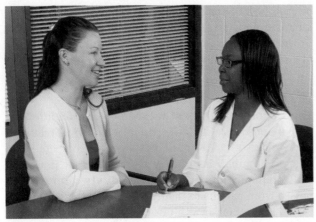

Figure 16-2 Conduct the patient interview in a private office or exam room. (Reprinted from Kronenberger J, Ledbetter J. *Jones & Bartlett Learning's Comprehensive Medical Assisting.* 4th ed. Burlington, MA: Jones & Bartlett Learning, LLC; 2013.)

protected with password protection and limited access by authorized individuals. The patient may give specific permission for persons involved in the patient's care to access the record.

Interview Communication

The medical assistant must collect accurate and useful information during the interview. A number of interviewing skills help with this process.

Reflecting

Reflecting is repeating back what the patient said, using open-ended statements. For example, you might say, "So, you were saying your heartburn is bad when…"

Paraphrasing

Paraphrasing means rephrasing what the patient said in your own words. For example, you might say, "It sounds as if you're saying you have had heartburn and sour stomach for the past week."

Asking for Examples

Asking the patient for an example allows you to clarify what the patient told you. For example, you might say, "Can you describe exactly the pain from the heartburn?"

Asking Questions

Asking questions can help you get more information or details about what the patient has said. For example, you might ask, "Does the heartburn seem to happen after eating certain meals or at a particular time of day?"

Summarizing

Summarizing, or recapping, the main points of what the patient said helps to make sure you understood the patient. For example, you might say, "Let me see if I have

understood you correctly…" and then give a summary of what the patient told you.

Allowing Silence

Allowing silence, or a pause, can be helpful during a conversation. It gives the patient a chance to think about what to say next.

Active Listening

Throughout the interview process, the medical assistant will utilize active listening skills to show that you are interested in what the patient is saying. Active listening can be shown through words (verbal) or body language (nonverbal).

Verbal. Show you are listening by occasionally using encouraging words or sounds such as "yes," "mm-hmm," or "ah."

Nonverbal. Your body language shows you are listening when you nod your head, smile, or make frequent eye contact with the patient.

Case Question

Mr. Foster was seen in the emergency room for abdominal pain a few days ago and is now being seen for the first time in the physician's office as a follow-up. In order to obtain the most complete information about his condition, what questions should the medical assistant ask him?

Before the Interview

In order for the patient to feel comfortable and relaxed during the interview, there are steps to take prior to meeting. Here are two items that need to be planned prior to the interview:

- *Be prepared.* Make sure you're familiar with the medical history form and any previous medical history provided by the patient. New patients will have filled out a new patient questionnaire. For an established patient, review and update the chart with any new information.
- *Find the right location.* To keep patient information confidential, a private area is necessary to conduct the interview. Avoid public areas such as the reception area where others might hear the patient's answers. A good location might be a private office or examination room. Besides ensuring privacy, you will be avoiding distractions and interruptions. Interview the patient alone unless he wishes family members to be present.

Begin the Interview

At the beginning of the interview, put the patient at ease. Begin every patient interview by identifying your name and title. Make sure to mention your credentials when talking to patients so they don't get the false impression that you are a nurse or physician. Explain the purpose of the interview and how long it will take. Also tell the patient that all information will be kept confidential.

For example, you might say something like this: "Good morning, Mr. Foster. My name is MaryAnn, and I am Dr. Kauffman's medical assistant. I would like to ask you a few questions that will take about 15 minutes and help the doctor diagnose and treat you. Please be assured that all your responses will be kept in strict confidence."

First Impressions

You may be the first person in the medical office the patient sees or talks with. The impression you make is critical to the patient's overall opinion of the medical practice. The words and manners you use should communicate respect as well as concern for the patient. This professional but caring attitude will help you gain the patient's confidence. Some patients may not share information until that feeling of trust has been established.

Communication Barriers

Sometimes, patients may have difficulty expressing themselves. You also may have a hard time understanding a patient. As you speak to patients, assess whether there are any barriers to communication—things that will get in the way of each of you understanding the other. Here are some common communication barriers.

- The patient has difficulty speaking, reading, or understanding English.
- The patient has impaired vision or hearing.
- The patient has a mental or psychological limitation.

There are several ways to help patients understand what you are saying. You can help keep communication flowing by:

- Avoiding highly technical or medical terminology
- Paying attention to the patient's nonverbal behavior
- Adjusting your questions to suit the situation
- Maintaining good eye contact
- Having a family member or caregiver accompany the patient

Assessing the Patient

During the patient interview, listen carefully as the patient describes his medical problems. Pay attention to the signs and symptoms, as well as the patient's behavior.

- **Signs** are objective information. That means they can be observed or seen by someone other than the patient. Some examples of signs are rash, bleeding, or coughing. Other signs may be found during the physician's examination.
- **Symptoms** are subjective information. They reflect changes in the body sensed by the patient. Symptoms are not usually evident to anyone other than the patient. Examples include patient complaints such as headache, leg pain, nausea, or dizziness.
- Acknowledge the patient's feelings using techniques such as reflecting or paraphrasing. Saying something like, "I understand that makes you feel worried," will reassure the patient that you're attentive to his concerns.
- Respond with facts, rather than reacting with emotions. You may feel impatient with a patient's questions or behavior, but the patient needs you to be both professional and calm.

Sometimes, signs may indicate patient symptoms. A facial expression, such as wincing, may be a sign that a patient is in pain. If the patient is holding onto furniture or walls while walking, it could be a sign that the patient is feeling dizzy.

Making Observations

A good interview involves observation. This means noticing things about the patient's appearance or behavior. When you write your observations in the patient's medical record, make sure you include only what you saw and heard. You should not record any judgments, opinions, or conclusions you might have made about what you observed. For example, you would not write that someone must have hit the patient because there were signs of bruising. Avoid making these assumptions. Some examples of observations you might make of physical and mental status information are as follows:

- Pale or flushed skin
- Visible bruises or injuries
- Lethargy or tiredness
- Crying
- Confusion

Chief Complaint and Present Illness

After recording the patient's medical history, you need to find out why the patient has come to see the physician. To do this, you must determine the patient's chief complaint (**CC**) and present illness (**PI**).

- The chief complaint is the reason the patient is visiting the doctor. It's one statement describing the signs and symptoms that led the patient to seek medical care—for example, "I've had a headache for the past 3 days." The chief complaint is recorded for every visit, even if it is for a checkup or annual exam.
- The present illness is a more specific account of the chief complaint. It includes an order of events, such as when the symptoms began, and any remedies the patient may have tried prior to the appointment.

Determining the Chief Complaint

Prior to the interview, review the patient's medical history form to become familiar with the patient and help you get complete information.

Asking open-ended questions usually will lead the patient to reveal a chief complaint. Open-ended questions are those that encourage the patient to respond with more than one or two words. Some examples are, "What's the reason for your visit today?" or "Can you describe what's been going on?" Make sure you maintain eye contact so the patient knows you're listening actively.

Closed-ended questions most often require only a yes or no answer. These types of questions will not provide many details about the patient's condition. For example, "Do you have pain?" doesn't provide much information. However, you can use closed-ended questions to get specific information about the present illness, such as, "When did the pain first start?"

You should document the chief complaint (CC) on the progress report form in the patient's record. Use the patient's own words in quotation marks whenever you can. Make sure the progress report includes the date, time of day, and your signature and credentials.

Detailing the Present Illness

Once you have recorded the patient's chief complaint, you need to get more details about the patient's present illness (PI). It is important to establish the chain of events associated with the illness.

For example, you must find out if the patient has tried any over-the-counter medications. These are medications that do not require a prescription. They include aspirin, decongestants, antihistamines, and many others. They also include vitamins, natural drugs such as herbs, and some homeopathic medications.

Homeopathic medications are tiny doses of substances that would, in normal doses, produce the symptoms of the disease being treated. For example, Allium cepa, which is made from onions, is a homeopathic remedy for a cold. It is used because onions make your nose run and eyes water when you cut them, just like a cold does. In order to get more information about the patient's present illness, these are some questions that you can ask:

- Chronology—How and when did this problem first begin?
- Location—Can you explain or show me where the pain or problem is?
- Severity—Can you describe the pain? Is the pain constant? When did the pain first begin? Are there times or movements that make the pain occur? Some medical offices have patients rate the severity of the pain on a scale of 1 to 10, with ten being the worst pain they can imagine.
- Self-treatment—What medications (both prescriptions and over the counter) and herbs have you taken? Have they helped?

- Quality—Does anything you do make the symptoms better? Worse?
- Duration—Have you had these symptoms before? If so, when and under what circumstances?

When you are trying to get accurate information, take care to keep your questions general. If you include details, patients may use your words instead of their own in their responses. Follow these tips for getting the information you need:

- Do not suggest answers by the way you ask questions. If you say, "Is the pain worse when you walk?" patients may say *yes* because they think that is what they're supposed to say.
- Do not coax patients by suggesting other symptoms. You may have an idea of what symptoms a patient is experiencing based on the chief complaint. But it is better to hear what the patient has to say than to make suggestions. Some patients will agree to the symptoms you describe, because they think they "should" be experiencing them.
- Use closed-ended questions to get specific information but avoid feeding the patient too much detail such as asking "Is the pain sharp?" Some patients might agree to everything you say. Ask these questions only after the patient has answered open-ended questions. For example, you might say, "How long have you had this pain?"

Cultural Connection

With the increase of new immigrants to the United States, it is important for the first time appointment with the physician to request that the patient bring all medications, herbal and supplemental products, and any other preparations they may have been prescribed or used when in their country of origin. The Federal Food and Drug Administration (FDA) may not recognize or have approved all preparations that other countries allow for use. In some countries, pharmacists still customize preparations for patients based on a written formula provided by the physician. Also, the FDA generally does not allow travelers to import medications that cannot be legally prescribed in the United States, and prescription drugs purchased outside the United States might not be allowed even if the medication could be prescribed in the United States. For example, travelers must have a prescription from a US doctor to bring back prescription medicine from another country, even if the drug is authorized in the United States and the traveler has a prescription from a physician in the foreign country. Thus, travelers wishing to purchase less expensive medicine while traveling in another country may require a prescription from a US doctor and, if required by the foreign country, a foreign doctor as well.

ANTHROPOMETRIC MEASUREMENTS

In addition to collecting information about the patient's medical history, you may need to take physical measurements. Medical assistants obtain **anthropometric** measurements or physical measurements of the patient's body. Typically, medical assistants measure the patient's height and weight. All measurements are recorded in the patient's medical record.

Measurements taken at the first visit are recorded as baseline data. Baseline data are used as a reference point to compare measurements at later visits. Usually, an adult's height is only recorded on the first visit and then once a year. The weight and vital signs are taken and recorded at each visit.

Weight (Wt)

The patient's weight is measured and recorded at each office visit. Weight can be measured in pounds or kilograms, depending on the practices in your medical office. It is especially important to monitor the weight for the following patients:

- Infants
- Children
- Elderly patients
- Pregnant patients

Other patients may need special monitoring if they are trying to lose or gain weight or if they are on medications that are calculated according to body weight.

Certain diseases also require special monitoring. Most medical offices have only one scale. It should be placed in a private location to keep patients from feeling uncomfortable when being weighed. Several types of scales, as shown in Figure 16-3, are used to measure weight:

- Balance beam scales
- Digital scales
- Dial scales

Balance Beam Scale

Here are the steps to follow when weighing a patient using a balance beam scale:

1. Wash your hands.
2. Make sure the scale is properly balanced at zero.
3. Ask the patient to remove their shoes and any heavy outerwear or purses that could distort the reading. Have a place for the patient to sit while removing shoes.
4. Place a paper towel on the scale before the patient steps on. Because the patient will be standing in bare feet or stockings, the paper towel will prevent the spread of microorganisms.
5. Make sure the patient is facing forward on the scale without touching or holding onto anything if possible.
6. Slide the counterweights on the bottom and top bars from zero to the approximate weight of the patient. Always begin with the heavier weight bar (bottom). Each counterweight should rest securely in a notch with an indicator mark.
7. Adjust the counterweights by small amounts until the balance bar hangs freely at the exact midpoint.

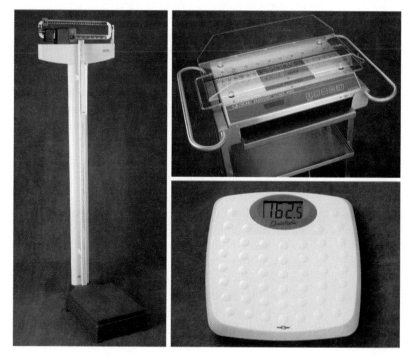

Figure 16-3 The three types of scales used in medical offices include the digital, dial, and balance beam scale. (Reprinted from Kronenberger J, Ledbetter J. *Jones & Bartlett Learning's Comprehensive Medical Assisting.* 5th ed. Burlington, MA: Jones & Bartlett Learning, LLC; 2016.)

8. To calculate the patient's weight, add the top reading to the bottom one. For example, if the heavier bottom counterweight reads 100 and the lighter upper one reads 16 plus 3 small lines, the patient's weight is 116.75 pounds.

9. Help the patient off the scale if necessary. You should stay close to the patient while he is on the scale. Anyone can lose his balance when getting on and off the scale, regardless of age.

10. Discard the paper towel. It also might be necessary to wipe the platform of the scale with a cleaning disinfectant.

11. Record the weight in the patient's medical record. Be sure to include the date, time, your signature, and your credentials. If you are measuring the patient's height at the same time, you can record them together.

Digital and Dial Scales

The same steps for using the balance scale are used with a digital or dial scale; however, there are some differences. A digital or dial scales do not have any counterweights to slide. When you weigh a patient on a digital scale, read and record the weight displayed on the digital screen. If you weigh a patient on a dial scale, an indicator arrow will rest at the patient's weight. Be sure to read the number from directly above the arrow. If you take the reading from an angle, you will not see the correct measurement.

Height (Ht)

Most balance beam scales have a moveable ruler at the back for measuring height. In some offices, a graph ruler is mounted on the wall. More accurate measures are obtained when a parallel bar is moved down to rest against the top of a patient's head. Height is measured in inches or centimeters, depending on the physician's preference.

Follow these steps to measure a patient's height using a scale with a ruler or on a wall mount device:

1. If this procedure is not performed at the same time as the weight measurement, wash your hands first. Have the patient sit down and remove his shoes. Place a paper towel on the scale before the patient steps on.

2. Be sure the patient is standing straight with heels together and eyes straight ahead. The patient's posture must be erect for an accurate measurement. The best measurement of height is made with the patient's back to the ruler on the scale, but it is also acceptable for the patient to face the ruler.

3. Hold the measuring bar perpendicular (at a right angle) to the ruler.

4. Lower the measuring bar until it firmly touches the patient's head. Press lightly if the patient's hair is full or high. You do not want to include full hair in the height measurement.

5. Read the measurement at the point where the bar slides out of the scale. If measurements are in inches, convert them to feet and inches. For example, if the bar reads 65, the patient is 5 foot and 5 inches (60 inches equals 5 feet). If the measuring bar falls between two full inches, the height is measured to the nearest ¼, ½, or ¾ of an inch based on the smaller lines between the inch markers.

6. When you are finished measuring the patient's height, assist the patient off the scale if necessary. Watch for signs that the patient is unsteady.

7. Have a place for the patient to sit to put on his shoes.

8. Record the patient's height in the medical record.

9. Discard the paper towel and wipe the platform of the scale with a cleaning disinfectant.

Physical Measurements of Children

An infant's length (height) and weight are measured at every routine visit. You may also need to measure an infant's chest and head circumference. These measurements help the physician monitor the infant's growth and development.

Procedures for measuring an infant's weight and length are somewhat different from those for older children and adults. Pediatric (infants and children) weights and heights are often recorded on a growth chart as well as in the patient's medical record. The growth chart provides a graph of the child's growth patterns and the percentile the child falls within. Charts are available based on the child's age and gender. Figure 16-4 shows a growth chart that would be used to record measurements for a female child from birth to 36 months.

Measuring Infant Length

To measure infant length, you need an examining table with clean table paper and a tape measure. Always wash your hands first. Explain the procedure to the parent. Ask the parent to remove the infant's clothing, except for the diaper. Follow these steps for measuring infant length:

1. Wash your hands.

2. Place the infant on a firm examination table covered with clean table paper. You need a firm surface for accurate measurements. If you are using a measuring board, it should be covered with clean paper.

3. Hold the infant's head at the midline. Fully extend the infant's body by grasping the knees and pressing them flat onto the table. Most infants stay in a flexed position, so you need to extend the legs to get an accurate measurement. Be gentle, but firm. If you need help, ask the parent or a coworker to help you. A footboard against the soles of the infant's feet will give the most accurate measurement.

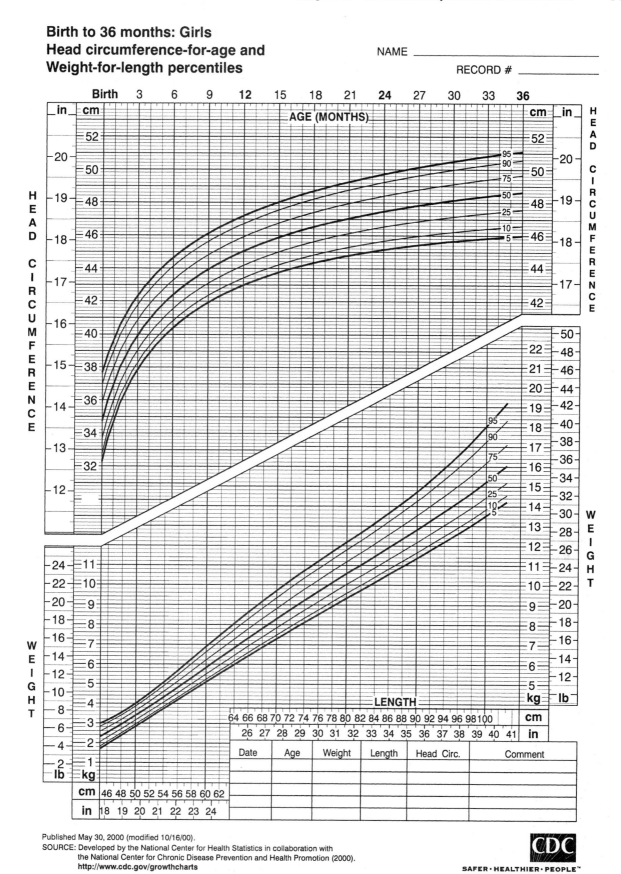

Birth to 36 months: Girls
Head circumference-for-age and
Weight-for-length percentiles

NAME _____

RECORD # _____

Published May 30, 2000 (modified 10/16/00).
SOURCE: Developed by the National Center for Health Statistics in collaboration with
the National Center for Chronic Disease Prevention and Health Promotion (2000).
http://www.cdc.gov/growthcharts

CDC
SAFER · HEALTHIER · PEOPLE™

Figure 16-4   Growth chart. Birth to 36 months, girls. (Reprinted from Kronenberger J, Ledbetter J.
Jones & Bartlett Learning's Comprehensive Medical Assisting. 5th ed. Burlington, MA: Jones & Bartlett
Learning, LLC; 2016.)

4. Mark the table paper with your pen at the top of the infant's head. Make a second mark on the paper at the infant's heel.
5. Using the measuring tape, measure between the marks on the paper.
6. Record the length in the infant's medical record and on the growth chart.
7. Clean the area and wash your hands.

Measuring Infant Weight

Infant weight is measured using a scale designed for infants. Follow these steps to obtain the infant's weight:

1. Wash your hands.
2. Place protective paper on the scale and balance the scale. The balance beam must be centered before each use.
3. Remove the infant's diaper just before placing the infant on the scale. For the most accurate weight, infants should be weighed without any clothing. Cool air against the infant's skin may cause voiding (urination) so be sure to cover the genital area of infant boys. In some offices, the infant is weighed in a diaper, as long as it is dry and clean. If so, you need to note that the infant wore a dry clean diaper.
4. Lay the infant on the scale. Keep one of your hands over or near the infant on the scale at all times. Larger infants who can sit may be weighed while sitting. Sitting can help to make the experience less frightening.
5. Quickly move the counterweights to balance the apparatus exactly.
6. Pick up the infant. Ask the parent to replace the infant's diaper if it was removed.
7. Record the weight in the infant's medical record and on the growth chart.
8. Clean the area and wash your hands.

Other Pediatric Measurements

You also may need to measure and record the head and chest circumference of an infant. Head circumference refers to the measurement around the largest part of the infant's head. Chest circumference is the measurement around the chest. You will use a flexible cloth or paper measuring tape. Follow these steps to obtain the head and chest circumference of an infant:

1. Wash your hands.
2. Lay the infant supine (lying on the back with face upward) on an examination table, or ask the parent to hold the infant.
3. Measure around the head above the eyebrow and posteriorly at the largest part of the occiput, the bone forming the back of the skull.
4. Record the infant's head circumference on the growth chart and in the infant's medical record.

5. Now measure around the chest (with clothing removed) at the nipple line. Be sure to keep the tape measure at the same level anterior and posterior (front and back). This ensures the most accurate reading.
6. Record the infant's chest circumference on the growth chart and in the infant's medical record.
7. When finished with both measurements, wash your hands and clean the equipment.

Study Skill

Most students use index (3 × 5″) cards to write information that they need to memorize; however, when you are trying to learn normal values such as vital signs, it might be better to design a memory box. This is a table or chart with information consolidated into columns and rows. The data can be sorted and easily accessed when needed. You can still use a 3 × 5″ card for this project. The memory box will help you visualize the relationships among data. You also get to decide what information is most important.

 ## VITAL SIGNS

In addition to anthropometric measurements, medical assistants may be required to measure patient vital signs, also known as cardinal signs. Vital signs are physical measurements of basic body functions that keep a person alive. See Table 16-1 for normal vital sign values by age.

- Temperature (**T**) is the internal heat produced by the body.
- Pulse rate (**P**) is the beating of the heart, felt in an artery and heard with a stethoscope.
- Respiratory rate (**R**) is the speed at which a patient breathes, heard with a stethoscope or observed.
- Blood pressure (**BP**) is the force of blood pressing on arteries as it circulates in the body.

Temperature

The body temperature reflects a balance between the heat produced by the body and the heat lost by the body. The body produces heat through:

- Body **metabolism**, the normal physical and chemical processes that occur inside the body
- Muscle movement, exercising
- Disease such as infection

The body loses heat through normal processes, such as:

- Respiration, or breathing
- Elimination of waste products
- Conduction, or transmission through the skin

Table 16-1	Normal Ranges for Vital Signs by Age

Age	Pulse (beats/min)	Respirations (breaths/min)	Blood Pressure— Systolic (mm Hg)	Blood Pressure— Diastolic (mm Hg)	Temperature (°F)
Newborn (0–4 wk)	120–160	40–60	>60		
Infant (1–12 mo)	100–120	25–30	70–95		97.5–100.4
Children (1–8 y)	80–100	15–30	80–110		97.0–99.7
Adolescents	60–100	12–20	118–132	70–82	97.8–99.1
Adults	60–100	12–20	80–130	60–90	
Elderly adults	55–70	12–20	80–130	70–90	96.4–99.5

The average body temperature is 98.6° Fahrenheit (F) or 37.0° Celsius (C). A patient with a normal temperature is **afebrile**, without fever. A patient with a temperature above 99.5° Fahrenheit is considered **febrile** or has a fever.

Measuring Body Temperature

Medical assistants need to be familiar with the different methods and sites for measuring body temperature.

- Oral—An oral thermometer is placed in the mouth under the tongue. This is the most commonly used method and thermometer.
- Rectal—A rectal thermometer is gently inserted in the rectum. This method is often used for infants.
- Axillary—To measure temperature, a thermometer is placed under the armpit.
- Tympanic—A tympanic thermometer is one that is inserted into the ear canal.
- Temporal scanner—The thermometer is placed lightly on the forehead, used for infants over 3 months.

Disposable thermometers are designed to be used once and then thrown away. These can be used in the mouth, under the arm, or on the forehead.

Temperature Comparisons by Method

	Fahrenheit	Celsius
Oral and tympanic	98.6	37.0
Rectal	99.6	37.6
Axillary	97.6	36.4

Temperature readings from different parts of the body are not equal. An average reading of 98.6°F is considered normal when obtained by mouth, but readings from other sites may be slightly different.

- Rectal temperatures are generally 1°F *higher* than oral temperatures. This is because of the blood supply and tightly closed environment of the rectum. A rectal

temperature of 101°F is the equivalent to an oral temperature of 100°F.
- Axillary temperatures are usually 1°F *lower* than oral temperatures. It's difficult for patients to keep the axilla, or armpit, tightly closed. An axillary temperature of 101°F is the equivalent of an oral temperature of 102°F.
- Tympanic thermometers give similar readings to oral thermometers as long as they are used properly.
- When you record a temperature in a patient's chart, you'll need to write where you took the measurement as well as the temperature itself—for example, *101°F, axillary.*

Glass Thermometers

Glass thermometers are used to measure oral, rectal, and axillary temperatures. They once contained liquid mercury, a hazardous material, but now are filled with nonhazardous mineral spirits or an alcohol-based substance. Figure 16-5 shows both the oral and rectal model thermometers with Celsius and Fahrenheit calibrations.

A disposable sheath may be used to cover the thermometer before using. Thermometers are cleaned and stored separately based on their use. The tip of the glass thermometers are shaped differently for oral and rectal use.

- Rectal thermometers have a rounded or stubbed bulb. The end opposite the bulb is usually color-coded red.
- Thermometers with a long, slender bulb are used for axillary or oral temperatures. They are often color-coded blue.

Reading a Glass Thermometer

When a glass thermometer is placed in position for a certain length of time, the patient's body heat expands the liquid in the tube. The liquid rises in the glass tube and stays there until you shake it back down into the bulb.

There are two main scales for glass thermometers.

- *Fahrenheit thermometer.* The glass stem of the Fahrenheit thermometer is calibrated with lines and numbers showing temperature readings in even

Centigrade

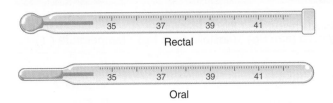

Rectal

Oral

Fahrenheit

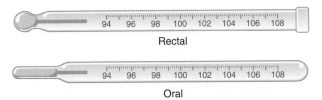

Rectal

Oral

Figure 16-5 The two-glass thermometers on the top are calibrated in the Celsius (centigrade) scale, and the two on the bottom use the Fahrenheit scale. Note the blunt bulb on the rectal thermometers and the long thin bulb on the oral thermometers. (Reprinted from Kronenberger J, Ledbetter J. *Jones & Bartlett Learning's Comprehensive Medical Assisting.* 4th ed. Burlington, MA: Jones & Bartlett Learning, LLC; 2013.)

degrees (94°, 96°, 98°, and so on). Uneven numbers (95°, 97°, 99°, and so on) are marked only with a longer line. Between both even and uneven numbers, four smaller lines show 0.2° increments of temperature. Looking at the level of the liquid in the thermometer will give you the temperature reading.

- *Celsius thermometer.* The glass stem of the Celsius thermometer has markings to show each degree. Between each degree, there are 10 smaller markings to show 0.1° increments. For example, if the liquid rises to the third small line past the line marked 37, the temperature reading to record is 37.3°C.

Electronic Thermometers

Electronic thermometers consist of a base unit and an attached temperature probe. The base unit is battery operated, so it can be carried to the location where you need to use it. Various models are available such as those shown in Figure 16-6. Store the electronic thermometer in a charging unit when it is not being used. Electronic thermometers have interchangeable temperature probes for different uses. The probes are color-coded red for rectal readings and blue for oral or axillary readings.

When the probe is positioned properly, it senses the body temperature. A digital readout shows in the window of the handheld base.

Before using an electronic thermometer, place a disposable probe cover over the probe. Be careful to not contaminate the probe cover by touching it or placing it on a surface. When you are done taking the patient's

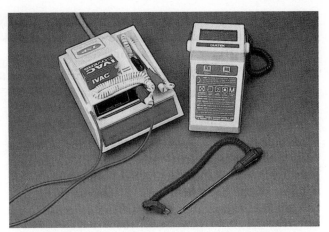

Figure 16-6 Two types of electronic thermometers and probes. (Reprinted from Kronenberger J, Ledbetter J. *Jones & Bartlett Learning's Comprehensive Medical Assisting.* 4th ed. Burlington, MA: Jones & Bartlett Learning, LLC; 2013.)

temperature, discard the probe cover in a biohazard waste container. Sanitize and disinfect the thermometer according to the office policy.

Tympanic Thermometers

These battery-powered thermometers are sometimes called aural thermometers, because they are inserted into the ear canal. The end of the thermometer is covered with a disposable cover. When it is in place, pressing a button emits infrared light inside the ear. The light bounces off the tympanic membrane, or eardrum. The technique for using a tympanic thermometer is shown in Figure 16-7.

A sensor in the thermometer measures the temperature of the blood in the tympanic membrane. The temperature reading is displayed on a digital screen on the unit within 2 seconds. If used correctly, this is a highly

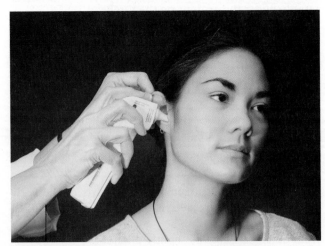

Figure 16-7 The tympanic thermometer in use. (Reprinted from Kronenberger J, Ledbetter J. *Jones & Bartlett Learning's Comprehensive Medical Assisting.* 5th ed. Burlington, MA: Jones & Bartlett Learning, LLC; 2016.)

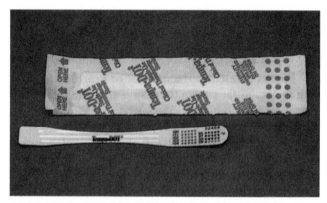

Figure 16-8 Disposable paper thermometer. The dots change color to indicate the body temperature. (Reprinted from Kronenberger J, Ledbetter J. *Jones & Bartlett Learning's Comprehensive Medical Assisting.* 5th ed. Burlington, MA: Jones & Bartlett Learning, LLC; 2016.)

reliable method for measuring temperature. However, you should not use a tympanic thermometer when the patient has a buildup of ear wax or an ear infection.

Disposable Thermometers

Disposable thermometers are designed for one use only (Fig. 16-8). They do not measure as exact or accurate as glass, electronic, or tympanic thermometers. They register temperature quickly by showing color changes on a strip. This makes them useful for simple screenings in settings such as schools or day care centers.

Other disposable thermometers for young children take the form of sucking devices or pacifiers. However, these are not used in the medical office setting.

How the Body Controls Temperature

A patient's temperature is influenced by heat produced or lost by the body. However, temperature is controlled by the hypothalamus, an area at the base of the brain.

When the body is too warm, the hypothalamus sets off vasodilation—a process where blood vessels widen or dilate. The result is that excess heat is carried to the surface of the body in the blood. The hypothalamus also signals

an increase in perspiration, or sweating. Perspiration cools the body as moisture evaporates from the skin.

If the body is too cool, the hypothalamus begins vasoconstriction, or the narrowing of blood vessels. Less blood reaches the surface of the body, reducing heat loss. The person may also begin shivering, a process that generates more heat. See Table 16-2, which lists the mechanisms of heat transfer.

Factors Influencing Temperature Control

Temperature changes may be a sign of illness or disease, but there are several other factors that cause temperatures to vary.

- Age—Children usually have higher temperatures than adults because of their increased metabolism. On the other hand, overall, elderly people have a lower metabolism and lower temperature. The temperatures of infants and the elderly are easily affected by the environment.
- Gender—Women have slightly higher temperatures than men, especially at time of ovulation.
- Exercise—When you exercise, you burn more calories for energy. That raises the body temperature.
- Time of day—Body temperature is usually lowest in the early morning, before you become physically active.
- Emotions—Temperature typically rises when you're under stress and falls when you're experiencing depression.
- Illness—Disease can cause high or low body temperatures.
- Heat or cold—Hot or cold beverages as well as a hot or cold environment can affect temperature.

Fever

Fever is a rise of body temperature. It often results from a disease process such as a bacterial or viral infection.

A fever of 102°F or higher (rectally) or 101°F or higher (orally) is referred to as **pyrexia**. An extremely high temperature, 105°F to 106°F, is called **hyperpyrexia**. Hyperpyrexia is considered dangerous because the intense body heat may destroy cells in the brain or other vital organs.

Table 16-2 Mechanisms of Heat Transfer

Mechanism	Definition	Example
Radiation	Diffusion or spreading out of heat by electromagnetic waves	The body gives off waves of heat from uncovered surfaces.
Convection	Heat is produced by motion between areas of unequal density.	An oscillating fan blows cool air across the surface of a warm body.
Evaporation	Liquid is converted to vapor.	Body fluid (perspiration) radiates from the skin.
Conduction	Heat is transferred during contact between two objects.	The body transfers heat to an ice pack, melting the ice.

A rise in body temperature also can result from exercise, anxiety, or dehydration—a loss of fluids from the body. However, these causes are unrelated to disease and are not considered fevers.

Stages of the Fever Process

The fever process has several well-defined stages.

1. Onset—The onset, or beginning of the fever, may be abrupt or gradual.
2. Course—The course is how long the fever lasts. It can range from a day or so to several weeks. There are several ways to describe a fever's course. If a fever is constant over its entire course, it is a sustained fever. If it occurs off and on over its course, it is known as a remittent fever. An intermittent fever is one that occurs at intervals. If after a period of normal readings the fever returns, it is a relapsing fever.
3. Resolution—The return to normal is the resolution. If the resolution occurs abruptly, it is a crisis. If the resolution is more gradually, it is lysis.

Patient Education on Fever

Understandably, patients are often concerned about fevers. When talking to a patient about a fever, explain that a rise in temperature is usually a natural response to disease. Therefore, a patient's attempts to "bring down a fever" may slow the disease recovery process. However, if the patient is uncomfortable or the fever is abnormally high, it should be brought down to about 101°F. The body's natural defenses may still be able to destroy the pathogen without extreme discomfort to the patient.

After consulting with the physician, you can instruct patients about several different comfort measures.

- Drink clear fluids, as tolerated, to rehydrate body tissues. (Patients should use caution when drinking clear fluids if nausea and vomiting are present.)
- Keep clothing and bedding clean and dry, especially after diaphoresis (sweating).
- Avoid becoming chilled. Chills cause shivering, which raises the body temperature.
- Rest and eat a light diet, as tolerated.
- Use antipyretics (fever-reducing agents) to stay comfortable.
- Do not give aspirin products to children under 18. Aspirin has been associated with Reye syndrome, a potentially fatal disorder, following cases of viral illnesses and varicella–zoster (chickenpox).

Pulse

The rate and power of the heartbeat is determined by measuring the pulse. As the heart beats, blood is forced through the arteries. This causes the arteries to expand. When the heart relaxes, the arteries relax as well. The expansion and relaxation of the arteries can be felt at different locations of the body called pulse points (Fig. 16-9)

The most commonly used pulse points are:

- Carotid
- Apical
- Brachial
- Radial
- Femoral
- Popliteal
- Posterior tibial
- Dorsal pedis

Taking a Pulse

For many pulse points, you can determine the pulse rate through palpation. Palpation is using the sense of touch to examine the patient. To palpate a pulse, place two or three fingers over one of the pulse points. You can use any of the following combinations of fingers:

- Index and middle finger
- Middle and ring finger
- Index, middle, and ring finger

Do not use your thumb to palpate a pulse because your thumb has its own pulse. If you used your thumb, you could be counting your own pulse and not the patient's pulse.

When you press on a pulse point with your fingers, each expansion of the artery counts as one heartbeat. You should be able to find a pulse in arteries supplying blood to the patient's arms and legs. A pulse in arteries supplying blood to one of the extremities tells you that oxygenated blood is flowing to that limb. Sometimes, you may use a stethoscope to help you listen for the heartbeat. For example, you will need a stethoscope to measure the apical pulse. Place the bell on the patient's body over the apex of the heart and listen for the pulse.

Pulse Characteristics

When you palpate the pulse, there are three different characteristics you should notice: rate, rhythm, and volume.

- Rate—The number of heartbeats per minute is the pulse rate. You can assess the rate by palpating the pulse and counting each heartbeat while watching the second hand of your watch. To get an accurate reading, you count the number of beats for a full minute. Another method is to count the number of beats for 30 seconds and multiply the number of beats by 2; however, this cannot be used when taking an apical

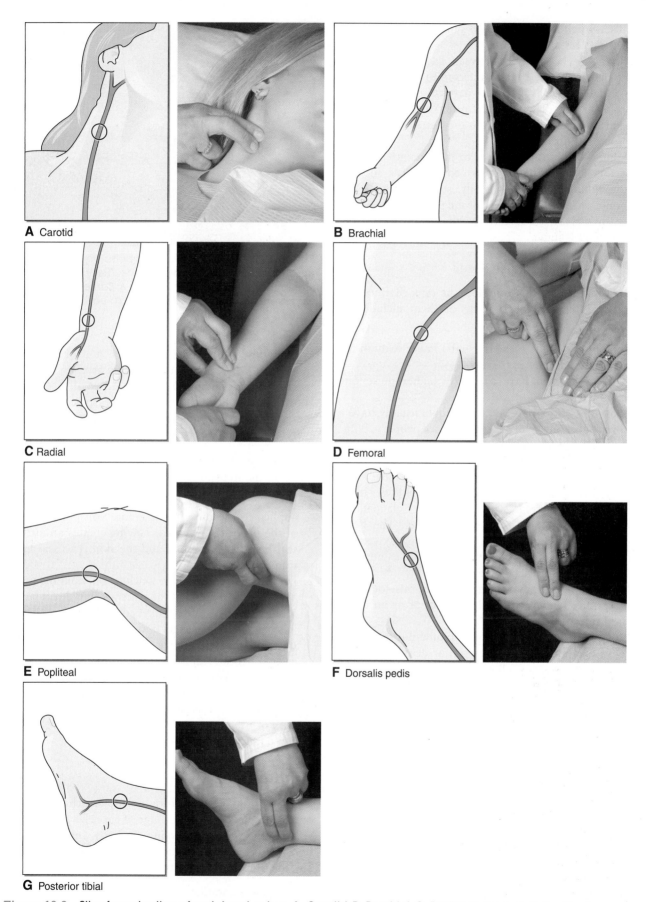

Figure 16-9 Sites for palpation of peripheral pulses. **A.** Carotid. **B.** Brachial. **C.** Radial. **D.** Femoral. **E.** Popliteal. **F.** Dorsalis pedis. **G.** Posterior tibial. (Reprinted from Kronenberger J, Ledbetter J. *Jones & Bartlett Learning's Comprehensive Medical Assisting.* 5th ed. Burlington, MA: Jones & Bartlett Learning, LLC; 2016.)

pulse. When taking an apical pulse, you must count the beats for a full minute.

- Rhythm—The interval between each heartbeat or the pattern of the beats is referred to as the rhythm. Normally, there is a regular pattern. Each heartbeat occurs at a regular, consistent rate. You need to document any irregular rhythm in the patient's chart and inform the doctor.
- Volume—The volume refers to the strength or force of the heartbeat. It is described in words such as soft, bounding, weak, thready, strong, or full. You should record a description of the pulse volume in the patient's chart. Be sure to tell the doctor about any abnormal volume.

Factors Affecting Pulse Rates

Many different factors can affect the rate, rhythm, and volume of the heartbeat. Some of them include the following:

- Time of day—The pulse is usually lower early in the morning than later in the day.
- Gender—Women have a slightly higher pulse rate than men.
- Body type and size—Tall, thin people usually have a lower pulse rate than shorter, stockier people.
- Exercise—Heart rate increases with exercise because blood needs to circulate faster in the body.
- Stress or emotions—Anger, fear, excitement, and stress will raise the pulse; depression will lower it.
- Fever—Fever increases the pulse rate. Cell metabolism increases in the presence of fever. The heart rate increases as the body works to supply oxygen and nutrients to cells. The pulse may rise as much as 10 beats/min for each degree of fever.
- Medications—Many medications may raise or lower pulse rates, either as a desired effect or as an undesired side effect.
- Blood volume—Loss of blood volume due to hemorrhage (a dramatic loss of blood) or dehydration can increase pulse rate. Cell metabolism increases, so the heart rate increases to supply more nutrients to cells.

When the Pulse Is Hard to Find

Medical assistants usually measure pulse rate from the radial artery in the arm. It is convenient for both the medical assistant and the patient. Sometimes, the radial pulse may be irregular or hard to palpate. The next best choice is to listen to the apical pulse.

Peripheral pulses, or pulses found in the arms or legs, are sometimes hard to detect. Another way to measure peripheral pulses that are hard to palpate is to use a Doppler unit.

The Doppler unit, shown in Figure 16-10, is a small electric device that is used to listen to the pulse. It has

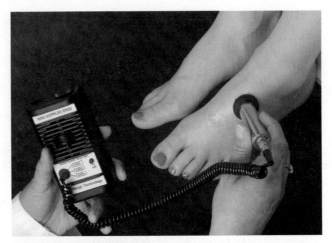

Figure 16-10 The dorsalis pedis pulse being auscultated using a Doppler device. (Reprinted from Kronenberger J, Ledbetter J. *Jones & Bartlett Learning's Comprehensive Medical Assisting.* 5th ed. Burlington, MA: Jones & Bartlett Learning, LLC; 2016.)

a main box with control switches, a probe, and an earpiece unit that plugs into the main box.

The probe contains a transducer—a device which allows you to hear the pulse. The earpiece resembles the earpiece of a stethoscope. It can be detached so that everyone in the room can hear the sounds, if desired.

Using a Doppler Unit

Here are the steps to follow in using a Doppler unit.

1. Apply gel—A coupling or transmission gel should be applied to the pulse point before you place the end of the probe on the area. The gel creates an airtight seal between the probe and the skin. The seal helps transmit the sound.
2. Find the pulse—With the machine on, hold the probe at a 90-degree angle to the patient's skin. Press lightly to make sure the probe makes contact. Move the probe in small circles in the gel until you hear the pulse. The Doppler unit will emit a loud pumping sound with each heartbeat. Adjust the volume control if necessary.
3. Clean up—After you assess the rate and rhythm of the heartbeat, clean the patient's skin with a tissue or soft cloth. Use a tissue or cloth to clean off the probe. Do not use alcohol or water to clean the probe as it can damage the transducer.

Respirations

You may think of respiration as just breathing. But the term also refers to the exchange of gases between the air you breathe and the blood in your body. During respiration, the body takes in oxygen and pushes out carbon dioxide. Respiration has two phases.

- External respiration involves exhalation, or breathing out, and inhalation, or breathing in. It is the process of moving air through the respiratory system. Air travels to the alveoli, tiny air sacs in the lungs. In the alveoli, oxygen is absorbed into the bloodstream and carbon dioxide exits the blood and is exhaled, as a waste product.

- Internal respiration is the exchange of gases between the blood and the cells that make up body tissues.

The Respiration Process

Respiration is controlled by the respiratory center in the brain stem. Chemoreceptors in the carotid arteries monitor the level of carbon dioxide in the blood. They provide feedback to the respiratory center.

The diaphragm is a muscle between the chest and abdomen that the body uses for breathing. As a patient breathes in, the diaphragm contracts and flattens out. The rib cage lifts and expands. Air flows into the lungs. The medical term for this inhalation process is inspiration.

During expiration, or exhalation (breathing out), the diaphragm relaxes, moving upward into a dome-like shape. This allows the rib cage to contract allowing air in the lungs to flow out of the chest cavity.

Normal Respiration Rates

Respiratory rates, like heart rates, change with age. They can also be affected by temperature. Patients with an elevated body temperature usually also have increased pulse and respiratory rates.

- Infants can have 25 to 60 respirations per minute, depending on their age.
- Children typically have a rate of 15 to 30 respirations per minute.
- Adults normally range from 12 to 20 respirations per minute.

Measuring Respirations

Respirations can be measured by observing the rise and fall of the patient's chest. This is usually done at the same time as you are measuring the pulse. Here are some things to keep in mind:

- Try not to make the patient aware that you are counting respirations. Patients often change their breathing action if they know they are being observed.
- Count the number of respirations (one inspiration and one expiration) in a full minute or for 30 seconds and multiply by 2.
- A stethoscope can also be used to listen to respirations if necessary.

Respiration Characteristics

There are three main characteristics of respirations:

- Rate—The number of respirations occurring in 1 minute is the respiration rate.
- Rhythm—The time or spacing between each respiration is referred to as the rhythm. Normally, respirations are

equal and regular. If the rhythm is abnormal, you need to document it in the patient's chart. You would write *irregular* after the respiration rate and notify the doctor.

- Depth—The depth refers to the volume of air inhaled and exhaled. When a person is at rest, the depth should be regular and consistent. There are normally no noticeable sounds other than those involved in the regular exchange of air.

Respirations that are abnormally deep or shallow must be documented in the patient's record. You also need to document any abnormal sounds, such as crackles (wet or dry sounds), popping sounds, or wheezes (high-pitched sounds). You must also inform the doctor of these abnormalities because they may indicate the presence of disease.

Describing Abnormal Breathing

Medical professionals use specific terms to describe respiration when they document abnormal breathing.

- Tachypnea—a respiratory rate that is much faster than normal
- Bradypnea—a respiratory rate that is much slower than normal
- Dyspnea—difficult or labored breathing
- Apnea—no respiration
- Hyperpnea—abnormally deep, gasping breaths
- Hyperventilation—a respiratory rate that greatly exceeds the body's oxygen demand
- Hypopnea—shallow respirations

Blood Pressure

Blood pressure is the measurement of the pressure of blood in an artery as it is forced against the artery walls. It is measured in two phases of the cardiac cycle, or heartbeat. The cardiac cycle lasts from the beginning of one heartbeat to the beginning of the next. There are two pressure phases in each cycle:

- Systolic pressure—The phase of the cardiac cycle when the heart muscle contracts is known as systole. As the heart contracts, it forces blood to move through chambers of the heart known as the atria and ventricles. The highest pressure level during contraction is recorded as the systolic pressure.
- Diastolic pressure—A second phase in the cardiac cycle occurs as the heart pauses to rest and refill. During diastole, the pressure in the arteries drops. The pressure level recorded during this phase is called the diastolic pressure.

Measuring Blood Pressure

To measure blood pressure, you need to use a stethoscope and a **sphygmomanometer**, a blood pressure cuff. You need to record both the systolic pressure and the diastolic pressure. These two numbers are written as a fraction, with the systolic pressure on top and the diastolic pressure on the bottom—for example, 120/80.

Three types of sphygmomanometers are commonly used in medical offices. They differ in terms of how readings are displayed.

- Aneroid sphygmomanometers display blood pressure readings on a circular dial (Fig. 16-11).
- Column sphygmomanometers display blood pressure readings using mercury-free liquid in a glass tube.
- Automated blood pressure monitors inflate the cuff when a button is pushed and show the results as numbers on a digital readout.

These blood pressure monitors are calibrated to measure blood pressure in millimeters of mercury (mm Hg). That means a blood pressure reading of 120/80 indicates the amount of force needed to raise a column of mercury to the 120-mm calibration mark on the tube during systole, contraction of the heart, and to 80 mm during diastole, relaxation of the heart.

Choosing the Correct-Size Sphygmomanometer

Before taking a patient's blood pressure, assess the size of the patient's arm and then choose the correct cuff size. Pediatric- and adult-sized cuffs are shown in Figure 16-12.

Different cuff widths are available for infants to obese adults. The width of the cuff should be 40% to 50% of the circumference of the arm. Figure 16-13 demonstrates how to measure the cuff to ensure the proper size is selected for use.

To determine the correct size, hold the narrow edge of the cuff at the midpoint of the upper arm. Wrap the width, not the length, of the cuff around the arm. The cuff width should reach not quite halfway around the arm.

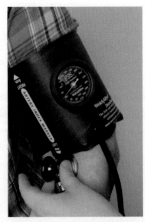

Figure 16-11 An aneroid sphygmomanometer. (Reprinted from Kronenberger J, Ledbetter J. *Jones & Bartlett Learning's Comprehensive Medical Assisting.* 5th ed. Burlington, MA: Jones & Bartlett Learning, LLC; 2016.)

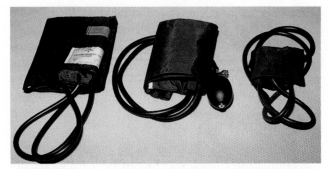

Figure 16-12 Three sizes of blood pressure cuffs (from left): a large cuff for obese adults, a normal adult cuff, and a pediatric cuff. (Reprinted from Kronenberger J, Ledbetter J. *Jones & Bartlett Learning's Comprehensive Medical Assisting.* 5th ed. Burlington, MA: Jones & Bartlett Learning, LLC; 2016.)

Obtaining a Blood Pressure Reading

The sphygmomanometer is attached to a cuff by a rubber tube. A second rubber tube is attached to a hand pump with a screw valve. After the cuff is wrapped around the patient's upper arm, use the hand pump to inflate the air bladder inside the cuff. The screw valve turned clockwise keeps the air from escaping.

As the cuff inflates, it presses against the brachial artery, the major blood vessel in the upper arm. This pressure stops blood from flowing through the artery. As you slowly turn the screw valve counterclockwise, the pressure decreases. Blood begins to flow through the artery again. With a stethoscope placed directly over the brachial artery, you listen to the sounds the blood makes as it begins flowing again.

Korotkoff Sounds

Different sounds indicate the systolic and diastolic pressures. These sounds are named for a Russian physician, Nicolai Korotkoff, who first described them. A different sound marks each phase as the cuff deflates. Only the sounds of phase 1 and phase 5 are recorded as blood pressure.

- Phase 1—faint tapping sound; this marks the systolic blood pressure.
- Phase 2—soft swishing sound.
- Phase 3—rhythmic, sharp, distinct tapping.
- Phase 4—soft tapping sound that becomes faint.
- Phase 5—the last sound heard; this is the patient's diastolic blood pressure.

All of the Korotkoff sounds are not recorded, only those sounds heard during phase 1 and phase 5.

Auscultatory Gap

In patients with a history of hypertension, or high blood pressure, you may experience an auscultatory gap during phase 2 of the Korotkoff sounds. An auscultatory gap is

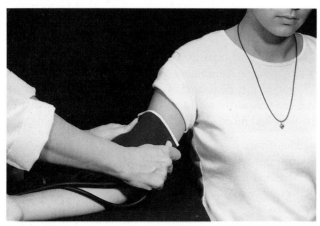

Figure 16-13 Choosing the right blood pressure cuff. (Reprinted from Kronenberger J, Ledbetter J. *Jones & Bartlett Learning's Comprehensive Medical Assisting.* 5th ed. Burlington, MA: Jones & Bartlett Learning, LLC; 2016.)

the loss of any sounds for a drop of up to 30 mm Hg after the first sound is heard.

You need to be aware of the possibility of this gap. It can lead to errors in blood pressure readings. The last sound heard at the beginning of the gap may be inaccurately recorded as the diastolic pressure. It is important to watch the dial or column liquid carefully until you are sure you have heard the last sound before noting the diastolic pressure.

Pulse Pressure

The difference between systolic and diastolic readings is called the pulse pressure. For the average adult blood pressure of 120/80, the pulse pressure is 40 (120 – 80 = 40).

The normal range for pulse pressure is 30 to 50 mm Hg. As a general rule, the pulse pressure should be no more than one-third of the systolic reading. If the pulse pressure is much larger or smaller, you need to notify the physician.

Patients with Shunts and Mastectomy

Some patients require special attention when taking blood pressure.

- A dialysis shunt is a surgically made access port that allows a patient with little or no kidney function to be connected to a dialysis machine. Taking blood pressure in the arm with the shunt could permanently damage the shunt. Do not use the arm that has an implanted shunt. If the shunt is damaged, the patient cannot receive dialysis until a surgeon puts in a new shunt.
- Patients who have had a mastectomy (surgery to remove a breast) should also not have blood pressure taken in the arm on the affected side. That side of the body may have impaired circulation because of the surgery.

Medical records of patients who have had a mastectomy or who have a dialysis shunt should clearly show that no blood pressure measurements or blood draws are to be performed on the designated arm. You should be able to use the other arm to measure blood pressure.

Most patients are aware of the importance of not taking blood pressure or specimens from the affected arm. Although they will probably alert you before you make a mistake, it is always best to check the medical record first.

Normal Blood Pressure

The average adult blood pressure is 120/80. Athletes may have a lower normal blood pressure because their cardiovascular systems are highly conditioned.

Sometimes, blood pressure drops suddenly when the patient moves from a sitting or lying position to a standing position. This drop is called postural hypotension or orthostatic hypotension. It can cause symptoms such as vertigo, or dizziness. It also may cause fainting. Be careful when asking patients to change from lying down to sitting or standing, and remind patients to move slowly.

Diseases Affecting Blood Pressure

Blood pressure readings depend on the elasticity of the artery walls, the strength of the heart muscle, and the quantity and thickness of the blood. Any diseases that affect these body structures will affect blood pressure readings. Some diseases affect the size and elasticity of the arteries.

- Arteriosclerosis refers to a number of diseases that cause narrowing and hardening of the artery lumen, the space inside the arteries. Arteriosclerosis causes artery walls to thicken and lose elasticity.
- Atherosclerosis is a specific type of arteriosclerosis in which plaque builds up in the linings of arteries. Plaque is deposits of fatty substances and cholesterol. These deposits cause arteries to narrow and harden, reducing blood flow.

How Health Affects Blood Pressure

Sometimes, a patient's family history can be a factor in a patient's blood pressure, but good general health practices can help keep the arteries and the heart healthy. Some general health practices and patient history that may affect blood pressure include the following:

- Dietary habits
- Alcohol use
- Tobacco use
- Exercise habits (amount and type of exercise)
- Previous heart conditions

Along with the patient's general health, there are many other factors that can affect blood pressure readings.

- Age—As the body ages, blood vessels begin to lose elasticity. More force is needed to expand artery walls. The buildup of plaque from the process of atherosclerosis also increases the force needed for blood flow.
- Activity—Exercise temporarily raises blood pressure. Inactivity or rest usually lowers the pressure.
- Weight—People who are obese, or even just overweight, are at increased risk for developing high blood pressure.
- Stress—During stress, the body releases a hormone called epinephrine (also known as adrenaline). This hormone increases the heart rate and raises the blood pressure.
- Body position—Blood pressure normally lowers when a person is supine, or lying down on her back.
- Medications—Some medications lower blood pressure and others may raise it.

So many factors can affect blood pressure. Physicians usually diagnose high blood pressure when there have been three or four elevated readings over a period of time.

What Can Go Wrong

As a medical assistant, you need to be concerned about getting accurate assessments of vital signs. If you do get a reading that is not within normal limits, recheck the blood pressure before reporting it. You might have made an error. There are many possible sources of errors in taking blood pressure readings. It is important to be aware of them—and to try to avoid them. Sources of errors include:

- Wrapping the cuff improperly.
- Failing to keep the patient's arm at the level of the heart while taking blood pressure readings.
- Failing to support the patient's arm on a stable surface while taking a blood pressure reading.
- Recording the auscultatory gap as the diastolic pressure.
- Failing to keep the pressure gauge at eye level.
- Applying the cuff over the patient's clothing and attempting to listen through clothing.
- Allowing the cuff to deflate too rapidly or too slowly.
- Failing to wait 1 to 2 minutes before rechecking the same arm.
- Using the wrong size cuff can cause an error as much as 30 mm Hg.

Newborn Vital Signs: The Apgar Score

The Apgar score is a method for describing the general health of newborns at 1 and 5 minutes after delivery. Vital sign measurements are part of the Apgar score. Obstetricians, pediatricians, and delivery room personnel use this score to assess newborns who may need to be watched more closely. Five signs are assessed:

- Heart rate
- Respiratory effort
- Muscle tone
- Response to a suction catheter in the nostril
- Color

A perfect score for each sign is two. A total absence of any sign is zero. A perfect Apgar score of 10 indicates all of the following things about a newborn:

- Heart rate is >100 beats/min.
- Respirations are good and the infant is breathing normally or the baby is crying.
- Muscle tone is good and the baby is active.
- Baby coughs or sneezes in response to the suction catheter.
- Skin is pink, with no acrocyanosis (blue color in the extremities).

Most babies have 1-minute scores of 7 to 9. Many may have a bit of acrocyanosis until their respiration is fully established. Babies with 1-minute scores of <4 usually require medical assistance. They often need oxygen to help them with their breathing.

Study Skill

Some students find that they learn material and have better retention of information when they develop their own quizzes. Write a few (4 to 5) questions based on information from the lesson or the chapter. Multiple-choice questions are the easiest to write. Give 4 or 5 possible answers with only one being the correct answer. Write each question on an index card. After completion of a few chapters, you will have a collection of questions you can use for your course exam, final exam, or national certification exam review. As you write these questions, you will be reinforcing the correct answer for future recall.

Procedure 16-1	Interviewing the Patient to Obtain a Medical History

1. Gather the supplies you need—a medical history form or questionnaire in electronic or paper format. If using paper format, you will also need a black ink pen.

2. Review the medical history form before you speak to the patient so that you are familiar with the order of the questions and the type of information needed.

3. Take the patient to a private and comfortable area of the office. You want to ensure confidentiality and prevent distractions.

4. Face the patient so you are both at the same eye level. Standing above the patient may make the patient feel threatened or uncomfortable.

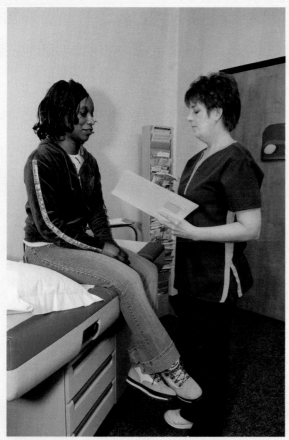

(Reprinted from Kronenberger J, Ledbetter J. *Jones & Bartlett Learning's Comprehensive Medical Assisting.* 5th ed. Burlington, MA: Jones & Bartlett Learning, LLC; 2016.)

5. Introduce yourself providing your name and title, and explain the purpose of the interview.

6. Ask the appropriate questions and document the patient's responses. Make sure you determine the CC and PI.
   - Be sure to use language and words the patient can understand.
   - No matter what the patient tells you, be professional.
   - Take care that your words and actions do not show judgmental attitudes. You want your patient to trust you.

7. Maintain frequent eye contact to show that you are listening. This reassures the patient you are interested in what she is saying.

8. If appropriate, explain to the patient what to expect during the medical examination or procedures. Keeping the patient informed may help decrease anxiety.

9. When the interview is finished, thank the patient for cooperating. Offer to answer any questions the patient may have.

| Procedure 16-2 | Document a Chief Complaint and Present Illness | |

1. Gather supplies, including the patient's medical record containing a cumulative problem list or progress note form.

2. Review the new or established patient's medical history form. Being as familiar as possible with the patient will help you get complete information about the CC and PI.

Professional Medical Associates – History Form

NAME: *Fred Smart*   DATE OF BIRTH: *09-15-1945*

What is the main reason for your visit to the doctor? *Physical Exam*

_____

Were you referred? *No*   if so, by whom? _____

PAST MEDICAL HISTORY:

Are you allergic to any medication? *Yes*

If so, list medications: *Penicillin*

List current medications, dosage, and how many times a day you take them:

Medication	Dose	Times A Day
Multivitamin	*1 tablet*	*every day*

Alcohol Consumption: What type? *Beer*   Amount *2-3*   How Often? *Every week*

History of Alcoholism? *No*

When was your last TB or Tine test? *I can't remember*

Have you ever had a positive test for tuberculosis? *No*

When was your last Tetanus shot? *Last year, I cut my finger when fishing.*

List all surgeries you have had in the past:

Date	Type of Surgery
1952-childhood?	*Tonsillectomy*

List all past hospitalizations (not involving surgeries above):

Date	Reason For Hospital Stay
Spring, 1999	*Pneumonia*

List all past problems with trauma (broken bones, lacerations, etc.):

Cut my finger while fishing last year. I had a broken leg from a car accident in 1984.

REVIEW OF SYSTEMS, PAST MEDICAL PROBLEMS:

If you have been told you have any of the problems listed below, or are having any of the problems listed below, please CIRCLE:

1. GENERAL: Weight loss, (weight gain) fever, chills, night sweats, hot flashes, tire easily, problems with sleep, crying spells, history of cancer.

2. SKIN: Rash, sores that won't heal, moles that are new or changing, history of skin problems.

3. HEENT: Headache, eye problems, hearing problems, sinus problems, hay fever, dizziness, hoarseness, sores in your mouth that won't heal, dental problems.

   Do you chew tobacco or dip snuff? *No*

4. METABOLIC/ENDOCRINE: Thyroid problems, diabetes or sugar problems, high cholesterol.

(Reprinted from Kronenberger J, Ledbetter J. *Jones & Bartlett Learning's Comprehensive Medical Assisting.* 5th ed. Burlington, MA: Jones & Bartlett Learning, LLC; 2016.)

5. <u>RESPIRATORY:</u> (Cough,) wheezing, breathing problems, history of asthma, history of lung problems.

   Do you smoke cigarettes or pipe? *Cigarettes* _____

   How much? *1 pack a day* _____ For how long? *20 years* _____

6. <u>BREAST (WOMEN):</u> Breast lumps, changes in nipples, nipple discharge, breast problems, family history of breast cancer. When was your last mammogram? _____

7. <u>CARDIOVASCULAR:</u> Heart murmur, rheumatic fever, high blood pressure, angina, heart problems, heart attack, abnormal heart rhythm, chest pain, palpitations, leg swelling, history of phlebitis or blood clots.

8. <u>GI:</u> Problems with appetite, swallowing, heartburn, nausea, vomiting, pain in the abdomen, constipation, diarrhea, blood in stool, history of ulcers, liver problems, hepatitis, jaundice, pancreas problems, gallbladder problems, or colon problems.

9. <u>REPRODUCTIVE (WOMEN):</u> Problems with irregular menstrual cycles, abnormal vaginal bleeding or discharge, history of sexually transmitted diseases, sexual problems.

   AGE OF FIRST MENSES (PERIOD) _____ AGE OF MENOPAUSE _____

   LAST PAP SMEAR _____ METHOD OF CONTRACEPTION _____

   Obstetric History (Women)

   NUMBER OF PREGNANCIES _____ PLEASE LIST AS FOLLOWS:

   Delivery Date   Pregnancy Complications   Type Delivery   Baby's Weight

   _____

   _____

   <u>MEN:</u> Problems with genital discharge, history of venereal diseases, sexual problems, prostate problems.

   METHOD OF CONTRACEPTION _____

10. <u>UROLOGIC:</u> Problems with painful urination, urinary frequency, blood in urine, weak urinary stream, history of bladder or kidney infections, or kidney stones.

11. <u>MUSCULOSKELETAL:</u> Arthritis, back pain, cramps in legs.

12. <u>NEUROLOGIC:</u> Seizures, stroke, arm or leg weakness or numbness, black-out spells, memory or thinking problems, depression, anxiety, psychiatric problems.

13. <u>HEMATOLOGIC:</u> Anemia, bleeding problems, enlarged lymph nodes.

   HAVE YOU EVER HAD A BLOOD TRANSFUSION? _____ DATE _____

FAMILY HISTORY:

List any medical problems that run in your family and which family members have these problems.

Grandmother had colon cancer; Father has high blood pressure _____

SOCIAL HISTORY:

MARITAL STATUS: *Married for 30 years* _____

OCCUPATION: *Mail Carrier* _____

EDUCATION: *Graduated high school 1963* _____

HOBBIES: *Fishing, camping* _____

WHAT DO YOU DO FOR ENJOYMENT? _____

(Reprinted from Kronenberger J, Ledbetter J. *Jones & Bartlett Learning's Comprehensive Medical Assisting.* 5th ed. Burlington, MA: Jones & Bartlett Learning, LLC; 2016.)

3. Greet the patient by name and escort him to the examination room. Using the patient's name helps develop rapport and may ease any patient anxiety. Correctly identifying the patient also can help prevent mistakes.

4. Use open-ended questions to find out why the patient is seeking medical care. Be sure to maintain eye contact so the patient is aware that you are actively listening.

5. Determine the PI using open-ended and closed-ended questions. Use several open-ended questions first. Then, use closed-ended questions to get more specific information.

6. Document the CC and PI on the cumulative problem list or progress report form. Include the date, time, CC, PI, and your signature (first initial, last name, and title). Use only correct medical terminology and approved abbreviations.

7. When you have finished asking questions, thank the patient for cooperating. Explain that the physician will be in soon for the examination. If you give a time frame about when the physician will arrive, be honest.

Procedure 16-3 | Measuring Oral Temperature Using a Mercury-Free Glass Thermometer

1. Gather the following supplies: a glass mercury-free oral thermometer with a blue top, a disposable plastic sheath, tissues or cotton balls, disposable exam gloves, a biohazard waste container, and disinfectant solution. Then, wash your hands and put on gloves.

2. Dry the thermometer if it has been stored in a disinfectant solution. To dry the thermometer, use tissues or cotton balls to wipe the thermometer from the bulb up the stem. A dry thermometer will slip easily into the sheath.

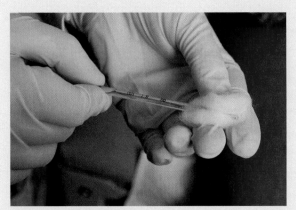

(Reprinted from Kronenberger J, Ledbetter J. *Jones & Bartlett Learning's Comprehensive Medical Assisting.* 4th ed. Burlington, MA: Jones & Bartlett Learning, LLC; 2013.)

3. Carefully check the thermometer for chips or cracks. A damaged thermometer could injure the patient.

4. Check the thermometer reading. Hold the stem at eye level and turn it slowly to see the liquid in the column.

5. If the reading is above 94°F, shake down the thermometer. The liquid inside must be below 94°F to provide an accurate temperature reading.
   - Grasp the thermometer carefully at the end of the stem using your thumb and forefinger.
   - Snap your wrist several times.
   - Be careful not to hit the thermometer against anything when snapping your wrist.

6. Insert the thermometer into the plastic sheath.

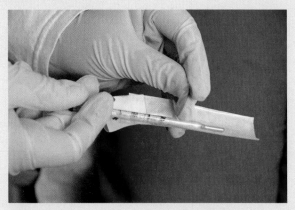

(Reprinted from Kronenberger J, Ledbetter J. *Jones & Bartlett Learning's Comprehensive Medical Assisting.* 4th ed. Burlington, MA: Jones & Bartlett Learning, LLC; 2013.)

7. Greet the patient by name. Explain the procedure and ask about any eating, drinking of hot or cold fluids, gum chewing, or smoking within the last 15 minutes.
   - Any of these could alter the oral reading.
   - Wait 15 minutes before taking the reading or choose another method.

8. Place the thermometer under the patient's tongue to one side of the frenulum, a small strip of tissue that connects the tongue to the floor of the mouth. This area has the highest blood flow and will give the most accurate reading.

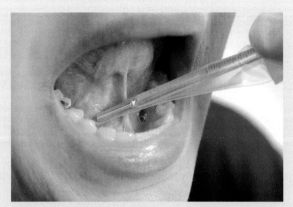

(Reprinted from Kronenberger J, Ledbetter J. *Jones & Bartlett Learning's Comprehensive Medical Assisting.* 4th ed. Burlington, MA: Jones & Bartlett Learning, LLC; 2013.)

Procedure 16-3 | Measuring Oral Temperature Using a Mercury-Free Glass Thermometer (*continued*)

9. Ask the patient to keep the mouth and lips closed. This prevents air from entering the mouth and causing an inaccurate reading. Remind the patient not to bite down on the thermometer.

10. Leave the thermometer in place for 3 to 5 minutes.
    - Three minutes is long enough if the patient has no evidence of fever.
    - If the patient is noncompliant and frequently talks or opens her mouth, the thermometer should be left in place for 5 minutes.
    - It also should be left in place for 5 minutes if the patient is febrile.
    - While you are waiting for a temperature reading, you can take the patient's pulse, respirations, and blood pressure.

11. When the time is up, remove the thermometer from the patient's mouth. Be sure to wear gloves.

12. Then, remove the sheath by holding the edge of the sheath with the thumb and forefinger of one hand and pulling down from the open edge over the length of the thermometer to the bulb. The soiled area should now be inside the sheath. Discard the sheath in a biohazard waste container.

13. Hold the thermometer horizontal at eye level. Note the level of liquid that has risen into the column.

14. Sanitize and disinfect the thermometer according to office policy. Remove your gloves and then wash your hands.

15. Record the temperature reading in the patient's medical record. Remember, procedures are not considered done if they are not recorded. The vital signs are usually recorded together.

Procedure 16-4 | Measuring a Rectal Temperature

1. Gather the following supplies: a glass mercury-free rectal thermometer with a red top, a disposable plastic sheath, tissues or cotton balls, disposable exam gloves, a biohazard waste container, lubricant, and disinfectant solution. Then, wash your hands and put on gloves.

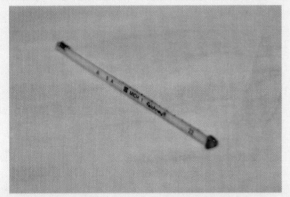

(Reprinted from Kronenberger J, Ledbetter J. *Jones & Bartlett Learning's Comprehensive Medical Assisting.* 4th ed. Burlington, MA: Jones & Bartlett Learning, LLC; 2013.)

2. Dry the thermometer if it has been stored in a disinfectant solution. To dry the thermometer, use tissues or cotton balls to wipe the thermometer from the bulb up the stem. A dry thermometer will slip easily into the sheath.

3. Carefully check the thermometer for chips or cracks. A damaged thermometer could injure the patient.

4. Check the thermometer reading. Hold the stem at eye level and turn it slowly to see the liquid in the column.

5. If the reading is above 94°F, shake down the thermometer. The liquid inside must be below 94°F to provide an accurate temperature reading.
    - Grasp the thermometer carefully at the end of the stem using your thumb and forefinger.
    - Snap your wrist several times.
    - Be careful not to hit the thermometer against anything when snapping your wrist.

6. Insert the thermometer into the plastic sheath.

7. Spread lubricant onto a tissue and then from the tissue onto the sheath of the thermometer. Do not apply lubricant directly onto the thermometer. Lubricant should always be used for rectal insertion to prevent patient discomfort.

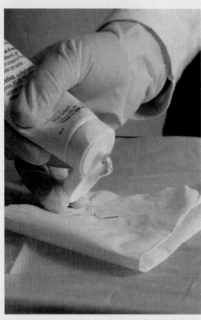

(Reprinted from Kronenberger J, Ledbetter J. *Jones & Bartlett Learning's Comprehensive Medical Assisting.* 4th ed. Burlington, MA: Jones & Bartlett Learning, LLC; 2013.)

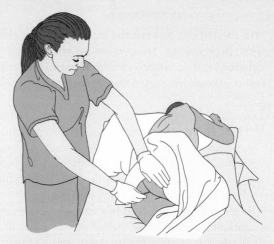

(Reprinted from Kronenberger J, Ledbetter J. *Jones & Bartlett Learning's Comprehensive Medical Assisting.* 4th ed. Burlington, MA: Jones & Bartlett Learning, LLC; 2013.)

8. Greet the patient by name and explain the procedure.

9. Ensure the patient's privacy by placing the patient in a side-lying position facing the examination room door, if possible. If the door is opened, a patient facing the door is less likely to be exposed. Drape the patient appropriately. The side-lying position facilitates exposure to the anus.

10. Visualize the anus by lifting the top buttock with your nondominant hand. Never insert the thermometer without first having a clear view of the anus.

11. Gently insert the thermometer past the sphincter muscle. The thermometer should be inserted about 1.5 inches for an adult, 1 inch for a child, and 0.5 inch for an infant.

12. Release the upper buttock and hold the thermometer in place with your dominant hand for 3 minutes. The thermometer will not stay in place if you do not hold it. Replace the drape to ensure the patient's privacy, but don't move your dominant hand.

13. After 3 minutes, remove the thermometer and sheath. Discard the sheath in a biohazard waste container. You need to remove the sheath before reading the thermometer to get an accurate reading.

14. Hold the thermometer horizontal at eye level and note the temperature reading.

15. Give the patient a tissue to wipe away excess lubricant.

16. Sanitize and disinfect the thermometer according to office policy. Then, remove your gloves and wash your hands.

17. Record the temperature reading in the patient's medical record. Be sure to mark the letter "R" next to the reading, to show the temperature was taken rectally. Temperatures are presumed to have been taken orally unless otherwise noted.

Note: Infants and very small children may be held in your lap or over your knees for this procedure. Hold the thermometer and the buttocks with your dominant hand while securing the child with your nondominant hand. If the child moves, the thermometer and your hand will move together, avoiding injury to the anal canal.

| Procedure 16-5 | Measuring an Axillary Temperature | |

1. Gather the following supplies: a glass mercury-free oral thermometer with a blue top, a disposable probe cover, tissues or cotton balls, disposable exam gloves, a biohazard waste container, and disinfectant solution. Then, wash your hands and put on gloves.

2. Dry the thermometer if it has been stored in a disinfectant solution. To dry the thermometer, use tissues or cotton balls to wipe the thermometer from the bulb up the stem. A dry thermometer will slip easily into the sheath.

3. Carefully check the thermometer for chips or cracks. A damaged thermometer could injure the patient.

4. Check the thermometer reading. Hold the stem at eye level and turn it slowly to see the liquid in the column.

5. If the reading is above 94°F, shake down the thermometer. The liquid inside must be below 94°F to provide an accurate temperature reading.
   - Grasp the thermometer carefully at the end of the stem using your thumb and forefinger.
   - Snap your wrist several times.
   - Be careful not to hit the thermometer against anything when snapping your wrist.

6. Insert the thermometer into the probe cover. Be careful not to contaminate the sheath by touching it or placing it down on any surface.

7. Explain the procedure to the patient. Expose the patient's axilla. Do not expose more of the patient's chest or upper body than is necessary. It's important to protect the patient's privacy at all times.

8. Place the bulb of the thermometer deep in the axilla. Bring the patient's arm down, crossing the forearm over the chest. This position provides the best skin contact with the thermometer. It also provides a closed environment. Drape the patient appropriately for privacy.

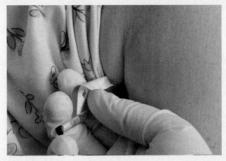

(Reprinted from Kronenberger J, Ledbetter J. *Jones & Bartlett Learning's Comprehensive Medical Assisting.* 4th ed. Burlington, MA: Jones & Bartlett Learning, LLC; 2013.)

9. Leave the thermometer in place for 10 minutes. Axillary temperatures take longer than oral or rectal ones. You shouldn't need to hold the thermometer in place unless the patient does not understand that the arm must stay down.

10. At the appropriate time, remove the thermometer.
    - Remove the probe cover by holding the edge of the cover with the thumb and forefinger of one hand and pulling down from the open edge over the length of the thermometer to the bulb. The soiled area should now be inside the cover.
    - Discard the probe cover in a biohazard waste container.

11. Hold the thermometer horizontal at eye level and note the temperature reading.

12. Sanitize and disinfect the thermometer according to office policy. Then, remove your gloves and wash your hands.

13. Record the temperature reading in the patient's medical record. Be sure to mark an *A* beside it. This indicates the reading was axillary. Temperatures are presumed to have been taken orally unless otherwise noted.

Procedure 16-6 — Measuring Temperature Using an Electronic Thermometer

1. Gather the following supplies: an electronic thermometer with an oral or a rectal probe, a disposable probe cover, lubricant, tissues, disposable exam gloves (for rectal temperature), and a biohazard waste container. Wash your hands and put on gloves.

2. Greet the patient by name and explain the procedure.

3. Choose the most appropriate method (oral, axillary, or rectal). Attach the appropriate probe to the battery-powered temperature unit.

4. Insert the probe into the probe cover. All probes fit into one size probe cover.
   - Covers usually are carried with the unit in a specially fitted box attached to the back of the unit.
   - If you use the last probe cover, be sure to attach a new box of covers to the unit to be ready for future patients.

5. Wait for the electronic unit to beep when it senses that the temperature is no longer rising. This usually occurs within 10 seconds.

6. After the beep, remove the probe. Note the temperature reading on the digital display screen on the unit.

7. Discard the probe cover in a biohazard container by depressing a button, usually on the end of the probe. Replace the probe in the slot on the unit, but make sure you have noted the temperature reading first. Most units automatically shut off when the probe is put back into the unit.

8. Remove your gloves if you are wearing them and wash your hands. Then, record the temperature in the patient's medical record. Record the reading in the same way as if you were using a glass thermometer. Indicate a rectal reading with an "R," an oral reading with an "O," and an axillary reading with an "A."

Procedure 16-7 — Measuring Temperature Using a Tympanic Thermometer

1. Gather the following supplies: a tympanic thermometer, disposable probe covers, and a biohazard waste container. Wash your hands.

2. Greet the patient by name and explain the procedure.

3. Insert the ear probe into the probe cover. Always put a clean probe cover on the ear probe before taking a temperature.

4. With your nondominant hand, straighten the patient's ear canal. Place the end of the ear probe in the patient's ear with your dominant hand.
   - For most patients, you straighten the ear canal by pulling the top posterior part of the outer ear up and back.
   - For children under 3 years of age, pull the outer ear down and back.

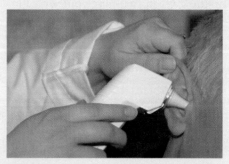

(Reprinted from Kronenberger J, Ledbetter J. *Jones & Bartlett Learning's Comprehensive Medical Assisting.* 5th ed. Burlington, MA: Jones & Bartlett Learning, LLC; 2016.)

5. With the ear probe properly placed in the ear canal, press the button on the thermometer. The reading will be shown on the digital display in about 2 seconds.

6. Remove the probe and note the reading. Discard the probe cover in a biohazard waste container. Probe covers are for one use only. Then, wash your hands.

7. Record the temperature on the patient's record in the same way that you record temperatures for a glass thermometer. Be sure to indicate that the tympanic temperature was taken.

Procedure 16-8 | Measuring the Radial Pulse

1. Wash your hands first. Have a watch or clock with a second hand available.

2. Greet the patient by name if you have not already done so and explain the procedure. In most cases, the pulse is taken at the same time as other vital signs.

3. Position the patient so the arm is relaxed. The arm should be supported either on the patient's lap or on a table. If the arm is not supported, or the patient is uncomfortable, it may be hard to find the pulse.

4. Use the index, middle, and ring fingers of your dominant hand to find the radial pulse. The pulse point is located on the patient's thumb side of the wrist.
   - Do not use your own thumb—it has a pulse of its own that can be confused with the patient's pulse.
   - You may place your thumb on the opposite side of the patient's wrist to steady your hand.

5. Press your fingers on the pulse point. Press firmly enough to feel the pulse. Pressing too firmly can cause the pulse to disappear.
   - If the pulse is regular, count it for 30 seconds, watching the second hand of your watch. Multiply the number of pulsations by 2 since the pulse is always recorded as the number of beats per minute.
   - If the pulse is irregular, count it for a full 60 seconds. Otherwise, the measurement may be inaccurate.

6. Record the pulse rate in the patient's medical record with the other vital signs. Make a note and notify the doctor if the rhythm is irregular and the volume is thready or bounding.

Procedure 16-9 | Measuring Respirations

1. Wash your hands. Have a watch or clock with a second hand available.

2. Greet the patient by name if you have not already.

3. Observe carefully for the easiest area to assess respirations. Some patients have abdominal movement instead of chest movement during respirations.

4. In most cases, respirations are measured at the same time as the pulse. After counting the radial pulse, continue to watch the second hand of your watch. Begin counting respirations. Count a complete rise and fall of the patient's chest as one respiration.
   - It is best not to inform the patient that you are counting respirations. A patient who is aware that you are counting respirations may alter his breathing pattern.

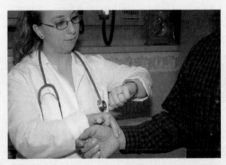

(Reprinted from Kronenberger J, Ledbetter J. *Jones & Bartlett Learning's Comprehensive Medical Assisting*. 5th ed. Burlington, MA: Jones & Bartlett Learning, LLC; 2016.)

5. If the breathing pattern is regular, count the respiratory rate for 30 seconds. Then, multiply by 2. If the pattern is irregular, count for a full 60 seconds. Otherwise, the measurement may be inaccurate.

6. Record the respiratory rate in the patient's medical record along with the other vital signs. Also, note the rhythm if irregular. Mark down any unusual sounds, such as wheezing.

Procedure 16-10   Measuring Blood Pressure

1. Wash your hands and gather a sphygmomanometer and a stethoscope.

2. Greet the patient by name and explain the procedure.

3. Position the patient with the arm to be used supported with the forearm on the lap or a table.
   - The arm should be slightly flexed, with the palm upward. This makes it easier to find and palpate the brachial artery.
   - The upper arm should be level with the patient's heart. If the upper arm is higher or lower than the heart, the reading may be inaccurate.

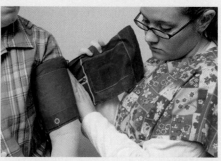

(Reprinted from Kronenberger J, Ledbetter J. *Jones & Bartlett Learning's Comprehensive Medical Assisting*. 5th ed. Burlington, MA: Jones & Bartlett Learning, LLC; 2016.)

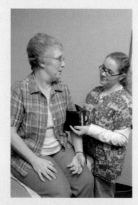

(Reprinted from Kronenberger J, Ledbetter J. *Jones & Bartlett Learning's Comprehensive Medical Assisting*. 5th ed. Burlington, MA: Jones & Bartlett Learning, LLC; 2016.)

4. Expose the patient's arm. Clothing over the area can block out the sounds you will need to hear. If the sleeve is pulled up, ensure it is not tight. A sleeve that is too tight can act as a tourniquet, decreasing the flow of blood and causing an inaccurate blood pressure reading. Make sure the patient's legs are not crossed and ask the patient to not talk during the procedure.

5. Palpate the brachial pulse in the antecubital area—the region of the arm in front of the elbow.
   - Center the deflated cuff directly over the brachial artery.
   - The lower edge of the cuff should be 1 to 2 inches above the antecubital area.
   - If the cuff is too low, it may interfere with placement of the stethoscope and cause noises that obscure the Korotkoff sounds.

6. Wrap the cuff smoothly and snugly around the arm. Secure the cuff with the Velcro edges.

7. Hold the air pump in your dominant hand, with the valve between your thumb and forefinger. Turn the valve screw clockwise to tighten it. The cuff will not inflate with the valve open.
   - Be careful not to make the valve screw so tight that it's hard to release. You need to be able to loosen it with one hand after the cuff is inflated.

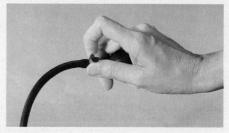

(Reprinted from Kronenberger J, Ledbetter J. *Jones & Bartlett Learning's Comprehensive Medical Assisting*. 5th ed. Burlington, MA: Jones & Bartlett Learning, LLC; 2016.)

8. First, determine a reference point for how far you need to inflate the cuff.
   - While palpating the brachial pulse with your nondominant hand, inflate the cuff.
   - Note the point or number on the dial or glass tube column at which you no longer feel the brachial pulse.
   - This will give you a reference point for reinflating the cuff when taking the blood pressure.

9. Deflate the cuff by turning the valve counterclockwise. Wait at least 30 seconds before reinflating the cuff. The waiting time allows blood circulation to return to the extremity.

10. Clean the earpieces of the stethoscope with an alcohol wipe. Place the stethoscope earpieces in your ears with the openings pointed slightly forward. Stand about 18 inches from the manometer with the gauge at eye level to reduce the chances of making an error while taking the reading.

Procedure 16-10 | Measuring Blood Pressure (*continued*)

11. Place the diaphragm of the stethoscope against the brachial artery and hold it in place with your non-dominant hand. Don't press too hard or you may obliterate the pulse. On the other hand, if you do not press firmly enough, you may not hear the sounds.
    - The stethoscope tubing should hang freely without touching or rubbing any part of the cuff. If the stethoscope rubs or touches any other objects, environmental sounds may make the Korotkoff sounds impossible to hear.

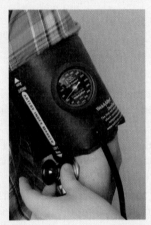

(Reprinted from Kronenberger J, Ledbetter J. *Jones & Bartlett Learning's Comprehensive Medical Assisting.* 5th ed. Burlington, MA: Jones & Bartlett Learning, LLC; 2016.)

12. With your dominant hand, turn the screw near the bulb just enough to close the valve. Inflate the cuff.
    - Pump the valve bulb to about 30 mm Hg above the number you noted during step 8.
    - Inflating more than 30 mm Hg above the baseline is uncomfortable for the patient and unnecessary. But if you don't inflate the cuff enough, the systolic reading may be inaccurate.

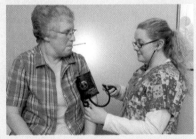

(Reprinted from Kronenberger J, Ledbetter J. *Jones & Bartlett Learning's Comprehensive Medical Assisting.* 5th ed. Burlington, MA: Jones & Bartlett Learning, LLC; 2016.)

13. Once the cuff is inflated appropriately, turn the valve counterclockwise. You want to release the air at about 2 to 4 mm Hg/sec.
    - Releasing the air too fast will cause missed beats.
    - Releasing it too slowly will interfere with circulation.

14. Listen carefully while watching the gauge. Aneroid and mercury-free measurements are always made as even numbers, because of the way the manometer is calibrated.
    - Note the point on the gauge at which you hear the first clear tapping sound. This is the systolic sound or Korotkoff phase 1.

15. Continue to listen and deflate the cuff. When you hear the last sound, note the reading, and quickly deflate the cuff.
    - The last sound heard is the Korotkoff phase 5 sound. It is recorded as the diastolic pressure or the bottom number.
    - If you are unsure of the reading, wait 1 to 2 minutes before repeating the procedure. Never immediately reinflate the cuff.

16. Remove the stethoscope earpieces from your ears. Remove the cuff and press any remaining air from the bladder of the cuff.
    - If this is the first reading or a new patient, the physician may also want a reading in the other arm or in another position.
    - In some patients, blood pressure varies between the arms or in different positions such as lying or standing.

17. When all readings are finished, put the equipment away and wash your hands.

18. Record the reading. The systolic pressure is always written as a fraction over the diastolic pressure (e.g., 120/80). Note which arm was used—RA for right arm, or LA for left arm. Record the patient's position if other than sitting.

Preparing for Externship

One of the tasks that medical assistants do in the One of the tasks that medical assistants do in the office is to collect the medical history of patients. This includes interviewing new patients and updating information for established patients. As an extern, you will observe the techniques used by the office staff to gather this information for the patient record. Take note of how the questions are stated and the way the patient responses are input into the medical record. Remember the externship experience is the "real world" and the scenarios you practiced in class are now playing out. What you hear from the patient, you must accurately document in the record for the physician or provider to read. Watch for spelling and grammar errors. You will become familiar with common phrases and ways to express what the patient says. You may want to review other entries made into the record on previous visits. This will help you to become familiar with proper charting styles. It will also allow you to see the level of detail necessary for proper and adequate documentation of the patient's visit.

Chapter Recap

- Medical assistants may need to collect information for the patient's medical history and medical assessment. The role of the medical assistant in collecting information depends on the policies of the medical office.
- The medical history provides the physician with a basis for asking questions during an examination. It also helps the physician understand how the patient's illness and lifestyle interact.
- During an assessment, patients are interviewed to establish signs and symptoms of illness. For each visit, a chief complaint and present illness are documented in the patient's record.
- Physical measurements also provide information about a patient's health. Medical assistants may collect anthropometric measurements and measure vital signs.
- Anthropometric measurements for adults typically include height and weight. Pediatric measurements may also include head and chest circumference.
- Body temperature reflects the balance between heat produced and heat lost by the body. The type of thermometer used for measuring temperature depends on the practices of the medical office.
- Four different methods for taking temperature are oral, rectal, axillary, and tympanic. The method must be documented in the patient's medical record, along with the reading.
- Pulse and respiration rates are often measured at the same time. Three important characteristics of the pulse are the rate, rhythm, and volume. Important characteristics of respirations are the rate, rhythm, and depth.
- Blood pressure is measured during two phases of the cardiac cycle called systole and diastole. Five phases of Korotkoff sounds can be identified with a stethoscope. The systolic pressure reading is measured during phase 1. The diastolic pressure reading occurs during phase 5.
- Measuring blood pressure can be tricky. By being aware of possible sources of errors, medical assistants can make sure their readings are accurate.

Online Resources for Students

Student Resources available on the text's online site include:
- Audio Glossaries
- Animations
- Competency Evaluation Forms
- Videos
- Anatomy & Physiology Module with Heart and Lung Sounds
- Weblinks
- Worksheets

Exercises and Activities

Certification Preparation Questions

1. Which of the following is part of the social history information on a new patient medical history form?

   a. Age
   b. Date of birth
   c. Prior surgical procedures
   d. Alcohol consumption
   e. Occupation

2. Which of the following supplies is required for obtaining a temperature on an infant?

   a. Tympanic thermometer
   b. Sterile exam gloves
   c. Digital thermometer with blue tip
   d. Biohazard sharps container
   e. Glass thermometer with red tip

3. Which of the following is an accurately recorded high blood pressure reading?

   a. 220/70 bpm
   b. 160/70 mm
   c. S190/D80
   d. 150/95
   e. 100/220

4. Which of these is the best response from the medical assistant if a patient refuses to provide information to complete the medical history form?

   a. I will need to obtain this information or the doctor will not be able to treat you today.
   b. We will reschedule your appointment until you can provide the needed information.
   c. I know this is difficult; however, the physician will need to have the information before he will see you.
   d. I will make a note on this form that you are refusing to provide any information.
   e. I will inform the physician that you are unable to provide the needed information.

5. What is the best location to obtain a radial pulse?

   a. Wrist on the little finger side
   b. Antecubital area of the arm
   c. Upper arm 2 inches above the elbow
   d. Wrist on the thumb side

   e. Midarm between the elbow and the hand

6. Which of the following is the first step in obtaining a blood pressure?

   a. Apply the blood pressure cuff.
   b. Pump the bulb on the gauge to ensure that it works.
   c. Check the size of the cuff to ensure it is appropriate for the patient.
   d. Locate the brachial artery and place the stethoscope over it.
   e. Determine the pulse pressure.

7. Which of these is a factor that a patient can change to affect their blood pressure?

   a. Age
   b. Gender
   c. Weight
   d. Family history
   e. Culture

8. Which of the following represents the blood pressure reading if the pulse pressure is 40?

   a. 110/60
   b. 122/82
   c. 130/94
   d. 160/100
   e. 90/58

9. If a patient's height registers 69 inches on the height meter, how tall is the patient?

   a. 6 feet 0 inches
   b. 5 feet 11 inches
   c. 5 feet 9 inches
   d. 5 feet 7 inches
   e. 4 feet 9 inches

10. Which of the following is not considered a sign?

    a. Coughing
    b. Rash
    c. Bleeding
    d. Headache
    e. Bruise

CareTracker Connection

>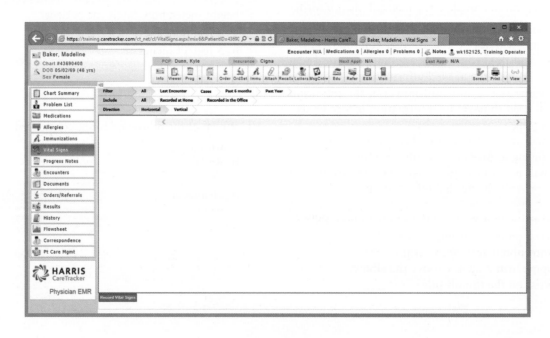
>
> **HARRIS** CareTracker Documenting Patient Health History and Assessment Findings
>
> *CareTracker Activities Related to This Chapter*
> - Case Study 4: Charting Patient Information

A patient's health information is some of the most valuable and sensitive data on the planet. It is often costly to obtain, essential in diagnosing and treating life-threatening diseases, and extremely personal. Collecting, documenting, managing, and protecting this information, therefore, are weighty responsibilities of the medical assistant. Fortunately for you, electronic health record systems, such as CareTracker, have revolutionized the documentation and management of patient data, making it possible to capture and organize a vast amount of complex data and make it accessible to health care professionals around the world while protecting the patient's privacy.

Tasks discussed in this chapter that can be performed in CareTracker include the following:

- Documenting the following patient health information:
  - Chief complaint
  - Present illness
  - Vital signs
    - Heart rate
    - Respiratory rate
    - Blood pressure
    - Temperature
  - Anthropometric measurements
    - Height
    - Weight
  - Allergies
  - Medications
  - Immunizations
  - Medical history
    - Diseases and conditions
    - Injuries
    - Hospitalizations
    - Surgeries
  - Social history
    - Diet
    - Exercise
    - Tobacco use
    - Alcohol use
    - Sexual and reproductive history
  - Family history

Many of these tasks are discussed in CareTracker Connection features in other chapters. A task we'll consider here is entering a patient's vital signs.

Some of the first data you will obtain during a patient visit are vital signs. In CareTracker, these data are entered into the Medical Record module, in the Vital Signs application.

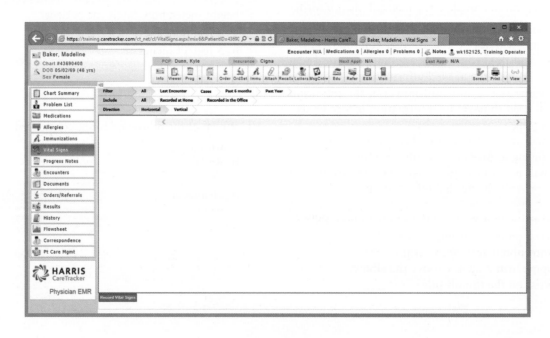

Within this application, clicking on the Record Vital Signs button causes the Vital Signs window to appear, where you may enter the patient's vital signs and chief complaint. Note that any measurements that are outside of normal parameters are automatically highlighted after the data are entered, such as the body mass index, shown in the figure below.

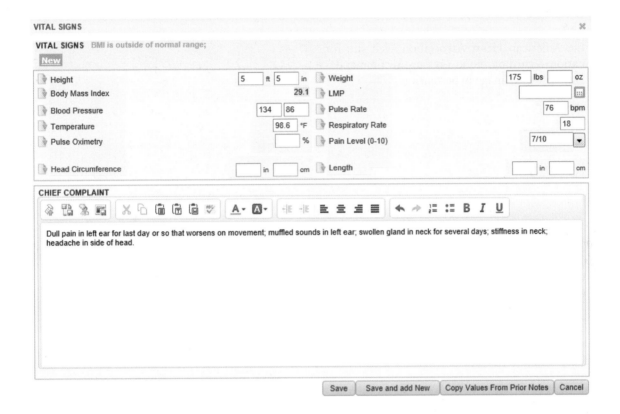

Once you save this information, a summary of the vital signs appears on the main Vital Signs screen. Again, abnormal measurements are highlighted.

	6/7/2017 (1)
Weight	175 lbs
Height	5 ft 5 in
Body Mass Index	29.1
Blood Pressure	134 / 86
Pulse Rate	76 bpm
Temperature	98.6 °F
Respiration Rate	18
Pulse Oximetry	
Pain Level ___(0-10)	7/10

These data are now available throughout the CareTracker system and may appear in other applications, such as the Progress Note. You'll get a chance to practice this task in Case Study 4: Charting Patient Information.

Internet Activities

1. Visit the American Heart Association Web site for information regarding blood pressure recommendations and how to manage hypertension.

2. Go to Web site for the Centers for Medicare and Medicaid Services (www.CMS.gov). Locate the site with information regarding HIPAA and the Medical Privacy of Protected Health Information.

17 Assisting with the Physical Examination

Chapter Objectives

- Identify the medical assistant's role in assisting with the physical examination.
- List the equipment and supplies needed in the patient examination room.
- Prepare and maintain patient examination and treatment areas.
- Explain the care and use of the equipment and instruments used in a physical examination.
- Describe six examination techniques used during the physical examination.
- Prepare patients for and assist with routine and specialty examinations.

- Describe the basic examination positions and explain their use.
- Understand the sequential process used by the physician to complete a physical examination.
- Explain how the physician evaluates a patient's posture, gait, and reflexes.
- Instruct patients how to recognize cancer warning signs and perform self-examinations of the breasts and testicles.
- List the guidelines for annual examinations, immunizations, and cancer screening.

CAAHEP & ABHES Competencies

CAAHEP

- Assist physician with patient care.
- Apply critical thinking skills in performing patient assessment and care.
- Use language/verbal skills that enable patients' understanding.
- Demonstrate respect for diversity in approaching patients and families.

- Explain the rationale for performance of a procedure to the patient.
- Document patient care.
- Respond to nonverbal communication.

ABHES

- General/physical examination
- Specialty examination
- Working with diverse populations

Chapter Terms

Accommodation	Inspection	Otorhinolaryngologist	Speculum
Asymmetry	Manipulation	Otoscope	Stethoscope
Auscultation	Mensuration	Palpation	Symmetry
Gait	Ophthalmoscope	Percussion	

Abbreviations

CC	PERRLA	PI	ROS
CPX	PAP	ROM	
ECG	PH		

Case Study

Medical assistant, Karen Stuart, escorts female patient, Rebecca Martin, to an examination room where she is scheduled for a complete physical examination. The patient tells Karen that it has been several years since she has had physical examination. The patient also shares with Karen that her mother died recently and she has had a very difficult time coping with the death of her mother. She decided to come to the office for a complete physical examination because she has been feeling very tired and depressed since the death of her mother. The patient states that she is afraid the physician may discover something that might be very serious or even terminal.

Study Skill

Students often overlook the value of the chapter objectives. After you have completed reading and studying the information in this chapter, write down each chapter objective. Give an answer or explanation for each objective based on the material included in the chapter. For example, the last objective states "List the guidelines for annual examination, immunization, and cancer screening." Write a list for each of these. This can be used as a review and study tool prior your course exam or national certification exam.

THE BASIC PHYSICAL EXAMINATION

The complete physical examination (**CPX**) is one of the most typical services provided in the physician's office. Patients may schedule to have a complete physical examination for various reasons including:

- Determining baseline information of a new patient
- Requirement for employment, attending school, and playing sports
- Approval for health or life insurance
- Periodic assessment of existing patients

A complete physical exam allows the physician to assess the patient's general state of health. Through the process of performing the examination, the physician does a review of systems (**ROS**) to detect signs and symptoms of disease. The complete physical examination process includes:

- Obtaining or updating the patient's medical history
- Performance of the actual physical examination
- Ordering laboratory tests
- Scheduling diagnostic tests

The medical assistant duties may vary according to the physician's preference and the practice's policies. Typically, the medical assistant will be responsible for:

- Preparing the examination room
- Assisting with or obtaining the patient's medical history
- Preparing the patient for examination
- Assisting the physician during the examination
- Collecting specimens for laboratory testing
- Performing or scheduling diagnostic tests
- Cleaning the examination room

The medical assistant may be required to be present in the patient examination room during the physical exam. The American Medical Association (AMA) recommends that a third party—someone other than the physician and patient—be present during a physical examination. Your presence provides a witness for the physician if there are any misunderstandings or accusations by the patient. The medical assistant hears and observes all the activity that occurs in the patient room during the physical exam. A patient may request that the medical assistant remain in the room if the physician does not require it.

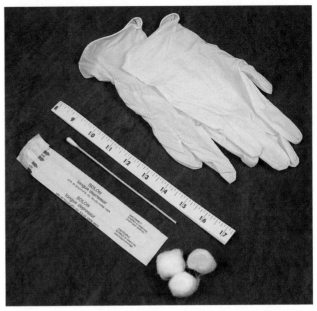

Figure 17-1 Common supplies used in adult physical examination: tape measure, gloves, tongue depressor, and cotton-tipped applicator. (Reprinted from Kronenberger J, Ledbetter J. *Jones & Bartlett Learning's Comprehensive Medical Assisting.* 5th ed. Burlington, MA: Jones & Bartlett Learning, LLC; 2016.)

 PHYSICAL EXAMINATION EQUIPMENT

Various instruments are used during the physical exam to help the examiner see, hear, or evaluate the areas of the patient's body that are being assessed. In most cases, the physician is the one who uses the instruments. The medical assistant needs to be familiar with the instruments and supplies, so you are prepared to assist the physician. Basic exam supplies are shown in Figure 17-1.

Instruments should be kept in a designated storage cabinet, drawer, or location in each examination room. The instruments and supplies used depend on the physician's preference. Some basic exam room supplies are always available during the physical examination and may include those listed in Table 17-1.

 PHYSICAL EXAMINATION INSTRUMENTS

Percussion Hammer (Reflex Hammer)

It is used to test neurological reflexes, the nervous system's response to specific stimuli.

The percussion hammer has a stainless steel handle and a hard rubber head (Fig. 17-2). The physician tests the patient's reflexes by striking the hammer over the tendons, the tough cords of tissue connecting muscle to bone.

The tip of the handle also may be used on the sole of the foot to assess the Babinski reflex—an abnormal reflex where stroking the sole of the foot causes the big toe to move upward. The Babinski reflex is a sign of brain or spinal cord injury (except in children under two where it is the normal response). Stroking the sole of the foot should result in the toes curling downward in the plantar reflex.

Table 17-1	Basic Exam Room Supplies	
Tape measure	Nondisposable	Take measurements of parts of the patient's body, chest, or head of an infant and measure size of a skin lesion. Units on the tape may be in inches or centimeters.
Gloves	Disposable	Latex and latex-free gloves are used whenever there may be contact with body fluids or broken skin.
Tongue depressors	Disposable	Wooden device used to press down the tongue during examination of the mouth and throat.
Cotton-tipped applicators	Disposable	Also called swabs. May be used to test sensory reactions and collect samples for laboratory testing.
Patient gown and drape	Disposable	Complete physical examination requires patient to disrobe and put on the gown. The drape is used to cover the patient's lap and legs.

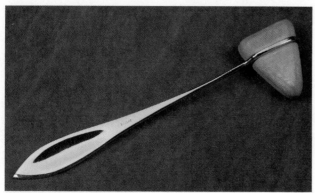

Figure 17-2 A reflex hammer. (Reprinted from Kronenberger J, Ledbetter J. *Jones & Bartlett Learning's Comprehensive Medical Assisting.* 5th ed. Burlington, MA: Jones & Bartlett Learning, LLC; 2016.)

Tuning Fork

A tuning fork is used to test hearing (Fig. 17-3).

It's a stainless steel instrument with two prongs at one end and a handle at the other. The examiner strikes the instrument against her hand, causing the prongs to vibrate. The vibrating prongs produce a humming sound. While it's vibrating, the examiner places its handle against a bony area of the patient's skull, near one of the ears. The patient is asked to describe what, if anything, he is hearing in that ear. The results of this test may lead the physician to order additional auditory tests.

Nasal Speculum

The nasal speculum is a stainless steel instrument, which is inserted into the nostril to help the examiner see inside (Fig. 17-4).

It also may be available in a disposable form. A speculum is a tool designed to allow examiners to investigate body cavities. Using the nasal speculum, the physician inspects:

- The lining of the nose
- The nasal membranes
- The septum, a thin wall between the nostrils that divides the two nasal cavities

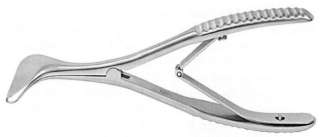

Figure 17-4 A nasal speculum. (Reprinted from Kronenberger J, Ledbetter J. *Jones & Bartlett Learning's Comprehensive Medical Assisting.* 5th ed. Burlington, MA: Jones & Bartlett Learning, LLC; 2016.)

Speculum

A **speculum** is a medical tool that enlarges and separates the opening of a body cavity so the examiner can see the interior structures and mucosa. A nasal speculum and vaginal speculum are routinely used during a complete physical examination.

Otoscope

The **otoscope** allows the examiner to see inside the ear canal and inspect the tympanic membrane (Fig. 17-5).

Also known as the ear drum, the tympanic membrane is a thin, oval membrane between the outer ear and middle ear. It transmits sound vibrations to the inner ear. The otoscope has a stainless steel handle at one end. At the other end is a head that consists of three parts, the light, magnifying lens, and cone-shaped hollow speculum.

A portable otoscope requires batteries to power the light source. An otoscope may be part of a unit attached to a wall. The unit is plugged into an electrical outlet to provide power. The speculum is covered with a disposable cover before it is placed in the ear canal.

Figure 17-6 shows an exam room wall unit otoscope with disposable ear pieces, an ophthalmoscope, and a blood pressure unit.

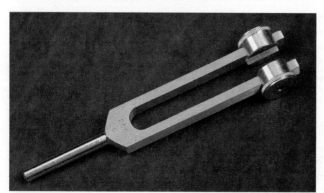

Figure 17-3 A tuning fork. (Reprinted from Kronenberger J, Ledbetter J. *Jones & Bartlett Learning's Comprehensive Medical Assisting.* 5th ed. Burlington, MA: Jones & Bartlett Learning, LLC; 2016.)

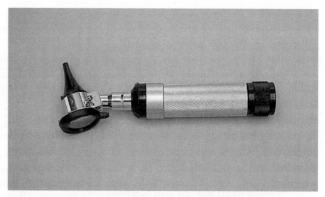

Figure 17-5 A portable otoscope. (Reprinted from Kronenberger J, Ledbetter J. *Jones & Bartlett Learning's Comprehensive Medical Assisting.* 5th ed. Burlington, MA: Jones & Bartlett Learning, LLC; 2016.)

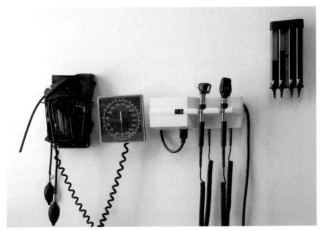

Figure 17-6 Wall-mounted examination instruments. From *left*: sphygmomanometer with cuff, otoscope, ophthalmoscope, and dispenser for disposable otoscope speculum covers. (Image from Shutterstock.com.)

Ophthalmoscope

An **ophthalmoscope** is a medical tool used to inspect the interior structures of the eyes. The ophthalmoscope allows the examiner to inspect the interior structures of the eyes. Like the otoscope, the ophthalmoscope has a handle at one end and a head with several parts including the light, magnifying lens, and an opening to view the eye.

A portable ophthalmoscope, shown in Figure 17-7, requires batteries to power the light source.

The portable unit also may have a common handle with interchangeable otoscope or ophthalmoscope head pieces that can be attached for examination of the eye and ear. The physician may use the otoscope light source to examine the nose and mouth.

Stethoscope

You are probably familiar with the **stethoscope**, an instrument used for listening to body sounds. It has a bell with a diaphragm at one end (Fig. 17-8).

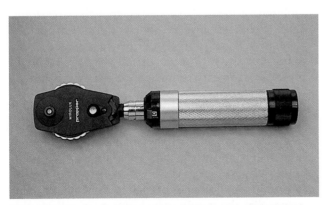

Figure 17-7 A portable ophthalmoscope. (Reprinted from Kronenberger J, Ledbetter J. *Jones & Bartlett Learning's Comprehensive Medical Assisting.* 5th ed. Burlington, MA: Jones & Bartlett Learning, LLC; 2016.)

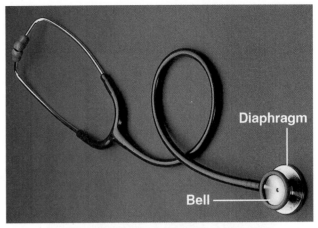

Figure 17-8 A stethoscope. (Reprinted from Kronenberger J, Ledbetter J. *Jones & Bartlett Learning's Comprehensive Medical Assisting.* 5th ed. Burlington, MA: Jones & Bartlett Learning, LLC; 2016.)

Flexible rubber tubing connects the bell to two earpieces. The earpieces have plastic or rubber tips that must be adjusted and directed inward before they are placed in the examiner's ears.

The diaphragm is placed on the patient's body, and the examiner listens to sounds through the earpieces. The stethoscope is typically used to listen to sounds of the heart, lungs, intestines, and carotid arteries.

PHYSICAL EXAMINATION LIGHTING

Special lights help the physician see more clearly during physical exams. It's your responsibility to make sure all these lights are in working order. Turn the light(s) on and off prior to the examination. If a light is battery operated, have additional batteries on hand. It is important to maintain a supply of replacement bulbs for all light sources.

- Overhead examination light—Some offices have an adjustable overhead examination light.
- Gooseneck lamp—This is a floor lamp with a movable stand that bends at the neck (Fig. 17-9). Some examination tables are equipped with a light source similar to the gooseneck light. The physician may use this lamp when overhead lighting is not good enough.
- Penlight—This small light is the size and shape of a ballpoint pen. It can be carried conveniently in a pocket. If no penlight is available, a small flashlight is a good substitute. These small lights provide extra light to a specific area, such as the eye, nose, or throat.

While assisting the physician, you may be asked to direct the examination light or the gooseneck lamp toward a specific area of the body. The physician usually holds the penlight.

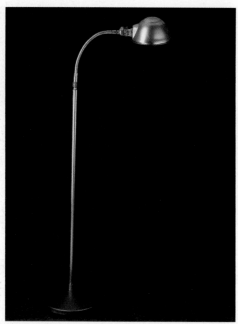

Figure 17-9   A gooseneck examination light. (Reprinted from Kronenberger J, Ledbetter J. *Jones & Bartlett Learning's Comprehensive Medical Assisting.* 5th ed. Burlington, MA: Jones & Bartlett Learning, LLC; 2016.)

SPECIALIZED MEDICAL EXAMINATIONS

Ear, Nose, and Throat Examinations

An **otorhinolaryngologist** is a physician who specializes in treating disorders and diseases of the ears, nose, and throat. During examinations, the physician may

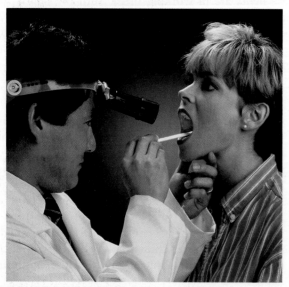

Figure 17-10   A head light. (Reprinted from Kronenberger J, Ledbetter J. *Jones & Bartlett Learning's Comprehensive Medical Assisting.* 5th ed. Burlington, MA: Jones & Bartlett Learning, LLC; 2016.)

wear a headband that has a light or mirror attached. A head light provides direct light to the area being examined.

A mirror reflects light from the examination light into the area being examined (Fig. 17-10).

Other special instruments used by the physician to visualize the throat and the larynx—the part of the throat that contains the vocal cords include the following:

- The laryngeal mirror is a stainless steel instrument with a long slender handle and a small round mirror. It's used to examine areas of the patient's throat and larynx that may not be directly visible.
- The laryngoscope consists of a handle and a head (Fig. 17-11).
- The handle is similar to the battery handle of an otoscope or ophthalmoscope. The head has a small light. Different blades can be attached to the head to help the examiner see the larynx or vocal cords. The blades may be curved or straight.

Study Skill

To assist in learning the equipment necessary for basic and specialty exams, draw a picture of a clinic that has many exam rooms. Assign each exam room a type of exam and write the type of physician that performs that type of exam and the equipment necessary for that type of exam. This activity will help you visualize an actual exam room and what you will need to set up the patient for the exam.

Special Roles for Clinical Medical Assistants

Clinical medical assistants who work in specialized medical offices may need to be familiar with other supplies and instruments. Some examples of specialized medical assistants include the following:

- Ophthalmic medical assistants help with eye care and assist ophthalmologists. Some duties may include testing eye muscle function or teaching patients how to use and care for contact lenses. They also maintain optical instruments related to eye examinations and eye care.
- Podiatric medical assistants assist podiatrists—physicians who care for and treat foot diseases and injuries. These medical assistants may need to make foot impressions and assist with foot surgery. The podiatrist may ask the medical assistant to take x-rays. It is the responsibility of the medical assistant to ensure that the state in which they work allows this task within the scope of practice for a medical assistant. Further education, training, and licensure are required.

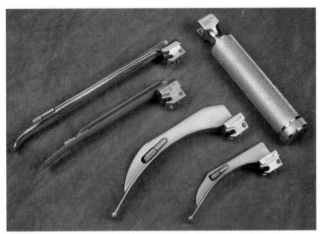

Figure 17-11 Laryngoscope handle and blades (straight and curved). (Reprinted from Kronenberger J, Ledbetter J. *Jones & Bartlett Learning's Comprehensive Medical Assisting.* 5th ed. Burlington, MA: Jones & Bartlett Learning, LLC; 2016.)

Gynecological Examinations

A gynecological examination pertains to the examination of the female reproductive system. A complete physical examination of a female patient may include a pelvic examination and a Papanicolaou (**PAP**) smear. A Pap smear is performed by scraping cells of the wall of the vagina and cervix—the part of the uterus that protrudes into the vagina. The smear is examined with a microscope to detect any abnormal cells, including cancer cells.

Gynecological Equipment

Vaginal Speculum
The vaginal speculum is an instrument that is either nondisposable stainless steel, which needs to be cleaned and sterilized, or it is made of disposable plastic. Figure 17-12 shows a disposable and a nondisposable speculum.

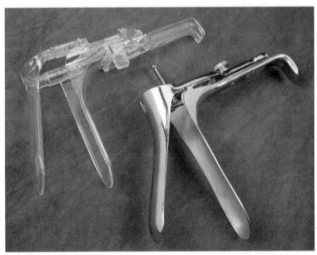

Figure 17-12 Vaginal specula. (Reprinted from Kronenberger J, Ledbetter J. *Jones & Bartlett Learning's Comprehensive Medical Assisting.* 5th ed. Burlington, MA: Jones & Bartlett Learning, LLC; 2016.)

The speculum is inserted into the vagina and is used to expand the vaginal opening. The physician can then examine vaginal canal and cervix. Cells from these structures can be obtained to submit to the laboratory to perform the Pap smear. Other equipment used during a gynecological examination may include the following.

Cotton-Tipped Applicator
A disposable applicator is larger than the small cotton-tipped swabs with which you may be familiar. Figure 17-13 shows a large swab, cervical scraper, and histobrush.

Often, it is used to remove excess vaginal secretions or to apply medications during gynecological examinations.

Lubricant
This is a water-soluble gel used to reduce friction. It is used to allow easier insertion of the vaginal speculum during examination of the vagina and as a lubricant on a gloved finger for manual examination of the vagina. It is also used for rectal examinations of female patients and to examine the rectum and prostate in male patients.

Ayre Spatula or Cervical Scraper
This disposable scraper is about 6 inches long and is made of plastic or wood. One end of the scraper has a tip with an irregular shape (Fig. 17-13). It is placed in the cervical opening and rotated to collect a specimen. The other end of the scraper has a rounded tip. This end may be used to collect a specimen from the vaginal wall.

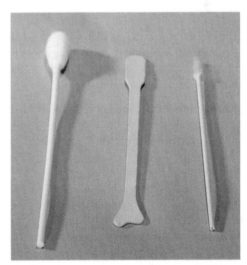

Figure 17-13 Cotton-tipped applicator (*left*), Ayre spatula (*center*), and histobrush (*right*). Cotton-tipped applicators of this size are frequently used to remove excess vaginal secretions or to apply medications during the gynecologic examination. (Reprinted from Kronenberger J, Ledbetter J. *Jones & Bartlett Learning's Comprehensive Medical Assisting.* 5th ed. Burlington, MA: Jones & Bartlett Learning, LLC; 2016.)

Histobrush

This disposable brush is made of nylon or plastic with soft bristles at one end. It may be used to obtain cells for a Pap smear (Fig. 17-13).

The conventional Pap smear was performed by transferring the collected cells to a glass slide, which is sprayed with a fixative and then sent to the laboratory for analysis. The more widely used, comprehensive, and more accurate method is called the ThinPrep Pap Test. The specimen for the ThinPrep method is collected using the brush or plastic spatula and the substance collected is rinsed into a vial of liquid. The vial is sent to the laboratory where the liquid is examined for any disease including cancer cells.

After the specimen is obtained for the Pap smear, a bimanual examination is performed. To perform this examination, two gloved, lubricated fingers from one hand are inserted into the vagina, while the other hand is placed on the abdomen. This allows the physician or practitioner to palpate internal structures in the pelvic cavity.

Case Questions

What should the medical assistant tell Rebecca Martin to reassure her about the physical examination process? What should the medical assistant relay to the physician prior to seeing the patient?

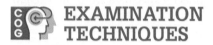 **EXAMINATION TECHNIQUES**

During the examination of a patient, the physician may use different techniques that will help the physician gather information about the patient's health. There are six basic examination techniques:

- **Inspection**—looking at areas of the body to observe physical features
- **Palpation**—touching or moving body areas with the fingers or hands
- **Manipulation**—moving a body part or joint
- **Percussion**—tapping or striking parts of the body with the hand or an instrument to produce sounds
- **Auscultation**—listening to body sounds
- **Mensuration**—the process of measuring

Inspection

The physician inspects the patient both with the naked eye and with instruments. Inspection may be done using room lighting or using a special light source. The physician reviews the patient's general appearance, including:

- Movements
- Color of skin and membranes
- Contours or shapes
- **Symmetry**, equality of size and shape, or **asymmetry**, inequality of size and shape
- Odors

Palpation

Palpation performed with both hands is called bimanual palpation. Palpation performed with the fingers only is a digital exam. The physician palpates areas of the body for several reasons:

- To determine pulse characteristics
- To detect the presence of growths, swelling, tenderness, or pain
- To assess the size, shape, and location of organs
- To assess skin temperature, moisture, texture, and elasticity

Manipulation

The physician moves the arms and legs at the joints to determine the patient's ability for extension and flexion. Extension is a movement of the joint that increases the angle between the bones at the joint. Flexion refers to bending a limb at the joint to decrease the angle between the bones. Extending and flexing the joints help the examiner determine the range of motion (**ROM**)—the ability of the joint to go through normal motions.

Percussion

Percussion allows the physician to determine the position, size, and density of the air or fluid that is inside a body organ or cavity. When performing percussion, the physician listens for sounds and feels the vibrations. Two types of percussion are performed with the hand:

- Direct percussion refers to striking the body with a finger.
- Indirect percussion is placing a finger on an area of the body and then striking the finger with a finger of the other hand.

Auscultation

The physician places a stethoscope or ear directly on areas of the patient's body including the heart, fetal heart tones, lungs, abdomen, intestines, and blood vessels.

Mensuration

The process of measuring body parts including the measurement of:

- The patient's height and weight
- The pressure of the patient's grip
- The flexion and extension in an extremity
- The size and depth of a wound
- The circumference of the head, chest, or waist
- The length and circumference of a limb
- The expansion of the uterus

 PREPARING THE EXAMINATION ROOM

Medical assistants are usually asked to prepare examination rooms. The room should be clean, well lighted, well ventilated, odor free, and at a comfortable temperature for the patient. Equipment and supplies should be prepared including the:

- Examination table—The table should be cleaned between patients with an approved disinfectant. You must remove used table paper and replace it with clean paper.
- Equipment—Ensure that the equipment is in working order at the beginning of each day. It should be clean and ready to use.
- Supplies—Make sure the room has a supply of gloves, cotton-tipped applicators, and other supplies needed during an examination.

 PREPARING THE PATIENT

After the room is ready, the medical assistant can escort the patient to the treatment area. Call the patient from the waiting area by name and confirm that it is the right patient. It is important to use good interpersonal skills when interacting with each patient. The goal is to put the patient at ease and ensure that the patient has confidence in you and the physician. Treat each patient as an individual. Speak clearly with a confident tone of voice as you ask questions and explain any procedures.

Cultural Connection

Patients from various cultural backgrounds may seek medical treatment in your medical facility. They may have very different expectations and reactions to treatment that come from their own cultural experiences. How can you make a good connection with patients from a culture that is different from yours? These are some tips to help you assist these patients and their families:

- Provide patients with detailed explanations about treatments. Details that are obvious to you may not be clear to the patient.
- Respect cultural practices and values that are different from yours.
- Listen carefully to the patient's concerns. If you do not understand what is being said, ask the patient to repeat it.
- Be aware that in some cultures, the husband speaks for his wife and she will not speak or answer directly to you.
- Individuals from certain cultures do not make direct eye contact.
- Touching or getting too close to the patient, or pointing with your finger, may be considered rude or disrespectful in specific cultures.
- Some patients may appear uncomfortable when asked to disrobe for an examination. Explain that the physician needs to visually examine the body and only that area will be uncovered.
- In some cultures, female patient's clothing may not be removed unless a female family member is present.
- Talk to the physician if the patient does not want to follow the instructions. The physician and the patient may be able to reach a compromise that will allow the examination to be performed.

 GETTING READY FOR THE EXAMINATION

Before the physician sees the patient, you may be responsible for recording the patient's past history (**PH**), chief complaint (**CC**), present illness (**PI**), and vital signs. A urine specimen may be indicated prior to a complete physical examination. Ask the patient to collect a specimen prior to the examination. When the patient's bladder is empty, it is easier for the physician to examine the abdomen. Escort the patient to the restroom and provide instructions for collecting the specimen.

In the examination room, give the patient instructions for disrobing. You'll need to explain which clothes to remove and how to put on an examination gown. Depending on the type of exam to be performed, patients may wear the gown with the opening in the front or the back. For example, a patient who needs a breast exam will wear the gown open in the front. To protect the patient's privacy, the medical assistant will leave the room while the patient undresses. Some patients may have special needs requiring your assistance, including:

- Elderly patients or patients with physical disabilities may use wheelchairs, walkers, or canes to move from place to place. In the examination room, they may need your help to disrobe, to move onto the examination table, and/or to move into different positions during the examination.
- Pregnant patients may require assistance to move onto the examination table or to assume different positions during the examination. Some examination positions may not be suitable for women in the later stages of pregnancy.

When the patient has put on the examination gown, you may have the patient sit on the examination table until the physician is ready to see the patient. If the patient is feeble or unsteady, the patient may not be safe sitting on the exam table unattended. You may have the patient sit in a chair in the exam room until the physician is ready to see the patient. Then you would assist the patient onto the exam table.

When a patient is sitting on the exam table in a gown, place a drape on the patient's lap to cover the legs. The patient is now ready to see the physician.

At all times, you want to respect and protect the patient's privacy. Here are some tips:

- Make sure the door is closed or that the patient is in a screened area when changing.
- Do not ask a patient who is wearing a gown to walk through public areas, such as the waiting room, to get to other rooms.
- Expose only the body parts that are needed for the examination. Use drapes to cover exposed body areas.

 ASSISTING THE PHYSICIAN

As a medical assistant, your responsibilities involve assisting the physician as well as the patient.

- Helping the physician—You may need to hand the physician instruments or supplies or direct an examination light. For legal reasons, you also may be required to remain in the room when a male physician examines a female patient or when a female physician examines a male patient. You will also be expected to help the patient into different examination positions.
  - Move the body slowly.
  - Watch for signs that the patient may be uncomfortable.
  - Provide a small pillow to help the patient feel more at ease.
- Helping the patient—You may need to assist the patient to move into the proper position for an

examination. You will assist the physician to adjust the drape to expose only the parts of the body being examined.

PATIENT EXAMINATION POSITIONS

Various patient examination positions may be required in order for the physician to appropriately examine the patient (Fig. 17-14). Table 17-2 is a list of exam positions: the body part examined using the position and the equipment, instruments, and supplies used for the examination.

As the patient changes positions, be sure to adjust the drapes to protect patient privacy. Patient examination positions include the following:

- Erect, standing, or anatomical position—Also known as anatomical position, the patient stands erect and faces forward with the arms at the sides.
- Sitting position—The patient sits erect at the end of the examination table. The feet are supported on a footrest or stool. Because the back is not supported, this position may be difficult for weak or elderly patients.
- Supine position—The patient lies on the back with arms at the sides. A pillow may be placed under the head for comfort. Most patients are comfortable in this position.
- Dorsal recumbent position—The patient is supine with the legs slightly separated, the knees bent, and the feet flat on the table. When the knees are bent, there is less stress on the back. Some elderly patients or patients with back pain may find this position more comfortable than the supine position.
- Lithotomy position—This position is similar to the dorsal recumbent position. The patient's legs are well separated and the patient's feet are supported in stirrups instead of flat on the table. The stirrups should be level with each other, about 12 inches out from the edge of the table. You may help patients move their feet in and out of the stirrups. Moving both feet at the same time prevents back strain. For patients who have difficulty getting into this position, the dorsal recumbent position may be used.
- Sims' position—The patient lies on the left side with the left arm and left shoulder behind the body. The right leg and arm are sharply flexed on the table. The left knee is slightly flexed. Patients who are uncomfortable lying on their sides, such as those with hip joint problems, may find this position difficult.
- Prone position—The patient lies on the abdomen with the head supported and turned to one side. The arms may be under the head or by the sides, depending on

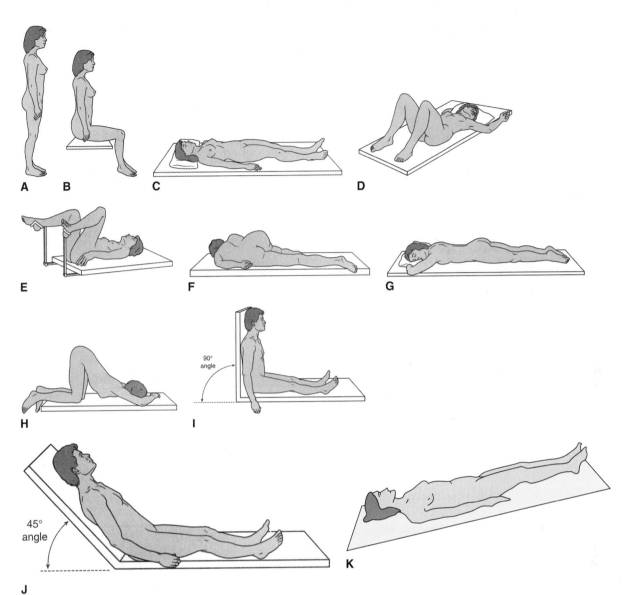

Figure 17-14   Patient exam positions. **A.** Erect or standing. **B.** Sitting. **C.** Supine. **D.** Dorsal recumbent. **E.** Lithotomy. **F.** Sims. **G.** Prone. **H.** Knee-chest. **I.** Fowler. **J.** Semi-Fowler. **K.** Trendelenburg. (Reprinted from Kronenberger J, Ledbetter J. *Jones & Bartlett Learning's Comprehensive Medical Assisting.* 5th ed. Burlington, MA: Jones & Bartlett Learning, LLC; 2016.)

which is more comfortable for the patient. This position is not used for an obese patient or a patient in the late stages of pregnancy. It may also be too uncomfortable for elderly patients or patients with breathing difficulties to be in this position.

- Knee-chest position—The patient kneels on the table with the arms and chest on the table. The patient's hips are elevated and back straight. The patient's head is turned to one side. You may need to help guide the patient into the correct position. Elderly patients, pregnant patients, or obese patients may find this position difficult.
- Fowler position—The head of the examination table is elevated 80 to 90 degrees. The patient is sitting with

the torso upright and the legs extended on the examination table.

- Semi-Fowler position—The examination table head is elevated 30 to 45 degrees. The patient is in a half-sitting position with the knees slightly bent.
- Trendelenburg position—The patient lies supine on the table. The lower end of the table is raised about 30 degrees so the head is lower than the feet and legs. This position is not used commonly in a medical office setting.
- Reverse Trendelenburg position—The patient lies supine on the table with the head higher than the feet and legs. The head of the table is elevated about 30 degrees to reach this position.

Table 17-2 | **Examination Positions and Their Uses**

Position	Body Parts Examined	Equipment, Instruments, and Supplies Used
Sitting	General appearance	
	Head, neck	Stethoscope
	Eyes	Ophthalmoscope, penlight
	Ears	Otoscope, tuning fork
	Nose	Nasal speculum, penlight, substances to smell
	Sinuses	Penlight
	Mouth	Gloves, tongue blade, penlight
	Throat	Gloves, tongue blade, penlight, laryngeal mirror, laryngoscope
	Axilla, arms	
	Chest	Stethoscope
	Breasts	
	Upper back	Stethoscope
	Reflexes	Percussion hammer
Supine	Chest	Stethoscope
	Abdomen	Stethoscope
	Breasts	
Lithotomy	Female genitalia and internal	Gloves, vaginal speculum, Ayre spatula, his-
Dorsal recumbent	organs	tobrush, lubricant, microscopic slide or liquid
Sims		preparation
	Female rectum	Gloves, lubricant, fecal occult blood test
Standing	Male genitalia and hernia	Gloves
	Spine, posture, gait, coordination, balance, strength, flexibility	
Dorsal recumbent	Male rectum	Gloves, lubricant, fecal occult blood test
Sims	Prostate	Gloves, lubricant
Prone	Back, spine, legs	
Knee-chest	Rectum	Gloves, lubricant, anoscope, proctoscope, or sigmoidoscope; fecal occult blood test
	Female genitalia	Glove, lubricant, vaginal speculum, Ayre spatula, histobrush
	Prostate	Gloves, lubricant
Fowler's	Head, neck, chest	Stethoscope
Trendelenburg	Chest, abdomen, pelvis, legs, feet	Stethoscope
Reverse Trendelenburg	Head, chest, abdomen, legs, feet	Stethoscope

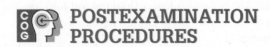

POSTEXAMINATION PROCEDURES

After the physician has completed the patient examination, the medical assistant has many responsibilities that include the following:

- Offering to help the patient return to a sitting position.
- Directing the patient to dress, assisting the patient as needed.
- Providing the patient with follow-up instructions.
- Escorting the patient to the front office to:
  - Check out and discuss any billing issues.

Table 17-3	Common Tests Associated with Complete Physical Examination		
Test	**Purpose**		**Medical Assistant's Role**
Complete Blood Count (CBC) Blood Chemistry	Blood tests are the most commonly performed medical tests. They provide information about the patient's general health status and can be used to detect various diseases, such as anemia and heart disease.		Draw specimens for blood tests ordered by the physician. If testing is not performed in the office, the medical assistant will process the specimen to be sent to the laboratory.
Urinalysis	A series of tests may be performed to examine the urine's appearance and acidity and the presence of proteins and sugars. These tests are used to detect infection and/or disease.		Medical assistants need to instruct the patient on various methods of urine collection. Some basic urine tests are performed in the office by the medical assistant.
Chest x-ray	Chest x-ray can be used to detect abnormalities of the lungs, heart, large blood vessels, ribs, and thoracic spine.		Only qualified x-ray technicians will obtain a chest x-ray. Medical assistants may need to provide directions to the office where the x-ray will be taken.
Electrocardiogram (ECG)	An electrocardiogram records the electrical activity of the heart. The report is used to determine if there are defects or disease of the heart.		The medical assistant may be trained to perform an electrocardiogram. Interpreting the ECG is the responsibility of the physician.

- Schedule a future appointment.
- Schedule follow-up treatment, tests, or procedures. See Table 17-3 for Common Tests Associated with Complete Physical Examination.

CLEANING THE EXAMINATION ROOM

The examination room cannot be used for the next patient until it has been cleaned and restocked with supplies. Disinfectant products are used to clean equipment that cannot be sterilized such as the otoscope and ophthalmoscope handles. The examination table is wiped clean with a disinfectant and table paper replaced. All disposable supplies that were used must be discarded. The waste receptacle in the room should be emptied.

THE SEQUENCE OF THE PHYSICAL EXAMINATION

The physician performs the physical examination in an orderly sequence. The medical assistant needs to know this sequence in order to best assist the physician during the examination. It is important that you anticipate the physician's needs. The sequence of examination is:

- Examination of specific areas of the body from head to toe—head and neck; eyes, ears, nose, and sinuses; mouth and throat; chest, breasts, abdomen, groin, genitalia, and rectum; legs
- Reflex testing
- Observation of posture, gait, and coordination; tests of balance and strength

EXAMINING THE BODY

Throughout the examination, the physician observes the patient's general appearance, behavior, speech, posture (the position of the body and its limbs), nutritional status, hair distribution, and skin. Now let's take a detailed look at the specific parts of the body the physician examines.

Head and Neck

The physician inspects the patient's skull, face, scalp, and hair. These structures also are palpated for size, shape, and symmetry. This includes looking for nodules, masses, and local trauma or injury. The patient may be asked to move his head in all directions to assess the range of motion. This allows the physician to check for any limitations of movement. Structures of the neck are also palpated.

- Trachea—This main airway for the passage of air to the lungs is sometimes referred to as the "windpipe."
- Lymph nodes or lymph glands—These small bean-shaped structures help fight infections. There are some lymph nodes located on the anterior neck.

- Thyroid—This gland is located in front of the neck below the larynx, the voice box. It produces substances that regulate metabolism and growth. The thyroid is palpated for size and symmetry. The patient may be asked to swallow to facilitate palpation.
- Carotid arteries—These are large blood vessels located on both sides of the neck. They supply oxygenated blood to the brain. The carotid arteries may be palpated and auscultated for abnormal sounds.

Eyes

The medical assistant often performs a visual acuity test with the patient before the physician's examination. A Snellen chart is usually used for this examination. For some patients, a color vision test may be performed. An Ishihara chart is used for this examination. It consists of a series of color plates or charts.

In addition to these vision tests, the physician will examine these structures of the eye.

- Sclera—The fibrous tissue that covers the eye. It is the white part of the eye. It is examined to be sure the color is normal.
- Pupil—The black, round opening in the center of the eye that allows light to pass through. The pupil will change size as more or less light is present. The physician uses a penlight to check that the patient's pupils are equal in size. The pupils will be examined to make sure they are round in shape and react normally to light. Normal pupil reaction is recorded as **PERRLA**, which means that the pupils are equal, round, and reactive to light and accommodation. **Accommodation** refers to the ability of the pupils to adjust when focusing on objects at different distances.
- Eye movement—The physician asks the patient to watch movements of her fingers to assess eye movements. Normal eye movement is documented as EOM, extraocular movement intact. Extraocular refers to outside the eye. This abbreviation indicates that that the eyes move appropriately to track moving objects.
- Peripheral vision—The ability to see things off to the side while looking straight ahead is known as peripheral vision.
- Retina—The light-sensitive area at the back of the eye. It may be viewed and assessed using the ophthalmoscope. The ophthalmoscope allows the physician to look inside the eye and examine the condition of the retina. The physician also looks at the blood vessels in the eye to check for any signs of disease.

Ears

The outer ear called the pinna or auricle is palpated for size, shape, and symmetry. The physician inspects the ear canal using an otoscope. Cerumen, ear wax, may be present in the ear canal. An accumulation of ear wax may lead to impaired hearing. The physician also examines the tympanic membrane, or eardrum. The tympanic membrane is evaluated for color and to ensure that it is intact with no tears. Normally, it appears pearly gray and concave. An infection of the ear may cause discoloration of the tympanic membrane. Accumulation of fluid behind the ear drum can cause the ear drum to bulge outward.

Nose and Sinuses

The physician may examine both the exterior and the interior of the patient's nose. The exterior is palpated for any abnormalities. The interior is inspected using a nasal speculum and light.

- Nasal septum—Checks the position of the nasal septum for deviation. The nasal septum is a thin wall that separates the nasal cavities. Sometimes, it can be displaced to the left or right as a result of injury. A damaged nasal septum can block the nasal passage.
- Nostrils—Check the color of the mucosa, the membrane lining the cavity. The nostrils are also examined for the presence of any discharge, lesions, obstructions, swelling, tenderness, or polyps. Polyps are soft growths on membrane linings. They may be benign (harmless) or malignant (cancerous).

The physician might test the patient's sense of smell. The patient closes his eyes and tries to identify a common substance such as alcohol, peppermint, lemon, or strawberry by smell alone. The physician also may inspect or palpate the paranasal sinuses. Sinuses are air-filled cavities in the bones of the skull and face. The paranasal sinuses are located near and are connected to the nose.

Mouth and Throat

The physician inspects the mucous membranes of mouth, gums, teeth, tongue, tonsils, and throat. Supplies and instruments used to examine these structures include the following:

- Disposable gloves
- A light source
- A tongue blade
- A laryngeal mirror, if necessary

The physician also assesses general dental hygiene and the functioning of salivary glands. The goal is to look for abnormalities in the oral cavity, such as abnormal color, ulcerations, or nodules.

Chest

The patient's gown is removed to the waist so the physician can examine the anterior chest. The general appearance and symmetry of the chest and breast area are evaluated. The respiratory rate and pattern are noted, as well as any obvious masses or swelling.

Examination of the chest includes palpation of the axillary lymph nodes and the area over the heart. The physician may use percussion to assess underlying structures. Using a stethoscope, the auscultation method of examination is used to evaluate lungs for abnormal breath sounds. During this examination, the patient may be asked to take several deep breaths. The physician also assesses heart sounds and the apical pulse.

The posterior chest is also inspected and palpated. The physician examines the muscles of the back and spine. Percussion of the back helps assess the lungs. With a stethoscope, the physician listens to posterior lung sounds. Again, the patient may be asked to take deep breaths to facilitate the examination.

Breast Examination

Breasts may be palpated in both male and female patients. The supine position is preferred for palpation. In this position, the breast tissue flattens out, making abnormalities easier to feel. The examination includes the:

- Breast tissue and nipple
- Tissue extending up to the clavicle, the collarbone
- Axillary tissue, the underarm or armpit
- Tissue down to the bottom of the rib cage

Patient Education

Teaching Breast Self-Examination for Female Patients

Your goal is to help your patient learn how to properly perform her own breast examination. Use a breast model if one is available or an instruction sheet containing illustrations. Teaching models should be sanitized with each use. Participants should do proper handwashing prior to touching the models.

1. Explain why the breasts should be examined regularly. Tell the patient that she needs to check for lumps, dimples, and thickened areas, as these could be signs of malignancy. She should be encouraged to examine her breasts at the same time each month, about a week after her menstrual period. Note that early detection leads to early diagnosis and treatment.
2. Tell the patient that her breast tissue needs to be examined in three different positions for the most thorough examination.
   - Explain that she should disrobe and inspect her breasts in front of a mirror. She needs to first place her hands on her hips and then raise her arms above her head. Tell the patient that she needs to look for any changes in the breast contour, or any swelling, dimpling of the skin, or changes in the nipple. Regular inspection will show her what is normal for her.
   - In the shower, the patient should feel each breast with her hands using the flat part of her first three fingers. Tell her to use her right hand to lightly press over all areas of her left breast. She should use her left hand to examine her right breast in the same way. Explain that she needs to check for any lumps, hard knots, or thickenings. Tell the patient that doing this in the shower will be easier because her hands will glide more smoothly over wet skin.
   - After showering, the patient should lie down and place a pillow or folded towel under her right shoulder. This helps distribute the breast tissue more evenly on the chest. Her right hand is placed behind her head. She should examine her right breast using the flat part of the fingers of her left hand. Describe how to use small, circular motions, beginning at the outermost top of the breast and moving clockwise around it. Remind the patient to palpate every part of the breast tissue, moving her fingers in toward the nipple. When she is finished, she will place the towel or pillow under the left shoulder and repeat the procedure, using her right hand to examine her left breast.
3. Tell the patient also to check for any abnormal discharge from her nipples. To do this, she should gently squeeze each nipple using her thumb and index finger. Tell her that she should report any abnormal knots, lumps, thickening, or discharge to the physician.
4. Provide the patient with a patient education instruction sheet or pamphlet for use at home.
5. Document your teaching in the patient's chart.

Abdomen and Groin

After examining the breasts, the drape is lowered to expose the body from the abdomen to the pubic area. The patient's chest is draped or gowned to just below the breasts.

The abdomen is inspected for contour, symmetry, and pulsations from the aorta—the main artery that carries blood from the heart to the body. The aorta extends from the heart down the center of the thoracic and abdominal cavities.

The physician uses a stethoscope to listen to bowel sounds. Percussion may be used to determine the outlines of the abdominal organs. Palpation is used to assess organ enlargement, masses, pain, or tenderness.

The lower abdomen and groin are palpated to assess enlargement of the inguinal lymph nodes. Inguinal means related to the groin region. Palpation also is used to determine the presence of a hernia. A hernia often results from a weakness or tears in the muscle allowing the underlying organ or structure to protrude through the opening. The physician also may palpate the femoral arteries, large arteries that pass through the right and left groin area and extend into the thigh.

Genitalia and Rectum: Male Patients

The physician follows a routine series of steps in examining the male genitalia and rectum.

1. The physician puts on clean, disposable gloves to examine the external male genitalia and the rectum. The genitalia are inspected to check for symmetry, lesions, swelling, masses, and hair distribution. The scrotal contents may be visualized using the transillumination technique in a darkened room. The scrotum is palpated for testicular size, contour, and consistency.
2. The patient is then asked to bear down as if having a bowel movement. The physician places a gloved index finger upward along the side of the scrotum in the inguinal ring to check for a hernia.
3. To check the anal region for lesions or hemorrhoids, the physician will have the patient stand and bend over the exam table or lie on the examination table in Sims position. The physician inserts a lubricated gloved finger into the anus and palpates the rectal sphincter muscle and prostate gland for size, consistency, and any masses. The prostate gland is a gland in men that produces the fluid part of semen.

After the rectal exam, an occult blood test, a test for hidden blood, may be performed on any stool obtained from the gloved finger. After the examination of these areas, provide the patient tissues to wipe off any excess lubricant.

Patient Education

Teaching Testicular Self-Examination for Male Patients

It will take about 10 minutes to teach a male patient how to perform a testicular self-examination. Using a testicular model or pictures, explain to the patient how to examine each testicle. Teaching models should be sanitized with each use. Participants should do proper hand washing prior to touching the models.

1. Tell the patient to gently roll each testicle between his fingers and thumb to check for lumps and thickenings. Tell him to roll each testicle in a horizontal motion and then in a vertical one. Both hands should be used to check each testicle to make sure all areas are palpated.
2. Explain that at the top of each testicle is a cord-like structure called the epididymis, which stores and transports sperm. The patient should be able to identify this structure to avoid mistaking it for an abnormal growth or lump.
3. Instruct the patient to report any abnormal lumps or thickenings to the physician.
4. Provide the patient with an instruction sheet to use at home.
5. Document your teaching in the patient's chart.

Genitalia and Rectum: Female Patients

The female genitalia and rectum usually are examined with the patient in the lithotomy position. One corner of the drape extends over the genitalia, and the other corner covers her chest. A light source is used to direct light on the vaginal area. There are several steps involved in this exam.

1. Wearing clean, disposable gloves, the physician inspects the external genitalia for lesions, edema or swelling, cysts, discharge, and hair distribution.
2. The physician inserts the vaginal speculum. This allows the physician to easily inspect the vaginal canal mucosa and cervix. A Pap smear from the cervix is obtained, and the speculum is removed.
3. The physician performs a bimanual examination to palpate internal reproductive organs. During this examination, the physician checks the organs for size, contour, consistency, and any masses.

A rectovaginal examination is performed to examine the posterior uterus and vaginal wall. The physician places a gloved index finger in vagina and a gloved and lubricated middle finger in rectum at same time.

The rectum is inspected and palpated for lesions, hemorrhoids, and sphincter tone. A stool specimen may be obtained from the gloved finger and tested for occult blood.

 GUIDELINES FOR WOMEN

There are several general guidelines for women, regarding gynecological and breast examinations.

- Pap smear—The first Pap smear is recommended at ages 18 to 20. After the first Pap smear, it's recommended that women have a Pap smear every year.

Breast examination—The physician should examine the breasts every 1 to 3 years for women ages 20 to 39 to detect lumps and thickenings that could be malignancies. For women age 40 and older, an annual breast examination is recommended. Patients also should perform regular breast self-examinations. They may detect abnormalities that should be reported to their physicians.

Mammogram—These x-rays of the breast are used to detect abnormalities or disease. Annual mammograms are recommended from the age of 40. If a patient is at risk for developing breast cancer, a physician may recommend mammograms earlier and more often.

Case Question

Knowing that the patient is anxious about the physical examination process, what can the medical assistant say to encourage Rebecca Martin to perform breast self-examination on a regular basis?

Legs

Visual inspection of the legs is performed to check for the presence of varicose veins. These are abnormally large, twisted blood vessels just below the skin that can cause pain, swelling, or itching. Peripheral pulse sites are palpated with the patient in the supine position. These sites may be palpated again when the patient is standing.

Posture, Gait, and Reflexes

With the patient standing, the physician will check the patient's general posture. The patient may be asked to walk or perform other movements so the physician can assess gait and coordination.

- **Gait** refers to the style or way in which a person walks.
- Coordination is the way the muscles and groups of muscles work together during movement.

The physician may ask the patient to do a balance test. The patient will stand with feet together and eyes closed. Normally, the patient will be able to maintain their balance. Other aspects of body movements that may be tested are range of motion and the strength of the arms and legs.

Reflexes

To test body reflexes, the patient needs to be in a sitting position. The physician strikes the tendon with a percussion hammer to observe the reaction of the body part. A tendon is a structure that attached a muscle to bone. The tendons that are usually tested include the following:

- Biceps tendon—A tendon of the large muscle on the front of the upper arm.
- Triceps tendon—The tendon of the muscle on the back of the upper arm that extends the elbow.
- Patellar tendons—Sometimes known as the patellar ligaments. Ligaments are similar to tendons. They are tough bands of tissue that connect bone to bone or cartilage. The patellar tendons connect the patella, or kneecap, to the leg bone known as the tibia.
- Achilles tendon—A large band of tissue connecting the gastrocnemius muscle on the back of the leg to the bone in the heel. This is the largest tendon in the human body.
- Plantar tendons—Several tendons on the sole (bottom) of the foot.

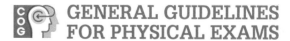

GENERAL GUIDELINES FOR PHYSICAL EXAMS

How often should patients have a complete physical examination? Physicians may vary in their recommendations, but here are some general guidelines.

- Ages 20 to 40, physical examinations may be performed every 1 to 3 years.
- Over 40, a physical examination every year is recommended.

Patients who are being treated for a medical condition may have a physical examination more frequently. At age 40, it is recommended that all patients have a baseline electrocardiogram (**ECG**)—a test that records the electrical activity of the heart.

Screening for Colon and Rectal Cancer

Beginning at age 50, patients should be tested for colon and rectal cancer. There are several different approaches recommended for colon and rectal cancer screening.

- Annual rectal examination and fecal occult blood test—Patients with increased risk for developing colon or rectal cancer may begin screening earlier or have screening more often.
- Flexible sigmoidoscopy—The physician examines the lining of the rectum and lower part of the colon with a flexible, lighted tube (Fig. 17-15).

This test is recommended every 5 years. It may be used in conjunction with annual fecal occult blood tests.

- Colonoscopy—The method of examining the colon—a test in which a long, flexible instrument with a light and lens on the end is inserted into the rectum and

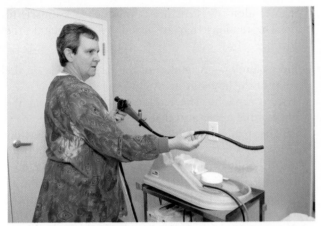

Figure 17-15 A flexible sigmoidoscope. (Reprinted from Kronenberger J, Ledbetter J. *Jones & Bartlett Learning's Comprehensive Medical Assisting.* 5th ed. Burlington, MA: Jones & Bartlett Learning, LLC; 2016.)

colon. It allows physicians to examine the lining of the colon and rectum for abnormalities. Some physicians recommend a colonoscopy at age 50. If the results are normal, this test is recommended every 10 years.

Patient Education

Teaching Warning Signs

You should take every opportunity to teach patients about signs that might signal health problems. Important signals that should not be ignored are frequent, severe headaches and persistent abdominal pain. Patient education also includes teaching patients to recognize the early warning signs of cancer. One way to help patients remember the signs is the acronym **CAUTION**:

C Change in bowel or bladder habits
A *A sore that does not heal*
U *Unusual bleeding or discharge*
T *Thickening, lumps, or changes in the shape of breasts or testicles*
I *Indigestion or difficulty swallowing*
O *Obvious change in a wart or mole*
N *Nagging cough or hoarseness of the voice*

Parents and guardians should also know the additional signs to watch for in children.

- Continual crying for no obvious reason
- Unexplained nausea and vomiting
- General failure to thrive
- Spontaneous bleeding or bleeding that does not stop
- Bumps, lumps, masses, or swelling anywhere on the body
- Frequent stumbling for no apparent reason

 # IMMUNIZATIONS FOR ADULTS

Immunizations are not just for children. Some immunizations are recommended for adults. The medical assistant should be familiar with the recommended schedule of immunizations for adults. The patient's immunization record should be reviewed annually to ensure that all immunizations are up to date.

- A tetanus booster should be given every 10 years or sooner if the patient has an open wound.
- One injection of pneumonia vaccine is recommended for all adults over age 65 years and one or two injections for younger adults with certain health problems.
- Adults born after 1957 should be vaccinated for mumps, measles, and rubella unless they are already immune to these diseases.
- Influenza vaccine for influenza A and B should be given annually after age 50 and after age 19 for persons with certain health problems.
- A series of three hepatitis B injections is recommended for adults who work in certain high-risk occupations or engage in certain high-risk activities.
- A series of two hepatitis A injections is recommended for adults who work in certain high-risk occupations, who engage in certain high-risk activities, or who have certain blood disorders or liver disease.

Case Question

 The medical assistant will need to provide a tetanus booster for Rebecca Martin. If the patient inquires about the reason for the injection, what can the medical assistant say to clearly explain why it is important that the patient receives this injection?

Procedure 17-1 | Cleaning and Preparing the Examination Room

Equipment: PPE, sharps container, gloves, paper towels, disinfectant, and biohazard waste container.

1. Wash your hands and put on clean, disposable gloves. If there's a chance of contact with soiled dressings, body fluids, or other contaminated items, put on personal protective equipment such as a disposable gown, protective eyewear, and shoe coverings.

2. Discard all disposable waste in the appropriate biohazard, sharps, or regular waste container.
   - Any broken glass requires special care. Use a dustpan and brush, or forceps if necessary, to pick up glass fragments and dispose of them properly. They may be contaminated.
   - Remove soiled examination table paper and linens.
   - Remove all soiled reusable instruments for disinfection or sterilization.

3. Remove the gloves and wash your hands. Put on a new pair of gloves to continue tasks. Using disposable paper towels, remove any visible soil from countertops, cabinets, or other surfaces in the room.

4. Wipe all surfaces with an approved disinfectant. Take care to clean every surface to prevent the spread of microorganisms.

5. Check the protective coverings on equipment in the office. If they are soiled, clean or replace them. Disinfect office equipment and allow it to air-dry before replacing any protective coverings.

6. Dispose of the paper towels in the biohazard waste container. Remove the gloves and discard them into the biohazard waste container. Wash your hands.

7. Check the supply of items that are kept in the examination room, such as cotton applicators, tongue blades, patient gowns, and instruments. Restock supplies.

8. Set up equipment and supplies needed for the next examination, including clean examination table paper.

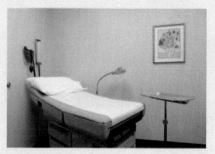

(Reprinted from Kronenberger J, Ledbetter J. *Jones & Bartlett Learning's Comprehensive Medical Assisting.* 5th ed. Burlington, MA: Jones & Bartlett Learning, LLC; 2016.)

9. Check equipment to ensure it is working properly, such as the otoscope and ophthalmoscope.

10. Select the proper gown for the patient and place it on the clean examination table. Set out any clean drapes needed for the examination.

11. Return any unused supplies and items to their proper places.

Procedure 17-2 | Preparing the Adult Patient for the Physical Examination

Equipment: Patient medical record, weight scale with height bar, spygmomanometer, stethoscope, Snellen eye chart, thermometer, and patient gown.

1. Wash your hands.

2. Greet the patient by name and escort him to the prepared examining room. Identifying the patient by name helps to prevent errors.

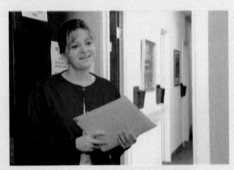

(Reprinted from Kronenberger J, Ledbetter J. *Jones & Bartlett Learning's Comprehensive Medical Assisting.* 5th ed. Burlington, MA: Jones & Bartlett Learning, LLC; 2016.)

3. Explain the procedure. This may help the patient feel less anxious.

4. Obtain and record the patient's medical history and chief complaint.

5. Measure and record the patient's vital signs, height, weight, and visual acuity. These measurements help give the physician an overall picture of the patient's health.

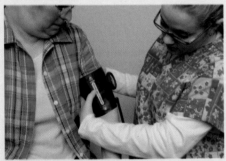

(Reprinted from Kronenberger J, Ledbetter J. *Jones & Bartlett Learning's Comprehensive Medical Assisting.* 5th ed. Burlington, MA: Jones & Bartlett Learning, LLC; 2016.)

6. If the physician requires it, instruct the patient to obtain a urine specimen. Even if a urine specimen is not part of the physical examination, an empty bladder makes abdominal and/or pelvic examinations more comfortable. Direct the patient to the bathroom.

7. When the patient returns to the examination room, provide instructions for disrobing and explain how to put on the gown, open in the front or the back.
   - The gown must open in the direction that provides the best accessibility for the examination.
   - Leave the room unless the patient needs help.
   - Elderly and disabled persons may need help disrobing and/or putting on the gown.

8. Assist the patient to sit on the end of the examining table. The sitting position is often the first position used by the physician. Cover the patient's legs with a drape.

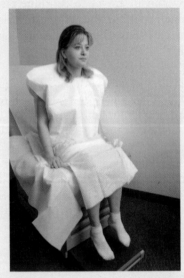

(Reprinted from Kronenberger J, Ledbetter J. *Jones & Bartlett Learning's Comprehensive Medical Assisting.* 5th ed. Burlington, MA: Jones & Bartlett Learning, LLC; 2016.)

9. Enter all information into the patient's electronic record or if a paper chart is used, place it in a secure area outside the examination room and notify the physician that the patient is ready.

Procedure 17-3 | Assisting with Patients in Wheelchairs

Equipment: Wheelchair and exam table.

1. Wash your hands and greet the patient by name. If you think you need help moving the patient, ask another staff member to assist you. Don't risk hurting yourself by trying to move the patient alone.

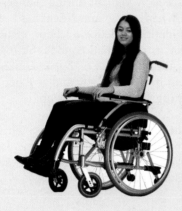

2. Bring the wheelchair as close as possible to the end of the examination table. Locate the wheelchair at a 90-degree angle to the table to minimize the distance for moving the patient.

3. Lock the wheels to stop the wheelchair from moving.

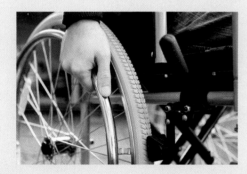

4. Check to make sure the patient is wearing shoes or slippers with nonskid soles. Lift the patient's feet off of the foot rests. Fold up the foot rests so the patient does not trip over them.

5. Keep your own feet in front of the patient's feet to prevent the patient from slipping.

6. For some patients, you may need to place a footstool in front of the table to support their feet.

7. If you are moving the patient yourself, face the patient and ask the patient to hold onto your shoulders. Your knees should be in line with the patient's knees. Bending your knees slightly will lower your body and make it easier for the patient reach you. It also helps to avoid injury to your back when you lift the patient.

8. Place your arms under the patient's arms and around the patient's body. Prepare the patient by explaining that you will count to three and then lift. If possible, the patient can help by supporting some of her body weight.

9. Count to three and lift the patient. Turn toward the examination table. The back of the patient's knees should touch the table.

10. Lower the patient onto the examination table. If the patient can't sit without support, help the patient into a supine position. Otherwise, keep the patient in a sitting position.

11. If someone else is helping you move the patient, decide which one of you will turn the patient toward the examination table during the transfer. The stronger person should perform this maneuver.

12. You and your helper should both face the patient with your knees slightly bent. Each of you should have one knee in line with the patient's knees. The patient will put one hand on each person's shoulder.

13. Place one of your arms around the patient. Your helper should do the same. Lock your wrists together to provide extra support. On the count of three, lift the patient together.

14. One person turns the patient toward the examination table then both of you will gradually lower the patient onto the table. You and the helper need to work together to make the move as smooth as possible for the patient.

15. After the patient is comfortable and safely positioned on the examination table, unlock the wheels on the wheelchair and move it back from the table to an area where it will not get in the way.

16. Provide the patient with a gown and drape. If necessary, help the patient disrobe.

Procedure 17-4 | Assisting with Pregnant Patients

Equipment: Spygmomanometer, stethoscope, weight scale with height bar, specimen container for urine, patient gown, and exam table.

1. Wash your hands.

2. Greet the patient by name, and escort her to the prepared examining room. Identifying the patient by name helps to prevent errors.

3. Prepare the patient for the examination as you would for any other adult patient explaining the examination procedure.

4. Measure and record vital signs, height, and weight.

5. Instruct the patient on collecting a urine sample. The physician may require a urine test.

6. Ask the patient if she has any specific questions regarding her pregnancy. Notify the physician of these questions prior to her examination. Provide the patient with education materials that may address her concerns.

7. Provide instructions for disrobing and explain how to put on the gown. Leave the room to give the patient privacy while disrobing. Ask if she needs any assistance.

8. Have the patient use a stool to step up to the examining table. Help her sit on the end of the table. Cover her legs with a drape and provide additional drapes as needed for privacy.

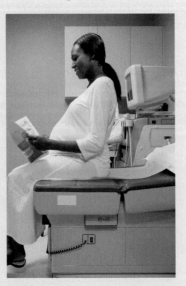

9. During the examination, take care when asking the patient to move into different body positions. Some body positions may not be suitable for pregnant women.

10. Watch for signs that the patient is uncomfortable. Be especially vigilant during changes in body position. When a pregnant patient has been lying on the examination table for a length of time, blood may collect in the pelvic regions. Sitting up suddenly can cause dizziness or hyperventilation. Help the patient to sit up slowly and give her time to adjust to sitting before she stands up.

11. At the end of the examination, help the patient down from the examination table. Leave the room to give her privacy while she dresses. Ask her if she needs assistance.

Procedure 17-5	Assisting with the Adult Physical Examination

Equipment: Stethoscope, ophthalmoscope, otoscope, penlight, tuning fork, nasal speculum, gloves, tongue blade, laryngeal mirror, patient gown, drape, lubricant, vaginal speculum, fecal occult blood test slide, and tissues.

1. Wash your hands and prepare the examination room and patient. When the physician is ready to begin the physical examination, you will assist by handing the physician the appropriate instruments and positioning the patient appropriately. Anticipating the physician's needs saves time and makes the procedure more efficient.

2. Begin by handing the physician the instruments necessary to examine different body areas. Although all physicians follow a systematic procedure, the order for examining different body areas may vary slightly depending on the physician. Instruments and supplies required to examine the different parts of the body are:
   - Head and neck—stethoscope.
   - Eyes—ophthalmoscope, penlight.
   - Ears—otoscope, tuning fork.
   - Nose—penlight, nasal speculum.
   - Sinuses—penlight.
   - Mouth—gloves, tongue blade, penlight. Pass the tongue blade by holding it in the middle. When it is returned to you, grasp it in the middle again so that you do not hold the end that was in the patient's mouth.
   - Throat—glove, tongue blade, laryngeal mirror, penlight.

3. Help the patient lower the gown to the waist for examination of the chest and upper back. The physician will use a stethoscope during the chest exam. Only the parts of the body being examined should be exposed. Maintain the patients' privacy by keeping them covered as much as possible.

4. Help the patient pull up the gown and remove the drape from the legs. Hand the physician the reflex hammer to test patient reflexes.

5. Help the patient into the supine position. Open the gown at the top to expose the chest again. Place the drape over the waist, abdomen, and legs. The physician will examine the breasts and may again listen to chest sounds.

6. Cover the patient's chest. Lower the drape to expose the abdomen. The physician will use a stethoscope to listen to bowel sounds.

7. Prepare and position the patient for examination of the genital and rectal areas.

For females:
   - Help the patient into the lithotomy position and drape appropriately.
   - Provide the physician with supplies and instruments used for examining genitalia and reproductive organs. These include gloves, lubricant, a speculum, microscope slides or prep solution, and a spatula or brush.
   - For the rectal examination, provide gloves, lubricant, and a fecal occult blood test slide.
   - After the examination, provide the patient with tissues to wipe off any excess lubricant.

For males:
   - Help the patient stand, if necessary. Have him bend over the examination table for a rectal and prostate examination.
   - For a hernia examination, provide gloves.
   - For a rectal examination, provide gloves, lubricant, and fecal occult blood test slide.
   - For a prostate examination, provide gloves and lubricant.
   - After the examination, provide the patient with tissues to wipe off any excess lubricant.

8. With the patient standing, the physician may assess legs, gait, coordination, and balance.

9. Help the patient sit on the end of the examination table. The physician often discusses findings with the patient at this time.

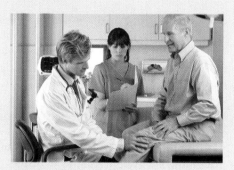

10. Perform or schedule any follow-up procedures or treatments.

11. Leave the room while the patient dresses unless the patient needs assistance. It is important to protect the patient's privacy.

Procedure 17-5 | Assisting with the Adult Physical Examination (continued)

12. Return to the examination room when the patient has dressed to answer any questions, reinforce instructions, and provide patient education. The patient's ability to follow the treatment plan depends on how well he understands it.

13. Escort the patient to the front desk. You can help clarify any appointment scheduling or billing issues.

14. Properly clean or dispose of all used equipment and supplies. Instruments, supplies, and equipment that came in direct contact with the patient must be cleaned, sterilized or disposed of appropriately.

15. Clean the counter surfaces of the room and the examination table with a disinfectant and prepare for the next patient.

16. Wash your hands and record any instructions from the physician in the patient's record. Note any test results, specimens taken for testing, and the laboratory where the specimens are being sent. Remember that if procedures and instructions are not recorded, they are not considered to have been done.

Procedure 17-6 | Measuring Distance Visual Acuity

Equipment: Snellen eye chart, eye occluder, and patient record for charting.

1. Wash your hands and prepare the examination area. Make sure the area is well-lighted.
   - A distance marker must be exactly 20 feet from the Snellen Eye Chart.
   - The chart must be at eye level.

2. Identify the patient by name and explain the procedure. Patients who understand the procedure are more likely to have accurate test results.

3. Position the patient at the 20-foot mark. The patient may be standing or sitting, as long as the chart is at eye level.

4. Note whether the patient is wearing glasses. If not, ask about contact lenses and record the information. Patients usually wear their corrective lenses during the visual acuity examination. The patient record must indicate if contact lenses or glasses were worn.

5. Have the patient cover the left eye with an eye occluder.
   - To maintain consistency, the test always starts with the left eye covered.
   - The patient's hand should not be used to cover the eye. Pressure against the eye or peeking can affect the results.
   - Instruct the patient to keep both eyes open, even though one is covered. Closing one eye can cause the other eye to squint, which can affect the results.

6. Stand beside the chart and point to each row as the patient reads it aloud. Begin with the first row, the 20/200 line. The line number is on the right side of the chart next to each line. If the patient can read these lines easily, move down to smaller figures. If the patient has difficulty reading the larger lines, you will need to notify the physician.

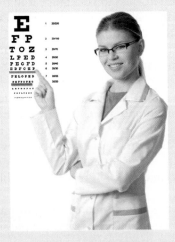

7. Record the smallest line the patient can read with no more than one error or according to office policy. Record the eye tested, the line number, and the errors. Use medical abbreviations. For example: OD 20/40—1 (OD means right eye).

8. Repeat the procedure with the right eye covered. Record the results using the abbreviation for the left eye, OS. For example: OS 20/20—0.

Procedure 17-6   Measuring Distance Visual Acuity (*continued*)

9. Repeat step 6 with both eyes uncovered. Record the results using the abbreviation for both eyes, OU. For example: OU 20/40—1.

10. A reading of 20/20 means that the person tested sees at 20 feet what the normal eye can see at 20 feet. 20/40 means that a person can see from 20 feet what the normal eye can see from 40 feet away.

11. Be sure to document the procedure in the patient's record. Procedures are not considered to have been done if they are not recorded.

Procedure 17-7   Measuring Color Perception

Equipment: Ishihara color plate book and gloves.

1. Wash your hands. Then put on gloves and get the Ishihara color plate book. In this case, you wear gloves to protect the color plates. Oils from your hands can alter the colors and interfere with testing.

2. Identify the patient by name and explain the procedure. Make sure the patient is seated comfortably in a quiet, well-lighted room.
   - Indirect sunlight is best. Sunlight should not shine directly on the color plates. The colors fade with exposure to bright lights.
   - Patients who wear glasses or contact lenses should keep them on. Corrective lenses don't interfere with the color perception test.

3. Hold the first plate in the book about 15 to 30 inches from the patient. The first plate should be obvious to all patients and serve as an example. Ask the patient if she can see the number formed by the dots on the plate.

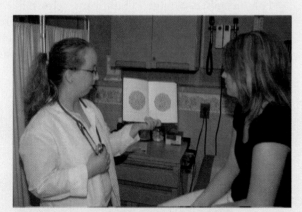

(Reprinted from Kronenberger J, Ledbetter J. *Jones & Bartlett Learning's Comprehensive Medical Assisting.* 4th ed. Burlington, MA: Jones & Bartlett Learning, LLC; 2013.)

4. Record the patient's results by noting the number of the figure the patient reports for each plate. Write the plate number followed by the patient's response.
   - If the patient cannot see the pattern, record the plate number followed by the letter *X*.
   - The patient should not take more than three seconds to read the plate and should not squint or guess. These behaviors indicate that the patient was unsure and the plate should be recorded as *X*.

5. Continue showing plates and recording patient responses for plates 1 to 10. Plate 11 requires the patient to trace a winding bluish-green line between two *X*'s. Patients with a color deficit will not be able to trace the line.
   - If 10 or more of the first 11 plates are read without difficulty, the patient does not have a color deficit. No additional testing is needed.
   - Plates 12, 13, and 14 are usually used to assess the degree of deficiency in patients with red-green color deficiencies.

6. Store the color plate book in a closed, protected area to protect the integrity of the colors. Remove your gloves and wash your hands.

Procedure 17-8   Assisting with the Pelvic Examination

Equipment:
- Gown and drape
- Vaginal speculum. If a metal nondisposable speculum is used, it can be warmed under running water, on a heating pad set on warm, or in a warming drawer found on some examination tables.
- Cotton-tipped applicators
- Pap smear collection materials
  - Ayre spatula or histobrush
  - Microscope slides with fixative solution or prepared solution for suspension of the sample
  - Laboratory requisition
- Water-soluble lubricant
- Examination gloves
- Examination light
- Tissues or wipes
- Basin or container for used instruments
- Biohazard waste container

1. Wash your hands and assemble required equipment and supplies.

2. If microscopic slides are used, label each slide according to the office or laboratory policy. A pencil is used to write on the frosted end of the slide. Each slide should be labeled *C* for cervical, *V* for vaginal, or *E* for endocervical, the region at the cervical opening into the uterus.

3. Greet the patient by name and explain the procedure. Identifying the patient by name prevents errors and may help put her at ease.

4. Ask the patient to empty her bladder and, if necessary, collect a urine specimen. An empty bladder makes the examination more comfortable.

5. Provide the patient with a gown and drape and ask her to disrobe. If she's also having a breast examination, she needs to disrobe completely. The gown should open to the front. If the patient is not having a breast exam, she need only disrobe from the waist down.

6. When the physician is ready, assist the patient into the lithotomy position. Her buttocks should be at the bottom edge of the table. This position may be embarrassing to the patient and may stress her back and legs. Explain that she won't need to stay in this position any longer than necessary for the examination.

7. Adjust the drape to cover the patient's abdomen and knees, exposing the genitalia. Adjust the light over the genitalia for maximum visibility.

8. Assist the physician with the examination by handing instruments and supplies as needed. Anticipating the physician's needs leads to a more thorough and efficient procedure.

9. After putting on examination gloves, hold the glass slides while the physician obtains and makes the smears.

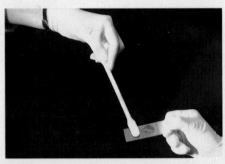

(Reprinted from Kronenberger J, Ledbetter J. *Jones & Bartlett Learning's Comprehensive Medical Assisting.* 4th ed. Burlington, MA: Jones & Bartlett Learning, LLC; 2013.)

10. Spray or cover each slide with fixative solution. Hold the slide 4 to 6 inches from the can and spray lightly once. Or carefully drop the fixative solution onto the slide.
    - The fixative preserves the cervical scrapings for analysis.
    - Spraying the solution too close may distort the cells or blow them off the slide.

11. When the physician removes the vaginal speculum, have a basin or other container ready to receive it.

12. Apply about 1 to 2 inches of lubricant across the physician's two fingers. Lubricant helps make the manual examination more comfortable. Don't place lubricant on the vaginal speculum before insertion. It can cause inaccurate Pap smear results.

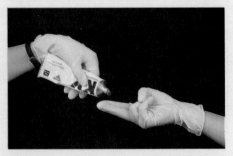

(Reprinted from Kronenberger J, Ledbetter J. *Jones & Bartlett Learning's Comprehensive Medical Assisting.* 4th ed. Burlington, MA: Jones & Bartlett Learning, LLC; 2013.)

Procedure 17-8 | Assisting with the Pelvic Examination (*continued*)

13. Encourage the patient to relax during the bimanual examination. Your support may help the patient feel less anxious.

14. After the examination, help the patient slide to the far end of the examination table. Then remove both feet from the stirrups at the same time.
    - Moving the patient away from the stirrups helps prevent strain and possible injury while removing her feet from them.
    - Removing both feet at the same time also puts less strain on the patient.

15. Offer the patient tissues to remove excess lubricant. Help her sit up if necessary. Watch the patient for signs of vertigo. Some patients, especially if elderly, may be dizzy when they sit up.

16. Ask the patient to get dressed and assist if needed. Respect the patient's privacy as she dresses.

17. Reinforce any instructions from the physician regarding follow-up appointments. The patient also will appreciate knowing when and how to get laboratory results from the Pap smear.

18. After the patient leaves, properly care for and dispose of equipment. Clean the room and remove gloves. Wash your hands. Document your responsibilities during the procedure, such as routing the specimen to the laboratory and patient education provided.

Preparing for Externship

At some point of the externship, you will probably be in the examination room with the physician or provider during an exam of the patient. You need to remember that you are there to assist the physician with whatever they may need and you are there to support the patient. Do not talk, unless the physician addresses you. Only answer and respond to what the physician is asking. Always anticipate what is going to happen next in the exam room before, during, and after the exam. As you witness more exams, you will become more comfortable and knowledgeable with expectations.

Chapter Recap

- The purpose of the physical examination is to assess general health and detect signs and symptoms of disease.
- During a physical examination, the medical assistant's duties may involve taking a medical history, preparing the patient for the examination, assisting during the examination, and processing collected specimens.
- Depending on office policies, the medical assistant may be asked to remain in the room during the examination to serve as a witness and provide legal protection for the physician.
- Medical assistants must be familiar with the instruments and supplies used for a general physical examination or a specialty examination.
- In preparing the examination room, the medical assistant should check the examination table, the equipment, and the supplies.
- The medical assistant has an important role in preparing the patient for the examination. Duties may include obtaining the medical history and chief complaint, checking vital signs, and processing specimens.
- The medical assistant ensures the patient's privacy at all times.
- As the physician examines different parts of the body, the patient may be asked to assume different positions. The medical assistant needs to be familiar with different examination positions to assist the patient if needed.
- Elderly, disabled, and pregnant patients may need extra assistance before, during, and after the examination. The medical assistant must be sensitive to patient needs.
- The physician follows a systematic order in examining the patient. The examination typically begins with the head and neck and progresses to the legs and feet.
- The physician uses six different techniques to gather information during a physical examination—inspection, palpation, manipulation, percussion, auscultation, and mensuration.
- The medical assistant will be required to assist with specialty procedures such as measuring distance visual acuity, measuring color perception, or assisting with pelvic examinations.
- After the examination, the medical assistant may need to help the patient dress, give further instructions, or perform follow-up procedures. The medical assistant is also responsible for cleaning the examination room and preparing it for the next patient.
- It is important to watch for opportunities to teach patients about warning signs that can indicate health problems. Medical assistants may provide patient education regarding procedures including breast self-examination and testicular self-examination.

Online Resources for Students

Student Resources available on the text's online site include:
- Audio Glossaries
- Animations
- Competency Evaluation Forms

- Videos
- Anatomy & Physiology Module with Heart and Lung Sounds
- Weblinks
- Worksheets

Exercises and Activities

Certification Preparation Questions

1. Which of the following examination methods is used to determine the patient's ability for extension and flexion?
   a. Inspection
   b. Palpation
   c. Manipulation
   d. Mensuration
   e. Percussion

2. Which instrument is used to determine the presence of cerumen in the ear canal?
   a. Nasal speculum
   b. Ophthalmoscope
   c. Percussion hammer
   d. Laryngoscope
   e. Otoscope

3. Which of the following is a nondisposable supply used during a physical examination?
   a. Patient gown
   b. Tongue depressor
   c. Tape measure
   d. Gloves
   e. Patient drape

4. Which of the following is a true statement regarding a Snellen chart vision exam?
   a. A person with 20/40 vision can see at 20 feet what a normal person can see at 20 feet.
   b. A person with 20/50 vision can see at 50 feet what a normal person can see at 20 feet.
   c. A person with 20/20 vision can see at 20 feet what a person with corrective lenses can see at 20 feet.
   d. A person with 20/200 vision can see at 200 feet what a normal person can see at 20 feet.
   e. A person with 20/70 vision can see at 20 feet what a normal person can see at 70 feet.

5. Which of the following would be used to detect abnormalities of the lungs, heart, large blood vessels, ribs, and thoracic spine?
   a. Complete blood count
   b. Electrocardiogram
   c. Urinalysis
   d. Chest x-ray
   e. Blood chemistry

6. Which of the following positions would be used to examine the female genitalia?
   a. Fowler's
   b. Lithotomy
   c. Trendelenburg
   d. Prone
   e. Supine

7. The purpose of the physical examination is to:
   a. update the patient's health history.
   b. comply with insurance company annual requirements.
   c. assess general health and detect signs and symptoms of disease.
   d. update immunizations.
   e. review the patient's health issues and surgeries performed.

8. Which of the following examination methods is used to evaluate the patient's skin condition?
   a. Inspection
   b. Palpation
   c. Manipulation
   d. Mensuration
   e. Percussion

9. Which of the following items is required to examine the ears?
   a. Penlight and ophthalmoscope
   b. Otoscope and tuning fork
   c. Ophthalmoscope and Snellen chart
   d. Laryngeal mirror and penlight
   e. Tuning fork and ophthalmoscope

10. Which of the following is not a responsibility of the medical assistant?
    a. Perform Snellen chart exam
    b. Interpret the electrocardiogram
    c. Use mensuration to obtain patient's height and weight
    d. Collect blood specimen for laboratory testing
    e. Chart patient data in the EMR system

 ## CareTracker Connection

Documenting Clinical Data Generated From a Physical Examination

 HARRIS CareTracker **CareTracker** Activities Related to This Chapter
- Case Study 5: Family Practice Patient Practicum
- Case Study 6: Pediatric Patient Practicum

The physical examination typically marks the point in an office visit when the primary care provider appears for the first time and takes charge of the patient. The medical assistant's role at this point is to assist in conducting the examination, document data that are generated from the examination, and order any medications or tests that the primary care provider requests. Once again, CareTracker provides the tools a medical assistant needs to carry out these tasks.

Tasks discussed in this chapter that can be performed in CareTracker include the following:

- Documenting the following patient clinical information:
  - Health history
  - Review of systems
  - Physical examination findings
  - Tests and procedures completed during the visit
  - Diagnoses
  - Treatment plan
- Ordering the following:
  - Medications
  - Laboratory tests
  - Diagnostic tests

Many of these tasks are discussed in CareTracker Connection features in other chapters. A task we'll consider here is entering physical examination findings.

The primary application in CareTracker for entering clinical data related to a physical examination is the Progress Note, which may be accessed from the Medical Record module. Although the primary care provider typically enters data into the Progress Note, medical assistants are sometimes required to do so.

The Progress Note contains many tabs, including those related to the chief complaint, health history, review of systems, physical examination, injections, tests and procedures, diagnoses, and treatment plan. Many data entered earlier in the patient's visit, such as the chief complaint, vital signs, and health history, appear now in the Progress Note—both as a narrative summary on the left side of the screen and within the corresponding tabs, as shown below.

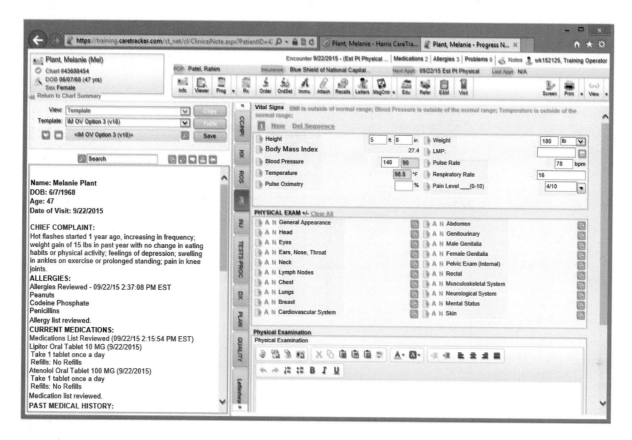

On the physical exam (PE) tab, you may indicate findings related to each region, system, or organ of the body examined, such as "N" for normal and "A" for abnormal.

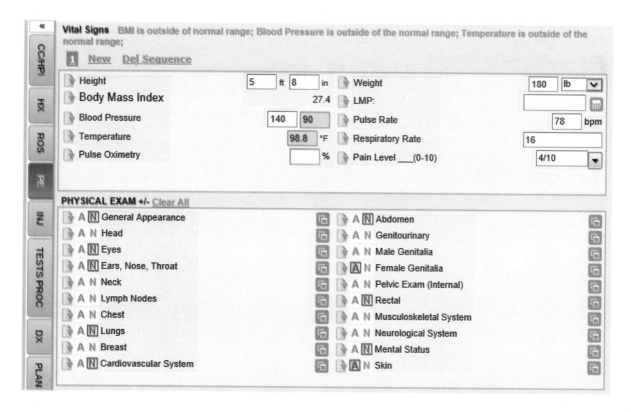

More detailed findings may be entered by clicking on the gray arrow icon to the left of each area, which causes a pop-up box to appear.

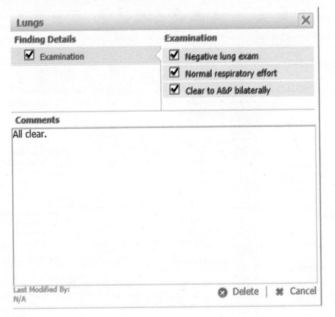

Internet Activities

Visit the Internet to access information from various Web sites for the following:

1. Recommended immunizations for infants, children, and adults, visit the Centers for Disease Control site at www.cdc.gov/vaccines/schedules
2. Images of a healthy and an infected ear drum

18 Assisting with Minor Office Surgery

Chapter Objectives

- Explain the principles and practices of surgical asepsis.
- Describe how to perform a surgical scrub.
- Wrap items for autoclaving.
- Perform sterilization techniques.
- List some of the surgical instruments commonly used in the medical office.
- Summarize how to care for and clean medical instruments.
- Explain how to prepare a treatment room for a surgical procedure, including how to open a sterile surgical pack.
- List possible indicators that a surgical pack has been contaminated.
- Explain how to apply surgical gloves.

- List strategies for maintaining a sterile field.
- Prepare patient for and assist with procedures, treatments, and minor office surgeries.
- Explain how to prepare the patient's skin for minor surgery.
- Identify different methods for wound closure and the necessary supplies.
- Outline the medical assistant's responsibilities in collecting specimens.
- List the responsibilities of the medical assistant following minor surgical procedures.
- Explain how to apply bandages and note the signs of impaired circulation.
- Identify the phases of wound healing and their main characteristics.

CAAHEP & ABHES Competencies

CAAHEP

- Differentiate between medical and surgical asepsis used in ambulatory care setting, indentifying when each is appropriate.
- Document patient care.
- Prepare items for autoclaving.
- Perform sterilization procedures.

ABHES

- Procedure/minor surgery.
- Perform specialty procedures including but not limited to minor surgery, cardiac, respiratory, OB-GYN, neurological, gastroenterology.

Chapter Terms

Approximation
Autoclave
Biopsy
Dehiscence
Dissect

Excise
Fenestrated drape
Forceps
Hemostat
Incision

Informed consent
Medical asepsis
Purulent
Retractor
Sanitizing

Scalpel
Sterile field
Sterilization
Surgical asepsis

Abbreviations

Bx   C&S   DSD   I&D

Case Study

Linda Bridges, a medical assistant, is registering Lloyd Barnes, a patient who has a laceration on his forearm due to a fall onto a glass coffee table. Ms. Bridges takes him into an exam room and is certain that Mr. Barnes will need sutures to repair the laceration. She knows that she will need to prep him for the minor office procedure. She will gather all the necessary equipment and supplies and then notify the physician to examine the patient.

As a medical assistant, you may need to assist with minor surgeries performed in the medical office. The types of surgeries performed in a medical office will depend on its medical specialty. But typical office procedures in a general medical practice include the following:

- Inserting or removing sutures; surgical stitches are used to hold body tissues together.
- Making incisions for drainage, a surgical process of cutting into the body to remove fluids and discharge from wounds or cavities.
- Performing sebaceous cystectomy—the removal of a cyst, an abnormal sac under the skin that is filled with fluid or fatty matter.

Study Skill

Learning the terms for surgical procedures can be challenging. Even if the procedure isn't done in the medical office, you may encounter the term during patient care. It's useful to keep in mind that root words (usually body parts) are often combined with suffixes or endings that indicate some kind of surgical action. Here are some common suffixes:

- *ectomy* refers to excision or removal. For example, a **cystectomy** is the removal of a cyst.
- *otomy* refers to incision or cutting. A **tracheotomy** is a procedure for cutting into the trachea, or windpipe, to create an airway.

- *plasty* means repair. A **rhinoplasty** is surgical reconstruction of the nose.
- *ostomy* is forming an opening. A **colostomy** is a surgical procedure to create a new opening for waste to pass from the colon.

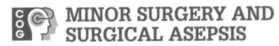

MINOR SURGERY AND SURGICAL ASEPSIS

The process for preparing the patient and setting up supplies and equipment is much the same, no matter what surgery is being performed. For any surgical procedure, medical assistants practice surgical asepsis, otherwise known as "sterile technique."

The difference between surgical asepsis and medical asepsis is **medical asepsis** stops microbes from spreading from one patient to another and surgical asepsis stops microbes from getting into the patient's body during an invasive procedure.

Surgical asepsis is a set of practices designed to keep areas or items free of microorganisms. Its purpose is to destroy organisms before they enter the body. Surgical asepsis is necessary:

- When handling sterile instruments that break the skin
- When performing or assisting with surgical procedures
- When changing wound dressings

Table 18-1	Comparing Medical and Surgical Asepsis	
	Medical Asepsis	**Surgical Asepsis**
Definition	Destroys microorganisms after they leave the body	Destroys microorganisms before they enter the body
Purpose	Prevents transmission of microorganisms from one person to another	Prevents entry of microorganisms into the body during invasive procedures
When to Use	During contact with a body part that is not normally sterile	During contact with normally sterile parts of the body
Handwashing Techniques	Hands and wrists are washed for 1–2 min.	Hands and forearms are washed for 5–10 min using a brush.
Cleaning Techniques	Typically use sanitation and disinfection	Requires sterilization

What Is Different about Surgical Asepsis?

Surgical asepsis requires the absence of microorganisms on instruments, equipment, and supplies. The procedures you will use for surgical asepsis are different from those you learned for medical asepsis. Even your handwashing technique will be different. Table 18-1 shows the differences between medical and surgical asepsis.

The Surgical Scrub

The goal of the surgical scrub is to remove microbes from the hands, nails, and forearms. This will minimize the risk of infection to the patient. The process requires a sink that has a foot or arm control for the running water. You will also need the following supplies:

- Surgical soap in a dispenser
- An orange stick or nail brush
- A sterile brush
- Sterile towels

The scrubbing procedure should take at least 5 minutes for each hand and arm. It is best to follow a systematic approach so you do not miss any areas.

 ## STERILIZATION TECHNIQUES AND EQUIPMENT

Sanitation and disinfection are the main ways medical assistants maintain medical asepsis. Sanitation is maintaining a healthful, disease-free environment. **Sanitizing** means reducing the microorganisms on a surface by using low-level disinfection practices.

Instruments and equipment used in surgical procedures must be sanitized first and then sterilized. **Sterilization** is the complete elimination or destruction of all microbes, including spores. Here are the most common sterilizing agents (Table 18-2 compares the various methods of sterilization.):

- Steam under pressure (autoclaving)
- Dry heat
- Ethylene oxide (gas used in sterilization)
- Liquid chemicals
- Microwave process

Steam is the most common method of sterilization in medical offices. One of the newest methods combines microwave radiation with the steam to shorten the

Table 18-2	Methods of Sterilization	
	Method of Sterilization	**Directions**
Heat	Moist heat (steam under pressure)	250°F (121°C) for 30 min
	Boiling	212°F (100°C) for 30 min or more
	Dry heat	340°F (171°C) for 1 h; 320°F (160°C) for 2 h
Liquids	Glutaraldehyde	Follow manufacturer's directions or OSHA requirements and guidelines.
	Formaldehyde	Follow manufacturer's directions or OSHA requirements and guidelines.
Gas	Ethylene oxide	450–500 mg/L at 122°F (50°C) for 1–3 h

sterilization process. The method you use will depend on what must be sterilized and the types of microbes that must be destroyed. Several types of equipment are used for sterilizing items in the medical office. Here is what you will need to know how to properly perform sterilization in your office:

- How the equipment works
- What the equipment is used for
- When to schedule preventive maintenance
- How to schedule service, if necessary
- What supplies to order so the equipment can operate properly

Sanitizing Comes First

Sanitization or disinfection is the first step in preparing instruments for sterilization. Two different methods are commonly used for sanitization.

- Hand cleaning instruments is especially appropriate for delicate instruments that can be damaged easily.
- Mechanical washing uses a machine. Mechanical washers can be used for cleaning most instruments. They are useful for cleaning sharp instruments that can cause injury when cleaned by hand.

Sanitizing Instruments

Before cleaning instruments by hand, be sure to put on heavy duty utility gloves, a gown, and eye protection. You need to protect yourself and your clothes from contaminants that might splash up during the procedure. See Figure 18-1.

Follow these key guidelines for sanitizing instruments:

1. Take any removable sections of an instrument or equipment apart. If the item can't be sanitized right away, soak the instrument or equipment in a solution of cold water and detergent so blood and other substances don't dry on the instrument.
2. Before you begin cleaning an instrument, check to make sure it works properly. Equipment that's broken should be repaired or discarded, according to office policy.
3. Rinse the instrument with cool water. Hot water can cause some contaminants to stick to the instrument. This will make it harder to clean.
4. Force streams of hot soapy water through any tubular or grooved instruments. You need to clean the inside as well as the outside.
5. Use a hot, soapy solution to dissolve fats or lubricants.
6. Next, place the instruments in a soaking solution, according to office policy. After soaking them for 5 to 10 minutes, use friction to clean them. Use a soft brush or gauze to wipe each instrument and loosen microorganisms. Don't use abrasive materials on delicate instruments and equipment. A soft brush works well on grooves and joints as shown in Figure 18-2.

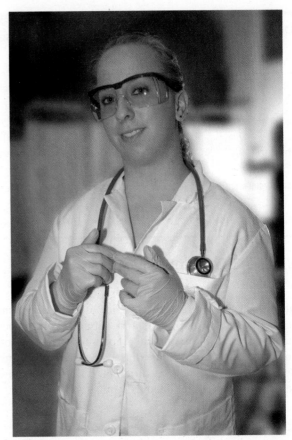

Figure 18-1 Always wear personal protective equipment when a splash may occur. (Reprinted from Kronenberger J, Ledbetter J. *Jones & Bartlett Learning's Comprehensive Medical Assisting.* 5th ed. Burlington, MA: Jones & Bartlett Learning, LLC; 2016.)

7. While cleaning, keep instruments immersed in the cleaning solution to avoid spreading microorganisms through the air.

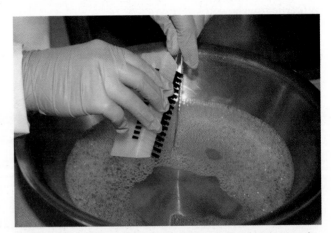

Figure 18-2 Soiled, contaminated surgical instruments are sanitized using a brush with soap and water prior to preparation for autoclaving. This process removes blood and tissue. Always wear utility gloves when cleaning the instruments. (Reprinted from Kronenberger J, Ledbetter J. *Jones & Bartlett Learning's Comprehensive Medical Assisting.* 5th ed. Burlington, MA: Jones & Bartlett Learning, LLC; 2016.)

8. Open and close the jaws of moveable instruments, such as forceps or scissors, several times to make sure all contaminants have been removed.
9. Rinse instruments well to remove soap residue and any remaining microorganisms.
10. Dry instruments thoroughly before sterilization. Excess moisture can interfere with the sterilization process. It also can cause instruments to rust or become dull.

Be sure to discard used brushes, gauze, and solution after sanitizing instruments and equipment. These items are considered grossly contaminated and cannot be reused.

The Autoclave

The **autoclave** is the most commonly used piece of equipment for sterilization. It is a device that uses steam heat under high pressure to sterilize objects. The autoclave consists of two chambers and a vent. See Figure 18-3A, B. Here is how it works.

- The outer chamber is the place where pressure builds. Distilled water is added to a reservoir. It is converted to steam when a preset temperature is reached.
- The inner chamber is where sterilization occurs. Steam is forced into the inner chamber. As the pressure inside the chamber increases, the temperature rises to 250°F or higher. This is much higher than the normal boiling point of water, which is 212°F or 100°C. The high temperature of the steam destroys all organisms, including viruses and spores.
- The air exhaust vent is located on the bottom of the autoclave. It allows air in the inner chamber to be pushed out and replaced by steam. When no air is present, the chamber seals and the temperature gauge starts rising.

Most autoclaves can be set to vent, time, turn off, and exhaust at preset times and levels. With older models, you may need to do this manually.

All manufacturers provide instructions for operating the machine. They also recommend the time needed to sterilize different types of loads. The autoclave instructions should be posted near the machine in a place where everyone can see them.

The autoclave is commonly used to sterilize:

- Minor surgical equipment and instruments
- Surgical storage trays and containers
- Some surgical equipment, such as bowls for holding sterile solutions

Autoclave Wrapping Material

Autoclave wrap may be double layers of cotton muslin, special sterilization paper, or plastic or paper pouches or bags. Many offices use a variety of materials. But whatever wrapping material you use, be sure it has these properties:

- Permeable to steam but not contaminants
- Resists tearing and puncturing during normal handling
- Allows for easy opening to prevent contamination of the contents
- Maintains the sterility of the contents during storage

Special Indicators

Items to be sterilized in the autoclave are wrapped before they are placed inside. But it is the special indicators that help ensure the items are properly sterilized. These special indicators include autoclave indicator tape, sterilization indicators, and the culture test. Examples of indicators are shown in Figure 18-4.

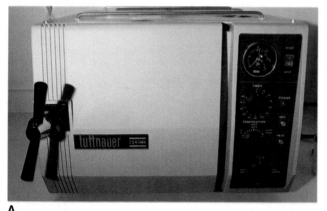
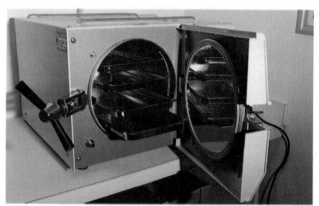

A   B

Figure 18-3   A. An autoclave that may be found in the medical office. **B.** The interior of the autoclave. (Reprinted from Kronenberger J, Ledbetter J. *Jones & Bartlett Learning's Comprehensive Medical Assisting.* 5th ed. Burlington, MA: Jones & Bartlett Learning, LLC; 2016.)

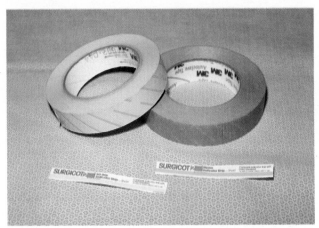

Figure 18-4 Autoclave tape (**top**: steam and gas tape) and sterilization indicators (**bottom left and right**). (Reprinted from Kronenberger J, Ledbetter J. *Jones & Bartlett Learning's Comprehensive Medical Assisting.* 5th ed. Burlington, MA: Jones & Bartlett Learning, LLC; 2016.)

Autoclave Tape

Autoclave indicator tape is a special tape placed on the outside of the wrap used to package equipment that is going into the autoclave. As you wrap the equipment, you should write on the tape what is inside the package and the date it is being autoclaved. Figure 18-5 shows the color change of the autoclave tape after sterilization.

Autoclave tape is designed to change color when it is exposed to steam. But the tape does not guarantee that items inside the package have been heated enough to be sterilized—only that the outside has been exposed to steam.

Sterilization Indicators

Sterilization indicators are placed inside the wrapped packs to show that proper temperature and pressure were reached during the sterilization process. They are placed inside the wrapping so you will know the steam penetrated the inner parts of the pack.

There are several different kinds of sterilization indicators. Some change colors at high temperatures. Others are tubes containing wax pellets. If the pellets melt, it shows that the required temperature was reached.

Culture Tests

The culture test is the best method for checking the effectiveness of the sterilization. Strips with heat-resistant spores are placed between packages in the autoclave load. When the sterilization process is finished, the strips are removed from the packets and placed in a broth culture for incubating. At the end of the incubation period, the culture is compared with a control to see if all the spores have been killed.

Loading an Autoclave

For effective autoclaving, steam needs to reach everywhere. The location of items in an autoclave can make a big difference in where the steam goes. Follow these tips for loading the items to be sterilized.

- Load the autoclave loosely to allow steam to circulate. If too many items are put in, enough steam may not get to and penetrate the packs in the center. See Figure 18-6.
- Place the packs on their sides for the best steam circulation. This applies to containers and bowls too. If a container or bowl is upright, air will settle into its interior. This will keep steam from circulating to the inner surfaces. Container lids should be wrapped separately.

Filling the Reservoir

Use only distilled water to fill the reservoir tank. Tap water contains chemicals and minerals that may coat the

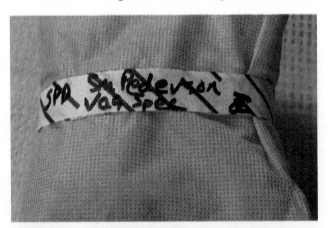

Figure 18-5 The stripes on autoclave tape change color, indicating that the pack has been exposed to steam. (Reprinted from Kronenberger J, Ledbetter J. *Jones & Bartlett Learning's Comprehensive Medical Assisting.* 5th ed. Burlington, MA: Jones & Bartlett Learning, LLC; 2016.)

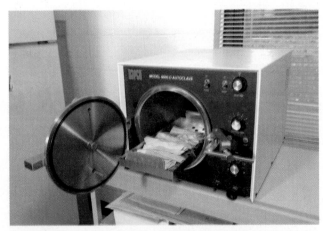

Figure 18-6 Properly loaded autoclave. (Reprinted from Kronenberger J, Ledbetter J. *Jones & Bartlett Learning's Comprehensive Medical Assisting.* 5th ed. Burlington, MA: Jones & Bartlett Learning, LLC; 2016.)

interior chamber and clog the exhaust valves. This can cause the autoclave to function improperly.

When filling the interior chamber with water from the reservoir, make sure the water level is up to the fill line. Adding too much water can make the steam saturated and less efficient. Too little water means there will not be enough steam produced. The sterilization process depends on getting the correct level of steam.

The Autoclave at Work

Besides steam, three other elements are critical for proper sterilization:

- Temperature
- Pressure
- Time

In general, 250°F at 15 pounds of pressure for 20 to 30 minutes is sufficient. However, the temperature, pressure, and time may vary depending on the items being sterilized. Solid or metal loads may take a little less time than soft, bulky loads. The office should have a policy regarding the proper settings to use for effective sterilization.

When the items have been in the autoclave at the right temperature for enough time, the timer will ring. It is important not to set the timer until the proper temperature has been reached. Some microbes are only killed if they are exposed to high enough temperature for a specific length of time. Be sure to vent the autoclave to allow the temperature to drop safely. Newer autoclaves vent automatically.

Do not handle or remove autoclaved items until they are dry. If the coverings are still moist, microorganisms from your hands might be drawn inside.

Storing Autoclaved Items

Once the items are completely dry, remove the packages from the autoclave. Store them in a clean, dry, and dust-free area. Packs that are sterilized on-site in an autoclave are considered sterile for 30 days. After 30 days, they must be sterilized again. You can avoid unnecessary work by placing recently autoclaved items toward the back of the cabinet. Move items that were previously autoclaved up to the front. Prior to reautoclaving packs, check the wrapping material to ensure it is not damaged or torn. Place new autoclave tape on the pack before reautoclaving.

Maintaining the Autoclave

You are responsible for performing routine maintenance on the autoclave. A schedule, or log, for maintenance should be posted near the machine. The log should include spaces for initials or a signature after the

maintenance has been performed. Weekly routine maintenance includes the following:

- Washing the interior of the chamber with a soft brush or cloth
- Drain the water from the autoclave and replace it with a cleaning solution
- Run the cleaning solution through a heat cycle for at least 20 minutes, then drain it and replace with a distilled water rinse.
- Run the rinse through a heat cycle for at least 20 minutes and drain
- Remove the shelves from the autoclave and scrub them. Also wipe the inside chamber clean
- Refill the autoclave with distilled water

From time to time, you also may need to check the performance of the autoclave using culture tests or other controls. It is important to keep good records of any tests done to check the autoclave's performance—and the results. If they show the sterilization process was not effective, you must report this fact in the log. Your report should include information about the problem and how it was resolved.

Cold Chemical Sterilization

Cold sterilization is used for items that are sensitive to heat, too large, or very delicate. For example, one instrument commonly sterilized this way is an endoscope. Endoscopes are long flexible tubes with an optical system that allows the physician to look inside body cavities.

Equipment and Supplies

Here is a list of items needed for chemical sterilization.

- Large container with tight-fitting lid—The container must be large enough to submerge the items in the chemical solution. It should be used only for the sterilization process. By covering the container, you ensure that the chemical solution will not evaporate during the process. The lid also prevents airborne microorganisms from entering the solution.
- Appropriate chemical solution—The sterilizing solution you will use depends on what your medical office prefers and the type of items being sterilized. Some chemicals, such as hydrogen peroxide or bleach, will corrode metal instruments. No matter what chemical is used, it is important to follow the manufacturer's instructions carefully when mixing the solution. If it's too diluted, the instruments will not be sterilized properly.
- Personal protective equipment—When using the chemical solution, you need to protect yourself. Wear heavy duty utility gloves, protective goggles, and an apron to cover your clothing. If the chemical comes

into contact with your skin, eyes, or mucous membranes, it can cause irritation or burns.

- Vent hood—The vent hood is used to remove unwanted fumes the chemicals may release into the air. For safety reasons, you need to use the vent hood when working with any chemical solutions.

The chemicals used are sometimes similar to those used for sanitizing. A key difference is the exposure time. The exposure time for the sterilization process varies for different chemicals.

Always check the instructions provided by the chemical manufacturer to find out the correct exposure time for sterilization. Also, you will need to make sure the chemical solution has not expired. The instructions should advise you on how long you can expect the chemical to remain effective.

After Chemical Sterilization

When the instruments have soaked in the chemical solution for the proper length of time, they can be removed. Because the items are now sterile, you must wear sterile gloves or use sterile transfer forceps to grasp and remove items from the solution. You will need to rinse the chemical solution from each instrument before it comes into contact with the patient. Rinse each item thoroughly using sterile water. Dry the item with a sterile towel.

Ultrasonic Cleaning

The ultrasonic cleaning unit is a method of machine washing that sanitizes items using high-frequency sound waves. Items are submerged in a tank of water and cleaning solution. Vibrations from sound waves create bubbles. Scrubbing action from the bubbles loosens soil from instruments. After the recommended amount of time, items are rinsed and dried in the unit. When they're removed, they're ready for sterilization.

 # SURGICAL INSTRUMENTS

To assist the physician with minor surgical procedures, you must be familiar with the surgical instruments. You also must know how to care for each instrument.

As a clinical medical assistant, you will need to know how to set up instruments and equipment for surgical procedures. You may be the one to pass instruments to the physician during the procedure as well.

The instruments used in minor surgery all have specific functions. The main functions are as follows:

- Cutting
- Dissecting
- Grasping
- Holding

- Retracting (pulling back body tissues to expose other areas)
- Suturing (the process of using stitches to close cuts made in body tissues)

Surgical instruments are designed with different shapes to suit their functions. They can be curved, straight, sharp, blunt, serrated (grooved), toothed, or smooth. Many are made of stainless steel and are reusable; some are disposable.

Common Surgical Instruments

The most widely used surgical instruments are:

- **Forceps** and clamps—These tools generally have two clamping blades and a handle. They are used for grasping and holding things.
- Scissors—Like common household scissors, surgical scissors consist of two cutting blades joined by a small screw.
- **Scalpel**—This small surgical knife has a straight handle and a straight or curved cutting blade.

Forceps and Clamps

Forceps and clamps form the largest group of surgical instruments. Both are used for the same tasks—to grasp, handle, compress, pull, or join tissue, equipment, or supplies.

They come in many kinds and sizes. Some have teeth or serrations. (A serration is a groove cut into the blade of an instrument to improve its grasp.) They can have curved or straight blades. Some have sharp tips. Others have ring tips or blunt tips.

Many forceps have ratchets in the handles. Ratchets are notched mechanisms that click into position to maintain tension. They work to hold the tips of the forceps tightly together. Some forceps have spring handles that are compressed between thumb and index finger to grasp objects. Various forceps are shown in Figure 18-7A–Q.

You need to learn the names and purposes of the basic types of forceps. This will help you know which instrument is needed when the physician asks for it. Here are some of the more common ones.

Hemostats

A **hemostat** is a surgical instrument with slender, straight, or curved jaws. Usually, it's used to grasp and clamp blood vessels to establish hemostasis (the stopping of blood flow or bleeding).

Kelly Hemostats

Kelly hemostats are larger than many other hemostats and they have serrations only on the tips of their blades. Those with long handles are used for grasping blood vessels. Like other hemostats, their blades can be straight or curved.

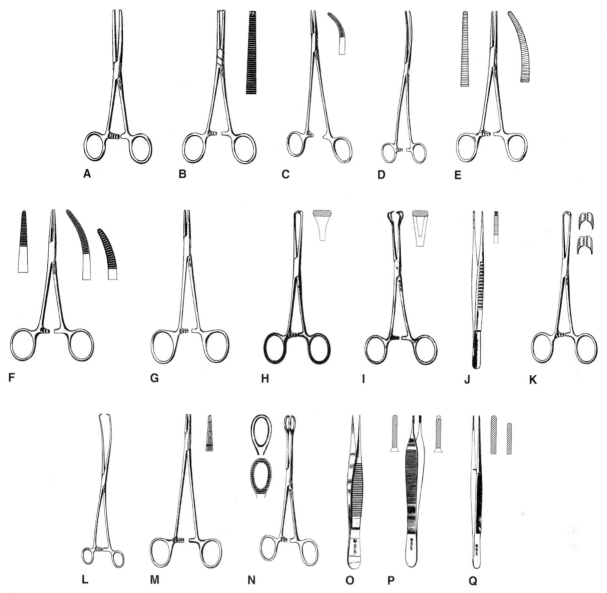

Figure 18-7 Forceps. **A.** Rochester-Pean forceps. **B.** Rochester-Ochsner forceps. **C.** Adson forceps. **D.** Bozeman forceps. **E.** Crile hemostat. **F.** Kelly hemostat. **G.** Halsted mosquito hemostat. **H.** Allis forceps. **I.** Babcock forceps. **J.** DeBakey forceps. **K.** Allis tissue forceps. **L.** Duplay tenaculum forceps. **M.** Crile-Wood needle holder. **N.** Ballenger sponge forceps. **O.** Fine-point splinter forceps. **P.** Adson dressing forceps. **Q.** Potts-Smith dressing forceps. (Reprinted from Kronenberger J, Ledbetter J. *Jones & Bartlett Learning's Comprehensive Medical Assisting.* 5th ed. Burlington, MA: Jones & Bartlett Learning, LLC; 2016.) (Courtesy of Sklar Instruments, West Chester, PA.)

Sterile Transfer Forceps

Sterile transfer forceps are used to transfer sterile supplies, equipment, and other surgical instruments to a sterile field. A **sterile field** is a specific area that is considered free of microbes.

Needle Holder

A needle holder is used to hold and pass a needle through tissue during suturing. It is sometimes called a suture forceps.

Spring or Thumb Forceps

This type of forceps helps the user grasp tissue for dissection or suturing. Tissue forceps and splinter forceps are types of spring forceps.

Towel Clamps

Towel clamps are used to hold sterile drapes in place. See Figure 18-8.

Sterile drapes are placed around the operative site to protect it from microbes. They expose only the part of

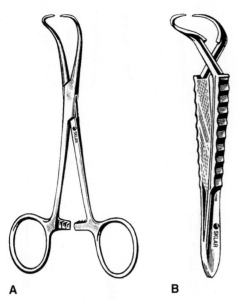

Figure 18-8 Towel clamps. **A.** Backhaus towel clamp. **B.** Jones cross-action towel clamp. (Courtesy of Sklar Instruments, West Chester, PA.) (Reprinted from Kronenberger J, Ledbetter J. *Jones & Bartlett Learning's Comprehensive Medical Assisting.* 5th ed. Burlington, MA: Jones & Bartlett Learning, LLC; 2016.)

the body where surgery is being performed. This helps maintain the sterile field. In some surgeries, such as during vasectomies, towel clamps are also used to clamp tissue.

Scissors

Surgical scissors are used for cutting sutures and bandages. Physicians also use them to **dissect** (cut apart) superficial, deep, or delicate tissues. The points on surgical scissors may be blunt, sharp, or both, depending on the function of the instrument. There are several kinds of scissors shown in Figure 18-9.

- Straight scissors cut deep or delicate tissue and sutures.
- Curved scissors dissect superficial and delicate tissues.
- Suture scissors have a straight top blade. The blunt bottom blade is curved out or hooked to fit under, lift, and grasp sutures for snipping. They are used to remove not insert sutures.

Bandage scissors are used for removing bandages. The bottom blade is flattened, blunt, and longer than the top blade. The longer blade fits safely under bandages. They are designed not to cut into the skin. The most common type is Lister bandage scissors.

Scalpels

Scalpels are another type of cutting tool. They consist of a reusable steel handle and a disposable blade as shown in Figure 18-10.

The handle can hold different blades for different surgical procedures. Many offices use scalpels with disposable handles and blades that are packaged as a one-piece sterile unit.

Scalpels have different uses.

- Scalpels with straight or pointed blades are used for **incision** (cutting into tissue) and to make a puncture into the skin for drainage procedures.
- Scalpels with curved blades are used to **excise**, or cut out, tissue.

Scalpel blades come in several sizes, with #10, #11, and #15 being the most common. Handles also come in different sizes. The larger the size number, the more delicate the handle. For example, a #3 handle would be a sturdier handle than a #7 handle.

Scalpel blades must be handled carefully before use to avoid contamination and damaging the blade. When using a nondisposable scalpel, a forceps or a needle holder is used to remove the scalpel blade from the

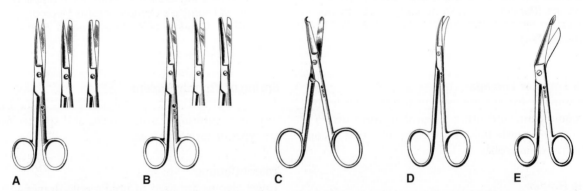

Figure 18-9 Scissors. **A.** Straight blade operating scissors. **Left to right:** S/S, S/B, B/B. **B.** Curved blade operating scissors. **Left to right:** S/S, S/B, B/B. **C.** Spencer stitch scissors. **D.** Suture scissors. **E.** Lister bandage scissors. S/S, sharp/sharp; S/B, sharp/blunt; B/B, blunt/blunt. (Courtesy of Sklar Instruments, West Chester, PA.) (Reprinted from Kronenberger J, Ledbetter J. *Jones & Bartlett Learning's Comprehensive Medical Assisting.* 5th ed. Burlington, MA: Jones & Bartlett Learning, LLC; 2016.)

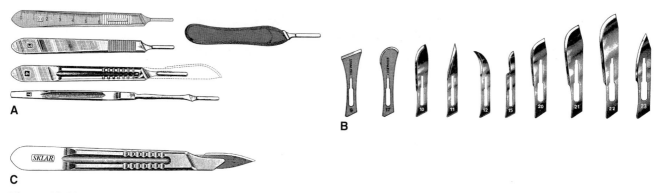

Figure 18-10   Scalpels. **A.** Scalpel handles. **B.** Surgical blades. **C.** Complete sterile disposable scalpel. (Courtesy of Sklar Instruments, West Chester, PA.) (Reprinted from Kronenberger J, Ledbetter J. *Jones & Bartlett Learning's Comprehensive Medical Assisting.* 5th ed. Burlington, MA: Jones & Bartlett Learning, LLC; 2016.)

packet and attach it to the scalpel handle. When you are finished, you should use forceps to remove the used blade to avoid injury. Scalpel blades removed from the handle and disposable scalpels are discarded into a sharps container.

Probes, Directors, and Retractors

Before performing a procedure, the physician may first explore a cavity or wound with surgical tools including probes, directors, and retractors.

Probe

A probe is a thin, flexible instrument that can help the physician examine the angle and depth of the cavity or wound. There are many different kinds of probes as those shown in Figure 18-11.

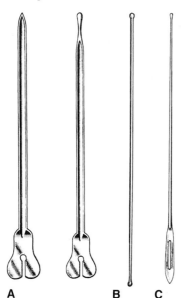

Figure 18-11   Probes. **A.** Director and tongue tie. **B.** Double-ended probe. **C.** Probe with eye.(Courtesy of Sklar Instruments, West Chester, PA.) (Reprinted from Kronenberger J, Ledbetter J. *Jones & Bartlett Learning's Comprehensive Medical Assisting.* 5th ed. Burlington, MA: Jones & Bartlett Learning, LLC; 2016.)

The physician's choice of probe depends on the area being explored.

Director

The director guides the knife or instrument once a procedure has begun. In surgical incisions, the director helps ensure correct depth and direction.

Retractor

Retractors are used to separate the edges of a wound and to hold open layers of tissue. Their main purpose is to expose areas beneath the surface tissues. Retractors come in different sizes and shapes. They may be plain or toothed. Toothed retractors may be sharp or blunt. Some retractors are designed to be held by an assistant during surgery. See Figure 18-12.

Self-retaining retractors can be screwed open and do not need to be held manually.

Other Surgical Instruments

Various medical specialties require different kinds of instruments for surgical procedures. Table 18-3 shows some of these surgical instruments and explains the use of each.

Care and Cleaning of Surgical Instruments

Typically, the medical assistant is responsible for taking good care of surgical instruments to help ensure that they will function properly. Follow these guidelines to keep surgical instruments in good working order.

- Rinse instruments as soon as possible—Rinse instruments right after minor surgical procedures to remove obvious contamination. When substances, blood and tissue, dry or harden on instruments, they are harder to clean. Make sure you follow OSHA standards to prevent contact with blood or body fluids. This definitely includes wearing gloves.

A   B   C

Figure 18-12 Retractors. **A.** Volkman retractor. **B.** Lahey retractor. **C.** Senn retractor. (Courtesy of Sklar Instruments, West Chester, PA.) (Reprinted from Kronenberger J, Ledbetter J. *Jones & Bartlett Learning's Comprehensive Medical Assisting.* 5th ed. Burlington, MA: Jones & Bartlett Learning, LLC; 2016.)

Table 18-3 | Commonly Used Instruments and Equipment Listed by Medical Specialty

Medical Specialty	Instruments	Use
Dermatology (disorders of the skin)	(A) Keyes cutaneous punch	Remove a small circle of skin for microscopic study; available in different sizes (2–8 mm); disposable or reusable
	(B) Schamberg comedone extractor	Remove blackheads or open pustules

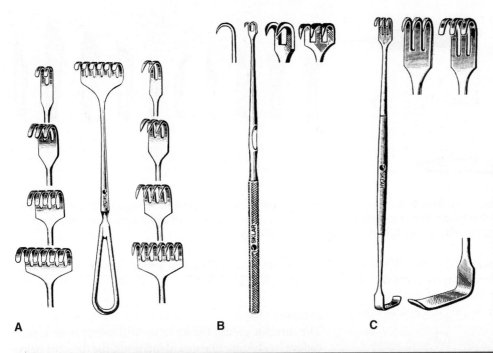

Obstetrics, gynecology	(A) Graves vaginal speculum (B) Pederson vaginal speculum	Widen the vaginal opening to view vaginal walls and/or the cervical os, or opening; available in various sizes; reusable or disposable plastic
	(C) Duplay tenaculum forceps (D) Schroeder tenaculum forceps	Grasp and hold tissue with its hook-like tips
	(E) Sims uterine sound (F) Simpson uterine sound, malleable (A sound is a long instrument for exploring or dilating body cavities or searching cavities for foreign bodies.)	Explore and dilate the uterus to assess its depth
	(G) Hand uterine dilator	
	(H) Hegar uterine dilator	Widen the cervical os, usually by 3–18 mm
	(I) Thomas uterine curettes, (J) Sims uterine curettes	Scrape endometrium (lining of uterus); may be blunt or sharp

Table 18-3	Commonly Used Instruments and Equipment Listed by Medical Specialty (*continued*)

Medical Specialty	Instruments	Use

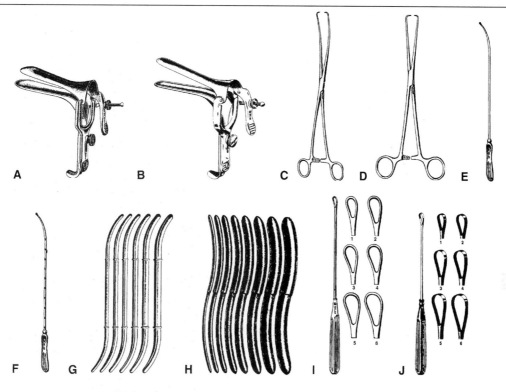

Ophthalmology	(A) Desmarres lid retractor, (B) Bailey foreign body remover	Hold eyelids open for removal of foreign bodies
	(C) Schiötz tonometer	Measure intraocular pressure to diagnose glaucoma

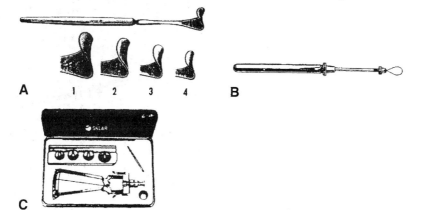

Otology (disorders of the ear, a subspecialty of otolaryngology); rhinology (disorders of the nose, a subspecialty of otolaryngology)	(A) Wilde ear forceps	Insert or remove materials from ear or nose canal
	(B) Lucae bayonet forceps	
	(C) Buck ear curet	Remove cerumen from deep ear canal
	(D) Vienna nasal speculum	Opens, extends nostrils for visualization of nasal passages

(*continued*)

Table 18-3	Commonly Used Instruments and Equipment Listed by Medical Specialty (*continued*)

Medical Specialty	Instruments	Use

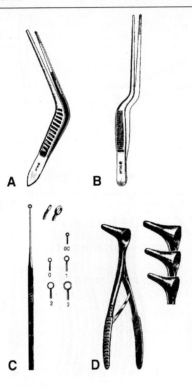

Orthopedics (disorders of the skeletal system, including the bones, joints, and spine)	(A) Oscillating plaster saw	Remove casts
	(B) Stille plaster shears	Remove casts
	(C) Hennig plaster spreader	Separates the edges of a cast that has been cut

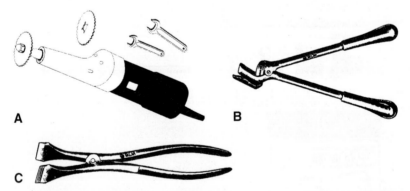

Proctology (disorders of the colon, rectum, and anus)	(A) Ives rectal speculum	Visualize lower intestinal tract; most have an obturator for ease of insertion. (An obturator is a smooth, rounded, removable inner portion of a hollow tube that allows for easier insertion.)
	(B) Pratt rectal speculum	
	(C) Hirschman anoscope, proctoscopes	
	Sigmoidoscope	Visualize lower sigmoid colon; may be rigid or flexible and has a fiber-optic light; some have a suction device
	Punch biopsy	Remove small, circular piece of tissue for study
	Alligator biopsy	Grasp and excise tissue with jaws of instrument

Table 18-3	Commonly Used Instruments and Equipment Listed by Medical Specialty (*continued*)

Medical Specialty	Instruments	Use

Urology (disorders of the urinary system)	(A) Otis-Dittel urethral sound	Explore bladder depth and direction; dilate urethral meatus (opening); comes in different sizes (Fr 8–26)
	(B) Dittel urethral sound	
	Prostate biopsy	Removes tissue for microscopic study

Images used with permission from Sklar Instruments.

- Discard disposable instruments promptly—Disposable scalpel blades should be removed from reusable handles and placed in sharps waste containers. If a disposable scalpel is used, the whole unit is placed in the sharps container. Syringes with needles attached and suture needles also must be discarded in the sharps container.
- Sanitize instruments before they are sterilized—Sterilization is more effective when instruments have been cleaned of visible contamination.
- Check instruments before sterilization—You need to make sure instruments stay in good working order. Watch for instruments in need of repair.

Checking Instruments

Surgical instruments should be checked carefully to make sure they are working properly. Here is what to look for.

- Blades or points should be free of bends and nicks.
- Instrument tips should close evenly and tightly.
- Instruments with box locks should move freely, but should not be too loose.
- Instruments with spring handles should have enough tension to grasp objects tightly.
- Scissors should close in a smooth, even manner with no nicks or snags. Scissors may be checked by cutting through gauze or cotton to be sure there are no rough areas.

Reducing Damage to Surgical Instruments

Surgical instruments are delicate. You can help minimize the chance of damage to instruments by following simple guidelines.

- Use instruments appropriately. Only use instruments for their specific purpose. For example, never use surgical scissors to cut paper or open packages. This could damage their cutting edges.
- Don't toss or drop instruments into a basin or sink. Blades or tips are easily damaged. Keep delicate instruments, such as tissue forceps or scissors, separate.
- Avoid stacking instruments in a pile. They may tangle and be damaged when separated.
- Always store sharp instruments separately. This helps prevent dulling or damaging sharp edges. It also helps prevent accidental injuries.
- Keep ratcheted instruments open when not in use. That way, the ratchet mechanism is less likely to be damaged.

Maintaining Surgical Equipment

You need to be familiar with the manufacturer's recommendations for each instrument or piece of equipment. Maintenance records should include any service provided by the manufacturer's representative. There also should be a place to record recommended or daily maintenance for keeping equipment in optimum working condition. Specific items in the maintenance record for each piece of equipment include the following:

- Date of purchase
- Model and serial number of equipment
- Time of recommended service
- Date service was requested
- Reason for the service request
- Name of the person requesting the service
- Description of the service performed and any parts replaced
- Name of the person performing the service and the date the work was completed
- Signature and title of the person who acknowledged completion of the work

Warranties and guarantees should be kept with the equipment records, along with the name of the manufacturer's contact person. You need to know whom to call if there's a problem.

Maintaining Surgical Supplies

Clinical medical assistants need to keep an up-to-date master list of all supplies, including purchases and replacements. Parts and supplies that are vital to the operation of the facility always should be kept on hand. Check instruction manuals for each piece of equipment when you order supplies for replacement or maintenance.

There are several factors to keep in mind when you decide which items to keep in inventory:

- Shelf life of the item
- Storage space available
- Time required to order and receive the item

If a piece of equipment cannot function without all of its components and some of the components have short lives, you need to have replacements on hand. For example, an ophthalmoscope without a light is basically useless.

Storage and Records

Clean and sterile supplies must be kept away from soiled items and waste. Sterile instruments, equipment, and supplies are usually kept in specific storage areas in the medical office. It is helpful if the storage area is near the rooms where the supplies will be used. The storage area should be kept neat and dust free.

Medical assistants are responsible for keeping accurate records of sterilized items and equipment. Typically, these records are kept in a log. The records include maintenance information about the equipment and load or sterilization information, including the following:

- Date and time of the sterilization cycle
- General description of the load
- Exposure time and temperature

- Name or initials of the operator
- Results of the sterilization indicator
- Expiration date of the load (usually 30 days)

GETTING READY FOR SURGERY

One of your responsibilities may be to prepare the treatment or examination room and the supplies needed for surgery. Many medical offices keep a box with index cards or a loose-leaf binder listing surgical procedures commonly performed in the office. It will include the items you will need to set up for the procedure.

Preparing the examination room and the supplies for surgery requires clean hands and careful technique to avoid contaminating the items inside the sterile area.

Case Question

What type of equipment, instruments, and supplies will the medical assistant, Ms. Bridges, need to gather in preparation of the suturing procedure to repair the laceration that Mr. Barnes has on his forearm?

Sterile Surgical Packs

Many of the basic supplies and equipment for a surgical procedure may be packaged together in a sterile surgical pack. Surgical packs may be prepared in the medical office or purchased from a commercial supplier. An example of a commercial pack is shown in Figure 18-13.

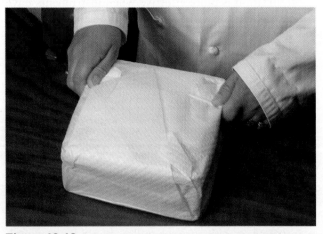

Figure 18-13 A wrapped sterile surgical package. (Reprinted from Kronenberger J, Ledbetter J. *Jones & Bartlett Learning's Comprehensive Medical Assisting.* 5th ed. Burlington, MA: Jones & Bartlett Learning, LLC; 2016.)

Packs Prepared in the Medical Office

Sterile setups are wrapped in a suitable wrapper and prepared in the office using autoclave sterilization. Packs are labeled according to the type of procedure. Each pack contains the general instruments needed for the procedure. Some basic supplies, such as gauze, cotton balls, and towels, also may be included before autoclaving.

Disposable Surgical Packs

Disposable surgical packs are popular because they are convenient and come with a variety of contents. They may contain one sterile item, such as a 4 × 4 sterile dressing, or a complete sterile surgical setup. Many are packaged with peel-apart wrappers. These wrappers have two loose flaps that can be pulled apart. They are designed to make it easy to drop the items carefully onto the operative field.

In some cases, the insides of the wrappers may be opened out and used as a sterile field. Some packages are enclosed in plastic and wrapped inside a barrier material that can be used as a sterile field.

Opening Surgical Packs

Labels for packs prepared in the office may only state the type of setup. However, labels on disposable sterile packs list the contents item by item. Disposable packs are generally more expensive than packages prepared in the office, so it is important to check that you have the right one for the procedure before you open it. You also need to check the expiration date on the package. If the pack has expired, don't use it. It may not be sterile.

Once a sterile pack has been opened, the procedure is similar whether the pack has been prepared commercially or in the office. Keep the following points in mind.

- Use clean hands to open the sterile items or packages.
- The outside surface of the outside wrapper is *not* sterile.
- Take care not to touch any sterile areas with your hands or other surfaces. The sterile area includes the inside surface of the outside wrapper, the inside wrapper (if any), and the contents of the package.
- If any sterile area or item does contact another surface, the pack is considered contaminated and must be replaced.
- Check the sterilization indicator inside the sterile pack. It indicates whether the items inside the package have been sterilized properly.

Maintaining a Sterile Field

Even in minor surgery, it's important to prevent pathogens from entering the patient's body during the procedure. This requires that the surgical area or field remains sterile. Remember that "sterile to sterile is sterile," and "sterile to unknown is contaminated." Here's what to do and what to avoid to maintain a sterile field.

1. Always face a sterile field. That way, you can be sure it hasn't been contaminated. If you need to turn your back or leave the area, cover the field with a sterile drape. Make sure you use sterile techniques.
2. Hold all sterile items above waist level. When sterile items aren't where you can see them, you'll have to presume they've become contaminated.
3. Place sterile items in the middle of the sterile field. A 1-inch border around the field is considered contaminated.
4. Don't spill any liquids, even sterile liquids, onto a sterile field. The surface below the field isn't sterile. Moisture can be wicked up into the field—along with microorganisms.
5. Don't cough, sneeze, or talk over the sterile field. Microbes from your respiratory tract can contaminate the field.
6. Never reach over the sterile field. Dust or lint from your clothing might enter the sterile field.
7. Don't pass soiled supplies, such as gauze or instruments, over the sterile field.
8. If you know or suspect the sterile field has been contaminated, alert the physician. Sterility must be established before the procedure can continue.

Watch for Signs of Contamination

When you work with sterile surgical items, you need to know when items are considered contaminated—even if they have not been used. Contaminated items must be repackaged and sterilized again if any of the following situations occur.

- Moisture is present on the pack. Microbes can be drawn into the package in liquid absorbed through its wrap. If a package sterilized in the medical office gets moist, it must be repackaged in a clean, dry wrapper and sterilized again. If a damp pack is disposable, it must be discarded.
- Items are dropped outside the sterile field. If an item touches a surface outside the sterile field, it is considered contaminated.
- Expired date. The date on the outside of the pack should not be over 30 days old for packs prepared in the office. Commercially prepared packs should not be used after the expiration date listed on the pack.
- The wrapper is damaged or torn. Damaged or torn wrappers could allow microbes into the package. Items should be discarded or rewrapped and sterilized again.
- When any area is known or thought to have been touched by a contaminated item.

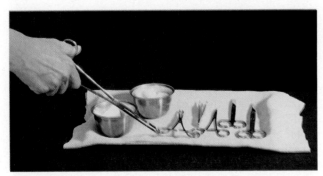

Figure 18-14 Sterile transfer forceps may be used to add or move items on the sterile field.

Using Sterile Transfer Forceps

One way to move sterile items or place them on the sterile field is to use sterile transfer forceps. When using sterile transfer forceps, the tips of the forceps and items being moved must stay sterile. See Figure 18-14. The handles of the forceps are considered medically aseptic, but not sterile, because they are touched by the bare hands of the person using them.

Storing Sterile Transfer Forceps

Sterile transfer forceps can be stored in one of three ways.

- In a dry, sterile container. The forceps and the container must be sanitized and autoclaved every day.
- In a wrapped sterile package. The wrapping protects the forceps from being exposed to microorganisms and maintains sterility.
- In a sterile solution in a closed container system. A closed container helps to protect tips of forceps from

contamination. The forceps and the container must be sterilized every day. Fresh solution must be added daily.

Peel-Back Packages and Solutions

Sometimes, the sterile pack will contain all the supplies needed for a procedure, including gauze squares or cotton balls. In other cases, additional supplies are required.

Usually, small supplies are provided in commercially prepared, peel-apart packages. These packages contain small or single items to add to the sterile field. The packaging is designed with two flaps. The flaps allow the package to be opened without contaminating its sterile contents as demonstrated in Figure 18-15.

To open the peel-pack package properly, you must use both hands. Here is how.

- Place your thumbs just inside the tops of the flaps' edges.
- Separate the flaps using a slow, outward motion of the thumbs and flaps.
- Keep in mind that the inside of the sealed package and its contents are sterile. When you open the pack, finger and airborne droplets from talking or sneezing can contaminate the pack rendering it unsterile.

Once the peel-back package is opened, there are three ways to add its contents to the sterile field.

- Using sterile transfer forceps. Once the package is opened, hold down the two edges. Lift the contents up and away with sterile forceps as demonstrated in Figure 18-16.

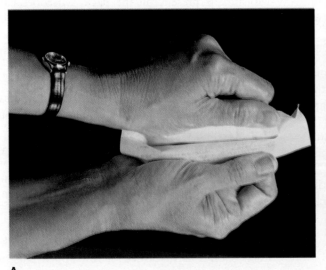

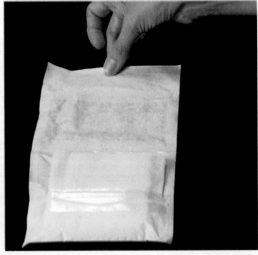

A   **B**

Figure 18-15 **A.** Open sterile packets by grasping the edges and rolling the thumbs outward. **B.** Opening the packet properly forms a sterile field. (Reprinted from Kronenberger J, Ledbetter J. *Jones & Bartlett Learning's Comprehensive Medical Assisting.* 5th ed. Burlington, MA: Jones & Bartlett Learning, LLC; 2016.)

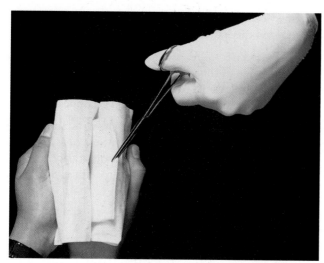

Figure 18-16 The physician may use sterile forceps to remove small supplies from peel-back packages. (Reprinted from Kronenberger J, Ledbetter J. *Jones & Bartlett Learning's Comprehensive Medical Assisting.* 5th ed. Burlington, MA: Jones & Bartlett Learning, LLC; 2016.)

- This process often requires two people—one to hold the package open and the other to remove the contents with the sterile forceps.
- Using a sterile gloved hand. This method requires two people. The medical assistant opens the package and holds the edges carefully to avoid touching the physician's gloves. The physician uses a gloved hand to remove the contents (Fig. 18-17).
- Flipping the contents onto the sterile field. To do this, you need to step back from the sterile field so that your hands and the outer wrapper of the package, which isn't sterile, don't cross the sterile field. Pull

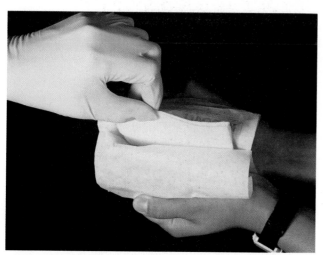

Figure 18-17 Sterile gloved hands may be used to remove sterile items. (Reprinted from Kronenberger J, Ledbetter J. *Jones & Bartlett Learning's Comprehensive Medical Assisting.* 5th ed. Burlington, MA: Jones & Bartlett Learning, LLC; 2016.)

the package edges down and away from the contents. Carefully drop or flip item onto the middle of the sterile field without touching the 1-inch border around the edge of the sterile field.

Most items in peel-back packages are disposable items. This means they cannot be resterilized after being opened. They must be discarded, even if they have not been used. Because they are relatively expensive, sterile packs of disposable items should not be opened until they are needed. You might place a small supply near the area where the procedure is being performed, to be opened only if necessary.

Some additional small items and solutions used during the surgical procedure must be added to the sterile field at the time of setup. Some procedures may require sterile water, saline, or an antiseptic solution such as Betadine. Solutions need to be poured into sterile basins or containers.

 PREPARING THE PATIENT FOR SURGERY

As a clinical medical assistant, you will play an important role in preparing the patient before the physician performs minor surgery. You may need to:

- Help obtain the patient's consent for the procedure
- Answer questions about instructions to the patient
- Position and drape the patient for the procedure
- Prepare the patient's skin

Cultural Connection

As we discover different cultures and beliefs, we must examine some of the religions of the world and the practices that need to be considered and respected as we provide health care to the followers. The Sikh faith was established in India in the 1400s. It is the fifth largest religion in the world. A true follower of the Sikh religion believes that body hair should be naturally preserved. When providing medical care to a Sikh, it is important to consult with the patient before cutting any hair or shaving any part of the body. To a Sikh, uncut hair represents spirituality. A Sikh may actually refuse to have medical treatment if required to cut or shave hair from the body. This is particularly important if the patient needs to have a surgical procedure that requires removing hair from the body.

Informed Consent

It is necessary to obtain informed consent from the patient before performing a surgical procedure in the medical office. An **informed consent** form is a legal document that explains the course of treatment, including the risks and benefits to the patient. This form may be signed on a visit prior to the day of surgery or on the day of the surgery. The procedure cannot go ahead unless the patient signs the form.

It's the physician's legal responsibility to give the patient a full explanation of any surgical procedure. By signing the informed consent document, the patient agrees that she has received this explanation. The document must state:

- The procedure
- The purpose of the procedure
- The expected results of the procedure
- Any possible side effects, risks, and complications

The form should have spaces for the date and signatures of the patient, physician, and witness or witnesses. By signing the document, the patient voluntarily accepts the risks involved and agrees to the procedure. See sample form in Figure 18-18.

SPECIAL CONSENT TO OPERATION OR OTHER PROCEDURE(S)

PATIENT _____   PATIENT NUMBER _____

DATE _____   TIME _____

1. I HEREBY AUTHORIZE DOCTOR _____ AND/OR SUCH ASSISTANTS AS MAY BE SELECTED BY HIM, TO PERFORM THE FOLLOWING PROCEDURE(S):

   _____

   ON _____
       (NAME OF PATIENT OR MYSELF)

2. THE PROCEDURE(S) LISTED ABOVE HAVE BEEN EXPLAINED TO ME BY DR. AND I UNDERSTAND THE NATURE AND THE CONSEQUENCES OF THE PROCEDURE(S).

3. I RECOGNIZE THAT, DURING THE COURSE OF THE OPERATION, UNFORESEEN CONDITIONS MAY NECESSITATE ADDITIONAL OR DIFFERENT PROCEDURES THAN THOSE SET FORTH. I FURTHER AUTHORIZE AND REQUEST THAT THE ABOVE NAMED SURGEON, HIS ASSISTANTS, OR HIS DESIGNEES PERFORM SUCH PROCEDURES AS ARE IN HIS PROFESSIONAL JUDGMENT NECESSARY AND DESIRABLE, INCLUDING, BUT NOT LIMITED TO, PROCEDURES INVOLVING PATHOLOGY AND RADIOLOGY. THE AUTHORITY GRANTED UNDER THIS PARAGRAPH SHALL EXTEND TO REMEDYING CONDITIONS NOT KNOWN TO DR. _____ AT THE TIME THE OPERATION IS COMMENCED.

4. I AM AWARE THAT THE PRACTICE OF MEDICINE AND SURGERY IS NOT AN EXACT SCIENCE AND I ACKNOWLEDGE THAT NO GUARANTEES HAVE BEEN MADE TO ME AS TO THE RESULTS OF THE OPERATION OR PROCEDURE.

5. TISSUE REMOVED DURING SURGERY SHALL BE SENT TO PATHOLOGY TO BE EXAMINED AND DISPOSED OF IN ACCORDANCE WITH THE RULES AND REGULATIONS OF THE MEDICAL STAFF OF THE SURGERY CENTER.

_____   _____
Procedure has been discussed with patient. (Surgeon's Signature)   SIGNATURE OF PATIENT

PATIENT IS UNABLE TO SIGN BECAUSE   ☐ HE (SHE) IS A MINOR _____ YEARS OF AGE

☐ OTHER (SPECIFY) _____

_____   _____
WITNESS   PERSON AUTHORIZED TO SIGN FOR PATIENT

_____
RELATIONSHIP OF ABOVE TO PATIENT

Figure 18-18 Sample consent form. (Reprinted from Kronenberger J, Ledbetter J. *Jones & Bartlett Learning's Comprehensive Medical Assisting.* 5th ed. Burlington, MA: Jones & Bartlett Learning, LLC; 2016.)

The medical assistant is not responsible for informing the patient, but often acts as a witness.

Answering the Patient's Questions

Although the physician is responsible for obtaining informed consent, the patient may ask you questions about the procedure—for example:

- How long will it take?
- What preparations are needed?
- Is fasting necessary?

You may answer these questions after verifying the information with the physician.

Prior to the day of surgery, the patient may be given instructions about how to prepare for surgery. The physician may prescribe medication for the patient to take at home before the procedure. It is good practice to give the patient written instructions to take home.

You need to notify the physician if the patient seems confused or does not understand the instructions. Encourage the patient to call the office if he thinks of questions later. Of course, the instructions should be documented in the patient's medical record.

Positioning the Patient

Before positioning the patient for a minor surgical procedure, ask the patient to void, or urinate, to help prevent discomfort during the procedure.

Here are some other ways you can make the patient more comfortable.

- Offer to help the patient remove whatever clothing is necessary to expose the operative site.
- Provide the patient with extra sheets or a blanket. If the office is air conditioned, it may be uncomfortably cool for the patient's exposed skin.
- Help the patient into a comfortable position on the examining table. While waiting for the physician, there is no need for the patient to stay in an uncomfortable position, such as the lithotomy or the knee-chest position.

When the physician is ready to begin, help the patient into a position that exposes the operative site and makes it accessible to the physician. You may give the patient pillows for support or comfort.

Types of Drapes

The procedure and the patient's position determine the type of drapes used to expose the operative site and cover the patient. Disposable paper drapes are commonly used in the medical office. They come in many sizes and shapes, depending on their specific use. Paper drapes can be used alone or in combination with separate drape sheets and towels.

Fenestrated drapes have an opening to expose the operative site while covering other areas. They also come in various sizes. Small fenestrated drapes may be used for procedures such as inserting sutures. Large fenestrated drapes might be used to cover the legs and lower abdomen while exposing the perineal area—the area between the anus and the genital organs.

Some sterile drapes are combined with adhesive-backed clear plastic. The plastic sticks to the patient's skin and eliminates the need for towel clamps.

Draping the Patient

After the surgical scrub has been done, follow these steps for draping a patient with a sterile drape:

1. Pick up the drape on the 1-inch border that's considered nonsterile. No gloves are needed.
2. Lift the drape over the surgical area without contaminating the drape.
3. Place the drape on the patient from his side farthest away to closest. This way you will not have to reach over the drape after you've placed it on the patient. See Figure 18-19.

To remove contaminated drapes from the patient after the procedure, put on clean examination gloves. You need to follow standard precautions when removing soiled sheets, towels, or drapes after minor surgery. They could be contaminated with blood or body fluids. Carefully roll the items away from your body, keeping the contaminated edges inside. By surrounding the dirtier areas of the drape with the cleaner areas, your clothing is less likely to be contaminated.

Preparing Skin

Before surgery, you need to remove as many microbes as possible from the patient's skin in the operative area.

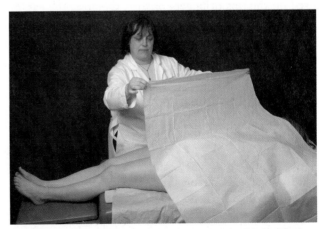

Figure 18-19 Applying a sterile drape. (Reprinted from Kronenberger J, Ledbetter J. *Jones & Bartlett Learning's Comprehensive Medical Assisting.* 5th ed. Burlington, MA: Jones & Bartlett Learning, LLC; 2016.)

Preparing the skin decreases the chance of wound contamination and infection. Skin preparations may include the following:

- Applying antiseptic solution
- Removing gross contaminants and hair

 # ASSISTING WITH SURGERY

During minor surgery, your role will be to assist the physician as needed. You may be asked to hold supplies for the physician, adjust the patient's drapes, pass instruments to the physician, or help collect specimens. As you become more experienced, you will find it easier to anticipate what is needed and have instruments and supplies ready before the physician asks for them.

Local Anesthetics

A local anesthetic is a substance that numbs the operative area to minimize pain or discomfort to the patient. Local anesthetic may be used occasionally if a wound contains embedded debris. The anesthetic is injected in the wound site to make the process of wound cleaning more comfortable for the patient.

Many different kinds of anesthetics are used in the medical office. A few examples are:

- Lidocaine (Xylocaine or Baylocaine)
- Mepivacaine (Carbocaine)
- Bupivacaine (Marcaine)

Sometimes, epinephrine is added to local anesthetics to cause vasoconstriction (the narrowing of blood vessels). It slows the absorption of the anesthetic by the body and lengthens its effectiveness. Epinephrine may be used when the physician expects a long procedure. But in some cases, vasoconstriction can damage body tissues. Anesthesia with epinephrine should never be used on the tips of fingers or toes, the nose, the ear, or the penis.

There are two methods for administering local anesthesia. The method used will depend on when the physician plans to administer the anesthesia.

Administering Anesthetic: Method 1

In the first method, you will draw the anesthetic as the physician's assistant.

- When you draw the anesthetic for the physician into a syringe, it is important to keep the vial beside the syringe for the physician's approval.
- When you draw the anesthetic, the outside of the syringe and needle unit are not sterile. The anesthetic is given to the patient before the physician puts on sterile gloves.

Administering Anesthetic: Method 2

In the second method, the physician draws the anesthetic. This method is used if the physician puts on sterile gloves before administering the anesthetic.

1. Include a sterile syringe and needle on the sterile field setup.
2. When the physician is ready to administer the anesthetic, show the physician the label on the vial. Then clean the rubber stopper of the vial with an alcohol swab.
3. You hold the vial while the physician draws the required amount into the syringe.

There are many ways to hold the vial securely while the physician draws the anesthetic. You and the physician will work together to develop a method that maintains surgical asepsis. See Figure 18-20 for the proper method of holding a vial for the physician.

Passing Surgical Instruments and Supplies

Passing instruments to the physician requires careful attention. You must maintain the integrity of the sterile field throughout the procedure. Tell the physician immediately if there is any possibility that the sterile field

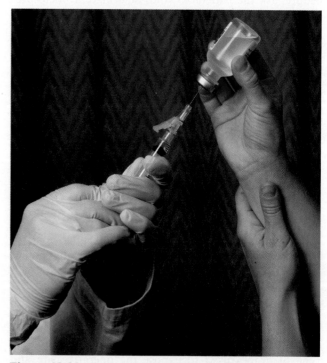

Figure 18-20 Hold the vial containing the anesthetic downward, supporting that wrist with the other hand. (Reprinted from Kronenberger J, Ledbetter J. *Jones & Bartlett Learning's Comprehensive Medical Assisting*. 5th ed. Burlington, MA: Jones & Bartlett Learning, LLC; 2016.)

has been contaminated. Here are some tips for passing instruments during minor surgery:

- Watch the procedure closely so you can anticipate the physician's needs. For example, if the physician is making an incision, have sterile sponges ready to soak up any blood.
- The physician may ask for an instrument verbally or show you what is needed with her hands. After you have worked together for a while, you will learn what the physician is likely to ask for during different parts of the procedure.
- When passing an instrument to the physician, grip the instrument firmly by its tips. Hold blades or sharp edges down for safety. The handle end should be directed toward the physician.
- Place the instrument gently but firmly into the physician's palm or fingers.
- Wait until you feel the physician grasp the instrument before you let go. You do not want the instrument to drop onto the floor—or onto the patient.

Wound Closure

Many types of wounds need to be closed in order to heal rapidly, with minimal scarring. This is accomplished by **approximation**, or bringing the edges of the wound as close together as possible to their original position. There are several methods and materials for closing wounds. The most common ones are:

- Sutures
- Adhesives
- Staples

Sutures

Sutures are sterile, surgical materials for connecting wounds and tissues. See examples in Figure 18-21.

Sometimes, incisions are necessary to bring tissue layers into close approximation. Sutures are inserted:

- To bring tissues together after the removal of a cyst or tissue sample
- To close lacerations
- To help skin surfaces heal

Some sutures are absorbed by the body, while others must be removed. In the medical office, suturing is the most common method for closing wounds.

Adhesives

Adhesive skin closures may be used to approximate the edges of a small wound if sutures are not needed. Strips are placed transversely across the line of the wound. In most cases, the strips are left in place until they fall off. Examples are shown in Figure 18-22A, B.

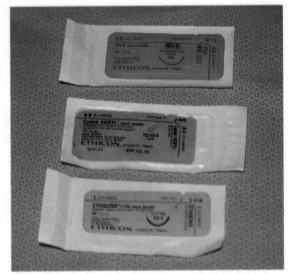

Figure 18-21 Suture material and needles are supplied in see-through packages with the size of the suture material and the type of needle listed on the packet. The inside of the packet is sterile. (Reprinted from Kronenberger J, Ledbetter J. *Jones & Bartlett Learning's Comprehensive Medical Assisting.* 5th ed. Burlington, MA: Jones & Bartlett Learning, LLC; 2016.)

In some cases, the physician may want them replaced or removed if they become soiled with drainage. Strips should not be pulled away from the wound. Tension on the wound site may disrupt the healing process.

Staples

Skin staples are sometimes used to close large incisions over areas where dehiscence can occur. **Dehiscence** is the separation of wound edges.

Sterile skin staples are commonly made of stainless steel. Areas where staples might be used include the knee, hip, or abdomen. Specialized staples made of sterling silver may be used in neurosurgery. Staples usually are not inserted in the medical office. They are removed when the wound is completely healed.

Suture Needles

The supplies used for suturing are needles and suture materials. There are several kinds of suture needles. Needles used for minor office surgery will depend on the type of surgery being performed.

Needles are classified in these ways: by shape, by point, or by eye.

Classified by Shape

Needles may be curved or straight. Curved needles usually are clamped in a needle holder before being handed to or used by the physician. Straight needles are not clamped in a needle holder. They are handed to the physician with the point up. Straight needles rarely are used in medical offices.

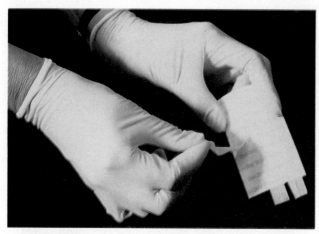
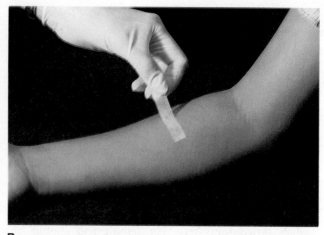

A   **B**

Figure 18-22 Adhesive skin closures. **A.** These lightweight lengths of porous tape are used for closing small wounds. **B.** Strips are placed transversely across a wound. (Reprinted from Kronenberger J, Ledbetter J. *Jones & Bartlett Learning's Comprehensive Medical Assisting.* 5th ed. Burlington, MA: Jones & Bartlett Learning, LLC; 2016.)

Classified by Point

Needle points are cutting, or round, and tapered. Cutting needles have sharp edges and are used to cut through tough tissues, such as skin. Straight cutting needles are called Keith needles. Noncutting tapered or round needles are used on subcutaneous tissue. Subcutaneous tissue is located below the skin. They also may be used on muscle or on the peritoneum, a thin membrane lining the body cavity and covering some organs.

Classified by Eye

Traumatic needles have an eye and can be threaded with any length of suture material. Atraumatic needles are eyeless and come with a specific length of suture thread attached. Atraumatic needles are also called swaged needles because the suture material is swaged, or fused, to the needle in the manufacturing process.

Atraumatic needles cause less damage than traumatic needles when they pass through body tissues. Needles with eyes have a double thickness of suture where the suture passes through the eye. This double thickness makes a larger opening when pulled through tissues, compared to the single thickness of suture in eyeless needles.

Choosing a Needle

The physician usually selects the suture and the needle. In medical offices, curved swaged needles are used far more often than any other type. Swaged needles are selected based on the size and length of the suture material and the needle gauge. The needle gauge, or needle diameter, is marked clearly on the packaging material. When a suture must be threaded through an eyed needle, both the needle gauge and the suture size must be selected.

Sutures, needles, and suture–needle combinations come in peel-apart packages. The packages are sterile on the inside. Sutures and needles can be added to the sterile field using sterile transfer forceps, a sterile gloved hand, or by carefully flipping them onto the field.

Types of Sutures

There are two main types of sutures: absorbable sutures and nonabsorbable sutures.

Absorbable sutures are broken down by the body and do not have to be removed. Here are some other useful facts about these sutures.

- These sutures are referred to commonly as catgut. This suture material is made from the intestines of sheep or cattle.
- The two forms of absorbable gut suture are chromic and plain. Chromic means the suture is chemically treated to delay absorption by the body. Plain absorbable suture is not treated and is absorbed more quickly.
- Absorbable sutures are used most often in hospital settings to hold deep tissue.

Nonabsorbable sutures either remain in the body permanently or are removed after healing.

They are made of natural fibers such as silk or cotton; synthetics such as nylon, Dacron, or polypropylene, or stainless steel wire.

Nonabsorbable sutures come in many different brands, lengths, sizes, and swaged needles, making them very versatile.

Common Office Surgical Procedures

Two of the most frequently performed minor surgeries in a general medical office are as follows:

- Removing skin lesions
- Draining abscesses

Biopsy (Bx), the removal of a tissue sample for diagnostic examination, is another procedure that's commonly performed in some medical offices. You must follow standard precautions when you assist with any of these procedures.

Excision of a Lesion

A lesion is a local area of diseased or abnormal tissue. Some lesions that may be removed in a medical office include the following:

- Mole
- Skin tag
- Lentigine, a small, flat, dark spot on the skin that resembles a freckle
- Keratosis, a horny growth, such as a wart or callus

To excise something is to cut it out. Physicians use several techniques to excise lesions or remove them in other ways.

- Standard method refers to the process of excising the lesion using a scalpel.
- Electrosurgery is a process where high-frequency electric current is used to excise the lesion or else destroy it.
- Laser surgery uses focused, intense beams of light to penetrate and remove tissue.
- Cryosurgery is a method that uses extreme cold to either excise or destroy diseased or abnormal tissue.

Some lesions may be desiccated or fulgurated (destroyed by drying up) by using electrosurgical or cryosurgical methods. However, in many cases, samples are sent to a pathology laboratory for diagnosis. If samples are required, the lesion is excised using one of the above methods.

Tissue Biopsy

Excision also can be used to remove tissue for biopsy. The tissue is sent to the laboratory and examined under a microscope to assist in diagnosis. Typically, only small samples of tissue are needed for examination. When a lesion is biopsied, however, the entire lesion is generally excised for evaluation. In a punch biopsy, a small section is removed from the center of the abnormal tissue. Although some biopsies are performed in a hospital, skin biopsies can be performed in the medical office.

Cervical Biopsies

Another procedure that may be performed in the medical office is the cervical biopsy. This is a procedure in which a small piece of tissue is removed from a female patient's cervix. The physician removes the tissue during a colposcopy—a visual examination of the cervix using an instrument with a magnifying lens and a light (colposcope).

Physicians usually perform this procedure when a patient's Pap smear shows abnormal results, or when the physician sees an abnormal area on the cervix during a routine examination.

Incision and Drainage

An incision and drainage (I&D) is performed to release pus from an abscess. An abscess is a collection of pus that has formed in a cavity surrounded by inflamed tissue. An abscess is the body's response to an infection, when pathogens have entered through a break in the skin. Abscesses may be referred to as boils, furuncles (a single lesion), or carbuncles (several lesions grouped closely together). Abscesses are very painful for the patient. The site of the abscess must be incised (cut into), and the infected material drained before healing can take place.

Specimen Collection

Many minor office procedures yield specimens that must be sent to a laboratory for examination. Specimens include samples of tissue, foreign bodies, and samples of wound exudate, or drainage. It is your job to choose a proper container with an appropriate preservative for the procedure being performed. The preservative helps to prevent the sample from breaking down or decaying before it can be examined.

The laboratory where the specimen is sent usually provides the appropriate containers with preservative. There should be a stock of them on hand in the medical office. You will need to assist the physician in collecting the specimen by holding the open container steady. The physician must drop the specimen directly into the preservative without touching the sides of the container. See Figure 18-23.

You will be responsible for attaching a label to the specimen. The label must contain the patient's name and

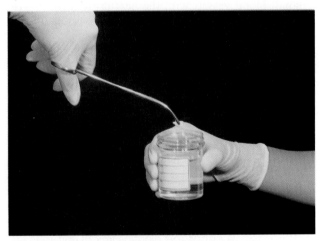

Figure 18-23 Tissue samples are placed in the preservative by the physician. (Reprinted from Kronenberger J, Ledbetter J. *Jones & Bartlett Learning's Comprehensive Medical Assisting.* 5th ed. Burlington, MA: Jones & Bartlett Learning, LLC; 2016.)

the date. You will also need to complete a laboratory request form to send with the specimen. Several pieces of information must be included on the form:

- The patient's name, age, and gender
- The patient's identification number or social security number
- The date the specimen was taken
- The type of specimen
- The location the specimen was taken from
- The type of examination requested
- The physician's name or laboratory contract number

Electrosurgery

Medical offices often use electrosurgery to remove moles, cysts, warts, and certain types of skin and cervical cancers. In electrosurgery, high-frequency alternating current is used to destroy or cut and remove tissue. One advantage of this method is that the electricity seals small bleeding vessels and reduces the blood and cell fluid lost in the process.

Electrosurgical units use disposable electrodes, or devices that carry electricity. An example is shown in Figure 18-24.

The tips on the electrodes have different shapes and sizes depending on their use. Electrode tips include blades, needles, loops, and balls. The following procedures are considered electrosurgery.

- Fulguration destroys tissue with controlled electric sparks. The physician holds the electrode tip 1 to 2 mm from the operative site. A series of sparks destroys superficial cells at the site.
- Electrodesiccation dries and separates tissue with an electric current. The electrode is placed directly on the site.
- Electrocautery causes quick coagulation or clotting of small blood vessels with the heat created by electric current. This process is also called electrocoagulation.

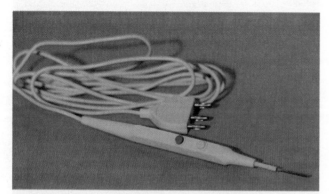

Figure 18-24 A disposable electrosurgical unit. The blade is designed either to cut or to cauterize. (Reprinted from Kronenberger J, Ledbetter J. *Jones & Bartlett Learning's Comprehensive Medical Assisting.* 5th ed. Burlington, MA: Jones & Bartlett Learning, LLC; 2016.)

- Electrosection is the incision or excision of tissue. Bleeding is minimal with this type of procedure. However, it may increase damage to the surrounding tissues.

During electrosurgery, you are responsible for the safety and comfort of the patient. You will need to hand the electrode to the physician as needed. Always pass the electrode with the tip pointing down.

Electrosurgery Safety

The physician will power on and operate the electrosurgical unit. However, you could cause injuries to the patient, the physician, and yourself if you do not follow proper procedures. Pay close attention to these safety measures when assisting with electrosurgery.

- Make sure all working parts are in good repair. The electrical current is carefully regulated. If the machine is defective, the patient might be seriously injured.
- Make sure all metal is removed from the patient. You also need to ensure the patient does not have any metal implants or a cardiac pacemaker. Metal conducts electricity and can cause serious burns. Metal implants may become very hot, and pacemakers can malfunction.
- Be sure the patient is grounded with a pad supplied by the manufacturer. Attach the pad to the patient at a site recommended by the manufacturer. Some manufacturers advise placing the pad near the operative site. Others recommend placing it far away. Know what the recommendations are for the device in your office. Improper placement of the pad can lead to injury.
- Place the grounding pad firmly and completely against the patient's skin. With some pads, you must apply a conducting gel to the pad and to the patient. Adhesive-backed pads facilitate conduction through the grounding pad. If areas of the skin under the pad do not have good contact with the pad, hot spots may occur. Hot spots can burn the patient.

Maintaining the Electrosurgical Unit

Here are some hints to maintaining the electrosurgical unit properly.

- The electrode tips for the unit are usually disposable. They should be discarded after use.
- Some medical offices may still use reusable electrode tips. These should be disinfected and processed in the autoclave according to the manufacturer's directions. Reusable tips must be polished with steel wool if they become dull.
- The surfaces of the electrosurgical unit should be kept clean and dry.
- Machines should be covered when not in use.
- Electrosurgical machines must be inspected from time to time to ensure they are working properly. Check

the operating manual for the regular maintenance to be performed by office staff. It also will contain information about how often routine inspections should be performed by trained technicians. A maintenance log should be kept.

Laser Surgery

Lasers also can be used to cut tissue and coagulate small bleeding vessels. Lasers are devices that focus high-intensity light in a narrow beam to create extreme heat and energy. Light from a laser usually is not visible. Colored filters illuminate the laser's target. This allows the physician to direct the laser beam to the surgical area.

There are many types of lasers, each with a specific medical use. The most common types of lasers used in the medical office are the:

- Argon laser, used for coagulation
- Carbon dioxide laser, used for cutting tissue
- Nd:YAG, used for coagulation and to separate warts and moles from surrounding tissues

You need to pay special attention when caring for and handling the laser. It is important to read and follow the maintenance schedules and procedures in the instruction manual. It is recommended that health care workers complete a training program before assisting with laser procedures. During a laser procedure, everyone in the room must wear goggles to protect their eyes—including the patient.

AFTER SURGICAL PROCEDURES

The medical assistant has several other important responsibilities once the surgery is complete.

- Applying dressings and bandages to surgical wounds. A dressing is a sterile material or cloth used to cover a wound and stop bleeding. A bandage is a material used to secure a dressing.
- Instructing the patient about postoperative wound care. This care includes observing the wound for changes that indicate infection or other problems with healing.
- Assisting with postoperative instructions such as prescriptions, medications, and scheduling return visits.
- Removing and caring for instruments, equipment, and supplies. You need to dispose properly of waste, including disposable items, sharps, and contaminated or unused supplies.
- Preparing the room for the next patient.

Most offices provide detailed written patient instructions prior to releasing the patient from the office. The instructions will help the patient remember what to do once they are home and assist in avoiding any postoperative problems.

Wound Care

Dry sterile dressings (DSD) and bandages protect wounds during the healing process. Sterile dressings have several purposes in wound care:

- To protect the wound from contamination
- To exert pressure on an open wound to control bleeding
- To absorb drainage such as blood, pus, or serum (a clear, sticky part of blood that remains after coagulation)
- To hold medications against the wound and facilitate healing
- To hide temporary disfigurement

Bandages are strips of woven material typically used with sterile dressings. The purposes of bandages are:

- To hold dressings in place
- To provide additional pressure to control bleeding
- To provide protection from contamination
- To keep an injured body part immobile during healing
- To support an injured body part
- To improve circulation

Sterile Dressings

A sterile dressing is considered contaminated if it is damp or outdated, if the wrapper is damaged, or if it has been improperly removed from the wrapper. Sterile dressings are items such as 4 × 4-inch absorbent gauze sponges and nonadhering dressings that are made for use on open wounds. They typically are prepackaged in small numbers. They come in various sizes and shapes, each for a specific use. You will choose the dressing to use based on the size of the wound and the amount of drainage. You must use sterile technique when handling dressings. A sterile dressing may be held in place by different kinds of bandages.

Changing Sterile Dressings

When you remove a sterile dressing or change an existing one, always wear clean examination gloves. Observe the wound carefully for any drainage or exudates. Note the characteristics of the wound drainage in the patient's chart.

It is normal to see serum or bloody drainage in small or moderate amounts immediately following the closure of a wound. If you notice **purulent** drainage—that is, drainage with a color other than pink—notify the physician while the wound is still uncovered. The physician can then examine the wound and make a decision about how well healing is progressing.

Wound Drainage

When observing wound drainage and documenting it in the patient's chart, be sure to note the color and amount as described below.

Color

- Serous drainage is clear.
- Sanguineous drainage is blood tinged.
- Serosanguineous drainage is pinkish, or a mixture of clear and red.
- Purulent drainage is white, green, or yellow tinged. It's usually accompanied by an unpleasant odor. This type of drainage is a sign of infection.

Amount

- Copious is a large amount.
- Medium describes a moderate amount.
- Scant refers to a small amount.

You also can quantify the amount by noting the size of the drainage (e.g., 2-inch diameter, entire 4 × 4 dressing saturated) or the size of the dressing.

Types of Bandages

There are several different types of bandages, including roller, elastic, or tubular gauze. A bandage may be used to hold a sterile dressing in place. The type of bandage used depends on the nature of the wound or injury.

Roller Bandages

These bandages are soft, woven materials packaged in a roll. They are available in various lengths and widths, from 1 to 6 or more inches. The bandage size used depends on:

- The part being bandaged
- The desired thickness of the completed bandage

Most bandages are made of a porous, lightweight material. Some may be sterile. Others are just clean. Gauze bandages conform easily to body surfaces. Stretchy gauze is made to adjust to body contours. It resists unrolling much better than plain types of gauze. Kling and Conform are two frequently used brands. Paper or surgical tape is used to hold the ends of the bandage in place.

Elastic Bandages

These are special bandage rolls with elastic woven through the fabric. They are generally brownish tan in color. Unlike other types of roller gauze, elastic bandages can be given to the patient to take home to be washed and reused many times. Ace is one brand of elastic bandage that is widely available.

Elastic bandages should be applied without wrinkling in partly overlapping layers. Some elastic bandages have adhesive backing, which helps keep the layers in place and provides a secure, snug, and comfortable fit. Adjust the bandage if it seems too loose or if the patient says it is uncomfortable or tight.

You must take care in applying this type of bandage because of the elastic fibers. The bandage must be applied snugly to give support to the injured part. But a bandage that is too tight can slow or cut off blood circulation.

The bandage should be wrapped in the direction of blood flow from the distal to proximal area of the limb. Never stretch or pull on an elastic bandage during application because you might apply it too tightly.

Ask the patient how tight the bandage feels as it is being applied. Instruct the patient on signs of impaired circulation. The patient should check an extremity (a limb such as an arm or leg) distal (farthest away) from the bandage for these signs:

- Increased swelling or pain
- Pale skin
- Cool skin when compared to the other extremity
- Bluish coloring to toenails or fingernails

Most manufacturers of elastic bandages have removed the separate metal clips that were used to hold the end of the bandage in place. These small clips are dangerous if they are lost and swallowed by a small child. Use paper or surgical tape to hold the bandage in place.

Tubular Gauze Bandages

Tubular gauze bandages are used to enclose rounded body parts. The bandage looks like a hollow tube and is very stretchy. These bandages come in various widths from 5/8 to 7 inches. They can be used to enclose the fingers, toes, arms, legs, and even the head and torso.

Tubular gauze is applied using a tubular, frame-like applicator. The applicator is made of metal or plastic and is available in various sizes. The size of the applicator should be slightly larger than the body part to be covered. This allows the gauze to slide easily over the body part. Applicators are marked according to a size number that corresponds to different sizes of tubular gauze.

Applying Bandages

When properly applied, bandages should feel comfortably snug. They should be fastened securely enough to remain in place until they are removed. Bandages may be fastened using safety pins or adhesive tape.

Here are the basic techniques to use when wrapping a gauze or elastic roller bandage.

- Circular turn—This technique is used mainly to anchor the bandage or to provide extra support. The bandage is wrapped around the body part two or more times, with each turn completely overlapping the previous turn.
- Spiral turn—After the circular turn anchors the bandage, the wrapping continues in a spiral manner up the body part. Each turn overlaps the previous one by one-half to two-thirds the width of the bandage. The spiral turn is a useful technique for bandaging parts like the wrist, fingers, and trunk.
- Reverse spiral turn—This wrapping technique also begins with a circular turn. Then each time the bandage

is spiral wrapped around the limb, it is twisted once. This method helps to fit limbs like forearms or lower legs that get larger as the bandaging continues.

- Figure-eight turn—This technique involves making slanting, overlapping turns that alternate moving up and down the limb in a crisscross pattern that looks like a figure eight. This is an effective method for bandaging joints, such as a knee, elbow, ankle, or wrist.

Steps for Applying Bandages

Here are some other important guidelines for applying bandages:

1. Observe the principles of medical asepsis. Surgical asepsis is not necessary. The bandage may be used to cover a sterile dressing or may be used alone if there is no open wound.
2. Keep the area to be bandaged and the bandage itself dry and clean. Moisture could wick bacteria into the wound. A moist bandage encourages the growth of pathogens.
3. Never place a bandage directly over an open wound. Apply a sterile dressing first. The bandage should extend approximately 1 to 2 inches beyond the edge of the dressing.
4. Never allow the skin surfaces of two body parts to touch each other under a bandage. Wound healing can cause opposing surfaces to stick together. This would lead to the formation of scar tissue. For example, burned fingers must be dressed separately then bandaged together. A gauze pad can also be inserted between digits before applying a bandage.
5. Pad joints and any bony prominences to help prevent skin irritation. Without padding, the bandage may rub against the skin over a bony area.
6. Bandage the affected body part in the normal position. Joints should be slightly flexed to avoid muscle strain, discomfort, or pain. Muscle spasms may occur if the part is bandaged in an unnatural position.
7. Apply bandages by beginning at the distal part and extending to the proximal part of the body. Bandage turns that extend distal to proximal (farthest to nearest) help to return venous blood to the heart. They also help to make the bandage more secure.
8. Always talk to the patient during bandaging. If the patient complains that the bandage is too tight or too loose, adjust the bandage. Instruct the patient to do the same at home. The bandage should fit snugly but not too tightly.
9. When bandaging hands and feet, leave the fingers and toes exposed whenever possible. Visible fingers and toes make it easier to check for impaired circulation. If the skin feels or looks cold or pale, the nail beds look cyanotic (bluish), or the patient complains of swelling, numbness, or tingling in the toes and fingers, remove the bandage immediately. Reapply it correctly.

Study Skill

You are more likely to learn new skills when you know why you are learning the skill and when you will use it in the medical field. Learning skills can be fun if you use the method of learning that was originally used for military training. It is the "See one, do one, teach one method." First you watch the procedure being performed so you can see how it is properly done. Then, you perform the procedure and repeat the process until you thoroughly understand how to correctly do the procedure and know the sequence of steps that are used to complete the skill. Now it is time for you to teach someone else how to do the procedure. You act as the instructor, demonstrating to a fellow classmate how to do the skill. You also answer any questions that student may have. If you can successfully teach someone else, you have mastered the procedure. Try writing procedures in the form of writing a recipe. You will have an easier time learning the proper sequence of steps.

Suture and Staple Removal

As a medical assistant, you may be the one who removes sutures from a wound. Keep the following points in mind if you are removing sutures.

- Explain to the patient that it is normal to feel a pulling sensation during suture removal, but there should not be pain.
- Cleanse the area with an antiseptic solution. Wear sterile gloves or use sterile transfer forceps. Clean the area using circular motions away from the wound or in straight wipes away from the suture line. The wipe should be discarded after each sweep. Use a new one for the next sweep across the area.
- Use a disposable suture removal kit or sterile reusable equipment. See example in Figure 18-25.

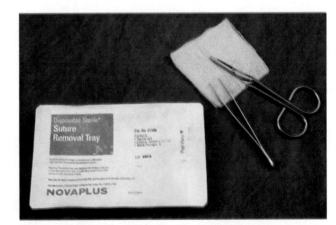

Figure 18-25 A disposable suture removal kit. (Reprinted from Kronenberger J, Ledbetter J. *Jones & Bartlett Learning's Comprehensive Medical Assisting.* 5th ed. Burlington, MA: Jones & Bartlett Learning, LLC; 2016.)

Metal staples may be used to close some incisions after hospital surgery. Patients often leave the hospital before the staples can be removed safely. They return later to the physician's office to have the staples removed.

Frequently, it will be your responsibility to remove staples. Most medical offices use staple removal kits that are similar to the kits supplied for suture removal. Instead of suture scissors, the kit will include a special instrument for removing staples.

Case Question

AFF When the physician is finished suturing Mr. Barnes arm, Ms. Bridges, medical assistant, begins to apply a dressing and bandage his arm. She instructs him that he needs to return in 7 to 10 days to have the sutures removed. He states that he will not be able to do that since he is going to be working out of town for some time. He then states that when he had stitches put in for a previous injury, he just took them out himself. How should the medical assistant handle his response and this situation?

The Healing Process

How a wound heals can depend on the type of wound and how it is treated. There are three classifications including primary, secondary, and tertiary intention. See examples in Figure 18-26.

Healing by Primary Intention

Healing by primary intention *is* the simplest form of healing. It occurs in wounds with edges that are closely approximated. Little or no bacteria enter the wound to complicate the healing process. Because the edges of the wound lie close together, new cells form quickly to bind the edges. Capillaries or tiny blood vessels grow across the tissue break to restore circulation to the tissues. Scarring is usually minimal.

Healing by Secondary Intention

In wounds where skin edges are not closely approximated, the edges of the wound cannot join directly. Rough, pink tissue forms between the wound edges. This process is called granulation. The tissue contains new cells and capillaries. Nerves may not rejoin across the wound, which results in decreased nerve stimulus in the area. A large scab forms to

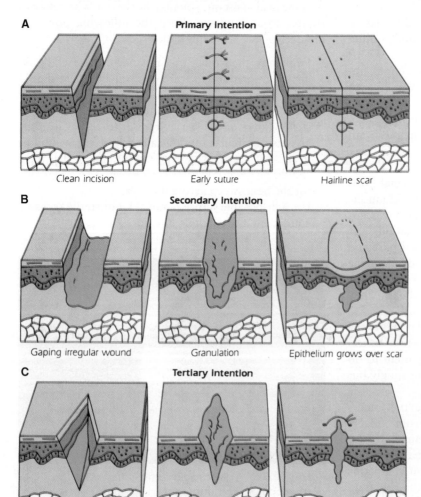

A   **Primary Intention**

Clean incision   Early suture   Hairline scar

B   **Secondary Intention**

Gaping irregular wound   Granulation   Epithelium grows over scar

C   **Tertiary Intention**

Wound   Increased granulation   Late suturing with wide scar

Figure 18-26   The wound healing process. Primary intention: the simplest form of healing **(A)**; Secondary intention: the edges of the wound do not come together, a scab forms and a more severe scar remains **(B)**; Tertiary intention: wound is left open for healing, large scar results **(C)**. (Reprinted from Kronenberger J, Ledbetter J. *Jones & Bartlett Learning's Comprehensive Medical Assisting.* 5th ed. Burlington, MA: Jones & Bartlett Learning, LLC; 2016.)

protect the area while healing occurs below it. Scarring is more severe than with primary intention healing.

Healing by Tertiary Intention

A wound may be left open at first if there is a possibility that it is already contaminated with microorganisms. Closing it would only trap microorganisms, increasing the likelihood of infection. Eventually, the open wound fills in with granular tissue. There is considerable scarring.

Phases of Wound Healing

Wound healing occurs in three main stages. The length of each phase may be different for different patients and different types of incisions.

1. Phase I (inflammatory, lag, or exudative phase). This phase usually lasts from 1 to 4 days.
   - The body attempts to heal itself by increasing circulation to the part and by beginning to repair or reroute blood vessels that supply the tissues.
   - The increased circulation brings more white blood cells to defend against pathogens.
   - Serum and red blood cells brought by the extra blood form a glue-like fibrin, a type of protein that works to block the wound.
   - As the fibrin dries, it pulls the edges of the wound closer together and forms a scab.

Signs that this phase is working include the following:

- Edema, or swelling from the tissue fluid
- Warmth from the extra blood
- Redness from the vasodilation
- Pain from the pressure on the nerve endings caused by the edema

2. Phase II (proliferative, healing, or granulation phase). This phase may last from several days to several weeks.
   - The blood vessels continue to repair themselves. If the damage is severe, they may reroute.
   - The scab from phase I continues to dry and pull the edges of the wound closely together.

3. Phase III (remodeling, maturation, or scarring phase). This phase may take from weeks to years, depending on how severe the wound is.

Patient Education Postoperative Instructions

After any surgical procedure, the patient should receive written and verbal instructions. They should include information about:
- Caring for the postoperative wound
- Taking prescribed medications correctly

- Returning to the office for follow-up visits, dressing changes, and suture removal
- Recognizing signs and symptoms of infection
- Contacting the medical office if there are any problems, including an after-hours number

The patient should be informed of the signs and symptoms of infections. You need to make sure the patient understands these warning signs:

- Excessive bleeding from the wound
- Throbbing pain, or tenderness in the wound area
- Pus or watery discharge collecting under the skin or draining from the wound
- Drainage that is yellow, green, or foul smelling
- A foul odor from the wound
- Redness, red streaks, or excessive swelling around the area
- Tender lumps or swelling in the armpit, groin, or neck
- Chills or fever

Patients also should be on the lookout for abnormal flushing of the skin, general pain or tenderness, heat in the area of the wound, and any loss of function or mobility.

Tell the patient to call the medical office if these symptoms occur. Also teach patients about how to stop any excessive bleeding by applying direct pressure or elevating the body area.

Patients who require follow-up care will need additional information about several things.

- Dressing and bandage changes. Tell the patient, per the physician's instructions, when to return to the office to have dressings or bandages changed, or how and when to change the dressings and bandages at home.
- Follow-up visits. Remind the patient to schedule follow-up appointments before leaving and provide a reminder card for each appointment.
- Showering or bathing. After consulting with the physician, tell the patient when she can take a shower or bath. Advise the patient on whether the surgical wound can get wet. This depends on the location and depth of the wound and the physician's preference.
- Laboratory results. If a specimen was taken for analysis, tell the patient when the results will be available and how he will be informed.
- Patient concerns. Answer any questions about postoperative experiences. Encourage the patient to call the office at any time if there's a problem.
- It may be necessary to ask permission to bring a caregiver into the room to hear these instructions, too. Some patients may not understand all of the directions immediately after the procedure.

Procedure 18-1   Performing a Surgical Scrub

Equipment: Sink, nail brush or orange stick, surgical soap, and sterile towel.

1. Remove any rings, watches, or bracelets. Jewelry provides hiding places for microbes. Don't let your clothing touch the sink.

2. Adjust the water to a comfortable temperature. If it's too hot, it can dry the skin, causing cracks and breaks. If it's too cold, the soap won't lather properly.

3. Hold your arms at or higher than waist level. (During surgical procedures, all areas below the waist are considered contaminated.) Keep your hands higher than your elbows. Otherwise, water may run down from unscrubbed areas of your arms and contaminate your hands.

4. Use an orange stick or nail brush to clean under each nail. Then discard the orange stick taking care not to touch the insides of the sink or the faucet.

5. Apply surgical soap and wash your hands thoroughly. Use a firm circular motion. Hold your fingers up and rub each side of each finger, between the fingers, and the back and front of each hand. This process should take about 5 minutes for each hand.

6. Keeping your hands higher than your elbows, wash your wrists and forearms thoroughly with soap. Rinse your arms and hands under running water without touching the sides of the sink or faucet.

7. Using more surgical soap and a sterile brush, scrub all the surfaces you just washed. As before, follow a systematic approach. Begin with your fingers, then scrub your hands, and finally your arms. Don't scrub too hard, as that could scratch your skin.

8. Discard the sterile brush and rinse your hands and arms by passing them through the running water in one direction—from the hand to the elbow. Remember to keep your hands higher than your elbows.

9. Turn off the faucet using the foot or arm mechanism.

10. Dry your hands using a sterile towel. Using one end of the towel, dry one hand, then the arm, then the forearm. Use the other clean end of the towel to dry the other hand, arm, and forearm. Avoid touching your clean hands with the part of the towel that comes into contact with your arms.

Procedure 18-2   Applying Sterile Gloves

To move sterile items or place them on the sterile field, you must use sterile gloves. Be sure to choose gloves that are the right size for your hands. Follow these steps to apply them.

Equipment: Sterile gloves.

1. Before you put on the gloves, remove any rings or other jewelry. Rings may pierce the gloves and contaminate the procedure.

2. Wash your hands before applying gloves. Wearing gloves isn't a substitute for handwashing.

3. Place the glove package on a clean, dry, flat surface. The cuffed end of the glove should be facing you.

4. Pull the outer wrapping apart to expose the sterile, inner wrap.

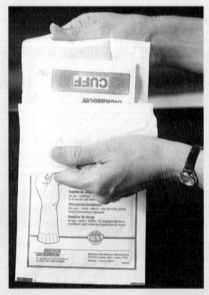

(Reprinted from Kronenberger J, Ledbetter J. *Jones & Bartlett Learning's Comprehensive Medical Assisting.* 5th ed. Burlington, MA: Jones & Bartlett Learning, LLC; 2016.)

Procedure 18-2 | Applying Sterile Gloves (*continued*)

5. With the cuffs toward you, fold back the inner wrap to expose the gloves.

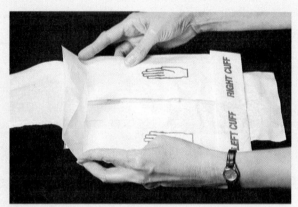

(Reprinted from Kronenberger J, Ledbetter J. *Jones & Bartlett Learning's Comprehensive Medical Assisting.* 5th ed. Burlington, MA: Jones & Bartlett Learning, LLC; 2016.)

6. Grasping the edges of the outer paper, open the package out to its fullest. Remember that the inner surface of the package is a sterile field.

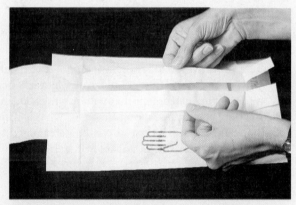

(Reprinted from Kronenberger J, Ledbetter J. *Jones & Bartlett Learning's Comprehensive Medical Assisting.* 5th ed. Burlington, MA: Jones & Bartlett Learning, LLC; 2016.)

7. Using your nondominant hand, pick up the dominant hand glove by grasping the folded edge of the cuff. Lift it up and away from the paper to avoid brushing an unsterile surface. (The folded edge of the cuff is contaminated as soon as it is touched with the ungloved hand.) Be very careful not to touch the outside surface of the sterile glove with your ungloved hand.

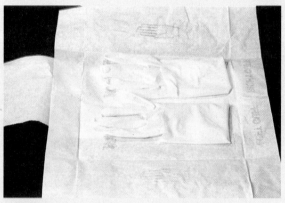

(Reprinted from Kronenberger J, Ledbetter J. *Jones & Bartlett Learning's Comprehensive Medical Assisting.* 5th ed. Burlington, MA: Jones & Bartlett Learning, LLC; 2016.)

8. Curl your fingers and thumb together and insert them into the glove. This prevents you from accidentally touching the outside surface of the glove. Straighten your fingers and pull the glove on with your nondominant hand still grasping the cuff.

9. Unfold the cuff by pinching the inside surface that will be against your wrist and pulling it toward your wrist. Only the unsterile portions of the glove will be touched by your hands.

10. Place the fingers of your gloved hand under the cuff of the remaining glove. Lift the glove up and away from the wrapper to prevent it from touching an unsterile surface. Slide your ungloved hand carefully into the glove with your fingers and thumb curled together.

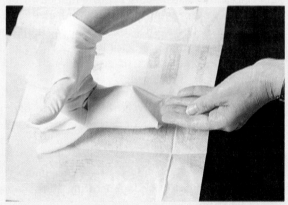

(Reprinted from Kronenberger J, Ledbetter J. *Jones & Bartlett Learning's Comprehensive Medical Assisting.* 5th ed. Burlington, MA: Jones & Bartlett Learning, LLC; 2016.)

Procedure 18-2	Applying Sterile Gloves (*continued*)

11. Straighten your fingers and pull the glove up and over your wrist by carefully unfolding the glove. Folding the cuffs out to their fullest allows the greatest area of sterility.

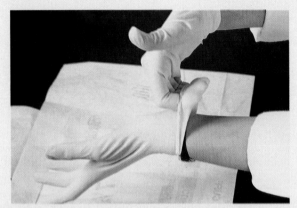

(Reprinted from Kronenberger J, Ledbetter J. *Jones & Bartlett Learning's Comprehensive Medical Assisting.* 5th ed. Burlington, MA: Jones & Bartlett Learning, LLC; 2016.)

12. Settle the gloves comfortably onto your fingers by lacing your fingers together and adjusting the tension over your hands. The gloves should fit snugly without wrinkles or areas that bind the fingers.

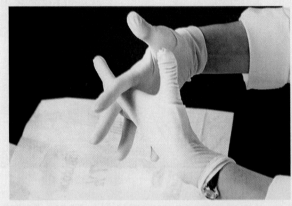

(Reprinted from Kronenberger J, Ledbetter J. *Jones & Bartlett Learning's Comprehensive Medical Assisting.* 5th ed. Jones & Bartlett Learning's Comprehensive Medical Assisting; 2016.)

Procedure 18-3	Wrapping Instruments for Sterilization in an Autoclave

Equipment: Gloves, autoclave wrapping material, autoclave tape, sterilization indicators, black or blue ink pen, and instruments for autoclave.

1. First, wash your hands and put on nonsterile gloves.

2. Check the instruments being wrapped to be sure they've been sanitized and disinfected and are dry. Also check that they're in working order. Instruments that are defective, broken, or in need of repair, sanitization, or disinfection shouldn't be wrapped or autoclaved.

3. Autoclave wrap may be double layers of cotton muslin, special paper, or appropriately sized instrument pouches. The wrapping material needs to have these properties:
   - Permeable to steam but not contaminants
   - Resists tearing and puncturing during normal handling
   - Allows for easy opening to prevent contamination of the contents
   - Maintains the sterility of the contents during storage

4. Tear off one piece of autoclave tape. Write the date, your initials, and the contents of the pack or the name of the instrument that will be wrapped. (After the item is wrapped, you cannot see what is inside.) The date is necessary so it can be determined later if the contents are still considered sterile.

5. Lay the wrapping material diagonally on a flat, clean, dry surface. Place the instrument in the center of the wrapping material.
   - Ratchets or handles should be open to allow steam to penetrate all surfaces.
   - Include a sterilization indicator.

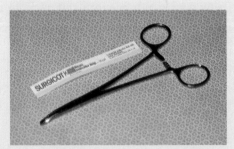

(Reprinted from Kronenberger J, Ledbetter J. *Jones & Bartlett Learning's Comprehensive Medical Assisting.* 5th ed. Burlington, MA: Jones & Bartlett Learning, LLC; 2016.)

Procedure 18-3	Wrapping Instruments for Sterilization in an Autoclave (*continued*)

6. Fold the flap at the bottom of the diagonal wrap up. Fold back the corner to make a tab. The tab allows the pack to be opened easily without contaminating the contents.

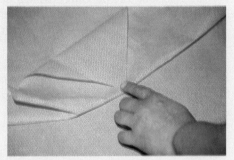

(Reprinted from Kronenberger J, Ledbetter J. *Jones & Bartlett Learning's Comprehensive Medical Assisting.* 5th ed. Burlington, MA: Jones & Bartlett Learning, LLCr; 2016.)

7. Fold the left corner of the wrap in to the center. Again, fold back the corner to make a tab. Do the same for the right corner of the wrap.

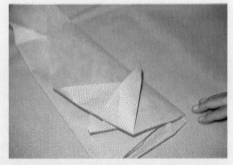

(Reprinted from Kronenberger J, Ledbetter J. *Jones & Bartlett Learning's Comprehensive Medical Assisting.* 5th ed. Burlington, MA: Jones & Bartlett Learning, LLC; 2016.)

8. Fold the top corner down, tucking the tab under the material.

9. Secure the wrapped instrument package with the labeled autoclave tape.

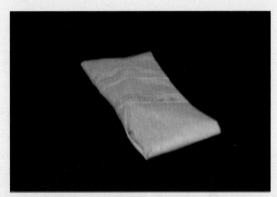

(Reprinted from Kronenberger J, Ledbetter J. *Jones & Bartlett Learning's Comprehensive Medical Assisting.* 5th ed. Burlington, MA: Jones & Bartlett Learning, LLC; 2016.)

Procedure 18-4	Operating an Autoclave

Equipment: Autoclave, distilled water, autoclave operating manual, and items wrapped for autoclaving.

1. Gather equipment and supplies.
   - Some medical offices will want you to include a separate, wrapped sterilization indicator with the autoclave load.
   - This allows you to check that the procedure was performed properly without opening a sterilized pack.

2. Check the water level in the autoclave reservoir. Add more distilled water if necessary.

3. Add water to the internal chamber of the autoclave. Make sure the water level is at the fill line.
   - Too little water means not enough steam will be produced.
   - Too much water can cause saturated steam, which extends drying time.

Procedure 18-4   Operating an Autoclave (*continued*)

4. Load the autoclave, following these guidelines:
   - Place trays and packs on their sides, 1 to 3 inches apart. Air cannot circulate if items are too tightly packed. Placing them vertically stops air from pooling in containers.
   - Put containers on their sides with lids off. Removing lids and placing containers on their sides improve air circulation.
   - In mixed loads, place hard objects on the bottom shelf and softer packs on the top racks. Otherwise, hard objects may form condensation, which can drip onto softer items.

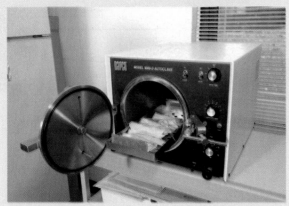

(Reprinted from Kronenberger J, Ledbetter J. *Jones & Bartlett Learning's Comprehensive Medical Assisting.* 5th ed. Burlington, MA: Jones & Bartlett Learning, LLC; 2016.)

5. Read the instructions for closing and operating the machine. Most machines require similar procedures, such as in the list below.
   - Close the door and secure or lock it.
   - Turn on the machine.

- When the temperature gauge reaches the required level (usually 250°F), set the timer. Many autoclaves can be programmed for the required time.
- When the timer indicates the cycle is over, vent the chamber.
- After releasing the pressure to a safe level, crack the door of the autoclave slightly to allow additional drying. Most loads dry in 5 to 20 minutes. Hard items dry faster than soft ones.

6. When the load has cooled, remove the items. Check the sterilization indicator, if one was included in the autoclave or in each pack.
   - If the indicator registers that the load or pack was properly processed, the items are considered sterile.
   - If not, the items are considered unsterile. They must be rewrapped and processed again.

7. Store the items in a clean, dry, dust-free area for 30 days. After 30 days, reprocessing is necessary. The pack must be rewrapped, taped with new tape with the current date, and autoclaved again.

8. Clean the autoclave according to the manufacturer's directions.

Typically, cleaning involves scrubbing the interior chamber with a soft brush and mild detergent.
- Pay attention to the exhaust valve. It can become blocked with lint accumulation.
- Rinse the machine thoroughly and allow it to dry.
- Record your maintenance procedures and the date they were performed in the maintenance and quality control logs.

Procedure 18-5   Performing Chemical Sterilization

Equipment: The sterilization chemical, the safety data sheet (SDS) for the sterilization chemical, personal protective equipment (PPE), heavy-duty utility gloves, a stainless steel or glass container with airtight cover, sterile water, a sterile basin, sterile transfer forceps, sterile towels, and the items to be sterilized.

1. Gather equipment and materials.

2. Put on disposable gloves, goggles, and other PPE. You need to protect your eyes, clothing, and exposed skin from possible harmful chemicals.

3. Scrub and sanitize the items to be sterilized to remove debris and body fluids.

4. Rinse and dry the items. They must be dry when placed in the chemical sterilization solution in order to avoid diluting the solution.

5. Check the expiration date on the container of the sterilization chemical. If the chemical is used past its expiration date, it may not be as effective.

Procedure 18-5   Performing Chemical Sterilization (*continued*)

6. Read the manufacturer's instructions on the container of the sterilization chemical and review the SDS for the chemical being used. This step minimizes the risk of injury from mishandling of the chemical and provides first-aid information should an accident occur.

7. Put on the heavy-duty utility gloves over the disposable PPE gloves. These gloves will protect your disposable gloves from punctures by sharp instruments and exposure to harsh chemicals that might damage your skin.

8. Mix or prepare the solution according to the manufacturer's directions on the label. This will ensure that the solution used is the correct strength.

9. Pour the solution into a glass or stainless steel container with an airtight lid. The solution should be left covered in order to avoid loss of potency through evaporation or injury from splashes or inhalation of fumes.

10. Carefully place the dry sanitized items into the container in order to avoid splashing, making sure they are completely covered by the solution. Replace the container's airtight lid.

11. Label the lid with the name of the chemical, the date and time, and the length of time required for sterilization.

12. Leave the items in the solution for the required time. This may be from 20 minutes to 3 hours or more, depending on the chemical being used. Do not open the container or add more items during this time.

13. After the recommended processing time has expired, open the container and remove each item from the solution using sterile transfer forceps. With the sterile forceps, hold the item over a sterile basin and pour large amounts of sterile water over and through it. This will remove all traces of the chemical solution from the item.

14. Continue to hold the item over the sterile basin for a moment to allow the excess water to drain off. Then place the item on a sterile towel.

15. After all the items have been removed from the container, rinsed, and transferred onto sterile towels, dry them with another sterile towel. Take care to avoid touching the instruments or the side of the towel being used to dry them.

16. Use the sterile transfer forceps to place the items in storage for future use according to your office procedures.

Note: Change the solution in the sterilization container every day or according to the manufacturer's instructions.

Procedure 18-6   Opening Sterile Packs

Equipment: Sterile surgical pack, Mayo or surgical stand, and sterile drape.

1. Verify the procedure to be performed and remove the appropriate surgical pack (tray or item) from the storage area. Check the label for the contents and expiration date. Packs that are past the expiration date should not be used.

2. Check the package for tears, stains, and moisture, which would suggest contamination.

3. Place the package, with the label facing up, on a clean, dry, flat surface, such as a Mayo or surgical stand. Although the field will be protected by the barrier below it, using a clean surface keeps microorganisms to a minimum. The surgical stand makes it easy to move the field as needed.

4. Wash your hands. Carefully remove the sealing tape. Take care not to tear the wrapper. For commercial packages, carefully remove the outer wrapper. Many disposable packages are wrapped in clear plastic film that will become the sterile field when properly opened.

Procedure 18-6 | Opening Sterile Packs (*continued*)

5. Loosen the first flap of the folded wrapper by pulling it up, out, and away from you. Let it fall over the far side of the table or stand. Then you will not need to reach across the sterile field again.

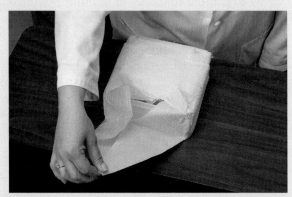

(Reprinted from Kronenberger J, Ledbetter J. *Jones & Bartlett Learning's Comprehensive Medical Assisting.* 5th ed. Burlington, MA: Jones & Bartlett Learning, LLC; 2016.)

6. Open the side flaps in a similar manner to minimize your movements over the sterile field. Use your left hand for the left flap and your right hand for the right flap. Touch only the outer surface (which is not sterile). Do not touch the sterile inner surface.

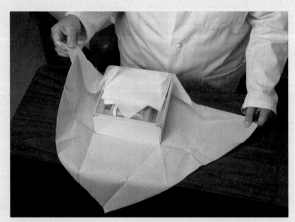

(Reprinted from Kronenberger J, Ledbetter J. *Jones & Bartlett Learning's Comprehensive Medical Assisting.* 5th ed. Burlington, MA: Jones & Bartlett Learning, LLC; 2016.)

7. Grasp the outer surface of the remaining flap. Pull it down and toward you. The outer surface of the wrapper should now be against the surgical stand. The sterile inside of the wrapper forms the sterile field.

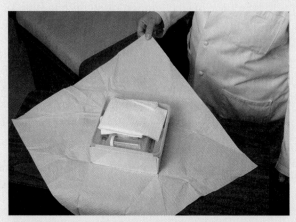

(Reprinted from Kronenberger J, Ledbetter J. *Jones & Bartlett Learning's Comprehensive Medical Assisting.* 5th ed. Burlington, MA: Jones & Bartlett Learning, LLC; 2016.)

8. Some packages have a second inside wrapper. Repeat steps 5 to 7 to open the second wrapper. It also will provide a sterile field.

9. If you need to leave the area after opening the sterile field, cover the tray and its contents with a sterile drape. Here is how.
   - Without leaving or turning your back on the sterile area, open the sterile drape.
   - Carefully lift it out of the package by the edges. Take care not to touch the drape to any surfaces.
   - Place the drape over the sterile field working from your body outward so that your arms do not cross the uncovered sterile field. Your arms can cross the drape that is covering the tray.

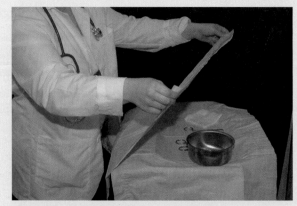

(Reprinted from Kronenberger J, Ledbetter J. *Jones & Bartlett Learning's Comprehensive Medical Assisting.* 5th ed. Burlington, MA: Jones & Bartlett Learning, LLC; 2016.)

Procedure 18-7 | Using Sterile Transfer Forceps

Equipment: Sterile transfer forceps, sterile tray set up, items to be transferred to sterile tray.

1. Sterile forceps often are stored in a container with sterilization solution. When you need to use them, slowly lift the forceps straight up and out of the

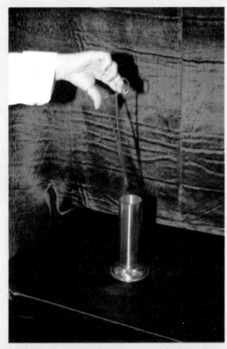

(Reprinted from Kronenberger J, Ledbetter J. *Jones & Bartlett Learning's Comprehensive Medical Assisting.* 5th ed. Burlington, MA: Jones & Bartlett Learning, LLC; 2016.)

container. Do not touch the outside of the container or the inside of the container above the level of the solution. These areas are not considered sterile.

2. Hold the forceps with the tips down at all times. This prevents contamination by preventing the solution from running up toward the unsterile handles and then down to the grasping blades and tips. Keep the forceps above waist level to avoid accidental or unnoticed contamination.

3. Use the forceps to pick up items to be transferred onto the sterile field. Drop the items carefully onto the field.
   - Do not let the forceps contact the sterile field. They may be moist from the soaking solution. Drops of solution on the sterile field could wick microorganisms from below.
   - Transfer forceps that have been wrapped and autoclaved may be placed with their tips on the sterile field and their handles extending beyond the 1-inch border that is considered contaminated. This allows you to move objects easily around the sterile field.

4. When finished moving items, carefully place the forceps back into the sterilization solution. The solution keeps the tips of the forceps sterile for future use. The solution should be changed at least daily, or according to office policy.

Procedure 18-8 | Adding Sterile Solution

Equipment: Sterile tray set up on sterile field, sterile bowl or cup, solution to pour in bowl.

1. Place a sterile bowl or cup on the sterile field using sterile transfer forceps. Identify the correct solution by carefully reading the label. The label should be checked three times to prevent errors. Check the label:
   - When taking the container from the shelf
   - Before pouring the solution
   - When returning the container to the shelf

2. Check the expiration date on the solution label. Don't use the solution if:
   - The solution is out of date
   - The label can't be read
   - The solution appears abnormal

Out-of-date solutions may have changed chemically or deteriorated. They are not considered sterile.
   - Sterile water and saline bottles must be dated when opened.
   - If not used within 48 hours, they should be discarded.

3. If you're adding medication, such as lidocaine, to the solution, show the medication label to the physician. This allows the contents to be verified.

4. Remove the cap or stopper on the bottle. Hold the cap with your fingertips, with the opening facing down to prevent contamination.

Procedure 18-8   Adding Sterile Solution (*continued*)

- If you must put the cap down, place it on a side table (not the sterile field) with the open end up.
- If you'll be pouring the entire contents of the bottle into the sterile bowl or cup, you can discard the cap.
- Keep the bottle so you can note the amount added to the field and for charting later.

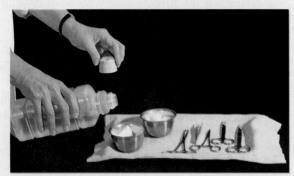

(Reprinted from Kronenberger J, Ledbetter J. *Jones & Bartlett Learning's Comprehensive Medical Assisting.* 5th ed. Burlington, MA: Jones & Bartlett Learning, LLC; 2016.)

5. Grasp the container with the label against the palm of your hand (known as palming the label). That way, if solution runs down the side of the bottle, it won't obscure the label.

(Reprinted from Kronenberger J, Ledbetter J. *Jones & Bartlett Learning's Comprehensive Medical Assisting.* 5th ed. Burlington, MA: Jones & Bartlett Learning, LLC; 2016.)

6. Pour a small amount of the solution into a separate container or waste receptacle. The lip of the bottle is considered contaminated. Pouring off this small amount cleanses the lip.

7. Without reaching across the sterile field, carefully and slowly pour the desired amount of solution into the sterile container.
   - Pouring slowly reduces the chances of splashing and overfilling.
   - Hold the bottle no more than 6 inches and no <4 inches above the container. The bottle of solution should never touch the sterile container or tray.
   - Solution poured too quickly from an improper height may splash. Spilled solution may lead to wicking of contaminants from the field below.

8. After pouring the solution, recheck the label for the contents and expiration date. Replace the cap carefully, without touching the bottle rim with any unsterile surface of the cap. This ensures the contents will remain sterile.

9. Return the solution to its proper storage area or discard the container after checking the label again.

Procedure 18-9   Performing Hair Removal and Skin Preparation

Equipment: Nonsterile gloves; shaving cream, lotion, or soap; a new disposable razor; gauze or cotton balls; warm water; antiseptic solution; and sponge forceps.

1. Wash your hands.

2. Gather the equipment.
   - A new razor must be used for each patient to prevent the spread of microorganisms.
   - The new blade also will ensure the closest possible shave.

3. Greet the patient by name and explain the procedure. Answer any questions the patient may have.

4. Put on gloves. Standard precautions must be observed when contact with blood or body fluids is possible.

5. Prepare the patient's skin. If shaving is required:
   - Apply shaving cream or soapy lather to the area to reduce friction.
   - Pull the skin taut and shave by pulling the razor across the skin in the direction of hair growth. This gives the closest shave, while reducing the chance of nicking the skin.
   - When all hair is removed from the operative area, rinse to remove soap residue and hair.
   - Thoroughly dry the area by patting with gauze square.
   - Using gauze squares picks up stray hairs that might have been left behind during rinsing.

6. If shaving isn't necessary, wash and rinse the patient's skin with soap and water. Dry the skin thoroughly.

7. Apply antiseptic solution of the physician's choice to the skin surrounding the operative area. Here's how it should be done.
   - Use sterile gauze sponges or sterile cotton balls to apply the solution, or use antiseptic wipes.
   - Hold the gauze or cotton ball in sterile sponge forceps.
   - Wipe the skin in circular motions, beginning at the operative site and working outward. Discard each sponge after a complete sweep has been made to prevent contamination.
   - If the area is large or circles are not appropriate, the sponge may be wiped straight outward from the operative site. Use a fresh sponge after every pass over the skin. Repeat the procedure until the entire area has been thoroughly cleaned.
   - A wipe that has been passed over the skin should never be returned to the cleaned area or to the antiseptic solution.

8. Holding dry sterile sponges in the sponge forceps, thoroughly pat the area dry. In some instances, the area may be allowed to air dry. Moist skin may moisten the sterile drapes, causing wicking and contamination.

9. Tell the patient not to touch or cover the prepared area to avoid contaminating the operative site.

10. Inform the physician that the patient is ready for the procedure. Drape the prepared area with a sterile drape if the physician will be delayed for more than 10 or 15 minutes.

Procedure 18-10   Assisting with Excisional Surgery

Equipment: A basin for solutions, gauze sponges and cotton balls, antiseptic solution, a sterile drape, sterile syringes and needles for local anesthetic, dissecting scissors, a disposable scalpel, a blade of the physician's choice, mosquito forceps, tissue forceps, a needle holder, a suture and needle of the physician's choice, sterile gloves, local anesthetic, antiseptic wipes, adhesive tape, sterile dressings, and a specimen container with a completed laboratory request form.

1. Wash your hands and gather the equipment and supplies.

Procedure 18-10 | Assisting with Excisional Surgery (*continued*)

2. Greet the patient by name and explain the procedure. Answer any questions the patient may have.

3. Set up a sterile field on a surgical stand with the at-the-side supplies and equipment close at hand. Cover the field with a sterile drape until the physician arrives.

4. Position the patient appropriately to expose the operative site.

5. Put on sterile gloves or use sterile transfer forceps and cleanse the patient's skin. When you're finished, remove your gloves and wash your hands. (Some physicians prefer to cleanse the skin themselves using supplies on the field. Always follow the preferences of the physician in your medical office.)

6. If the physician asks you, assist during the procedure.
   - You may need to add supplies, watch for opportunities to assist the physician, and comfort the patient.
   - You don't need to wear sterile gloves unless you'll be handling sterile instruments or supplies.

7. If the lesion is to be sent to pathology for analysis, you'll need to assist in specimen collection. Follow standard precautions and wear examination gloves when handling specimens. Have the container ready to receive the specimen.

8. At the end of the procedure, wash your hands and dress the wound using sterile technique. The wound must be covered to protect the incision from contamination.

9. Thank the patient and provide instructions for postoperative care, including dressing changes, postoperative medications, and follow-up visits.

10. Wearing gloves, clean the treatment room and prepare it for the next patient. Follow standard precautions.

11. Record the procedure. Documentation should include postoperative vital signs, care of the wound, instructions on postoperative care, and processing any specimens.

Procedure 18-11 | Assisting with Colposcopy and Cervical Biopsy

Equipment: Specimen container, laboratory request form, sterile gloves, a gown and drape, a vaginal speculum, a colposcope, a specimen container with preservative (10% formalin), sterile cotton-tipped applicators, sterile normal saline solution, sterile 3% acetic acid, sterile povidone-iodine (Betadine), silver nitrate sticks or ferric subsulfate (Monsel solution), sterile biopsy forceps or punch biopsy instrument, a sterile uterine curet, sterile uterine dressing forceps, sterile 4 × 4 gauze, a sterile towel, a sterile endocervical curet, a sterile uterine tenaculum, a sanitary napkin, examination gloves, an examination light, tissues, and biohazard container.

1. Label a specimen container with the patient's name and date. Prepare a laboratory request. Verify that the patient has signed the consent form. Colposcopy with biopsy is an invasive procedure that requires written consent.

2. Wash your hands.

3. Gather the equipment and supplies.

4. Check the light on the colposcope to make sure it's functioning properly.

5. Set up the sterile field using sterile technique. Items that can be placed on the sterile field include the sterile cotton-tipped applicators and sterile containers for the solutions.

Procedure 18-11	Assisting with Colposcopy and Cervical Biopsy (*continued*)

6. Pour sterile normal saline and acetic acid into their sterile containers. Cover the field with a drape to maintain sterility as you prepare the patient.

7. Greet the patient by name and explain the procedure, answering any last-minute questions from the patient.

8. When the physician is ready, assist the patient into the dorsal lithotomy position. If you are going to be assisting the physician from the sterile field, put on sterile gloves after you position the patient.

9. Hand the physician the applicator immersed in normal saline followed by the applicator immersed in acetic acid. Acetic acid swabbed on the area improves visualization of abnormal tissue.

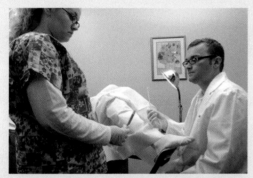

(Reprinted from Kronenberger J, Ledbetter J. *Jones & Bartlett Learning's Comprehensive Medical Assisting.* 5th ed. Burlington, MA: Jones & Bartlett Learning, LLC; 2016.)

10. Hand the physician the applicator with the antiseptic solution (Betadine). The area to be sampled for biopsy must be swabbed to reduce microorganisms and pathogens.

11. If you didn't apply sterile gloves to assist the physician, apply clean examination gloves. Receive the biopsy specimen into the container of 10% formalin preservative.

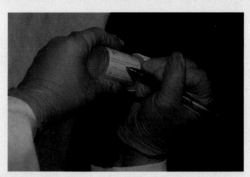

(Reprinted from Kronenberger J, Ledbetter J. *Jones & Bartlett Learning's Comprehensive Medical Assisting.* 5th ed. Burlington, MA: Jones & Bartlett Learning, LLC; 2016.)

12. If necessary, provide the physician with Monsel solution or silver nitrate sticks to stop any bleeding. Monsel solution and silver nitrate act as coagulants.

13. When the physician is finished, remove your gloves and wash your hands. Assist the patient from the stirrups and into a sitting position. Explain to the patient that a small amount of bleeding may occur (a small sanitary pad should be sufficient). Have a sanitary napkin available.

14. Ask the patient to get dressed and assist as needed. Allow the patient privacy for dressing.

15. Reinforce any instructions from the physician regarding follow-up appointments. Tell the patient how to obtain the biopsy findings.

16. Wearing gloves, properly care for or dispose of equipment and clean the examination room. Remove your gloves and wash your hands.

17. Document the procedure, including routing the specimen and patient education.

Procedure 18-12 | Assisting with Incision and Drainage

Equipment: See items listed in bullets under Step #1.

1. Wash your hands and gather the equipment as described below.
   - On the sterile field, you'll need a basin for solutions, gauze sponges and cotton balls, antiseptic solution, a sterile drape, sterile syringes and sterile needles for local anesthetic, a commercial I&D (incision and drainage) sterile setup *or* scalpel, dissecting scissors, hemostats, tissue forceps, sterile 4 × 4 gauze sponges, and a probe (optional).
   - At the side, you'll need sterile gloves, local anesthetic, antiseptic wipes, adhesive tape, sterile dressings, packing gauze, and a culture tube if the wound may be cultured.

2. The steps for this procedure are similar to those in the Hands On procedure for assisting with excisional surgery.

- You're expected to prepare the surgical field and the patient's surgical area as instructed or preferred by the physician.
- After the procedure, the wound must be covered to avoid further contamination and to absorb drainage.
- The exudate is a hazardous body fluid requiring standard precautions.
- Although a culture and sensitivity (**C&S**) may be ordered on the drainage from the infected area, no other specimen is usually collected.
- Label the specimen container and prepare a laboratory request if a culture and sensitivity has been ordered.

Procedure 18-13 | Applying a Sterile Dressing

Equipment: Sterile gloves, sterile gauze dressings, scissors, bandage tape, medication to be applied to dressing.

1. Wash your hands and gather your supplies.

2. Greet the patient by name and ask about any tape allergies. Some patients are sensitive to certain tape adhesives. Hypoallergenic tape should be available.

3. Depending on the size of the dressing, cut or tear lengths of tape to secure the dressing. Set the tape strips aside in a convenient place, such as affixing the end of each piece to a nearby countertop where it can be removed easily and applied. Having tape cut and prepared saves time and may prevent the dressing from slipping while tape is cut.

4. Explain the procedure and instruct the patient to remain still. The patient should avoid talking, sneezing, or coughing until the procedure is complete. You don't want droplets of moisture containing microorganisms to contaminate the sterile field or the wound.

5. Open the dressing pack to create a sterile field, leaving the sterile dressing on the inside of the opened package. Observe the principles of sterile asepsis.

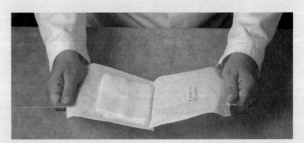

(Reprinted from Kronenberger J, Ledbetter J. *Jones & Bartlett Learning's Comprehensive Medical Assisting.* 5th ed. Burlington, MA: Jones & Bartlett Learning, LLC; 2016.)

6. Use sterile technique to prevent wound contamination. Put on sterile gloves if you won't be using sterile transfer forceps to apply the dressing.

| Procedure 18-13 | Applying a Sterile Dressing (*continued*) |

7. If a topical medication is needed, apply it to the sterile dressing that will cover the wound directly. Take care not to touch the medication bottle or tube to the dressing. Allow the medication to free fall onto the sterile dressing. The outside end of the medication container may not be sterile.

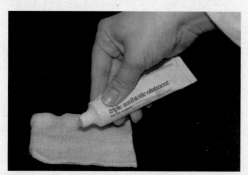

(Reprinted from Kronenberger J, Ledbetter J. *Jones & Bartlett Learning's Comprehensive Medical Assisting*. 5th ed. Burlington, MA: Jones & Bartlett Learning, LLC; 2016.)

8. Using sterile technique, apply the number of dressings necessary to cover and protect the wound. Sterile dressings must be placed carefully on the wound. Dragging them over the skin can lead to contamination from microorganisms on the surrounding skin.

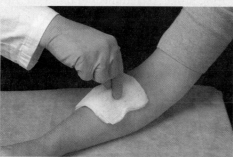

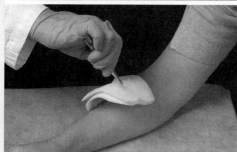

(Reprinted from Kronenberger J, Ledbetter J. *Jones & Bartlett Learning's Comprehensive Medical Assisting*. 5th ed. Burlington, MA: Jones & Bartlett Learning, LLC; 2016.)

9. Apply the previously cut lengths of tape over the dressing to secure it. When the wound is completely covered,

you may remove your gloves (discarding them appropriately) or keep them on to tape the dressing.
   - Avoid overuse of tape. Tape is used only to keep the dressing in place.
   - Too much tape can cause perspiration that will dampen the dressing and compromise its sterility. And keep in mind that too much tape may cause unnecessary discomfort to the patient when it has to be removed.
   - Tape shouldn't obstruct blood circulation.

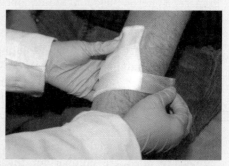

(Reprinted from Kronenberger J, Ledbetter J. *Jones & Bartlett Learning's Comprehensive Medical Assisting*. 5th ed. Burlington, MA: Jones & Bartlett Learning, LLC; 2016.)

10. Apply a bandage if necessary to hold the dressing in place, add support, or immobilize the area.

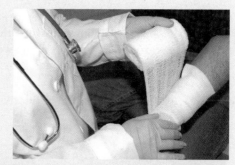

(Reprinted from Kronenberger J, Ledbetter J. *Jones & Bartlett Learning's Comprehensive Medical Assisting*. 5th ed. Burlington, MA: Jones & Bartlett Learning, LLC; 2016.)

11. If the patient needs to change dressings at home, instruct the patient on how to do so.
   - Dressings should be kept clean and dry.
   - They need to be changed if they become wet or soiled, or as instructed by the physician.
   - Instruct the patient about wound care and signs of infection.

12. Return reusable supplies (unopened sterile gloves or dressings, tape) to their storage areas. Properly discard contaminated supplies or waste.

13. Record the procedure in the patient's chart.

Procedure 18-14 | Changing an Existing Dressing

Equipment: Sterile gloves, nonsterile gloves, sterile dressing, prepackaged skin antiseptic swabs or sterile antiseptic solution in a sterile basin and sterile cotton balls or gauze, tape, and biohazard waste containers.

1. Wash your hands and gather your supplies.

2. Greet the patient by name and explain the procedure. Answer any questions the patient may have.

3. Prepare a sterile field, including opening sterile dressings. Follow the guidelines below when preparing the sterile field.
   - If using a sterile container and solution, open the package containing the sterile basin. Use the inside of the wrapper as the sterile field for the basin.
   - Flip the sterile gauze or cotton balls into the basin. Pour in the appropriate amount of antiseptic solution.
   - If using prepackaged antiseptic swabs, carefully open an adequate number for the size of the wound. Set them aside using sterile technique to avoid contamination.

4. Instruct the patient not to talk, cough, sneeze, laugh, or move during the procedure in order to prevent contamination of the sterile field.

5. Wearing clean gloves, carefully remove the tape from the wound by pulling it toward the wound. Pulling away from the direction of the wound may pull the healing edges of the wound apart.

6. Remove the old dressing. Never pull on a dressing that doesn't come off easily.

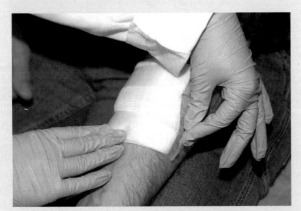

(Reprinted from Kronenberger J, Ledbetter J. *Jones & Bartlett Learning's Comprehensive Medical Assisting.* 5th ed. Burlington, MA: Jones & Bartlett Learning, LLC; 2016.)

- If the dressing is difficult to remove because of dried blood, soak it in sterile water or saline for a few minutes to loosen it.
- Gently pull the edges of the dressing toward the center.
- If this procedure doesn't loosen the dressing or causes undue discomfort to the patient, notify the physician.

7. Discard the soiled dressing in a biohazard waste container. Don't pass the dressing over the sterile field—it may shed microorganisms.

8. Before cleaning, inspect the wound for degree of healing, amount and type of drainage, and appearance of wound edges. If you inspect the wound after cleaning, most of the exudate will have been removed.

9. Remove and discard your gloves using medical aseptic practices.
   - The physician may want to inspect the wound before you remove exudates or drainage to assess the status of the healing process.
   - If a culture is ordered, the specimen must be taken before the wound is cleaned.

10. Using proper technique, put on sterile gloves. Clean the wound with the antiseptic solution ordered by the physician.
    - Clean in a straight motion with cotton or gauze and antiseptic solution or with prepackaged antiseptic swabs.
    - Discard the wipe after each stroke and use a fresh sterile one to continue.
    - Never return the wipe to the antiseptic solution or to the skin after one sweep across the area.

11. Remove your gloves and wash your hands. Change the dressing using the procedure for sterile dressing application.

12. Record the procedure.

Procedure 18-15   Removing Sutures

Equipment: Skin antiseptic, sterile gloves, prepackaged suture removal kit or thumb forceps, suture scissors, and gauze.

1. Wash your hands and apply clean examination gloves.

2. Check the chart before you begin the procedure to see how many sutures or staples were applied. This way you can be certain that you have removed them all.

3. Greet the patient by name and explain the procedure. Answer any questions the patient may have.

4. If dressings are still in place, remove them and dispose of them in biohazard waste containers. Remove your gloves and wash your hands.

5. Wearing clean examination gloves, cleanse the wound with antiseptic, such as Betadine. Use new antiseptic gauze for each swipe down the wound. The wound should be as free of pathogens as possible to prevent contamination.

6. Open the suture removal kit using sterile asepsis technique or set up a sterile field.

7. Put on sterile gloves. Suture removal is a sterile procedure.

8. The knots of the suture will be tied so that one tail of the knot is very close to the surface of the skin. The other will be closer to the area of suture that is looped over the incision. Here's how to cut and remove the sutures.
   - With the thumb forceps, grasp the end of the knot closest to the skin. Lift it slightly and gently up from the skin (A).
   - Cut the suture below the knot as close to the skin as possible (B). Cutting close to the skin frees the knot at an area that hasn't been exposed to the outside surface of the body. The only part of the suture that will pull through the tissues

will be suture that was under the skin surface. This helps to avoid contamination by microorganisms from the outside skin surface.
   - Use the thumb forceps to pull the suture out of the skin with a smooth, continuous motion (C). Keep the forceps at a slight angle to the wound to prevent tension on the healing tissue.

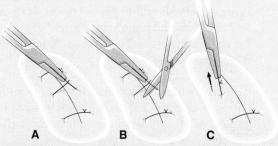

(Reprinted from Kronenberger J, Ledbetter J. *Jones & Bartlett Learning's Comprehensive Medical Assisting.* 5th ed. Burlington, MA: Jones & Bartlett Learning, LLC; 2016.)

9. Place the suture on the gauze sponge. Repeat the procedure for each suture to be removed. By setting the sutures on the gauze sponge, you can easily count the number removed. If six sutures were inserted and are to be removed, there should be six sutures on the gauze sponge at the end of the procedure.

10. Clean the site with an antiseptic solution. Cover it with a sterile dressing if the physician has directed you to do so. Some wounds still need to be protected; others have healed well enough to be left uncovered.

11. Thank the patient and properly dispose of equipment and supplies. Make sure you follow standard precautions. Clean the treatment area, remove your gloves, and wash your hands.

12. Record the procedure. Documentation must include the time, location of sutures, number removed, and the condition of the wound.

Procedure 18-16 Removing Staples

Equipment: Antiseptic solution or wipes, examination gloves, sterile gloves, sponge forceps, gauze squares, and prepackaged sterile staple removal instrument.

1. Wash your hands and gather your supplies.

2. Greet the patient by name and explain the procedure. Answer any questions the patient may have.

3. If the dressing is still in place, put on clean examination gloves and remove it. Dispose of it in a biohazard waste container. Remove your gloves and wash your hands.

4. Clean the wound with antiseptic. Pat dry with sterile gauze sponges. The wound should be as free of pathogens as possible to prevent contamination.

5. Put on sterile gloves. Staple removal is a sterile procedure.

6. Gently slide the end of the staple remover under each staple to be removed.
   - Press the handles together to lift the ends of the staples out of the skin.
   - The remover is designed to open the staple so the ends will lift free with minimal discomfort to the patient.

7. Place each staple on a gauze square as it is removed. This helps in counting the staples at the end of the procedure.

8. When all the staples have been removed, gently clean the site with antiseptic solution.
   - Pat dry and dress the site if the physician has ordered you to do so.
   - The area must be dry before the new dressing is applied to avoid wicking microorganisms.
   - The wound may be healed well enough to be left uncovered.

9. Thank the patient and properly dispose of equipment and supplies. Make sure you follow standard precautions. Clean the treatment area, remove your gloves, and wash your hands.

10. Record the procedure. Documentation must include the time, location of staples, number removed, and the condition of the wound.

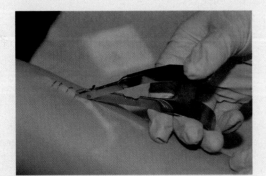

(Reprinted from Kronenberger J, Ledbetter J. *Jones & Bartlett Learning's Comprehensive Medical Assisting*. 5th ed. Burlington, MA: Jones & Bartlett Learning, LLC; 2016.)

Preparing for Externship

If your externship experience is in a practice where they perform minor surgical procedures, you need to review your clinical procedures specific to this area. Review the techniques and principles of surgical asepsis and be able to recognize the surgical instruments used for each procedure. Usually the medical practice has a schedule of procedures for the next day so it is easy for you to do your homework the night prior to ensure you are prepared to assist the physician, if necessary. After each procedure, write down notes of what was new, different or interesting so you will remember the next time you see the procedure.

Chapter Recap

- In assisting with minor surgical procedures, surgical asepsis is essential. Surgical aseptic techniques include sterilization and the surgical scrub. Before sterilization, equipment must be sanitized by hand or by using a mechanical washer. Handle medical instruments very carefully when cleaning them. Check to ensure instruments are in good working order.

- The autoclave uses steam heat under high pressure to sterilize instruments. Items must be wrapped carefully before they're placed in the autoclave. Special indicators help to ensure the items are properly sterilized. Loading the autoclave requires careful attention to item positions so steam can penetrate. Time, pressure, and temperature are three factors that affect sterilization.

- Cold chemicals may be used to sterilize delicate instruments, instruments that are sensitive to heat, or instruments that are too large to fit into the autoclave.

- The medical assistant is responsible for setting up instruments and equipment for surgical procedures. It's important to learn the names of commonly used instruments. Some basic instruments are scissors, scalpels, forceps, and clamps. Different medical specialties have specialized instruments for surgical procedures.

- Supplies and equipment for specific surgical procedures are often packaged together in a sterile surgical pack. Surgical packs may be prepared in the medical office or purchased from a commercial supplier. Do not use surgical packs that show any signs of contamination.

- Careful attention is required to maintain the sterile field. Don't talk, cough, sneeze, or reach across the sterile field. Small supplies and solutions may be added using sterile techniques. Use sterile gloves or sterile transfer forceps to move sterile items. The physician must be informed if there is any possibility the sterile field has become contaminated.

- Before surgical procedures, the medical assistant may help to obtain informed consent and to reinforce preoperative instructions. When the patient is gowned, surgical drapes are provided to expose the operative area. The patient's skin is cleansed and shaved, if necessary.

- During minor surgery, the medical assistant may be asked to hold supplies for the physician, adjust the draping of the patient, pass instruments to the physician, and help collect specimens.

- Common surgical procedures performed in a medical office are excision of lesions and incision and drainage (I&D). If a specimen is collected, the medical assistant is responsible for providing an appropriately labeled container, preparing a laboratory request form, and sending the specimen to the laboratory.

- In the medical office, wounds usually are closed using sutures. The physician chooses atraumatic or traumatic needles in the appropriate size or gauge. Sutures may be absorbable or nonabsorbable. Nonabsorbable sutures need to be removed after healing.

- When the surgical procedures are complete, the medical assistant is responsible for applying dressings and bandages to surgical wounds. The medical assistant usually performs suture and staple removal as well. Sterile technique is necessary for infection control.

- The medical assistant reinforces the physician's instructions for postoperative wound care and tells the patient how to observe the wound for changes that indicate infection or problems with healing.

- After minor surgery, the medical assistant is responsible for removing and caring for instruments, equipment, and supplies. Standard precautions need to be followed in cleaning and disposing of waste.

Online Resources for Students

Student Resources available on the text's online site include:

- Audio Glossaries
- Animations
- Competency Evaluation Forms

- Videos
- Anatomy & Physiology Module with Heart and Lung Sounds
- Weblinks
- Worksheets

Exercises and Activities

Certification Preparation Questions

1. Which of the following represents the process that kills all spores?

   a. Sanitation
   b. Disinfection
   c. Sterilization
   d. Boiling
   e. Chemical soaking

2. Which of these would not be included in an informed consent?

   a. Type of procedure
   b. Expected results of the procedure
   c. Purpose of the procedure
   d. Insurance reimbursement for the procedure
   e. Possible risks of the procedure

3. To maintain a sterile field you need to:

   a. avoid talking when you reach over the sterile field.
   b. keep your hands above waist level.
   c. never pour liquids directly into sterile containers on the sterile field.
   d. maintain a ½″ border around the field which is considered contaminated.
   e. keep your back to the field so you don't accidently touch it.

4. Which of the following is an absolute way of ensuring all microorganisms have been killed?

   a. Use autoclave indicator tape
   b. Perform culture testing
   c. Use a sterilization indicator
   d. Double wrap all surgical packs
   e. Reautoclave surgical packs

5. What are the three critical elements to ensure proper sterilization?

   a. Temperature, pressure, and time
   b. Pressure, size of load, and autoclave paper quality
   c. Time temperature, and sterilizer indicators
   d. Type of machine, steam, and drying time
   e. Type of items autoclaved, time, and autoclave indicator tape

6. Which of the following is not a feature of absorbable suture?

   a. It is removed after healing of the wound.
   b. It can be chemically treated to delay absorption.
   c. There are two forms available, chromic and plain.
   d. Type of suture can be made from sheep intestine.
   e. It is used to close deep tissues.

7. An I&D would be indicated to:

   a. excise a mole.
   b. incise an abscess.
   c. destroy tissue with electric sparks.
   d. perform a cervical biopsy.
   e. cut tissue and coagulate blood vessels.

8. What is the recommended storage time for sterile packs?

    a. 14 days
    b. 21 days
    c. 30 days
    d. 45 days
    e. 60 days

9. An instrument used for grasping is a:

    a. forceps.
    b. scalpel.
    c. probe.
    d. retractor.
    e. director.

10. Which of the following is not considered one of the main functions of surgical instruments?

    a. Cutting
    b. Dissecting
    c. Grasping
    d. Retracting
    e. Removing

Reference

Health Care and Religious Beliefs, Loma Linda University Health System, www.lomalindahealth.org

19 Pharmacology and Drug Administration

Chapter Objectives

- List the different ways patients receive medications from the physician.
- Identify the three different names associated with most medications.
- Describe the Schedule of Controlled Substances and provide an example of each.
- Explain how to monitor the office inventory of controlled substances.
- Maintain medication records.
- Describe how to prepare a written prescription as directed by a physician.
- Define what is meant by local effect and systemic effect for drug action.
- Discuss the four general processes involved in pharmacokinetics.
- Describe the main factors that influence a drug's effect on the body.
- List resources for finding out more about medications.
- List safety guidelines to follow when administering medications.
- Identify three measuring systems used for medications.
- Explain how to calculate adult and child medication doses.
- Apply pharmacology principles to prepare and administer oral and parenteral medications, excluding IV administration.
- List the different types of injections, their appropriate needle lengths, and their sites of administration.
- Explain what to do in the case of a medication error.
- List the seven rights to check for reducing the risk of medication errors.

CAAHEP & ABHES Competencies

CAAHEP

- Prepare proper dosages of medication for administration.
- Verify ordered doses/dosages prior to administration.
- Select proper sites for administering parenteral medication.
- Administer oral medications.
- Administer parenteral (excluding IV) medications.
- Demonstrate knowledge of basic math computations.
- Apply mathematical computations to solve equations.
- Identify measurement systems.
- Define basic units of measurement in metric, apothecary, and household systems.
- Convert among measurement systems.
- Identify both abbreviations and symbols used in calculating medication dosages.

ABHES

- Identify drug classification, usual dose, side effects, and contraindications of the top most commonly used medications.
- Demonstrate accurate occupational math and metric conversions for proper medication administration.
- Identify parts of prescriptions.
- Identify appropriate abbreviations that are accepted in prescription writing.
- Comply with legal aspects of creating prescriptions, including federal and state laws.
- Properly utilize Physician's Desk Reference (PDR), drug handbook, and other drug references to identify a drug's classification, usual dosage, usual side effects, and contraindications.

Chapter Terms

Allergy	Generic	Parenteral	Subscription
Ampule	Inhalation	Pharmacokinetics	Synergism
Anaphylaxis	Inscription	Potentiation	Transdermal
Antagonism	Instillation	Sublingual	Vial
Diluent	Interaction		

Abbreviations

BNDD	IM	OTC	SC
BSA	IV	PDR	SQ
DEA	NKA	PO	STAT
FDA	NPO	Rx	TB
ID			

Case Study

Mr. William Stevens and his wife, Betty, are retired senior citizens who are new patients of the clinic. Marjorie Adams, medical assistant, is completing the patient health history form for William, and when she questions him about any medications he is taking, he states that his wife brought their "bag" of pills. The medical assistant, Ms. Adams, will go through each container of medication to determine which drugs each of them is currently taking. In addition to the prescribed medication, it is important to find out what over-the-counter drugs and preparations are also used. The drugs will be documented in the patient chart for review by the physician.

Pharmacology is the study of drugs, their actions, dosages, and side effects. A drug is a chemical substance that affects how the body functions. Many drugs are used as medications. Medications are legal drugs that are used to treat illness according to established medical guidelines.

PHARMACOLOGY AND THE MEDICAL ASSISTANT

Patients receive medications in different ways. Medications may be:

- Administered—The medication is given to the patient in the office by an allied health professional or given by self or family member at home.
- Dispensed—The medication is supplied to the patient in the office for later use or given by a pharmacist at a pharmacy.

Case Question

 Why is it important to ask the patient about over-the-counter drugs that he may be taking?

- Prescribed—A written order given to the patient and taken to a pharmacist to be filled.

As a clinical medical assistant, you may be responsible for administering medications under the physician's supervision. You also may need to educate patients on how to use different kinds of medications that are dispensed or prescribed. It's important that you know different types of medications, their uses, and their potential abuses. For each medication, you'll need to be familiar with:

- The range of dosages
- The methods of administration
- Any adverse, or unwanted, effects

Types of Medications

There are two general types of medications—over-the-counter (**OTC**) and prescription-only.

- Over-the-counter medications are usually available in pharmacies and supermarkets without any restrictions. Some drugs may be released as over-the-counter medications at a lower strength, while a higher level of the drug requires a prescription. This can be confusing for patients, so you need to stay aware of the latest information about drug releases.
- Prescription-only medications must be prescribed or ordered by a physician, physician's assistant, or nurse practitioner. The prescription is a written order to the pharmacist. A physician, physician's assistant, or nurse practitioner must sign the prescription, or it cannot be filled.

Cultural Connection

When physicians order medications for patients, assumptions are made that the patient will accept the prescription and take the medication as ordered. Specific cultures may have a different view regarding the dosages and oral medications prescribed. For example, in the Asian culture, some patients may adjust the dosage and not take the full prescribed dose believing that the medicines are overly potent. This might be due to the fact that many Asians tend to be smaller in stature than the typical Westerner. These patients might also totally discontinue taking a medication when their symptoms have subsided. Many treatment plans require the patient to take all prescribed medication even though they may start feeling better. For example, antibiotics are prescribed for a specific number of days or doses. A patient needs to be told to take the entire course of antibiotic, typically 5 to 10 days.

The Name Game

Most over-the-counter and prescription medications have three different names.

- Chemical name—The first name given to any medication identifying the chemical components of the drug. This name is used mainly by the researchers and will not be used in the medical office.
- **Generic** name—The name assigned to the drug during research and development. It refers to the chemical ingredients that make up the drug. Generic drug names are usually made up of combinations of root words, prefixes, and suffixes that describe a certain type of drug or part of the body. Medical professionals often use the generic name in the medical office.
- Trade name—The name given the drug when it is ready for commercial use and distribution by the manufacturer. It's also known as the *brand name*. The trade name is registered by the U.S. Patent Office. After it is registered, the trademark symbol (^{TM}) must follow the name.

After the patent on a medication expires, other companies may manufacture generic versions and give them their own trade names.

Table 19-1 provides some basic information on common drugs, how they are classified, and their uses. The table includes prescription and over-the-counter drugs. It also provides their generic names and, in some cases, common trade names.

Sources of Drugs

Drugs come from many natural sources, such as plants, minerals, and animals. They also may be synthetic or prepared in the laboratory by artificial means. See Table 19-2 for a list of common drugs and their sources.

Legal Regulations

Federal laws and rules protect consumers by regulating the production, prescription, and dispensation of medications. Two government agencies in particular are involved with controlling drugs and their use.

- Food and Drug Administration (**FDA**)—Established to regulate the manufacture and sale of drugs and food products. It ensures that the ingredients listed on the labels are accurate and that the drugs are safe to use.
- Drug Enforcement Agency (**DEA**)—A branch of the Department of Justice. Some drugs may result in dependency or abuse. These drugs are classified as controlled substances. Its mission is to control the use of all drugs listed as controlled substances by the Bureau of Narcotics and Dangerous Drugs (**BNDD**). The DEA sends out information about changes in laws and procedures. Make sure your office is on the DEA mailing list.

Table 19-1 Common Drugs and Their Uses

Therapeutic Classification	Effect, Action, Uses	Common Examples
Adrenergic blocking agents	Affect alpha or beta receptors of adrenergic nerves	Metoprolol tartrate (Lopressor); propranolol hydrochloride (Inderal); Hytrin; Coreg
Adrenergic agents	Mimic activity of sympathetic nervous system (the part of the nervous system over which a person has no conscious control)	Epinephrine (adrenaline); ephedrine sulfate
Analgesics	Relieve pain	Aspirin, acetaminophen (Tylenol), codeine
Antacids	Neutralize or reduce stomach acidity	Magnesia (milk of magnesia); calcium carbonate (Tums)
Anthelmintics	Kill parasitic worms	Piperazine citrate, mebendazole (Vermox)
Antianginal agents	Promote vasodilation	Nitroglycerin, diltiazem hydrochloride (Cardizem)
Antianxiety agents	Act on brain to relieve symptoms of anxiety	Alprazolam (Xanax); lorazepam (Ativan); chlordiazepoxide (Librium); diazepam (Valium)
Antiarrhythmics	Reduce or prevent irregular cardiac rhythms	Procainamide hydrochloride (Pronestyl); esmolol (Brevibloc); lidocaine; amiodarone
Antibiotics	Interfere with growth of or destroy microorganisms	Penicillin, lop cefaclor, tetracycline; erythromycin; Levaquin
Anticoagulants and thrombolytics	Prevent or dissolve blood clots	Heparin sodium, Coumadin, streptokinase (Streptase); Lovenox; Plavix
Anticonvulsants	Reduce excitability of brain	Phenobarbital, phenytoin (Dilantin); Depakote; Neurontin
Antidepressants	Prevent or reduce symptoms of psychological depression	Amitriptyline hydrochloride (Elavil); fluoxetine hydrochloride (Prozac); Paxil; Zoloft; Wellbutrin
Antidiarrheals	Decrease intestinal peristalsis (contractions)	Loperamide hydrochloride (Imodium A-D); Lomotil
Antiemetic agents	Prevent nausea and/or vomiting	Dimenhydrinate (Dramamine); promethazine hydrochloride (Phenergan); Zofran
Antifungals	Destroy or slow the growth of fungi	Ketoconazole (Nizoral): miconazole nitrate (Monistat 3 or 7); Flagyl
Antihistamines	Counteract effects of histamine on organs and structures	Chlorpheniramine maleate (Chlor-Trimeton); diphenhydramine hydrochloride (Benadryl); loratadine (Allegra, Alavert)
Antihypertensives	Increase size of arteries	Methyldopa hydrochloride (Aldomet); prazosin (Minipress)
Anti-inflammatory agents	Reduce irritation and swelling of tissues	Aspirin, ibuprofen (Motrin); naproxen (Naprosyn)
Antilipemic agents	Reduce serum cholesterol	Zocor; Lopid; Zetia
Antineoplastic agents	Slow tumor growth	Cyclophosphamide (Cytoxan)
Antipsychotics	Exact mechanism not understood; used to treat psychoses (mental state involving distorted perceptions of reality)	chlorpromazine (Thorazine); haloperidol (Haldol)
Antipyretics	Decrease body temperature	Aspirin, acetaminophen (Tylenol)
Antitussives, mucolytics, expectorants	Relieve cough, loosen respiratory secretions, aid removal of thick secretions	Codeine sulfate; dextromethorphan hydrobromide (Benylin); guaifenesin (Entex)
Antivirals	Inhibit viral replication	Acyclovir (Zovirax), AZT
Bronchodilators	Dilate bronchi (air passages leading from trachea to lungs)	Albuterol sulfate (Ventolin), Alupent

(continued)

Table 19-1	Common Drugs and Their Uses (*continued*)	
Therapeutic Classification	**Effect, Action, Uses**	**Common Examples**
Cardiotonics	Increase force of myocardium (heart muscle)	Digoxin (Lanoxin), Primacor
Cholinergic blockers	Affect autonomic nervous system (the part of the nervous system that regulates automatic functions such as blood flow, digestion, and temperature)	Atropine sulfate, scopolamine hydrobromide
Cholinergics	Mimic activity of parasympathetic nervous system (the part of the nervous system that regulates automatic functions to conserve body energy, e.g., by slowing heart rate)	Neostigmine (Prostigmin); pilocarpine hydrochloride
Decongestants	Reduce swelling of nasal passages	Pseudoephedrine hydrochloride (Sudafed)
Diuretics	Increase secretion of urine by kidneys	Furosemide (Lasix); chlorothiazide (Diuril)
Emetics	Promote vomiting	Ipecacuanha (Ipecac syrup)
Histamine H_2 antagonists	Inhibit action of histamine at H_2 receptor cells of stomach	Cimetidine (Tagamet); ranitidine (Zantac); famotidine (Pepcid)
Hormones, female	Prevent symptoms of menopause	Estradiol (Estraderm, Premarin); medroxy-progesterone acetate (Provera)
Hormones, male	Therapy for testosterone deficiency	Androgen (Testamone)
Immunological agents	Simulate immune response to protect against disease	Vaccines against pneumococcus, influenza virus; diphtheria and tetanus toxoid
Insulin, oral hypoglycemics	Control diabetes	NPH, ultralente insulin; tolbutamide (Orinase); glipizide (Glucotrol)
Sedatives, hypnotics	Sedatives relax and calm; hypnotics induce sleep	Butabarbital sodium, Restoril
Stimulants	Increase activity of central nervous system	Doxapram hydrochloride (Dopram), amphetamine sulfate
Thyroid, antithyroid agents	Alter amount of thyroid hormone produced	Levothyroxine sodium (T4) (Levothroid)

Table 19-2	Common Drugs and Their Sources		
Source		**Drug**	**Use**
Plants	Cinchona bark	Quinidine	Antiarrhythmic
	Purple foxglove	Digitalis	Cardiotonic
	Opium poppy	Paregoric	Antidiarrheal
		Morphine	Analgesic
		Codeine	Antitussive, analgesic
Minerals	Magnesium	Milk of Magnesia	Antacid, laxative
	Silver	Silver nitrate	Placed in eyes of newborns to kill *Neisseria gonorrhoeae*, a bacteria that causes gonorrhea
	Gold	Solganal	Arthritis treatment
Animal proteins	Pork, beef pancreas	Insulin	Antidiabetic hormone
	Pork, beef stomach acids	Pepsin	Digestive hormone
	Animal thyroid glands	Thyroid, USP	Hypothyroidism
Synthetics		Demerol	Analgesic
		Lomotil	Antidiarrheal
		Gantrisin	Sulfonamide
		Humulin	
Semisynthetics	*Escherichia coli* bacteria, altered DNA molecules		Antidiabetic hormone

The Pure Food and Drug Act

The first federal law regulating medicine was the Pure Food and Drug Act. Here's a timeline of important milestones in the history of this law.

- The Pure Food and Drug Act was passed in 1906.
- In 1938, it was strengthened to require that a drug's safety be proved before being distributed to the public.
- In 1952, the Durham-Humphrey Amendment banned many drugs from being dispensed without a prescription.
- The Kefauver-Harris Amendment of 1962 required that prescription and nonprescription medications both be tested for their effectiveness before they are released for sale.

The Controlled Substances Act

In 1970, the Controlled Substances Act was passed to regulate the manufacture and distribution of dangerous drugs. This act requires that anyone who manufactures, prescribes, administers, or dispenses controlled substances register with the US government.

When a physician or practitioner registers, a number is issued to the physician called a DEA number. This registration limits which drugs that physician or practitioner can handle. The DEA number is active for 3 years. It also must be updated if the office moves or opens another location. It's the physician or nurse practitioner's responsibility, not the DEA's, to make sure the registration is kept up to date. As a medical assistant, you may be responsible for maintaining or reminding the physician or practitioner about registration with the DEA.

Controlled Substances in the Medical Office

The DEA is responsible for revising the list of drugs in the Schedule of Controlled Substances. Table 19-3 describes each of the five categories of controlled drugs. All the substances on the list have a potential for abuse and dependency. Drug dependence, also referred to as addiction, can be physical, psychological, or both.

- Physical dependence—Patients with a physical dependence on a drug will have mild to severe physiological symptoms. Symptoms gradually become more intense as the drug is stopped.
- Psychological dependence—Patients with a psychological dependence on a drug have developed a need for the feeling brought on by the drug.

Monitoring Inventory

A medical office must order controlled substances from Schedule II using a federal order form (DEA Form 222). One copy of the form is filed with the DEA by the supplier. In most states, controlled substances from Schedule II may be ordered through the drug supplier for your office. Orders of substances from Schedules III to V don't require the form. However, the physician or practitioner's DEA number is still required.

When controlled substances are received in the medical office, the delivery receipt should be signed by two office employees. Each controlled substance is then tracked on a special inventory form. The receipts and inventory forms must be kept for 2 years. They also must be available for inspection by DEA officials.

Table 19-3 Schedule of Controlled Substances

Schedule	Description	Examples
I	Highest potential for abuse; no accepted medicinal use in the United States; no accepted safety standards, although some are used in carefully controlled research projects	Opium, marijuana, lysergic acid diethylamide (LSD), peyote, mescaline
II	High potential for abuse; accepted medicinal use in United States but with severe restrictions. Abuse can lead to psychological or physiological dependence. Requires written prescription; prescription cannot be refilled or called in to pharmacy by medical office. Only in extreme emergencies may physician call in prescription; handwritten prescription must be presented to pharmacist within 72 h.	Morphine, codeine, cocaine, secobarbital (Seconal), amphetamines, hydromorphone (Dilaudid), methylphenidate (Ritalin)
III	Limited potential for psychological or physiological dependence. Prescription may be called in to pharmacy by physician and refilled up to five times in 6 months.	Paregoric, acetaminophen (Tylenol) with codeine, Fiorinal
IV	Lower potential for psychological or physiological dependence than those in Schedules II and III. Prescription may be called into pharmacy by medical office employee; may be refilled up to five times in 6 months.	Chlordiazepoxide (Librium), diazepam (Valium), propoxyphene (Darvon), phenobarbital
V	Lower potential for abuse than those in Schedules I to IV	Buprenorphine (Buprenex), codeine in cough preparations

Controlled substances are kept in a safe or secure locked box. The number of people with keys or access should be limited. Careful records must be kept of how and when controlled substances leave the inventory. Controlled substances leave the inventory when they are

- Administered
- Dispensed
- Disposed of as waste

When a controlled substance is administered or dispensed, you need to record the following information:

- Drug name
- Name of the patient who received the drug
- Dose given
- Date the drug was given
- Name of the physician who ordered the drug
- Name of the employee who handled the procedure

Federal law requires that every 2 years, the inventory of controlled substances must be reviewed and checked. The amount of each drug on hand is compared to the amounts ordered and the amounts dispensed to patients. Many facilities also inventory their controlled substances whenever a different staff member assumes responsibility for the locked cabinet's key. Other facilities account for their controlled substances at the end of each day.

If controlled substances are lost or stolen, notify local police immediately. It's the law.

Disposing of Controlled Substances

Sometimes, the physician may ask you to dispose of outdated medications or samples. You must follow federal, state, and local regulations when disposing of controlled substances. DEA Form 41 Registrants Inventory of Drugs Surrendered is completed in quadruplicate, and signed by the physician.

The information required for this form is similar to the information required for dispensing controlled substances. After completing the form, two copies are sent to the nearest DEA office. You'll then be notified about how to dispose of the drugs. Disposal methods may include incineration or shipping drugs to the DEA office by registered mail. Once the controlled substances are disposed of, the DEA will issue the physician a receipt. This receipt should be kept with the inventory records for controlled substances.

Prescribing Controlled Substances

In some cases, controlled substances are prescribed, not administered in the office. Some states require only that the prescription details be recorded in the patient's chart. Other states require that a separate file be kept in the medical office for copies of prescriptions for controlled substances.

Some states require the use of special prescription forms for controlled substances. They can be locked up until they are needed. The physician's DEA number should not be imprinted on this form so the physician will add it as it is signed.

Illegal Drug Use

If you suspect that a physician or any health care professional is diverting controlled substances illegally, it's your legal and ethical duty to report your suspicions.

- Gather and document evidence to back up your suspicions. You'll need to present this evidence and the reasons for your suspicions when you report them to the proper authorities.
- In most instances, you'll be allowed to remain anonymous.
- In most cases, you should contact the local police.
- If a physician is involved, you'll need to report the evidence to the DEA and the American Medical Association (AMA) as well.
- If the suspected health care worker is not a physician or nurse practitioner, report the evidence to your supervisor.

Most states have programs to help health care professionals get help to deal with addiction or dependency issues.

Electronic Prescribing

Electronic prescribing is a way for the physician or health care provider to send a prescription directly to the pharmacy electronically. This is a safe way of prescribing drugs. The patient does not have to wait for the pharmacy to fill the prescription. An electronic prescription is easier for the pharmacist to read and fill. There is also less chance for an error in the prescription.

Prescriptions in the Office

The physician or nurse practitioner may ask you to fill out a prescription form for his or her signature. When you write a prescription, you must follow established guidelines. This includes using a traditional prescription form. There are several important pieces of information you must fill in on the form:

- Date—Prescriptions must be filled within 6 months of the date they are issued.
- Patient's name and address—The pharmacist needs this information to fill the prescription.
- **Inscription**—Located below or beside the symbol Rx, you write the name of the medication, the desired form (e.g., liquid, tablet, capsule), and the strength (e.g., 250 mg, 500 ml).
- **Subscription**—This information tells the pharmacist how much of the drug to dispense. This could be the total number of tablets. For a liquid, it could be the total amount of the drug in milliliters.

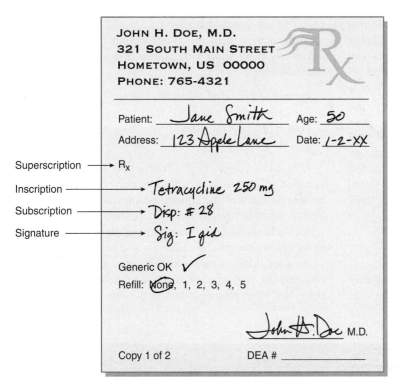

JOHN H. DOE, M.D.
321 SOUTH MAIN STREET
HOMETOWN, US 00000
PHONE: 765-4321

Patient: _Jane Smith_   Age: _50_
Address: _123 Apple Lane_   Date: _1-2-XX_

Superscription ⟶ R$_x$

Inscription ⟶ Tetracycline 250 mg

Subscription ⟶ Disp: # 28

Signature ⟶ Sig: I qid

Generic OK ✓
Refill: None, 1, 2, 3, 4, 5

John H. Doe M.D.

Copy 1 of 2   DEA # _____

Figure 19-1   Prescription form. (Reprinted from Kronenberger J, Ledbetter J. *Jones & Bartlett Learning's Comprehensive Medical Assisting.* 5th ed. Burlington, MA: Jones & Bartlett Learning, LLC; 2016.)

- Signature—This section is not where the physician signs. It refers to the instructions for patients about taking the medication (e.g., with meals, three times a day, four times a day). Sometimes, this section is used for the abbreviation Sig.
- Refills—The number of times a prescription can be refilled is indicated on the prescription. This is generally no more than five or six times within 6 months. If no refills are desired, the word "none" should be circled, or 0 should be written in.
- Physician's signature—The physician must sign the prescription. The physician is responsible for all prescriptions written in his or her office.
- Generic—Some physicians and insurance companies allow generic substitutes for some medications. This is noted on the prescription whether generic substitutions can be made. If the physician does not want a

medication substituted with a generic version, write DAW on the prescription, dispense as written.
- DEA number—The physician's Drug Enforcement Administration (DEA) registration number should appear on every prescription as a way to track the delivery of controlled substances.

Figure 19-1 is an example of a traditional handwritten prescription. Electronic medical record software provides a printout of a prescription the physician orders.

The symbol Rx is always found at the top left of the prescription pad. It's called the superscription and means recipe, or "take thou."

All prescription medications must be documented in the patient's medical record. Figure 19-2 is an example of written documentation of a prescription as it would appear in the patient's record.

DATE	TIME	ORDERS
7/5/XX	1000	Prescription for ampicillin 250mg, p.o., qid x7 days as ordered by Dr. Smith
		Sally Smith, CMA

Figure 19-2   Documentation of a prescribed medication in the patient's medical record. (Reprinted from Kronenberger J, Ledbetter J. *Jones & Bartlett Learning's Comprehensive Medical Assisting.* 5th ed. Burlington, MA: Jones & Bartlett Learning, LLC; 2016.)

If electronic record is used, the same information will be documented. Electronic software programs may vary; however, documented information is the same. This includes prescriptions that are called in or faxed to the pharmacist. The patient's chart is a legal document and may be called into court in the event of legal action. If the medication order isn't recorded, it will be presumed that the medication was never ordered. When prescribing, administering, or documenting patient prescriptions, you need to use appropriate medical terminology and abbreviations. Table 19-4 lists common medical abbreviations used in pharmacology.

Prescriptions by Phone

Sometimes, the physician may ask you to phone a prescription order to a patient's pharmacy. It may be a new prescription order or a renewal. You'll need to provide the pharmacist with information that is similar to the information on the written prescription. This includes the following:

- Patient's name and address
- Prescription information
- Name of the prescribing physician
- Number of refills

You can't phone in a prescription for a controlled substance. In an urgent situation, the physician may do so. The amount of the controlled substance must be limited to what is needed for the situation. A written prescription must be sent to the pharmacist within 72 hours to follow up the phone call.

As a medical assistant, you also may need to deal with requests for prescription renewals that are phoned into the office from pharmacies and patients. These requests

Table 19-4 Common Medical Abbreviations

Abbreviation	Meaning	Abbreviation	Meaning
aa	of each	os	mouth
amp	ampule	oz	ounce
amt	amount	p	after
aq	aqueous	pc	after meals
bid	twice a day	pm, PM	afternoon or evening
$\bar{c}$	with	po, **PO**	by mouth
cap	capsule	qt	quart
g, gm	gram	R	right, rectal
gr	grain	**Rx**	take, prescribe
gt(t)	drop(s)	$\bar{s}$	without
h, hr	hour	Sig	label
Id, ID	intradermal	SL	sublingual
IM	intramuscular (into muscle)	sol	solution
IV	intravenous	SOS	once if necessary
kg	kilogram	sp	spirits
L, l	liter	ss	one-half
lb	pound	stat, **STAT**	immediately
m, min	minim	supp	suppository
mcg, μg	microgram	syr	syrup
mEq	milliequivalent	tab	tablet
ml, mL	milliliter	T, tb, tbs, tbsp	tablespoon
n	normal	t, tsp	teaspoon
NaCl	sodium chloride	tid	three times a day
NKA	no known allergies	tinc	tincture (a solution of a substance in alcohol)
noc	night		
NPO	nothing by mouth	ung	ointment
NS	normal saline		

must be handled on the day they're made. Be sure you receive accurate information from the caller about the following:

- Patient's name, address, and phone number
- Phone number of the pharmacy
- Name of the medication, dosage, and amount

Once you have all the information, check it against the patient's medical record. Then, show the request and the patient's medical record to the physician. You must have the physician's approval before you phone in a renewal of a prescription. After you call it in, it's a good idea to call the patient to explain that the physician has renewed his or her prescription. Always document any prescription renewals made by phone and conversations you have with the patient regarding prescriptions.

Case Question

The medical assistant completed the review of the bag of drugs that Mr. Stevens brought to the office. She noted that some of the medication containers were empty and outdated. When she questioned the Stevens, they stated that they were unable to afford a refill of all the drugs so they just decreased the amount of some drugs they took in each dose. For example, Mr. Stevens was directed to take two tablets of his high blood pressure medication each day and he only took one tablet every other day. What problem would this cause for his condition?

Patient Education

After patients receive a prescription in the office, you should provide verbal and written instructions for using the medication. Here's what the patients need to understand:

- How much medication to take
- When to take it
- Instructions for how to take the medication (e.g., with food or not)
- How the patient's body may react to the medication
- How long the medication should be taken for and why it's important to not stop taking some medications too soon
- Side effects such as drowsiness or nausea
- When to report adverse reactions

- Any safety precautions that should be taken, such as driving or operating machinery
- How the medicine should be stored
- How the medicine will react with alcohol and other medications, including over-the-counter drugs and herbs
- How to dispose of old and expired medicine

It's important to speak clearly and slowly while giving instructions about medications. Some elderly patients may have difficulty hearing you. You also should make sure the patient understands what you've said by watching for nonverbal cues and by having the patient repeat back the instructions.

Provide written instructions that include the name of the medication and directions for taking it. This helps to avoid confusion. Your medical office may have preprinted information sheets (from the American Medical Association) for common medications. Pharmacies also provide instruction sheets for patients. Encourage patients to call the medical office if they have any questions about taking their medication.

DRUG ACTIONS AND INTERACTIONS

Every patient responds to drugs differently. An **interaction** is the effect or action that occurs between drugs and the human body. To understand the actions and interactions of drugs and the human body, there are two main considerations.

- Pharmacodynamics refers to the ways drugs act on the body. This includes their actions on specific cells, tissues, and organs.
- **Pharmacokinetics** is how the drugs move through the body after they're swallowed or injected.

Table 19-5 provides a list of factors that influence drug actions in the body. Some of the common factors include age, weight, and gender of the patient.

Pharmacodynamics

Different drugs have different effects on the body. In pharmacodynamics, it's important to distinguish between the actions of drugs and the effects of those drugs.

- Drug action refers to the chemical changes the drug has on the body's cells. All drugs cause cellular change.
- Drug effect refers to the observable changes the drug has on the body. All drugs have some degree of physiological effect.

Table 19-5	Factors Influencing Drug Action
Factors	**Effects on Drug Action**
Age	Elderly people have slow metabolic processes. Age-related kidney and liver dysfunctions also extend breakdown and excretion times. You must monitor the cumulative effects of drugs in elderly patients. Children may have an immediate response to drugs. Therefore, you should assess them frequently.
Weight	Many medication dosages are calculated according to the patient's weight. As a general rule, the larger the patient, the greater the dose. However, you also need to take into account a person's sensitivity to a drug.
Gender	Women's reactions to certain drugs may be different from those of men because of the ratio of fat to body mass or differing hormone levels.
Time of day	The absorption of certain drugs is delayed by the presence of food in the stomach or small intestine. Other drugs may be tolerated better when food is in the patient's stomach.
Psychological state	Nervous or highly excited patients may need larger or smaller amounts of certain drugs to achieve the desired effect than calmer patients require.
Existing pathology	The process, absorption, distribution, metabolism, and excretion may be affected, when the body is compromised by a disease.
Idiosyncratic and immune responses	Some people may have unexpected, abnormal, or allergic reactions to some drugs. The body must build an immune response, so first exposures may or may not indicate a problem. However, later reactions to the same drug may be more severe.
Cumulation	The rate at which the body absorbs, breaks down, or excretes some drugs; can result in high concentrations and possible toxic effects if repeat doses are not adjusted for this factor.
Tolerance	Some medications given over a long period of time cause the body to become resistant to their effects. If this happens, larger doses may be required to get the desired result.

For example, the drug action of penicillin is to prevent bacteria from building up cell walls. The drug effect of penicillin is that it kills bacteria.

Local or Systemic Effects

The effect of a drug may be either local or systemic (affecting an entire system). A local effect is limited to the area of the body where it's administered. When an ointment or lotion is applied to the skin, the drug action is limited to that area. The effect of the drug is local.

A systemic effect means that the drug is absorbed into the blood and carried to other parts of the body. Antibiotic therapy for a urinary tract infection produces a systemic effect. Antibiotic tablets are taken orally. Once the drug is absorbed into the bloodstream, it's carried to the urinary bladder. The drug acts on any microorganisms in the urinary bladder and destroys them.

A systemic effect can be obtained by administering drugs in several different ways:

- Oral—By mouth and swallowed
- **Sublingual**—Under the tongue
- Buccal—Between the cheek and gum
- Rectal—Through the rectum
- By injection—Into the bloodstream
- **Transdermal**—Through the skin
- By **inhalation**—Through the lungs

Pharmacokinetics

The way the body reacts to the drug depends on the following:

- How it's administered
- How quickly it's absorbed
- How long it takes to act
- How quickly it's eliminated from the body

There are four general processes involved in pharmacokinetics.

- Absorption is the process of getting the drug into the bloodstream. The method of administration affects the absorption rate, or how fast the drug moves in the body. Two different drug products that contain the same active ingredients may be absorbed at different rates. Other ingredients in the product may affect the absorption rate.
- Distribution refers to the movement of the drug from the bloodstream into cells and tissues. Different drugs move into different types of body tissues at different speeds.
- Metabolism is the physical and chemical breakdown of drugs by the body. This often takes place in the liver. Patients with hepatic disease have problems with liver function and may not be able to break down a drug properly. This will affect the time it takes for the drug to act. It also may affect how long the drug will continue acting.

Excretion is the process where by-products of drugs are sent to kidneys to be removed from the body. Some drugs reach the kidneys largely unchanged. They can be detected in the patient's urine after excretion. But if the kidneys are compromised by disease, the medication may not be eliminated properly. Drugs that are not eliminated properly may build up in the body. This may lead to toxicity or poisoning.

Pharmacokinetics may cause a drug to be contraindicated, or not recommended for use, if a patient has certain medical conditions. On the drug box or insert, the drug manufacturer lists contraindications, situations when the drug should not be given.

Drug Interactions

When two drugs are taken at the same time, the drugs may act on each other. When this happens, it's called an interaction. The drugs' effects may increase, decrease, or cancel each other out. Drug interactions can occur with prescribed drugs, over-the-counter medications, or herbal or other natural supplements. Alcohol consumption also can cause a drug interaction.

Types of interactions include synergism, antagonism, and potentiation.

- **Synergism** means that two drugs work together.
- **Antagonism** is an effect in which one drug makes the other less effective.
- **Potentiation** occurs when one drug extends or multiplies the effect of another drug.

Physicians and nurse practitioners sometimes may prescribe two or more drugs that interact to cause a specific effect. For example, a physician might prescribe both a muscle relaxant and a pain medication to treat an injury to a muscle or muscle group.

Some drug interactions produce unwanted effects. Here are two examples:

- Taking antacids to relieve symptoms of indigestion may prevent the absorption of antibiotics such as tetracycline (antagonism).
- Sedatives and barbiturates taken together can depress the nervous system (synergism).

Food–Drug Interactions

Patients take many prescription and over-the-counter medications by mouth, so the drugs are absorbed through the digestive system. Food in the digestive system can affect the absorption of the drug.

- Some medications are best absorbed when taken 1 to 2 hours after a meal. Examples are ampicillin or nafcillin (Unipen), both antibiotics. The physician may recommend that some drugs be taken an hour before or 2 hours after eating.

- Some medications should be taken with food to decrease the chance of stomach upset—for example, ibuprofen (Motrin), amoxicillin (an antibiotic), and verapamil (Calan, a heart medication).

Case Questions

While reviewing Mr. and Mrs. Stevens' medications, the medical assistant found that some of the medications were outdated. She told the Stevens that those outdated drugs need to be discarded and asked if she could do that for them. Mr. Stevens said that he would just take them home in case he or his wife might need them at a later time. He said they paid good money for them and will not agree to discard them. What should the medical assistant tell them? If the outdated drugs were taken, what could be the consequences?

Drug-Related Terms

When working around drugs, you'll need to be familiar with specific terms related to pharmacology. The following represents some basic terms you should know.

- Therapeutic classification—States the purpose for the drug's use (e.g., a cardiotonic drug strengthens the heart and blood vessels; an *anti-infective* drug fights infection).
- Teratogenic category—The level of risk to fetal or maternal health, ranging from Category A to D (where D is most dangerous). Category X means that a drug should never be given during pregnancy.
- Indications—Diseases and conditions for which the particular drug is prescribed.
- Contraindications—Conditions or instances when the particular drug should not be used.
- Adverse reactions—Undesirable side effects of a particular drug.
- Hypersensitivity—Excessive reaction, known as a drug **allergy**; the body must build this response, so first exposures may or may not indicate a developing problem.
- Idiosyncratic reaction—An abnormal or unexpected reaction to a drug that's peculiar to an individual patient; not technically an allergy.

Other medications interact with specific types of food. Some nutrients in food can bind with drug ingredients and reduce absorption or decrease a drug's effectiveness. Here are some common medications that interact with food.

- Atorvastatin (Lipitor)—A medication for reducing blood cholesterol levels; interacts with grapefruit juice.

- MAO inhibitors—Medications for treating depression can interact with some foods such as cheese or alcohol. The interactions can result in severe headaches or dangerous increases in blood pressure.
- Tetracycline—Absorption of this antibiotic is less effective when taken with calcium or foods containing calcium.
- Warfarin (Coumadin)—Green, leafy vegetables such as spinach or kale, which are high in vitamin K, may decrease the effectiveness of this blood thinner.

It's important to learn as much as you can about medications prescribed often in your medical office. You may need to educate patients on how to avoid food and drug interactions.

Patient Education

It is important to tell patients to take the medication prescribed by the physician. If a patient says that he or she prefers to use a herbal remedy or over-the-counter medication instead, how should you reply? You must caution the patient that treating self with an herbal remedy or over-the-counter medication isn't a substitute for the medication the physician has prescribed.

OTC medications may not offer enough benefits to treat the illness. In some cases, they can cover up symptoms or even aggravate the problem. They might even interact with other medications that the patient is already taking.

Encourage the patient to follow the physician's instructions. Reassure that if the patient has any questions while using the prescribed medication, he or she can call the office. You also should remind the patient not to mix OTC medications or herbal remedies with prescription medications. Mixing medications can create a new set of problems, including unwanted drug effects.

Allergic Reactions and Side Effects

When gathering information for the patient's medical history, it's important to ask about allergies of any sort, but especially allergies to medications. A drug allergy is a reaction such as hives, dyspnea (labored breathing), or wheezing. **Anaphylaxis** is a severe allergic reaction that can be life threatening. Allergic reactions can be immediate or delayed by 2 hours or longer. If the medication is administered by injection, any allergic reaction usually occurs within minutes.

If the patient reports allergies to a medication, you need to interview the patient carefully about the symptoms. Medications that produce true allergic symptoms need

to be noted in the patient's medical record. Drug allergies always should be noted prominently on the front of the patient's medical record and on each page of the medication record. Patients who've had an allergic reaction to a medication in the past shouldn't be given the medication again. It might cause an anaphylactic reaction.

If a patient is receiving allergy medication or any medication that has a high incidence of allergic reactions (such as penicillin for example), the patient should wait for 20 to 30 minutes and be rechecked before leaving the office. Some offices require that all patients who receive injections wait a specific amount of time (usually 15 to 20 minutes) before leaving. Once the patient is checked, be sure to document in the chart that there were no complaints or difficulties. Always follow the policies in your medical office regarding administering injections.

A patient may state she has an allergy to a medication, when the reaction was really a side effect. Side effects are predictable reactions to medications that occur in some patients. Manufacturers note expected side effects on the medication insert or container. Some common side effects include the following:

- Nausea
- Dryness of the mouth
- Drowsiness

Side effects often are annoying, but they're not usually life threatening. They don't need to be noted on the patient's allergy list.

Drug Information References

There are several resources medical assistants can use to find out more about medications. In addition to hard copy books, many references are available electronically.

- Physician's Desk Reference (**PDR**)—This resource includes the drug's chemical name, brand name or names, and generic name. It lists properties, indications, side effects, contraindications, dosages, and includes pictures of various medications. The physician must purchase this book.
- United States Pharmacopeia Dispensing Information (USPDI)—Two paperback volumes provide information about drug sources, physical properties, tests for identity, storage, and dosage. The USPDI does not contain photographs of medications. The physician must purchase these books.
- American Hospital Formulary Service (AHFS)—This is distributed to practicing physicians. It provides concise information arranged according to drug classifications.
- Compendium of Drug Therapy—This annual publication is distributed to physicians. It includes photographs of drugs and phone numbers of major pharmaceutical companies and poison control centers.

ADMINISTERING MEDICATIONS

You should be familiar with any medication the physician orders before you administer it. You also should know the procedures for administering the drug accurately and safely. If you're not familiar with a drug, look up its classification, usual dosage, and route of administration.

Safety First

As a medical assistant, you must follow important safety guidelines when administering medications. Following this list of guidelines will protect you and your patients.

1. Know your office's policies regarding the administration of medications.
2. Give only the medications the physician has ordered in writing. Don't accept verbal orders.
3. Check with the physician if you have any doubt about a medication or order.
4. Avoid conversation and other distractions while preparing and administering medications. Be attentive.
5. Work in a quiet, well-lighted area.
6. Check the label three times—once when taking the medication from the shelf, again when preparing the medication, and a third time when replacing the medication on the shelf or disposing of the empty container. Figure 19-3A, B, shows examples of medication bottles with typical labels indicating the medication and the strength of the drug.
7. Place the order and the medication side by side to compare for accuracy.
8. Check the strength of the medication (e.g., 250 as opposed to 500 mg) and the route of administration.
9. Read labels carefully. Don't quickly look at the label or medication order.
10. Check the patient's medical record for allergies to the medication or its components before giving it.
11. Check the medication's expiration date.
12. Be alert for color changes, precipitation, odor, or any indication that the medication properties have changed. If the medication has changed in consistency, color, or odor, discard it appropriately.
13. Measure exactly. There should be no bubbles in liquid medication.
14. Stay with the patient while he or she takes oral medication. Watch for any reaction and record the patient's response.
15. Never return a medication to the container after it's been poured or removed.
16. Put on gloves for all procedures that might result in contact with blood or body fluids.
17. Never recap, bend, or break a used needle.

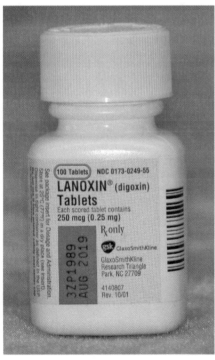

A

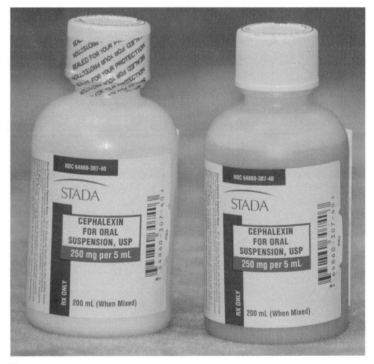

B

Figure 19-3 Medication labels provide the name of the drug and the dose per unit such as tablets and milliliters. **A.** 0.25 mg per tablet. **B.** 250 mg per 5 mL. (Reprinted from Kronenberger J, Ledbetter J. *Jones & Bartlett Learning's Comprehensive Medical Assisting.* 5th ed. Burlington, MA: Jones & Bartlett Learning, LLC; 2016.)

18. Have sharps containers as close as possible to the area of use.
19. Never give a medication that was poured or drawn up by someone else. Never prepare or draw up medication for someone else.
20. Always lock the medication cabinet when it's not in use.
21. Never give the keys for the medication cabinet to an unauthorized person. Limit access to the medication cabinet by limiting access to the cabinet keys.

Systems for Measuring

The most common system of measurement used in the medical office is the metric system.

While working in the clinical setting, you may need to calculate a dose in one system of measurement using mathematical equations. Also, you may need to convert a measurement from one system to another. It's important to understand the commonly used systems of measurement before trying to calculate doses.

Metric System

The metric system is used in the United States and throughout the world. Because it's based on multiples of 10, it uses decimals, not fractions. In the metric system:

- Meter (m) is the base unit of length.
- Gram (g or gm) is the base unit of weight.
- Liter (L or l) is used to measure fluid volume.

Prefixes are used in the metric system to show a fraction of the base unit or a multiple of it. With the base unit of a liter (1 L = approximately 1.06 quarts),

fractional measurements are in milliliters (ml or mL). Also, 1 cubic centimeter (cc), a solid, is equal to 1 ml. The Joint Commission (TJC) has identified the "cc" abbreviation on the do not use list. This abbreviation is dangerous to use since it is easily mistaken when written, thus causing an error. The abbreviation "ml" is used for this measurement. Decagrams and centigrams are not used in medication administration. See Table 19-6 for a list of the commonly used metric prefixes.

Apothecary System

This older system of measurement is used less now than in the past. It's gradually being replaced by the metric system. However, some physicians may continue to use this system. In the apothecary system of measurement, liquid measurements include the following:

- Drop (gt) or drops (gtt)
- Minim (min or m)
- Fluid dram (fl dr)
- Fluid ounce (fl oz)
- Pint (pt)
- Quart (qt)
- Gallon (gal)

Some measurements for solid weights are as follows:

- Grain (gr)
- Dram (dr)
- Ounce (oz)
- Pound (lb)

When writing drug doses, physicians may use Roman numerals to express numbers. See Table 19-7 for the conversion of Arabic numbers to Roman numerals.

Table 19-6 Commonly Used Metric Prefixes

Meaning	Value	Abbreviation	Example of Use	Example's Meaning
millionth of	0.000001	mc	8 mcg	8 micrograms (8 millionths of a gram) (0.000008 g)
thousandth of	0.001	m	3 ml	3 milliliters (3 thousandths of a liter) (0.003 L)
hundredth of	0.01	c	7 cm	7 centimeters (7 hundredths of a meter) (0.07 m)
tenth of	0.1	d	4 dL	4 deciliters (4 tenths of a liter) (0.4 L)
thousand times	1000.0	k	5 kg	5 kilograms (5 thousand grams) (5,000 g)

Table 19-7	Roman Numeral
Roman Numeral	**Arabic Number**
I	1
V	5
X	10
L	50
C	100
D	500
M	1,000

Household System

The household system of measurement is used most often by patients. It includes measures commonly used for cooking, such as:

- Teaspoon (tsp)
- Tablespoon (tbsp)
- Ounce (oz)
- Cup (c)
- Pint (pt)
- Quart (qt)
- Pound (lb)

Even though this system isn't used in the medical office for calculating doses, you may need to instruct patients on the proper household measurements for taking medications ordered in the metric system. For example, 5 ml is equal to 1 teaspoon (tsp). When converting from one measurement system to another, it is important to know the approximate equivalents. See Table 19-8 for a comparison between systems.

Converting Between Systems of Measurement

Sometimes, you'll need to calculate the conversion from one system to another. Here are the medicine-related conversions you're most likely to need in a medical office.

Converting Apothecary to Metric:
- To change grains to grams, divide the number of grains ordered by 15.

  Example: 30 gr ÷ 15 = 2 g

- If the amount of grains is < 1, change the grains to milligrams and multiply the grains by 60.

  Example: ¼ gr × 60 = 15 mg

Converting Household to Metric:
- To change fluid ounces to milliliters, multiply the number of ounces by 30.

  Example: 4 oz × 30 = 120 ml

Table 19-8	Most Commonly Used Approximate Equivalents	

Approximate Volume Equivalents

Metric	Apothecary	Household
0.06 ml	1 m	1 drop
1 ml	15 m	0.2 tsp
5 ml	1 fl dr	1 tsp (60 drops)
15 ml	0.5 fl oz (4 fl dr)	1 tbsp
30 ml	1 fl oz	2 tbsp
500 ml	16 fl oz	1 pt
1,000 ml	32 fl oz	1 qt

Approximate Weight Equivalents

Metric	Apothecary	Household
1 gm	15 gr	
30 gm	1 oz	1 oz
450 gm	1 lb	1 lb
1 kg (1,000 gm)	2.2 lb	2.2 lb

Approximate Length Equivalents

Metric	Apothecary	Household
1 cm (10 mm)		0.4 in
2.5 cm (25 mm)		1 in
30.5 cm (300 mm)		1 ft
90 cm (900 mm)		1 yd
1 m (100 cm)		3.25 ft (40 in)

- To change pounds to kilograms, divide the pounds by 2.2.

  Example: 44 lb ÷ 2.2 = 20 kg

Converting Metric to Household:
- To change milliliters to fluid ounces, divide the number of ml by 30.

  Example: 150 ml ÷ 30 = 5 oz

- To change kilograms to pounds, multiply the kilograms by 2.2.

  Example: 50 kg × 2.2 = 110 lb

Converting Within the Metric System

In the metric system, it's sometimes necessary to convert measurements to the same unit. For example, the physician may order 0.5 g of medication, and the medication label may read 500 mg. Note the use of a zero in front of the decimal point in the 0.5 g example. Never write a number less than a whole number without using a zero before the zero. This practice will help eliminate medication errors. These rules will help you make conversions within the metric system:

Check your conversion calculations twice. It's better to take the time to check your answers than to make a mistake.

Study Skill

Are you one of those people who do not like math? If you are struggling solving the math problems involved with medication calculations, it helps to do more problems. The more you practice, the better you will understand the methods used to accurately calculate medication dosages to administer to patients. Ask your instructor for additional problems to work on, or, if there is someone in your class that understands the math calculations, have the student write some problems that you can attempt to solve. Practice makes perfect! Before you administer any medication, you need to make sure you understand the accurate calculation of dosages. You will find that as you successfully complete problems, you will build your confidence.

Milligrams and Grams:

- To change grams to milligrams, multiply the number of grams by 1,000 (or move the decimal point three places to the right).

  Example: 0.5 g × 1,000 = 500 mg

- To change milligrams to grams, divide the number of milligrams by 1,000 (or move the decimal point three places to the left).

  Example: 500 mg ÷ 1,000 = 0.5 g

Milligrams and Micrograms:

- To change milligrams to micrograms, multiply the milligrams by 1,000 (move the decimal three places to the right).

  Example: 5 mg × 1,000 = 5,000 micrograms

- To change micrograms to milligrams, divide the micrograms by 1,000 (move the decimal three places to the left).

  Example: 500 micrograms ÷ 1,000 = 0.5 mg

Liters and Milliliters:

- To change liters to milliliters, multiply the liters by 1,000 (move the decimal three places to the right).

  Example: 0.01 L × 1,000 = 10 ml

- To change milliliters to liters, divide the milliliters by 1,000 (move the decimal three places to the left).

  Example: 100 ml ÷ 1,000 = 0.1 L

Calculating Adult Doses

Administration of medication is an exact science. Calculation errors can be fatal. Although the physician is the one who orders the amount of medication to administer, you may be the one to calculate the amount to withdraw into a syringe or to pour into a medicine cup.

Before you can calculate the correct dosage, make sure the measurements are in the same system (metric, apothecary, household) and units. Here are some examples of when this could be a problem.

- The physician uses the apothecary system when ordering medication. But the medication is packaged according to the metric system. So, you'll need to convert the amount ordered by the physician to the metric system.
- The physician orders a medication in grams. When the medication arrives, it's packaged in milligrams. You'll need to convert the physician's order to milligrams.

Once the measurement units are the same, there are two methods that can be used to calculate medication dosages for adults, the ratio method and the formula method.

The Ratio Method

In this method, two ratios are created using the information on the medication label and the desired dose in the physician's order. The proportion, or relationship between the ratios, should be the same. This allows you to calculate the amount of medication to administer. To calculate a dose using the ratio method, set up your problem like this:

$$\frac{\text{dose on label}:}{\text{quantity on label}} = \frac{\text{dose ordered}:}{\text{quantity to administer}}$$

OR

$$\frac{\text{dose on label (known)}}{\text{dose desired (known)}} = \frac{\text{quantity on label (known)}}{\text{quantity to administer (unknown)}}$$

Example 1: The physician orders erythromycin 250 mg. The label on the package reads erythromycin 100 mg/ml.

First, determine the proportion.

$$\frac{100 \text{ mg}}{250 \text{ mg}} = \frac{1 \text{ mL}}{x}$$

Follow these steps to calculate x (the amount to administer).

1. Cross multiply: $100 \times x = 100x$
2. Cross multiply: $250 \times 1 = 250$
3. The proportion is now: $100x = 250$
4. Divide both sides by 100 to find x. So, $x = 250 \div 100$, $x = 2.5$.

In this example, you need to administer 2.5 ml of the erythromycin for the patient to receive the dose (250 mg) ordered by the physician.

Example 2: The physician orders phenobarbital 25 mg. On hand are 12.5-mg tablets.

First, determine the proportion.

$$\frac{12.5 \text{ mg}}{25 \text{ mg}} = \frac{1 \text{ tablet}}{x}$$

Then calculate the quantity to administer.

1. Cross multiply: $12.5 \times x = 12.5x$
2. Cross multiply: $25 \times 1 = 25$
3. Now write: $12.5x = 25$
4. To find x, divide both sides by 12.5.
5. $25 \div 12.5 = 2$, $x = 2$. Therefore, the quantity to administer is two tablets.

The Formula Method

Another way to calculate the dose to administer is to use this formula:

(desired dose ÷ dose on label) × quantity on label = quantity to administer

Example 1: The physician orders ampicillin 0.5 g. On hand, you have ampicillin 250-mg capsules. How much ampicillin should be administered?

1. Remember, both doses should be in the same unit of measure. First, convert grams to milligrams. Multiply the grams by 1,000 (move the decimal point three places to the right). The result is 0.5 g = 500 mg. Therefore, the desired dose (0.5 g) is the same as 500 mg.
2. Put the information you know into the problem:

$(500 \div 250 \text{ mg}) \times 1 = $ quantity to administer
$2 \times 1 = 2$

3. The quantity to administer is two capsules.

Example 2: The physician orders 0.35 g of a medication and you have on hand a liquid of 700 mg/L. How many ml do you prepare to administer?

1. First, make sure both doses are in equal units. Change 0.35 g to milligrams by multiplying as in Example 1 ($0.35 \text{ g} \times 1,000 = 350 \text{ mg}$).
2. Put the information you know into the problem:

$(350 \text{ mg} \div 700 \text{ mg}) \times 1 = 0.5 \text{ ml} = $ quantity to administer

You may use either the ratio method or the formula method to calculate the dose to administer. Just be sure to follow the exact calculations for whichever method you choose—and check your work!

Calculating Pediatric Doses

Sometimes, you may know the adult dosage of a medication, but you need to know what the dosage would be for a child. Several formulas are used to calculate children's doses:

- Body surface area (**BSA**) method
- Young rule
- Clark rule
- Fried rule

The BSA Method

This is the most accurate method for children up to 12 years of age and for adults who are below normal body weight. It requires a scale called a nomogram (Fig. 19-4).

This chart uses the patient's height and weight to estimate the body surface area (BSA) in square meters.

A straight line is drawn from the patient's height in inches or centimeters (in the left column) to the patient's weight in kilograms or pounds (in the right column). The place where the line intersects the middle column is the patient's BSA, or body surface area (Fig. 19-5).

After you have determined the patient's estimated BSA, use this formula to calculate the child's dose:

(BSA × adult dose) ÷ 1.7 = child's dose

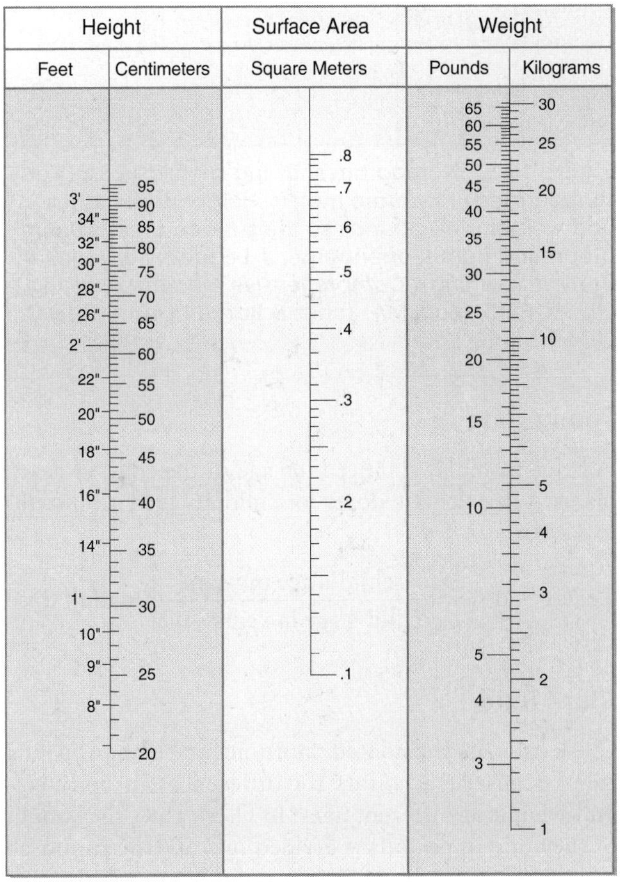

Figure 19-4 Nomogram for estimating surface area of infants and young children. Plot the child's height and weight to determine the surface area in square meters. (Reprinted from Kronenberger J, Ledbetter J. *Jones & Bartlett Learning's Comprehensive Medical Assisting.* 5th ed. Burlington, MA: Jones & Bartlett Learning, LLC; 2016.)

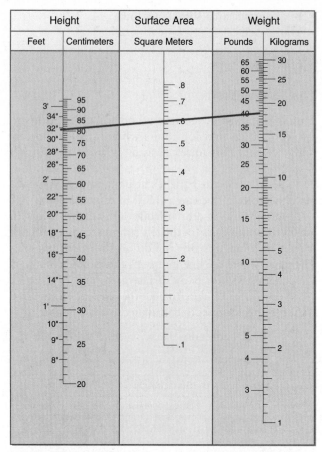

Height		Surface Area	Weight	
Feet	Centimeters	Square Meters	Pounds	Kilograms

Figure 19-5 Nomogram showing a child's BSA (body surface area) in square meters. Height is 32 inches and weight is 40 pounds so the surface area is 0.6 m². (Reprinted from Kronenberger J, Ledbetter J. *Jones & Bartlett Learning's Comprehensive Medical Assisting.* 5th ed. Burlington, MA: Jones & Bartlett Learning, LLC; 2016.)

Young Rule

For this formula, you need the age of the child in years. It's used to calculate doses for children aged 12 months to 12 years.

$$\text{Pediatric dose} = \frac{\text{child's age in years}}{(\text{child's age in years} + 12)} \times \text{adult dose}$$

Clark Rule

Clark rule is considered more accurate than Young rule because it accounts for differences in body size and weight at different ages. In Clark rule, the weight of the child in pounds is divided by 150 (the supposed weight of an average adult in pounds) and multiplied by the average adult dose to figure out the child's dose.

$$\text{Pediatric dose} = \frac{\text{child's weight in pounds}}{150 \text{ pounds}} \times \text{adult dose}$$

Fried Rule

Fried rule is used for calculating doses for infants < 2 years of age. It bases the calculation on the child's age in months. The number 150, included in this formula, represents the age in months of a 12.5-year-old child. The thinking is that a 12.5-year-old child would be eligible for an adult dose.

$$\text{Pediatric dose} = \frac{\text{child's age in months}}{150 \text{ months}} \times \text{adult dose}$$

Other Calibrations

Many medications that require careful calibration (adjustments) are dosed per kilogram of body weight. Instructions for calculating the amount to administer are included in the package insert that comes with the medication.

For example, the insert may state, "For adults and children over 25 kg (55 lb), give 500 mg. For children <25 kg, give 25 mg/kg." If the child who needs the medication weighs 20 lb, this weight must be converted to kg. Since 1 kg = 2.2 lb, this child weighs 9 kg. The equation for calculating the child's dosage is then:

$$25 \text{ mg} \times 9 \text{ kg} = 225 \text{ mg}$$

 # ADMINISTRATION ROUTES

There are many ways, or routes, for administering medication. The physician chooses the route of administration. The choice of the route can depend on three things:

- Cost
- Safety
- Absorption rate

The many routes of administration can be divided into two main groups—enteral and **parenteral**. The enteral routes are all related to the digestive tract in some way. These routes include medications taken in the following ways:

- Oral—Chewed, swallowed whole, or dissolved sublingually or buccally
- Rectal—Inserted into the rectum
- Nasogastric—A tube placed through the nose into the stomach or small intestine
- Gastric—A tube placed through the mouth into the stomach or surgically implanted through the abdominal wall into the stomach

Parenteral routes include any route other than the enteral ones—for example, injections, intravenous administration, and vaginal application.

There are many reasons to use parenteral methods of administration. Here are some of the most common ones:

- Some patients can't take oral medications.
- Some medications can't be absorbed through the gastrointestinal system.
- A patient's condition may require fast absorption of the drug.

Some drugs can be administered by one route only. This may be due to their form or chemical composition. Some may be toxic if given by a certain route. Some drugs may be absorbed only through one particular route. Others are effective when administered in a variety of ways. The different routes for drug administration are:

- Oral (by mouth)
- Sublingual (under the tongue)
- Injection
- Intravenous (directly into a vein)
- Inhalation
- Topical (on the skin)
- Instillation (eye, ear canal, or nose)
- Rectal
- Vaginal
- Intradermal

There are advantages and disadvantages to the oral and parental routes of administration. Several of these are listed in Table 19-9.

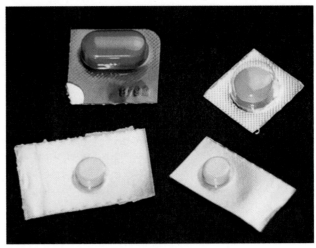

Figure 19-6 Unit dose packets. (Reprinted from Kronenberger J, Ledbetter J. *Jones & Bartlett Learning's Comprehensive Medical Assisting.* 5th ed. Burlington, MA: Jones & Bartlett Learning, LLC; 2016.)

Medication by Mouth

Patients often are given a medication to swallow in the form of a tablet, capsule, pill, or liquid. This method is preferred by many patients and is the easiest to administer. Drugs given orally in the medical office usually come in unit dose packs that contain a premeasured single dose of the drug. See examples of single dose packets in Figure 19-6.

Table 19-9	Oral versus Parenteral Medication Administration
Oral Medications	**Parenteral Medications**
Advantages:	**Advantages:**
• Easily administered	• Rapid response time to medication
• Economical to administer	• Accuracy of dosage
• Administered with a high degree of safety	• Ability to concentrate the medication in a specific body area, such as a joint
	• Ideal for patients who cannot take medication by mouth because of an illness or because the stomach acids would destroy the medication
Disadvantages:	**Disadvantages:**
• Objectionable taste and odor	• Rapid allergic reactions
• Discoloration of the teeth, mouth, and tongue	• Injury to bone, soft tissue, nerves, or blood vessel caused by needle
• Irritation to the stomach	• Needle breakage in tissue
• Poor absorption rate due to illness or nature of medicine	• Accidental injection into the vein instead of the soft tissue
• Failure of patient to take medicine	
• Less predictable effects on the body than when given by an injection	
• Patient may be unable to swallow pill, tablet, or capsule	

Table 19-10	Forms of Oral Medications	
Form	**Types**	**Description**
Solids	Buffered caplet	Medication has an added agent to decrease stomach acidity and prevent stomach irritation.
	Capsule	Medication is powdered or granulated in a gelatin sheath. Sheath is designed to be dissolved by gastric enzymes or high in the small intestine.
	Enteric-coated tablet	Dry, compressed medication coated to withstand stomach acidity and dissolve in the intestines. Never crush or break enteric-coated tablets.
	Gelcap	Oil-based medication in a soft gelatin capsule
	Chewable	Tablet chewed completely before swallowing in order to release the medication more quickly into the system
	Lozenge	A firm, compressed form of medication, usually for a local effect in the mouth or throat. Caution patients to let lozenges dissolve slowly and avoid drinking fluids after taking a lozenge
	Powder	Medication is in a finely ground form that may be difficult for some patients to swallow.
	Spansule, or time-release capsule	Medication is inside a gelatin capsule that will dissolve over time rather than all at once. Never open a time-release capsule unless recommended by the manufacturer.
	Tablet	Medication is shaped or colored for easy identification. Tablets usually dissolve high in the GI tract. They may be broken in half only if scored (marked with a line or groove) for that purpose.
Liquids	Syrup	A very sweet form of medication frequently used for children. It's usually flavored in addition to having a high sugar content.
	Elixir	Medication is dissolved in alcohol and flavored. It's less sweet than syrups and is usually preferred by adults. Not appropriate for alcoholics or diabetics.
	Emulsion	Medication is combined with water and oil. The emulsion must be shaken thoroughly to disperse the medication evenly.
	Extract	Highly concentrated form of medication made by evaporating volatile plant oils (oils that vaporize readily). It may be administered as drops and is usually given in a liquid to disguise the strong taste.
	Gel	Medication is suspended in a thin gelatin or paste.
	Suspension	Particles of medication are dissolved in a liquid. Must be shaken well before use

Oral medications are absorbed through the walls of the gastrointestinal tract. However, medications taken this way usually are slow to take effect. Also, not every patient can take medications by this method. See Table 19-10 for the various forms of oral medications.

The oral route is not suitable for patients who:

- Are unconscious
- Have nausea and/or vomiting
- Have been ordered to take nothing by mouth

Under the Tongue and Beside the Cheek

Some medications may be placed in the mouth, but they aren't meant to be swallowed. They're absorbed into the body through the mucous membranes of the mouth rather than digested in the stomach.

- Sublingual medication—The medication is placed under the patient's tongue. It must not be swallowed. The drug is dissolved by the saliva in the patient's mouth. It's absorbed directly into the bloodstream through the mucous membranes covering the sublingual blood vessels. Caution the patient not to eat or drink until the medication is dissolved. One of the most common sublingual medications is nitroglycerin, taken by patients with heart-related chest pain.
- Buccal medication—Medication is placed between the patient's cheek and gum at the side of the mouth. The drug is then absorbed through the vascular oral mucosa. Not many medications are manufactured for this route. The patient should not chew or swallow the medication or eat or drink until it's absorbed. Many lozenges are designed to be absorbed buccally.

Injections

Injection is the most efficient method of parenteral drug administration. However, it also can be the most hazardous. The effects are quite rapid, and once injected,

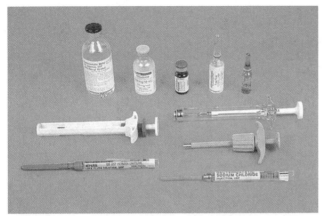

Figure 19-7 Ampules, vials, prefilled cartridges, and holders. (Reprinted from Kronenberger J, Ledbetter J. *Jones & Bartlett Learning's Comprehensive Medical Assisting.* 5th ed. Burlington, MA: Jones & Bartlett Learning, LLC; 2016.)

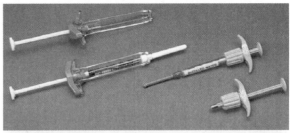

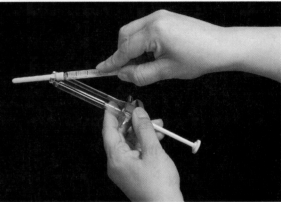

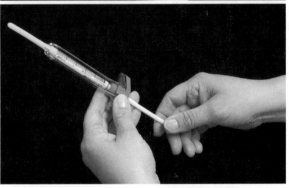

Figure 19-8 Prefilled medication cartridges and injector devices, inserting the cartridge into the injector device and ready for injection. (Reprinted from Kronenberger J, Ledbetter J. *Jones & Bartlett Learning's Comprehensive Medical Assisting.* 5th ed. Burlington, MA: Jones & Bartlett Learning, LLC; 2016.)

the medication can't be retrieved. Because the skin is broken, infections can develop if strict aseptic technique isn't followed.

Medications for injections are sometimes supplied in an **ampule**. These are small glass containers that must be broken at the neck of the ampule. Once they're broken, the solution is aspirated or removed by suction. You must use a filter needle when getting medication from an ampule to prevent small pieces of glass from being drawn up. All medication inside must be either used or discarded.

Medications for injections also may be supplied as vials or prefilled cartridges (Fig. 19-7).

Prefilled Cartridges

Prefilled syringes contain a premeasured amount of medication in a disposable cartridge with a needle attached. Figure 19-8 shows the preparation of a prefilled cartridge.

The prefilled cartridge and needle are placed in a holder for administration. After a cartridge and holder are used, the cartridge should be discarded in a sharps biohazard container. The holder is reusable, but it must be cleaned first. This is often done by wiping it thoroughly with an alcohol swab. Some offices also have containers filled with alcohol into which the holder can be placed after use.

Vials

A **vial** is a glass or plastic container that is sealed at the top by a stopper. Vials may be single-dose or multiple-dose containers. The contents of vials may be in the form of a solution or a powder. Powders must be reconstituted—mixed with a specific amount and type of diluting agent. The **diluent**, or diluting agent, usually

is sterile water or saline. Certain drugs, such as phenytoin (Dilantin), an anticonvulsant, require a special diluent supplied by the manufacturer.

When a powdered drug is reconstituted in a multiple-dose vial, you must write some information on the label:

- Date of reconstitution
- Initials of the person who reconstituted the drug
- Diluent used
- Strength of the medicine that was produced

Vials intended for multiple doses may hold up to 50 ml. They may be used repeatedly by inserting a needle through the self-sealing stopper to remove some of the solution. Unit dose vials usually contain 1 to 2 ml. All the solution is removed for a single injection.

Reconstituting Dry Medication

To reconstitute dry medication in a vial, follow these steps:

1. Check the vial label or manufacturer's instructions to find out how much diluent to add to the powder.
2. Wipe the top of the vial containing the diluent with an alcohol pad before inserting the needle. Then, withdraw the correct amount of diluent using aseptic technique.
3. Add the diluent to the vial containing the powder. Wipe the top of the vial with an alcohol pad before inserting the needle.
4. Replace the vial stopper. Roll the vial between your palms until the powder is dissolved. Don't shake the vial. Shaking can cause unnecessary bubbles, which make it hard to measure the exact amount of medication needed.

The concentration of the mixture will depend on how the medication will be given. The instructions from the drug's manufacturer usually tell how much diluent to add to the powder if the medication is to be given intravenously (IV), injected into the muscle (IM), or injected under the skin (SQ).

You must be sure that the concentration of the mixture is right for the method of administration. A dosage that's too strong for the method of administration may harm the patient's tissues. If the dose is too weak for the method of administration, the medicine may not have the proper effect.

Syringes and Needles

The choice of syringe and needle depends on the type of injection and the size of the patient. The 3 ml hypodermic syringe is the most commonly used. In a medical office, syringes that hold 5 ml or more usually are used for irrigation—the process of flushing a wound, cavity, or medical instrument with water or other fluid to clean it. Examples of syringes are shown in Figure 19-9.

Syringes have three main parts (Fig. 19-10):

* The plunger
* The body or barrel
* The needle

Needle lengths vary from 0.375 to 1.5 inch for standard injections. The needle gauge refers to the diameter of the needle lumen, or opening. Needle gauge varies from 10 (large gauge) to 33 (small gauge). Manufacturers package hypodermic needles separately in color-coded packages or in color-coded envelopes with the syringe attached. The size is written on the package (Fig. 19-11A, B).

The rule is the smaller the number the larger the lumen of the needle; the larger the number, the smaller the lumen of the needle.

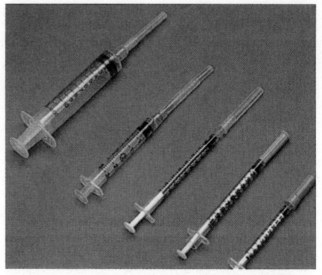

Figure 19-9   Syringes from largest on top to smallest on bottom: 10, 3, and 1 mL or tuberculin, insulin, and low-dose insulin. (Reprinted from Kronenberger J, Ledbetter J. *Jones & Bartlett Learning's Comprehensive Medical Assisting.* 5th ed. Burlington, MA: Jones & Bartlett Learning, LLC; 2016.)

When choosing a needle, you need to select the right needle length and gauge for the route of the injection and the type of medication. The needle length depends on the route of the injection.

An adult intramuscular injection, or injection into muscle tissue, requires a needle length of 1 to 3 inches. Some factors that affect the choice of needle length are the size of the patient, the muscle being used, and the fat to muscle ratio. The gauge varies from 20 to

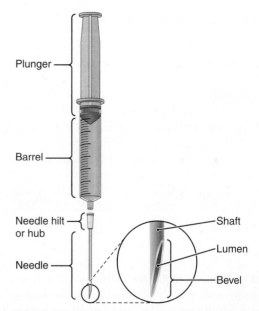

Figure 19-10   Parts of a syringe and needle. (Reprinted from Cohen BJ. *Medical Terminology: An Illustrated Guide.* 6th ed. Burlington, MA: Jones & Bartlett Learning, LLC; 2011, with permission.)

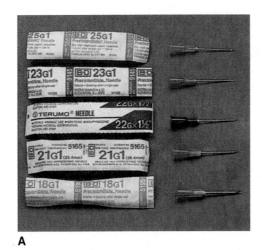

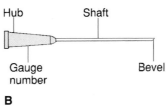

Figure 19-11 Needles. **A.** Different gauges and lengths. **B.** Parts of a needle. (Reprinted from Kronenberger J, Ledbetter J. *Jones & Bartlett Learning's Comprehensive Medical Assisting.* 5th ed. Burlington, MA: Jones & Bartlett Learning, LLC; 2016.)

25, depending on the thickness of the medication to be administered. A small-gauge needle, such as 25 or 27, would make it difficult to draw thick medications into a syringe or inject them into a patient. Examples of thick medications are penicillin and hormones. A subcutaneous injection (injection into the fatty layer just below the skin) is usually given with a short, small-gauge needle, such as 25 gauge (0.625 inch) or 23 gauge (0.5 inch).

When preparing an injection, the syringe tip, inside of the barrel, shaft of the plunger, and the needle must be kept sterile.

Types of Syringes

All hypodermic syringes are marked with calibrations showing milliliters and smaller divisions, depending on the size of the syringe. The other side of the syringe may be marked in minims (m), a very small fluid measure equaling about a drop.

Two special types of syringes used to administer medications are tuberculin syringes (1 ml) and insulin syringes.

- Tuberculin (**TB**) syringes are narrow and have a total capacity of 1 ml. Each syringe has 100 calibration lines. TB syringes are used for newborn and pediatric doses, for intradermal skin tests, and any time small amounts of medication are to be given.
- Insulin syringes are used only for administering insulin. The insulin syringe has a total capacity of 1 ml but uses a different calibration system than other syringes. The 1-ml volume is marked as 100 units (U). The units represent the strength of the insulin per milliliter. Most of the insulin that is used today is U-100, which means that it has 100 units of insulin per milliliter. On the syringe, large lines mark each group of 10 units. Five smaller lines divide the 10 units into groups of 2. Each small line represents 2 units.

Types of Injections

Different medications may be injected into different places in the body. The three main types of injections are:

- Intradermal (**ID**)
- Subcutaneous (**SC** or **SQ**)
- Intramuscular (**IM**)

The prefix <u>intra</u> means into or within. <u>Intradermal</u> means "into the skin." <u>Intramuscular</u> means "into the muscle." Figure 19-12 demonstrates the proper angle of

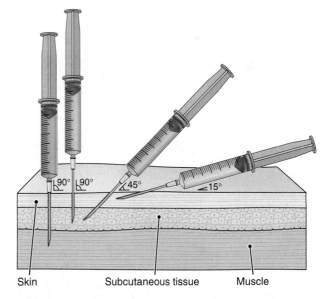

Figure 19-12 Required angles of insertion for intramuscular, subcutaneous, and intradermal injections. (Reprinted from Cohen BJ. *Medical Terminology: An Illustrated Guide.* 6th ed. Burlington, MA: Jones & Bartlett Learning, LLC; 2011, with permission.)

insertion for intramuscular, subcutaneous, and intradermal injections. It is critical to use the proper angle of insertion so the medication is delivered into the appropriate layer of tissue.

Intradermal Injections

These injections are administered into the dermis, or skin. Recommended sites for intradermal injections are the anterior forearm and the back. Intradermal injections are used to administer different kinds of skin tests for allergy testing and tuberculosis (TB) screening.

The needle is inserted at angle of 10 to 15 degrees, almost parallel to the skin surface.

When administered correctly:

- The needle tip and lumen are slightly visible under the skin.
- The bevel of the needle must be up.
- A small bubble known as a wheal is raised in the skin.

TB Tests. Two tests are used for the routine screening of TB—the tine test and the Mantoux test. Both use purified protein derivative (PPD) from a live tuberculin bacillus culture to test for tuberculin antibodies.

- Tine test—The applicator consists of small tines that contain PPD. After cleansing the forearm, press the applicator firmly into the intradermal layer of the skin. This test is not considered as useful for diagnostics as the Mantoux test. A positive tine test usually is followed by a Mantoux test. Figure 19-13 shows the technique used to administer a time test.
- Mantoux test—An injection containing PPD is made into the intradermal layer of skin. A positive Mantoux test indicates only the possibility of exposure to TB. It does not indicate that the patient has TB. The Centers for Disease Control and Prevention (CDC) prefers the Mantoux test and considers it the most accurate TB test.

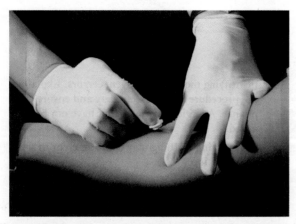

Figure 19-13 Administering the tine test for tuberculosis screening. (Reprinted from Kronenberger J, Ledbetter J. *Jones & Bartlett Learning's Comprehensive Medical Assisting.* 5th ed. Burlington, MA: Jones & Bartlett Learning, LLC; 2016.)

Both tests must be read within 48 to 72 hours. A positive Mantoux reaction has induration (a hard, raised area over the injection site) that is larger than 10 mm. A patient with a positive reaction will require a complete medical history and further testing, including a chest x-ray. Induration of <10 mm in a patient with no known risk factors is considered a negative result.

Subcutaneous Injections

Subcutaneous injections (SQ or SC) are given into the fatty layer of tissue below the skin. You should position the needle and syringe at a 45-degree angle. This method is chosen for drugs that may not be absorbed as rapidly through intramuscular or other routes. Common sites for subcutaneous injections include the following:

- Upper arm
- Thigh
- Back
- Abdomen

Intramuscular Injections

Injecting medication into a muscle requires positioning of the needle and syringe at a 90-degree angle to the skin. Absorption is fairly rapid because of the rich vascularity (blood supply) of muscle. If slower absorption is desired, the medication is mixed with an oil-based diluent rather than saline or water.

As previously noted, a 1- to 3-inch needle is needed to give an intramuscular (IM) injection to an adult. The length of the needle depends on the muscle chosen for the injection and the size of the patient.

The muscle chosen for the injection depends on the preferences of the medical assistant, the patient, and the amount of medication to be administered. Drug manufacturers also recommend sites for injecting specific drugs. You should try to follow their recommendations. Table 19-11 lists the recommended sites for intramuscular injections.

Figure 19-14 demonstrates the deltoid injection site in the upper arm. Figure 19-15 shows the location of the dorsogluteal site in the upper, outer area of the posterior hip. Figure 19-16 shows the location on the side of the hip that is called the ventrogluteal site. Figure 19-17 shows the location of the vastus lateralis on the side of the thigh. Figure 19-18 demonstrates the location of the rectus femoris injection site.

Z-Track Method. Some medications administered intramuscularly may stain and discolor skin and irritate or damage tissues if they leak back along the line of injection. The Z-track method prevents leakage by sealing off layers of skin along the route of the needle.

In the Z-track method, the skin is pulled to one side, and the needle is inserted. After the solution is injected and the needle is withdrawn, the skin is allowed to return

Table 19-11	Recommended Sites for Intramuscular Injections	
Injection Site	**Locating the Muscle**	**Cautions**
Deltoid	The deltoid muscle is located by palpating the lower edge of the acromial process. At the midpoint, in line with the axilla on the lateral aspect of the upper arm, a triangle is formed. Medications are administered within the triangle.	No more than 1 ml should be injected into this muscle in an adult.
Dorsogluteal	The dorsogluteal site is lateral and slightly superior to the midpoint of a line drawn from the trochanter to the posterior iliac spine.	The site must be identified correctly to avoid damage to the sciatic nerve. No more than 3 ml should be injected into an adult. Children < 2 years of age should never receive injections into the gluteal muscle. It's not well developed until the child is walking.
Ventrogluteal	The ventrogluteal site is located by placing the palm on the greater trochanter and the index finger toward the anterior superior iliac spine. The middle finger is then spread posteriorly away from the index finger as far as possible. A V or triangle is formed by this maneuver. Make the injection in the middle of the triangle.	No more than 3 ml should be injected into an adult.
Vastus lateralis	The vastus lateralis site is identified by dividing the thigh into thirds horizontally and vertically. The injection is given in the outermost third.	The site is preferred for children under 2 years of age and may be used for adults. The quantity of the injection should not exceed 2 ml.
Rectus femoris	The rectus femoris site is located on the anterior of the thigh.	Use this site only when other sites are contraindicated.

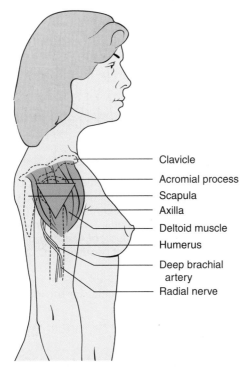

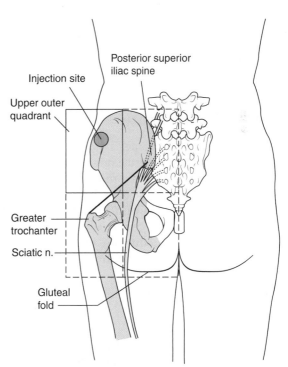

Figure 19-14 Deltoid muscle IM injection site. Located by palpating the lower edge of the acromial process. At the midpoint in line with the axilla on the lateral aspect of the upper arm, a triangle is formed. Medication is injected within this triangle. (Reprinted from Kronenberger J, Ledbetter J. *Jones & Bartlett Learning's Comprehensive Medical Assisting.* 5th ed. Burlington, MA: Jones & Bartlett Learning, LLC; 2016.)

Figure 19-15 Dorsogluteal IM injection site. Located lateral and slightly superior to the midpoint of a line drawn from the trochanter to the posterior superior iliac spine. This site minimizes the possibility of accidentally damaging the sciatic nerve. (Reprinted from Kronenberger J, Ledbetter J. *Jones & Bartlett Learning's Comprehensive Medical Assisting.* 5th ed. Burlington, MA: Jones & Bartlett Learning, LLC; 2016.)

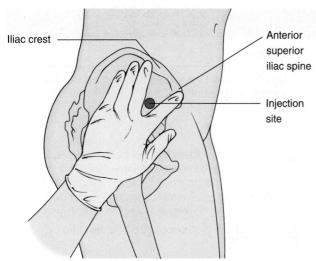

Iliac crest

Anterior superior iliac spine

Injection site

Figure 19-16 Ventrogluteal IM injection site. Located by placing the palm on the greater trochanter and the index finger toward the anterior superior iliac spine. The middle finger is then spread posteriorly away from the index finger as far as possible. A "V" or triangle is formed between the fingers, which is the location for this injection. (Reprinted from Kronenberger J, Ledbetter J. *Jones & Bartlett Learning's Comprehensive Medical Assisting.* 5th ed. Burlington, MA: Jones & Bartlett Learning, LLC; 2016.)

to its normal position. This blocks the solution from escaping from the muscle tissue. If the medication is very caustic, the instructions may require that you change the needle after drawing up the solution. Figure 19-19 shows the Z-track technique used to administer irritating medications.

The Intravenous Route

For the intravenous (**IV**) route, a sterile solution of a drug is injected through a needle or catheter into a vein by venipuncture. A catheter is a thin, flexible tube that carries fluids into or out of the body. Venipuncture is the process of puncturing a vein with a needle.

Medication acts quickly when administered by IV because it enters the bloodstream immediately. Only drugs intended for IV administration should be given using this route. Figure 19-20 is an example of IV equipment including the fluid and tubing.

Starting an IV

In most cases, the nurse or physician administers IV medication. However, in some states, medical assistants in ambulatory care centers must set up equipment and fluids for an IV, perform the venipuncture, and regulate IV fluids as directed by a physician or nurse practitioner. Medical assistants are not legally authorized to perform intravenous medication administration. You need to be aware of the state laws and training requirements for performing any IV procedures. If the medication

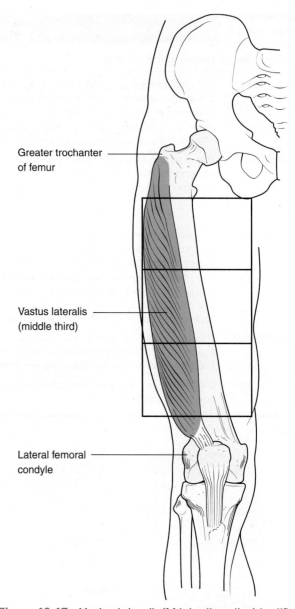

Greater trochanter of femur

Vastus lateralis (middle third)

Lateral femoral condyle

Figure 19-17 Vastus lateralis IM injection site. Identified by dividing the thigh into thirds horizontally and vertically. The injection is given in the outer middle third. (Reprinted from Kronenberger J, Ledbetter J. *Jones & Bartlett Learning's Comprehensive Medical Assisting.* 5th ed. Burlington, MA: Jones & Bartlett Learning, LLC; 2016.)

instructions recommend a specific site for injection, use that site.

If you are legally permitted to start an IV, you need the following equipment:

- Fluids, as determined by the physician
- IV catheter
- Tubing that connects to the catheter with a valve to regulate the flow of fluids

Once the IV is started, fluids are administered through the vein. These fluids either replace fluids lost by the patient or are used to administer medication through

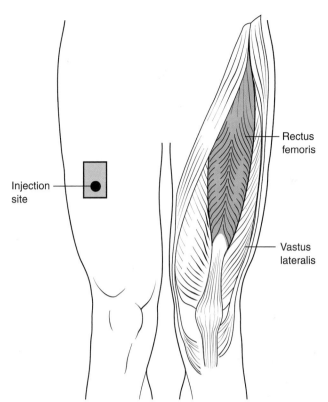

Figure 19-18 Rectus femoris IM injection site is used only when other sites are contraindicated. (Reprinted from Kronenberger J, Ledbetter J. *Jones & Bartlett Learning's Comprehensive Medical Assisting.* 5th ed. Burlington, MA: Jones & Bartlett Learning, LLC; 2016.)

special ports in the tubing. Some examples of fluids that come prepackaged for use in IV therapy are:

- Ringer lactate (RL)
- Dextrose 5% and water (D₅W)
- 0.9% normal saline (NS)
- 0.45% normal saline (NS)
- Combinations of the above (D₅NS, D₅RL)

The physician or nurse practitioner chooses the type and amount of fluid to be administered. An administration set (tubing) is used. The end of the tubing with the drip chamber is inserted into the IV fluid bag. The other end is inserted into the IV catheter after it's in the vein.

IV Problems

You must watch the IV fluids and the site of venipuncture carefully. Infiltration occurs when IV fluid infuses into tissues surrounding the vein. This usually happens because the catheter has been displaced.

You usually can prevent this problem by carefully securing the IV catheter and IV tubing. If infiltration occurs, stop the flow of the fluids. Remove the catheter and notify the physician. Signs of infiltration are:

- Swelling and pain at the IV site
- Slow or absent flow rate into the drip chamber when the roller clamp is open

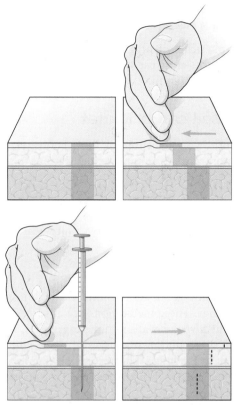

Figure 19-19 Z-track technique for IM injection of medications that are irritating to subcutaneous tissue. The skin is pulled to one side, the needle is inserted, and the solution is injected after careful aspiration. When the needle is withdrawn and the displaced tissue is allowed to return to its normal position, the solution is prevented from escaping from the muscle tissue. (Reprinted from Kronenberger J, Ledbetter J. *Jones & Bartlett Learning's Comprehensive Medical Assisting.* 5th ed. Burlington, MA: Jones & Bartlett Learning, LLC; 2016.)

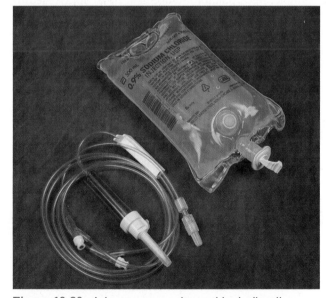

Figure 19-20 Intravenous equipment including the fluid and tubing. (Reprinted from Kronenberger J, Ledbetter J. *Jones & Bartlett Learning's Comprehensive Medical Assisting.* 5th ed. Burlington, MA: Jones & Bartlett Learning, LLC; 2016.)

No blood return or back up into the tubing when the fluid bag is placed below the level of the heart

If the physician or practitioner orders that the IV be reinserted, you must use the other arm or a site above the level of infiltration.

Other Medication Routes

Besides orally, by injection, or intravenously, there are several more ways to administer medications to patients.

- By inhalation
- On or through the skin
- By instillation into the eyes, ears, and nose
- By insertion into the rectum or vagina

Inhalation

Some medications are administered through inspiration into the lungs. These medications are absorbed quickly through the alveolar walls into the capillaries. The alveolar walls are found in small sacs of tissue where air is exchanged in the lungs. The absorption rate for inhaled medications may be difficult to predict for patients with lung diseases.

Patients with chronic pulmonary disorders may self-administer medications. They use a handheld nebulizer, or inhaler. Both devices produce a spray of medicated mist that's inhaled directly into the lungs through the mouth or through the mouth and nose.

Most nasal medications are administered by sprays or nasal inhalers. Some nasal medications have a local effect, such as relieving nasal congestion or preventing allergy symptoms. Others have a systemic effect. For example, butorphanol (Stadol) is a nasal spray used to relieve moderate to severe pain.

Skin Medications

There are two general types of medications applied to the skin.

- Topical medications include creams, lotions, ointments, and sprays. They produce local effects.
- Transdermal medications typically are administered using a patch that's placed on the skin. They produce systemic effects. Medication administered transdermally is delivered to the body through absorption by the skin. Delivery is slow and a steady, stable level of medication is maintained in the body.

Never cut a transdermal patch—The rate of absorption of the medication would then be changed. Transdermal patches may be placed in several locations:

- Chest
- Back
- Upper arm
- Behind the ear

Eyes, Ears, and Nose

Some medications may be designed for administration through the eyes, ears, or nose. You may need to administer these medications in the office or instruct patients on how to administer them at home. A common method of administration for these medications is **instillation**, the administration of a liquid drop by drop.

Ophthalmic medications are used to treat eye infections and to soothe eye irritation. They also may be used to dilate the pupils for diagnostic purposes. Eye medications usually are supplied as an ointment or a liquid and have a local effect. The label should state clearly that the medication is formulated for use in the eyes.

Otic medications, or ear medications, relieve ear pain and swelling, treat infections of the ear canal, or soften cerumen (ear wax). Ear medications typically come in the form of liquid drops and have a local effect.

Nasal medications can be administered by instillation. They usually are in the form of drops or sprays. Their most common use is to reduce swelling or drainage in nasal passages in patients suffering from colds or allergies. Some hormones also are administered nasally.

Rectal Administration

Rectal medications are available in suppository or liquid form. Suppositories have a cocoa butter or glycerin base that melts at body temperature. They need to be stored in the refrigerator. Liquid form is administered as an enema—a procedure where liquid is introduced into the bowel through a tube. Rectal medications can provide a local effect or be absorbed through the rectal mucosa for a systemic effect. Rectal medications may be used for patients who are NPO (allowed nothing by mouth) or who have nausea and vomiting. They are never used for patients who have diarrhea.

Rectal medications rarely are administered in the medical office. However, you may be asked to instruct patients on the proper technique for administering them at home. Both enemas and rectal suppositories should be retained by the patient for 20 to 30 minutes before elimination.

Figure 19-21 shows examples of suppositories and method used for rectal insertion.

Vaginal Administration

Vaginal medications include creams, tablets, suppositories, and solutions for douches. Medications prescribed for the vaginal route typically have local effects. Examples include hormonal creams or antifungal preparations (Fig. 19-22).

Instruct the patient to remain lying down for a while after the insertion of vaginal medications. For comfort, the patient may want to wear a light pad to absorb any drainage.

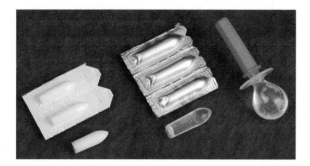

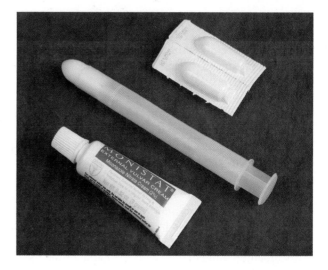

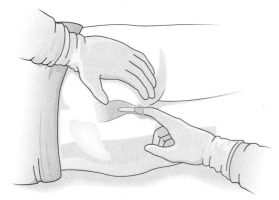

Figure 19-21 Examples of suppositories and the proper method used to insert a rectal suppository into the anus well beyond the internal sphincter. (Reprinted from Kronenberger J, Ledbetter J. *Jones & Bartlett Learning's Comprehensive Medical Assisting.* 5th ed. Burlington, MA: Jones & Bartlett Learning, LLC; 2016.)

Medication Errors

There are many steps for calculating, measuring, and administering medications. You need to perform each step carefully to avoid making errors that could harm your patients. Even so, all human beings occasionally make mistakes. If you notice that you've made a medication error, it's important that you report it to the physician as soon as possible.

Some medication errors might include the following:

- Giving the wrong medication to the patient
- Giving a medication to the wrong patient
- Giving the wrong amount of a medication
- Giving the medication using the wrong route of administration

Medication errors and corrective actions must be documented in the patient's medical record. You'll also need to fill out an incident report to file in the office. The incident report verifies that all possible precautions were taken for the patient. It also can be reviewed to determine if steps can be taken to make sure similar errors don't happen in the future.

You can avoid medication errors by preparing and administering medications carefully. By observing seven

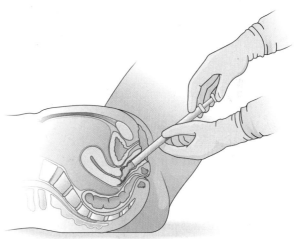

Figure 19-22 Example of vaginal suppository and applicator. Insertion of vaginal cream using an applicator. (Reprinted from Kronenberger J, Ledbetter J. *Jones & Bartlett Learning's Comprehensive Medical Assisting.* 5th ed. Burlington, MA: Jones & Bartlett Learning, LLC; 2016.)

"rights" when giving any medication, you'll eliminate the possibility of many errors. Here's the "right" list to follow:

1. Right patient—Ask the patient to state her name. Some patients may answer to any name. So if you simply say the name, it won't ensure you have the right patient.
2. Right time—Medications ordered to be given in the office must be given before the patient leaves. Some patients may have to be told when the next dose is due.
3. Right dose—Check doses carefully. Many medications come in various strengths.
4. Right route—Medications are administered by a variety of routes. Check the physician's order to ensure the proper route for a particular medication: oral, intramuscular, or topical medication.

5. Right drug—Many medication names are very much alike. For instance, Orinase and Ornade may be confused if you're not careful. Always look up unfamiliar medications in a drug reference book such as the *Physician's Desk Reference* (PDR).

6. Right technique—Check how the medication needs to be given, such as orally with or without food. Intramuscular, subcutaneous, and intradermal injections should be given only after carefully choosing a site and using the right procedure.

7. Right documentation—The medical record is a legal document. Make sure the medication is documented *after* it's administered, not before. Check to be sure you're documenting it in the right medical record. All medications given in the medical office must be documented immediately with the name of the medication, dose, route, and site (if injected). Don't forget your signature. When appropriate, the patient's response should be charted as well.

Documenting Errors

You've been working hard all day. Suddenly, you realize you made an error in the medication you gave to a patient. What should you do?

Even if you're extremely careful, you may make an error when administering a medication. Don't try to hide the mistake or solve the problem on your own. Report the error to the physician right away. If you've given too much or given an incorrect medication, it might harm the patient.

If you report the error right away, immediate action can be taken to resolve the problem. For example, if you've given the wrong medication or the wrong amount, the physician may want you to monitor the patient for adverse reactions. If the patient didn't receive the intended medication, you may need to administer it.

You'll need to document the error and all the actions taken to correct it in the patient's medical record. You also must complete an incident report. The report is kept on file in the medical office.

Procedure 19-1   Administering Oral Medications

Equipment: Physician's order, correct oral medication, disposable calibrated cup, glass of water, and patient's medical record.

1. Wash your hands and gather your supplies.

2. Check the medication label and compare it to the physician's order. Note the expiration date. Remember to check the medication label three times—when taking it from the shelf, when measuring, and when returning it to the shelf.

3. If necessary, calculate the correct dose.

4. For a multidose container, remove the cap from the container. Touch only the outside of the lid to avoid contaminating the inside. Single, or unit dose, medications come individually wrapped. Packages may be opened by pushing the medication through the foil backing or by peeling back a tab on one corner.

5. According to your calculations and the label, remove the correct dose of medication.
   A. For solid medications:
      • Pour the correct dose into the bottle cap to prevent contamination.

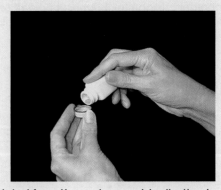

(Reprinted from Kronenberger J, Ledbetter J. *Jones & Bartlett Learning's Comprehensive Medical Assisting.* 5th ed. Burlington, MA: Jones & Bartlett Learning, LLC; 2016.)

   • Transfer the medication to a disposable cup.

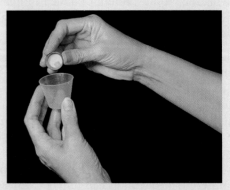

(Reprinted from Kronenberger J, Ledbetter J. *Jones & Bartlett Learning's Comprehensive Medical Assisting.* 5th ed. Burlington, MA: Jones & Bartlett Learning, LLC; 2016.)

Procedure 19-1   Administering Oral Medications (*continued*)

B. For liquid medications:

- Open the bottle and put the lid on a flat surface. The open end of the lid should face up to prevent contamination of the inside of the cap.
- Palm the label to prevent liquids from dripping onto the label. You don't want the label to become unreadable.
- With the opposite hand, place your thumbnail at the correct calibration on the cup. Holding the cup at eye level, pour the proper amount of medication into the cup. Use your thumbnail as a guide.

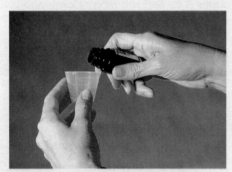

(Reprinted from Kronenberger J, Ledbetter J. *Jones & Bartlett Learning's Comprehensive Medical Assisting.* 5th ed. Burlington, MA: Jones & Bartlett Learning, LLC; 2016.)

6. Greet and verify the patient's name to avoid errors. Explain the procedure. Ask the patient about any medication allergies that may not be noted on the chart.

7. Give the patient a glass of water to wash down the medication, unless contraindicated (as in the case of lozenges or cough syrup). Hand the patient the disposable cup containing the medication.

8. Remain with the patient to be sure all the medication is swallowed. Observe any unusual reactions and report them to the physician.

9. Thank the patient and give any additional instructions as necessary.

10. Wash your hands and record the procedure in the patient's medical record.

Procedure 19-2   Preparing Injections

Equipment: Physician's order, medication for the injection in an ampule or vial, antiseptic wipes, a needle and syringe of appropriate size, a small gauze pad, a biohazard sharps container, and the patient's medical record.

1. Wash your hands and gather your supplies. Choose the needle and syringe according to the route of administration, type of medication, and size of the patient.

2. Review the medication order and compare it to the label on the medication container. Check the expiration date. Remember to check the medication label three times—when taking it from the shelf, while drawing it up into the syringe, and when returning it to the shelf.

3. Calculate the correct dose, if necessary.

4. Open the needle and syringe package. Assemble if necessary. Make sure the needle is attached firmly

to the syringe by grasping the needle at the hub and turning it clockwise on the syringe. A needle that isn't firmly attached may come off during the procedure.

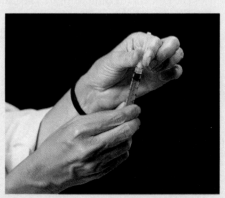

(Reprinted from Kronenberger J, Ledbetter J. *Jones & Bartlett Learning's Comprehensive Medical Assisting.* 5th ed. Burlington, MA: Jones & Bartlett Learning, LLC; 2016.)

Procedure 19-2 | Preparing Injections (*continued*)

5. Withdraw the correct amount of medication.
   A. From an ampule:
      - With the fingertips of one hand, tap the stem of the ampule lightly to remove any medication in or above the neck.
      - Wipe the neck of the ampule where the break will occur with an alcohol wipe. Wrap a piece of gauze around the neck to protect your fingers from broken glass. Snap the stem off the ampule with a quick downward movement of the gauze. Be sure to aim the break away from your face. Dispose of the ampule top in a biohazard sharps container.

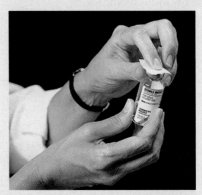

(Reprinted from Kronenberger J, Ledbetter J. *Jones & Bartlett Learning's Comprehensive Medical Assisting.* 5th ed. Burlington, MA: Jones & Bartlett Learning, LLC; 2016.)

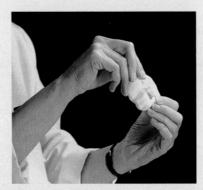

(Reprinted from Kronenberger J, Ledbetter J. *Jones & Bartlett Learning's Comprehensive Medical Assisting.* 5th ed. Burlington, MA: Jones & Bartlett Learning, LLC; 2016.)

- After removing the needle guard, insert a filtered needle into the ampule. The needle lumen should be below the level of medication.
- Withdraw the medication by pulling back on the plunger of the syringe. Take care not to touch the needle to the contaminated edge of the broken ampule. After you've withdrawn the correct amount, discard the ampule in the biohazard sharps container.
- Hold the syringe with the needle up. Remove any air bubbles by gently tapping the barrel of the syringe until the bubbles rise to the top. Draw back on the plunger to add a small amount of air. Then, gently push the plunger forward to eject the air from the syringe. Be careful not to eject any medication.

   B. From a vial:
      - Cleanse the stopper of the vial with an antiseptic wipe.

- Remove the needle guard. Pull back on the plunger to fill the syringe with a small amount of air equal to the amount of medication to be removed from the vial.

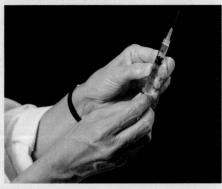

(Reprinted from Kronenberger J, Ledbetter J. *Jones & Bartlett Learning's Comprehensive Medical Assisting.* 5th ed. Burlington, MA: Jones & Bartlett Learning, LLC; 2016.)

- Insert the needle into the vial through the center of the cleansed vial top. Inject the air from the syringe into the vial above the level of the medication so that you don't make bubbles or foam in the medication. Injecting air into the vial prevents a vacuum from forming in the vial, which would make it difficult to withdraw the medication.

Procedure 19-2 | Preparing Injections (*continued*)

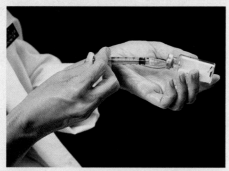

(Reprinted from Kronenberger J, Ledbetter J. *Jones & Bartlett Learning's Comprehensive Medical Assisting.* 5th ed. Burlington, MA: Jones & Bartlett Learning, LLC; 2016.)

- With the needle inside the vial, invert the vial, holding the syringe at eye level. Aspirate, or withdraw, the desired amount of medication into the syringe.

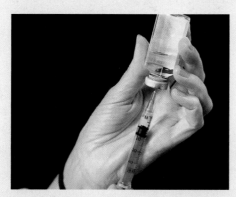

(Reprinted from Kronenberger J, Ledbetter J. *Jones & Bartlett Learning's Comprehensive Medical Assisting.* 5th ed. Burlington, MA: Jones & Bartlett Learning, LLC; 2016.)

- Gently tap the barrel of the syringe with your fingertips to displace any air bubbles. Remove the air by pushing the plunger slowly and forcing the air into the vial.

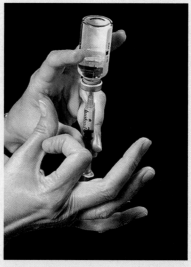

(Reprinted from Kronenberger J, Ledbetter J. *Jones & Bartlett Learning's Comprehensive Medical Assisting.* 5th ed. Burlington, MA: Jones & Bartlett Learning, LLC; 2016.)

6. Place the needle guard on a hard, flat surface. Without contaminating the needle, insert the needle into the cap and scoop up the cap with one hand. Recapping the needle protects the sterility of the needle until you administer the medication. You should use one hand to recap the needle to prevent needlestick injuries.

Procedure 19-3 | Administering an Intradermal Injection

Equipment: Physician's order, medication for the injection in an ampule or vial, antiseptic wipes, a needle and syringe of appropriate size, a small gauze pad, a biohazard sharps container, clean examination gloves, and the patient's medical record.

1. Wash your hands and gather supplies.

2. Review the physician's order and select the correct medication. Check the order carefully against the medication label. Make sure the expiration date

hasn't passed. Remember to check the medication label three times—when taking it from the shelf, while drawing it up into the syringe, and when returning it to the shelf.

3. Prepare the injection according to the steps in Procedure 19-2.

4. Greet and identify the patient. Explain the procedure and ask the patient about any known medication allergies.

Procedure 19-3	Administering an Intradermal Injection (continued)

5. Select the appropriate site for the injection. Recommended sites are the anterior forearm and the middle of the back.

6. Prepare the site by cleansing with an antiseptic wipe. Use a circular motion, starting at the injection site and working toward the outside. The circular motion will carry microorganisms away from the site. Don't touch the site after cleansing.

7. Put on gloves. You must follow standard precautions for your protection.

8. Remove the needle guard. Using your nondominant hand, pull the patient's skin taut. Stretching the patient's skin allows the needle to enter with little resistance and secures the patient against movement.

9. With the bevel of the needle facing upward, insert the needle at a 10- to 15-degree angle into the upper layer of the skin. This angle ensures that penetration occurs within the dermal layer.

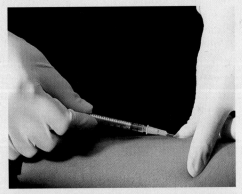

(Reprinted from Kronenberger J, Ledbetter J. *Jones & Bartlett Learning's Comprehensive Medical Assisting.* 5th ed. Burlington, MA: Jones & Bartlett Learning, LLC; 2016.)

- The bevel of the needle must be facing up for a wheal to form.
- Stop inserting the needle when the bevel of the needle is under the skin. The needle should be slightly visible below the skin.

10. Inject the medication slowly by depressing the plunger.
    - A wheal will form as the medication enters the dermal layer of the skin.

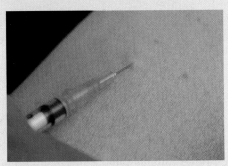

(Reprinted from Kronenberger J, Ledbetter J. *Jones & Bartlett Learning's Comprehensive Medical Assisting.* 5th ed. Burlington, MA: Jones & Bartlett Learning, LLC; 2016.)

- Hold the syringe steady; moving the needle will be uncomfortable for the patient.

11. Remove the needle from the skin at the angle of insertion.
    - Don't use an antiseptic wipe or gauze pad when withdrawing the needle.
    - Don't press or massage the site. Pressure on the wheal may press the medication into the tissues or out of the injection site.
    - Don't apply a bandage—it may cause redness or swelling that could result in an inaccurate reading of the test.

12. To reduce the risk of an accidental needlestick, don't recap the needle. If a safety device is attached to the needle, engage it according to manufacturer directions to cover the needle. Dispose of the needle and syringe in a biohazard sharps container.

13. Remove your gloves and wash your hands.

14. Depending upon the type of skin test administered, the length of time required for a reaction, and the policies of your medical office, perform one of the following:
    - Read the test results. Inspect and palpate the site for the presence and amount of induration.
    - Tell the patient when to return (date and time) to the office to have the results read.

15. Document the procedure, site, and results. Document any instructions to the patient.

Procedure 19-4 | Administering a Subcutaneous Injection

Equipment: Physician's order, medication for the injection in an ampule or vial, antiseptic wipes, a needle and syringe of appropriate size, a small gauze pad, a biohazard sharps container, clean examination gloves, an adhesive bandage, and the patient's medical record.

1. Wash your hands and gather supplies.

2. Review the medication order, select the correct medication, and compare it to the label on the medication container. Check the expiration date. Remember to check the medication label three times—when taking it from the shelf, while drawing it up into the syringe, and when returning it to the shelf.

3. Prepare the injection according to the steps in Procedure 19-2.

4. Greet and identify the patient. Explain the procedure and ask the patient about any known medication allergies.

5. Select the appropriate site for the injection. Recommended sites include the upper arm, thigh, back, and abdomen.

6. Prepare the site by cleansing with an antiseptic wipe. Use a circular motion starting at the intended injection site and working toward the outside. The circular motion will carry microorganisms away from the site. Don't touch the site after cleansing.

7. Put on gloves. You must follow standard precautions for your protection.

8. Remove the needle guard. Using your nondominant hand, hold the skin surrounding the injection site in a cushion fashion.

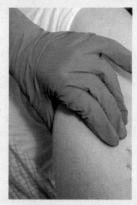

(Reprinted from Kronenberger J, Ledbetter J. *Jones & Bartlett Learning's Comprehensive Medical Assisting.* 5th ed. Burlington, MA: Jones & Bartlett Learning, LLC; 2016.)

9. With a firm motion, insert the needle into the tissue at a 45-degree angle to the skin surface. Make sure the bevel of the needle is facing upward. Hold the barrel between the thumb and index finger of the dominant hand and insert the needle completely to the hub. A quick, firm motion is less painful to the patient.

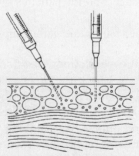

(Reprinted from Kronenberger J, Ledbetter J. *Jones & Bartlett Learning's Comprehensive Medical Assisting.* 5th ed. Burlington, MA: Jones & Bartlett Learning, LLC; 2016.)

10. Remove your nondominant hand from the skin. Holding the syringe steady, pull the syringe (aspirate) gently.

- If blood appears in the hub or the syringe, you've entered a blood vessel. If this happens, don't inject the medication. Injecting the medication into a blood vessel means that the medication may be absorbed too quickly. Remove the needle and prepare a new injection.
- If blood doesn't appear, you may continue with the procedure.

Procedure 19-4 | Administering a Subcutaneous Injection (*continued*)

11. Inject the medication by slowly pressing down on the plunger. If you press down on the plunger too quickly, the pressure will cause discomfort and possibly tissue damage to the patient.

12. Place a gauze pad over the injection site and remove the needle at the angle of insertion. With one hand, gently massage the injection site with the gauze pad and with the other hand, discard the needle and syringe into the sharps container. Don't recap the used needle. If available, engage the safety device on the needle. Apply an adhesive bandage, if needed.

13. Remove your gloves and wash your hands.

14. An injection for allergy desensitization means the patient must stay in the office for at least 30 minutes so you can observe any reaction the patient might have. Note: If a patient has any unusual reaction after any injection, let the physician know immediately.

15. Document the procedure, site, and results, as well as any instructions to the patient.

Procedure 19-5 | Administering an Intramuscular Injection

Equipment: Physician's order, medication for the injection in an ampule or vial, antiseptic wipes, a needle and syringe of appropriate size, a small gauze pad, a biohazard sharps container, clean examination gloves, an adhesive bandage, and the patient's medical record.

1. Wash your hands and gather supplies.

2. Review the medication order and select the correct medication. Check the order carefully against the medication label. Make sure the expiration date hasn't passed. Remember to check the medication label three times—when taking it from the shelf, while drawing it up into the syringe, and when returning it to the shelf.

3. Prepare the injection according to the steps in Procedure 19-2.

4. Greet and identify the patient. Explain the procedure and ask about any known medication allergies.

5. Select the appropriate site for the injection. Recommended sites include the deltoid, vastus lateralis, dorsogluteal, and ventrogluteal areas. Take into account the patient's age and size, as well as the medication, when choosing a site.

6. Prepare the site by cleansing with an antiseptic wipe. Use a circular motion starting at the injection site and working toward the outside. The circular motion will carry microorganisms away from the site. Don't touch the site after cleansing.

7. Put on gloves. You must follow standard precautions for your protection.

8. Remove the needle guard. Choose one of the following ways to hold the skin surrounding the injection site.
   - Using your nondominant hand, hold the skin surrounding the injection site taut with the thumb and index or middle fingers. This makes the needle easier to insert in an average or overweight individual.

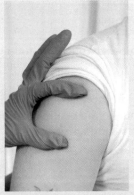

(Reprinted from Kronenberger J, Ledbetter J. *Jones & Bartlett Learning's Comprehensive Medical Assisting.* 5th ed. Burlington, MA: Jones & Bartlett Learning, LLC; 2016.)

   - Using your nondominant hand, grasp the muscle. This produces a deeper mass for the injection in a person who is very thin with little body fat.

Procedure 19-5	Administering an Intramuscular Injection (*continued*)

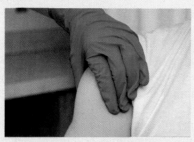

(Reprinted from Kronenberger J, Ledbetter J. *Jones & Bartlett Learning's Comprehensive Medical Assisting.* 5th ed. Burlington, MA: Jones & Bartlett Learning, LLC; 2016.)

9. Hold the syringe like a dart. Use a quick, firm motion to insert the needle into the tissue at a 90-degree angle to the surface. Hold the barrel between the thumb and index finger of your dominant hand and insert the needle completely to the hub. This way, the medication will go into the muscle tissue.

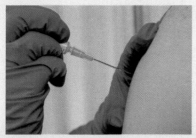

(Reprinted from Kronenberger J, Ledbetter J. *Jones & Bartlett Learning's Comprehensive Medical Assisting.* 5th ed. Burlington, MA: Jones & Bartlett Learning, LLC; 2016.)

10. Remove your nondominant hand from the skin. Holding the syringe steady, pull back the syringe (aspirate).
    - If blood appears in the hub or the syringe, you've entered a blood vessel. Don't inject the medication. Injecting the medication into a blood vessel means the medication may be absorbed too quickly. Place a gauze pad over the injection site and remove the needle. Prepare a new injection.
    - If blood doesn't appear, you may continue with the procedure.

11. Inject the medication by slowly pressing down on the plunger. If you press down on the plunger too quickly, the pressure will cause discomfort and possibly tissue damage to the patient.

12. Place a gauze pad over the injection site. Remove the needle at the angle of insertion. With one hand, gently massage the injection site with the gauze pad. Massaging helps to distribute the medication. If needle has a safety device, engage it then, discard the needle and syringe into the biohazard sharps container. Don't recap the needle.

13. Apply an adhesive bandage to the site, if needed. Remove your gloves and wash your hands.

14. Observe the patient for any reactions. If the patient has any unusual reactions, let the physician know immediately.

15. Document the procedure, site, and results, as well as any instructions to the patient.

Procedure 19-6	Administering an Intramuscular Injection Using the Z-Track Method

Equipment: Physician's order, medication for the injection in an ampule or vial, antiseptic wipes, a needle and syringe of appropriate size, a small gauze pad, a biohazard sharps container, clean examination gloves, an adhesive bandage, and the patient's medical record.

1. Follow steps 1 to 7 as described in Procedure 19-5. The ventrogluteal, vastus lateralis, and dorsogluteal sites work well for the Z-track method, but the deltoid does not.

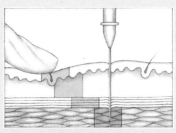

(Reprinted from Kronenberger J, Ledbetter J. *Jones & Bartlett Learning's Comprehensive Medical Assisting.* 5th ed. Burlington, MA: Jones & Bartlett Learning, LLC; 2016.)

Procedure 19-6 Administering an Intramuscular Injection Using the Z-Track Method (*continued*)

2. Remove the needle guard. Rather than pulling the skin taut or grasping the muscle tissue, pull the top layer of skin to the side and hold it with the non-dominant hand throughout the injection.

3. Hold the syringe like a dart and use a quick, firm motion to insert the needle into the tissue at a 90-degree angle to the skin surface. Hold the barrel between the thumb and index finger and insert the needle completely to the hub.

4. Aspirate by withdrawing the plunger slightly. If no blood appears, push the plunger in slowly and steadily. Count to 10 before withdrawing the needle. This allows time for the tissues to begin absorbing the medication.

5. Place a gauze pad over the injection site. Remove the needle at the same angle at which it was inserted while releasing the skin. Don't massage the area. Engage the safety device, if available, and discard the needle and syringe into the biohazard sharps container.

6. Apply an adhesive bandage to the site, if needed. Remove your gloves and wash your hands.

7. Observe the patient for any unusual reactions. Note: If a patient has any unusual reaction after any injection, let the physician know immediately.

8. Document the procedure, site, and results, as well as any instructions to the patient.

Procedure 19-7 Applying Transdermal Medications

Equipment: Physician's order, the medication, clean examination gloves, and the patient's medical record.

1. Wash your hands and gather supplies.

2. Review the medication order and select the correct medication. Check the order carefully against the medication label. Make sure the expiration date hasn't passed. Remember to check the medication label three times—when taking it from the shelf, when opening the medication package, and when returning it to the shelf.

3. Greet and identify the patient. Explain the procedure and ask about any known medication allergies.

4. Select the appropriate site for the medication. The usual sites are the upper arm, the chest or back, and behind the ear. These sites should be rotated.

5. Perform any necessary skin preparation. Make sure the skin is clean, dry, and free from any irritation. Trim any hair close with scissors, but don't shave areas with hair. Shaving may wear away the skin and cause the medication to be absorbed too quickly.

6. Open the medication package by pulling the two sides apart. Don't touch the area of medication. It may be absorbed into your skin, causing an unwanted reaction.

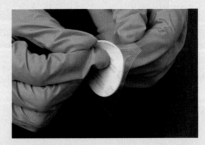

(Reprinted from Kronenberger J, Ledbetter J. *Jones & Bartlett Learning's Comprehensive Medical Assisting.* 5th ed. Burlington, MA: Jones & Bartlett Learning, LLC; 2016.)

7. Apply the medicated patch to the patient's skin following the manufacturer's directions. Starting at the center, press the adhesive edges down firmly all the way around. Starting at the center eliminates air spaces. If the edges do not stick, fasten with tape.

8. Wash your hands and document the procedure, including the site of the patch.

Procedure 19-8   Instilling Eye Medications

Equipment: Physician's order, correct medication, sterile gauze, tissues, and gloves.

1. Wash your hands and gather your supplies. Check the medication label three times. The medication label must specify ophthalmic use. Medications formulated for other uses may be harmful to the eyes.

2. Greet the patient and verify the patient's name. Explain the procedure. Ask the patient about any allergies not recorded in the chart.

3. Position the patient comfortably in a lying or sitting position with the head tilted slightly back. The level of the affected eye should be slightly lower than the unaffected eye. This will keep the medication from running into the unaffected eye.

4. Put on gloves. You may come into contact with fluids from the patient's eye.

5. Using sterile gauze, pull down the lower eyelid to expose the conjunctival sac (the space between the membrane covering the eye and the membrane inside the eyelid). Ask the patient to look up. Looking away from the medication will reduce the blink reflex.

6. Check the medication label for a second time to be sure it's the right medication. Instill the medication.

- *Ointment.* Discard the first bead of ointment from the container onto a tissue. It's considered contaminated. Do not touch the tissue because the tissue can contaminate the tip. Moving from the inner canthus (inner corner) outward, place a thin line of ointment across the inside of the eyelid. Placing the ointment in the sac avoids touching the eye with the tip of the ointment tube. Twist the tube slightly to release the ointment.
- *Drops.* Hold the dropper about half an inch from the conjunctival sac, not touching the patient. Release the proper number of drops into the sac. Discard any medication left in the dropper to prevent contamination of the rest of the container.

7. Release the lower eyelid. Ask the patient to close the eye and gently roll it to disperse the medication.

8. Wipe off any excess medication with the tissue. Instruct the patient to apply light pressure to the puncta lacrimalis (the opening in the eyelid where tears drain) for several minutes. This prevents the medication from running into the nasolacrimal sac and duct (tear duct).

9. Properly care for and dispose of equipment and supplies. When disposing of or putting away the medication, check the label for a third time. Clean the work area and wash your hands.

10. Document the procedure.

Procedure 19-9   Instilling Ear Medications

Equipment: Correct otic medication and cotton balls.

1. Wash your hands and gather your supplies. Check the medication label to be sure it's the right medication three times. The label should specify otic preparation.

2. Greet the patient and verify the patient's name. Explain the procedure.

3. Ask the patient to sit with the affected ear tilted upward. This position helps the medication flow through the canal to the tympanic membrane.

4. Check the medication label again. Draw up the amount of medication ordered.

5. Straighten the ear canal.
- *Adults.* Pull the auricle (outer ear) slightly up and back.
- *Children.* Pull the auricle slightly down and back.

6. Insert the tip of the dropper without touching the patient's skin. This avoids contamination. Let the medication flow along the side of the ear canal. The medication should flow gently to avoid discomfort.

7. Ask the patient to sit or lie with the affected ear up for about 5 minutes after the instillation. The medication should rest against the tympanic membrane for as long as possible.

Procedure 19-9 | Instilling Ear Medications (*continued*)

8. If the medication is to be retained in the ear canal, gently insert a moist cotton ball into the external auditory meatus (opening in the ear). The cotton ball keeps the medication in the canal. Because it is moist, it won't wick the medication out.

9. Properly care for and dispose of equipment and supplies. Check the medication label again. Clean the work area and wash your hands.

10. Document the procedure in the patient's chart.

Procedure 19-10 | Instilling Nasal Medications

Equipment: Gloves, correct nasal medication, and tissues.

1. Wash your hands and gather your supplies. Check the medication label three times to be sure it's the right one. It must be formulated for nasal instillation.

2. Greet the patient and verify the patient's name. Explain the procedure. Tell the patient that the procedure may be uncomfortable, but it shouldn't be painful. Ask about any allergies not recorded in the chart.

3. Position the patient in a comfortable, recumbent (lying down) position. Extend the patient's head beyond the edge of the examination table or place a pillow under the shoulders. Support the patient's neck to avoid strain as the head tilts back. Tilting the head back allows the medication to reach the upper nasal passages.

4. Put on gloves. Administer the medication.
   - *Drops.* Hold the dropper upright just above the nostril. Dispense one drop at a time without touching the patient. Keep the patient recumbent for 5 minutes to allow the medication to reach the upper nasal passages.
   - *Spray.* Place the tip of the bottle at the naris opening without touching the patient's skin or nasal tissues. Ask the patient to take a deep breath; spray as the patient is inhaling. If the patient breathes out while the medication is being sprayed, it won't reach the nasal passages.

5. For the patient's comfort, wipe away any excess medication from the skin with tissues.

6. Properly care for and dispose of equipment and supplies. Check the medication label as you do so. Clean the work area, remove your gloves, and wash your hands.

7. Record the procedure in the patient's chart.

Preparing for Externship

Regardless of the type of medical facility where you perform your externship, more than likely you will encounter information regarding drugs and drug terms. This can be difficult for most new students to grasp, understand, and remember. The drug names are usually long and unfamiliar. Start writing down the various drugs you encounter during the externship and research information on each one. You can use the Internet to locate information including the purpose for the drug, side effects, route of administration, and typical dose. Use individual index cards for each drug and write this information. These cards will become a quick way to refresh your memory and you will be amazed how soon the drugs will become more familiar to you.

Chapter Recap

- Medical assistants must be knowledgeable about different medications, their uses, side effects, and potential abuses. The medical assistant may need to administer medications under a physician's supervision and educate patients about using them correctly.

- Most over-the-counter and prescription medications have a chemical name, a generic name, and a trade name. Drugs are manufactured from natural sources and from synthetic materials.

- The Controlled Substances Act of 1970 regulates the manufacture and distribution of dangerous drugs. Physicians who prescribe or administer controlled substances must obtain a registration number from the U.S. Drug Enforcement Agency (DEA).

- Special documentation is required for controlled substances in the medical office. Careful records must be kept of drug purchases, prescriptions, and disposal. Separate dispensing records must be kept for all Schedule II drugs. Federal law requires that an inventory of controlled substances be taken every 2 years.

- Medical assistants sometimes prepare prescriptions for the physician's signature. They also may phone prescription orders to pharmacies or handle prescription requests from patients. The medical assistant may not sign off on refill requests and it must be seen and initialed by the physician unless there are written standing orders.

- Patients should receive written and verbal instructions regarding their medications. Patients should be encouraged to call the medical office if they have any questions.

- A medication may have a local effect or a systemic effect. The body's reaction depends on the route of administration, the absorption rate, drug metabolism, and excretion. Factors influencing drug effects are age, weight, sex, existing illnesses, and degree of tolerance.

- Drug interactions can occur with other prescribed drugs, over-the-counter medications, herbal supplements, alcohol, and food. In some cases, interactions can produce unwanted effects.

- To calculate dosages, medical assistants may need to convert between different systems of measurement.

- The most commonly used systems of measurement are the metric system and the household system. The household system is only used by patients at home.

- The ratio method and the formula method can be used to calculate medication dosages for adults. Several formulas are used to calculate children's dosages.

- Medication administration can be divided into two main groups—enteral and parenteral. Enteral routes include medication taken by mouth and medication administered rectally. Parenteral routes include any route other than the enteral ones—for example, injections, intravenous administration, and vaginal application.

- Strict aseptic technique must be followed when administering medication by injection. The three main types of injections are intradermal, subcutaneous, and intramuscular.

- The medical assistant must select the right needle length and gauge for the injection type. Different types of injections have different injection sites and different angles of insertion.

- Intravenous medications are injected through a catheter into the patient's bloodstream. In some cases, medical assistants must set up equipment and fluids for IV. They need to watch for infiltration of the IV fluid into the tissues surrounding the vein.

- Some medications are inhaled using an inhaler or nebulizer. Others are absorbed by the skin through a transdermal patch. Many eye, ear, and nasal medications are instilled drop by drop to produce a local effect.

- Rectal medications are packaged in the form of suppositories or enemas. They are rarely administered in the medical office. They may have local or systemic effects. Vaginal medications usually have local effects.

- Steps for preparing and administering medications must be performed carefully to avoid making errors. Checking the seven "rights" is a good way to reduce the possibility of errors. Any medication errors should be reported to the physician immediately and documented in the patient's chart.

Online Resources for Students

Student Resources available on the text's online site include:

- Audio Glossaries
- Animations
- Competency Evaluation Forms
- Videos
- Anatomy & Physiology Module with Heart and Lung Sounds
- Weblinks
- Worksheets

Exercises and Activities

Certification Preparation Questions

1. Which of these is a parenteral method of administration of medication?
   a. Oral
   b. Subcutaneous
   c. Topical
   d. Sublingual
   e. Rectal

2. Which of these drug classifications is associated with medications used to treat infections and kill bacteria in the body?
   a. Anticonvulsant
   b. Antibiotic
   c. Antifungal
   d. Anticoagulant
   e. Antiemetic

3. How many milliliters are equal to 0.01 L?
   a. 0.1 ml
   b. 1 ml
   c. 10 ml
   d. 100 ml
   e. 1,000 ml

4. Which of these is the abbreviation for the organization that issues a registration number to a health care provider in order to prescribe controlled drugs?
   a. BSA
   b. FDA
   c. DEA
   d. CIA
   e. NKA

5. How much medication would you give a patient if the physician orders 750 mg and the drug strength is 0.5 g per tablet?
   a. ½ tablet
   b. 1 tablet
   c. 1 ½ tablets
   d. 2 tablets
   e. 3 tablets

6. Which of these is an injection site located in the thigh?
   a. Deltoid
   b. Ventrogluteal
   c. Vastus lateralis
   d. Dorsogluteal
   e. Gluteus medius

7. Which of these is the process of getting the medication into the bloodstream?
   a. Secretion
   b. Metabolism
   c. Distribution
   d. Administration
   e. Absorption

8. Which of these locations is appropriate for the instillation of medication?
   a. On the skin
   b. In the rectum
   c. In the vagina
   d. In the eyes
   e. Under the tongue

9. A primary reason to administer medication using the parenteral method is that:
   a. it is easier to administer.
   b. it costs less than using the oral method.
   c. there is a rapid response time to the medication.
   d. there is a possibility of accidental injection into a vein.
   e. there is a rapid allergic reaction.

10. Which levels of controlled substance drugs are limited to refills of up to five times in a 6-month period and can be called into the pharmacist?
    a. I and II
    b. II and III
    c. III and IV
    d. IV and V
    e. V only

 ## CareTracker Connection

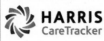 **HARRIS** CareTracker — Entering Prescriptions and Documenting Patient Medications

CareTracker Activities Related to This Chapter
- Case Study 12: Create and Print Prescriptions

NOTE: Case Study 12 has prerequisite cases (in addition to Cases 1 to 11), which must be completed first.

Many patients today are on multiple prescription medications. Accurately documenting a patient's medications and entering prescriptions for new ones is a major responsibility of the medical assistant. CareTracker facilitates these tasks by including a Medications application within the patient's medical record, in which current medications may be recorded and new ones may be ordered electronically.

Tasks discussed in this chapter that can be performed in CareTracker include the following:

- Documenting a patient's current medications
- Adding new medications to the patient's record
- Documenting the administration of medications performed during an office visit

- Reordering current medications
- Entering new medication prescriptions on the basis of a primary care provider's order

Many of these tasks are discussed in CareTracker Connection features in other chapters. A task we'll consider here is entering a new prescription.

New prescriptions may be entered in the Medications application of a patient's Medical Record module. (Note, however, that the student training version of CareTracker, which you are using, does not allow actual faxing or electronic transmission of prescriptions.)

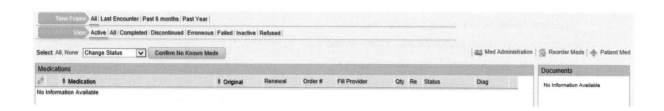

Clicking on the **+ *Patient Med*** icon causes a new window will appear.

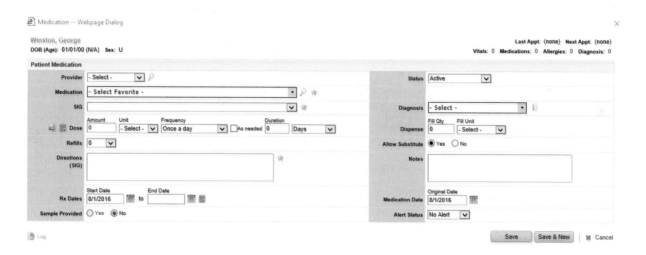

You would then select the name of the patient's provider and click on the search icon next to the Medications field, which causes the Medication Search window to appear. In this window, you would enter the medication desired (such as "Glucophage" in this example) into the Search Text field and set other parameters as indicated in the image below. On clicking Search, a list of related medications will appear.

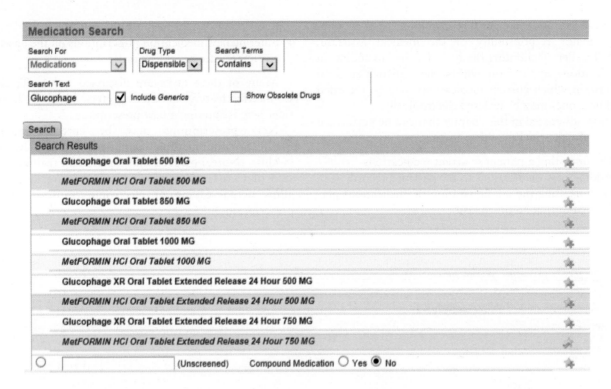

You would then select the desired medication, such as "*MetFORMIN HCl Oral Tablet Extended Release 24 Hour 750 MG.*" This will cause the Drug Interaction box to appear. After examining the information, you would select any relevant drug interactions and enter any needed notes, as shown below.

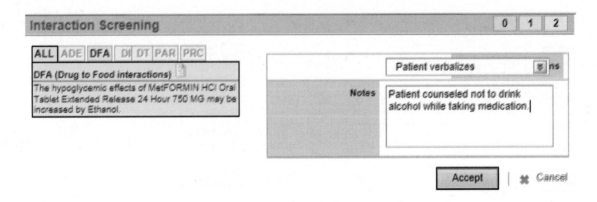

Back in the main Medication Order screen, you would enter the number of units, form, duration, number of refills, dispense fill quantity and unit, and prescription start and end dates, as shown below.

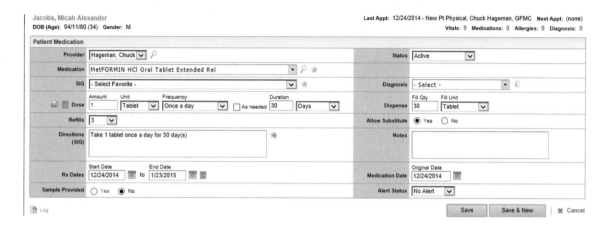

When done, you would click Save. The medication would now appear in the patient's clinical record, as shown below.

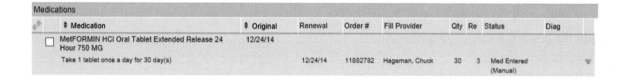

20 Diagnostic Testing

Chapter Objectives

- Explain the difference between radiolucent and radiopaque, using examples.
- List ways to protect patients and yourself from radiation hazards.
- Describe how to prepare patients for routine x-ray examinations.
- Discuss how to teach patients about contrast examinations.
- List the general steps in a routine radiographic examination.
- Compare and contrast fluoroscopy, MRI, and CT scans.
- List three typical uses for sonography.
- Describe the medical assistant's role in radiographic procedures.
- Explain how to handle and store radiographic film.

- Contrast invasive and noninvasive techniques for cardiological diagnosis.
- Describe the placement of electrocardiogram electrodes.
- Perform electrocardiography.
- Identify the main wave forms used for interpretation on an electrocardiogram tracing.
- Discuss three types of electrocardiogram artifacts and how to prevent them.
- Describe how to apply a Holter monitor.
- Define tidal volume and forced expiration.
- Perform basic respiratory testing.
- Briefly describe bronchoscopy and arterial blood gas tests.
- Explain how to teach a patient to use a peak flowmeter.

CAAHEP & ABHES Competencies

CAAHEP

- Prepare a patient for procedures and/or treatments.
- Schedule patient admissions and/or procedures.
- Perform within scope of practice.
- Perform electrocardiography.
- Perform pulmonary function testing.

ABHES

- Identify diagnostic and treatment modalities as they relate to each body system.
- Comply with federal, state, and local health laws and regulations as they relate to health care settings.
- Schedule of inpatient and outpatient procedures.

Chapter Terms

Artifact	Dyspnea	Radiography	Rhythm Strip
Cardiologist	Echocardiogram	Radiologists	Spirometer
Cassette	Fluoroscopy	Radiology	Teleradiology
Contrast medium	Murmurs	Radiolucent	Ultrasound
Dosimeter	Radiographs	Radiopaque	X-rays

Abbreviations

ABG	GI	PACS	SOB
ALARA	MI	PAT	SPECT
COPD	MRI	PET	
CT	NPO	PTCA	
ECG	PAC	PVC	

Case Study

Melissa Barber, a 42-year-old female patient, is experiencing mild chest discomfort and shortness of breath. The physician orders an electrocardiogram. She has never had an ECG performed and is worried about the procedure as well as the results of the test. Ms. Barber's father died of a heart attack at the age of 45, and she is afraid that she might be having a heart attack. David Carter, the medical assistant, reassures Ms. Barber about the procedure and that the physician will see her after the ECG to explain the results of the test.

 ## DIAGNOSTIC TESTING

Sometimes, a physician orders specific medical tests to help diagnose a patient's illness. As a medical assistant, it's likely that you'll have to assist with or help educate patients about several different types of diagnostic tests, such as:

- **Radiology**, which is a medical specialty that uses different imaging techniques to diagnose and treat diseases
- Cardiovascular tests, which are used to diagnose disorders of the heart
- Pulmonary (respiratory) tests, which are used in the diagnosis and treatment of respiratory conditions

You also may be responsible for screening and following up test results after the procedures have been performed.

 ## RADIOLOGY AND THE MEDICAL ASSISTANT

Among the most common diagnostic tests are those that create a visual image of internal body structures. Because of changing technology, new procedures are continually being developed to help visualize body structures. Physicians who specialize in interpreting these images are called **radiologists**.

Probably the most common radiology technique is the radiograph. **Radiographs** are shadow-like images of internal structures. They're digital or processed on a type of film similar to photography film. The images are created using **x-rays**—invisible, high-energy waves that can penetrate dense objects. The process of making these films is called **radiography**. Figure 20-1 shows a radiograph of the chest.

The process of radiography and the radiographs themselves are commonly referred to as x-rays. Patients

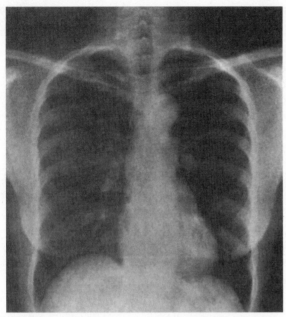

Figure 20-1 Radiograph of chest. (Reprinted from Kronenberger J, Ledbetter J. *Jones & Bartlett Learning's Comprehensive Medical Assisting*. 5th ed. Burlington, MA: Jones & Bartlett Learning, LLC; 2016.)

usually more frequently understand the term x-ray instead of radiograph. It is important to use terminology that patients can comprehend.

In some states, a medical assistant is allowed to take and process simple images such as chest x-rays or x-rays of bones. The training required to do this varies. In other states, only licensed radiographers may take and process x-rays. You should be familiar with your state laws and comply with any regulations. Although you may not perform radiological diagnostic procedures, you have an important role in preparing and educating the patient. Your responsibilities may include

- Preparing patients for radiology procedures
- Performing basic x-ray procedures in the medical office (where permitted by law)
- Assisting in educating patients about general radiology processes
- Scheduling the procedures

The medical community is making an effort to have procedures and treatments performed on an outpatient basis. Some medical offices have on-site x-ray equipment. Outpatient diagnostic imaging centers also have been created to offer a variety of radiology services. Some companies even specialize in providing basic x-ray services to patients in long-term care facilities or in patients' homes.

X-rays and X-ray Machines

X-rays are produced by electricity of extremely high voltage inside an x-ray tube. The x-rays exit the tube in one direction as a beam and pass though a device designed to control the beam's size. During an x-ray, a beam of light also shines on the patient. This light is not part of the x-ray beam. It's a guide to help the x-ray technician direct and position the x-ray beam.

Many modern x-ray machines are designed to work with computers to produce digital images of the body. Most permanently installed radiography units include a special table. Some tables can be electronically rotated from the horizontal to the vertical to help position the patient.

Before x-ray film is used, it's placed in a special x-ray film holder called a **cassette** to protect it from light. The cassette slides into a slot or opening in the table. Once the film inside the cassette has been exposed to x-rays, the cassette is placed in a special machine that removes the film and processes it. The processed film is the radiograph, or x-ray.

X-rays and the Body

Images form as the x-rays either pass through the body and strike the film or are absorbed by body tissues.

- **Radiolucent** substances allow x-rays to pass through them. These structures are not dense and don't absorb much radiation. They show up as black on the film. An example is the air in the lungs.
- **Radiopaque** substances don't allow x-rays to pass through them. Some tissue is dense and absorbs much of the radiation beam instead. Such tissue appears white on x-ray film. For example, bone is a radiopaque tissue that absorbs radiation. It shows up as white on an x-ray.
- Other body substances vary in density. Examples are muscle, fat, and fluid. They appear as different shades of gray on a radiograph, because of the way each substance absorbs the x-rays.

Patient Positions

A radiograph is a two-dimensional image. However, the human body is a three-dimensional structure. For this reason, x-ray exams usually require at least two exposures taken at 90-degree angles to each other. For example, a chest x-ray generally involves one exposure from the back and another from the side. Chest x-rays can help in the diagnosis of pulmonary problems, such as pneumonia, lung cancer, emphysema, tuberculosis, and pulmonary edema, or fluid in the lungs.

Other exams may require three or more x-rays from different angles. The projection refers to the body's position in relation to the x-ray beam and the film. Table 20-1 demonstrates the standard projections used in x-ray exams.

Each projection requires the patient to be placed in a specific position. If you are legally allowed to position patients for x-rays, you should be familiar with positioning terms:

- Erect—standing
- Recumbent—lying down
- Supine—lying on the back
- Prone—lying face down
- Anterior—on the front
- Posterior—on the back
- Lateral—on the side

Table 20-1	Standard Projections Used in X-Ray Exams	
Projection (Medical Abbreviation)	**Body Position**	**Illustration (*Arrows* Show the Direction of Motion of the X-rays)**
Anteroposterior projection (AP)	Patient is erect or supine, with back to the film.	Anteroposterior projection
Posteroanterior projection (PA)	Patient is erect, facing the film.	Posteroanterior projection
Right lateral projection (RL)	Patient is erect, with right side of body nearest to the film.	Right lateral projection
Left lateral projection (LL)	Patient is erect, with left side of body nearest to the film.	Left lateral projection
Right posterior oblique projection (RPO)	Patient is erect or recumbent, rotated so the right back is nearest to the film.	Right posterior oblique projection
Left posterior oblique projection (LPO)	Patient is erect or recumbent, rotated so the left back is nearest to the film.	Left posterior oblique projection
Right anterior oblique projection (RAO)	Patient is erect or recumbent, rotated so the right front is nearest to the film.	Right anterior oblique projection
Left anterior oblique projection (LAO)	Patient is erect or recumbent, rotated so the left front is nearest to the film.	Left anterior oblique projection

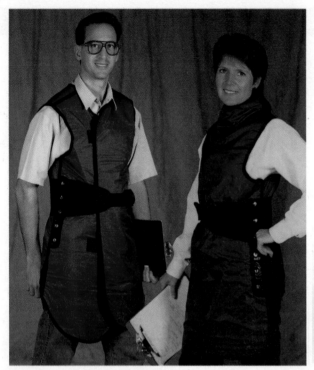
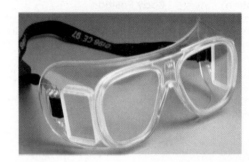
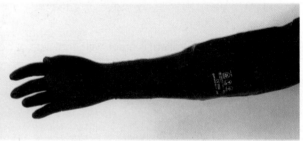

Figure 20-2 *X-ray protection equipment.* (Reprinted from Kronenberger J, Ledbetter J. *Jones & Bartlett Learning's Comprehensive Medical Assisting.* 5th ed. Burlington, MA: Jones & Bartlett Learning, LLC; 2016.)

Radiation Safety for Patients

Exposure to x-rays can damage the body's cells and genes. The harmful effects are most extreme for cells that reproduce quickly. The results of this damage may not show up for several years, however.

Pregnant women, children, and the reproductive organs of adults are at the highest risk from x-rays. It's important to follow these safety procedures to protect patients.

- Minimize the amount of exposure.
- Avoid unnecessary x-rays.
- Limit the area of the body that's exposed to radiation.
- Shield sensitive body parts, such as the gonads (organs that produce reproductive cells) and the thyroid (a gland in the neck that regulates the body's metabolism).
- Always ask female patients if they could be pregnant before taking x-rays (physician may order a pregnancy test to determine or confirm).

Radiation Safety for Clinical Staff

Patients need to be protected from radiation exposure, and the clinical staff needs to be protected also. Stay safe by following the **ALARA** principle: Do whatever is necessary to keep radiation exposure <u>a</u>s <u>l</u>ow <u>a</u>s <u>r</u>easonably <u>a</u>chievable. Here are some safety steps you and all clinical staff should follow:

- Limit the amount of time you're exposed to x-rays.
- Stay as far away from the x-rays as possible during exposure. Most facilities have a barrier for the technician to stand behind when taking the x-ray. The x-ray machine is housed in a room with lead-lined walls.

- Shield yourself using appropriate protective equipment, such as lead aprons and gloves. Figure 20-2 is an example of x-ray protection equipment.
- Avoid holding patients during exposures. If necessary, young children may be assisted by a parent wearing a lead apron.
- Wear a **dosimeter**. This is a small device you should clip to the outside of your uniform. It records the amount of radiation to which you're exposed. Your employer should supply dosimeters. They're obtained from companies that specifically monitor radiation exposure for health care workers. Figure 20-3 is an example of a dosimeter badge.
- Ensure x-ray equipment is working properly by scheduling routine maintenance.

Patient Education

Calming Patient Fears about X-Rays

Patients may be concerned about the exposure to radiation from having x-rays taken. They may worry about the effects of radiation. The medical assistant can reassure them by letting them know that the amount of radiation involved is very small and the body's exposure will be limited. Remind these patients that they will benefit from the procedure because it provides the physician valuable information for diagnosis and treatment.

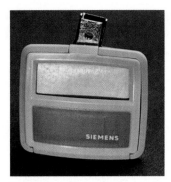

Figure 20-3 Dosimeter. (Reprinted from Kronenberger J, Ledbetter J. *Jones & Bartlett Learning's Comprehensive Medical Assisting.* 5th ed. Burlington, MA: Jones & Bartlett Learning, LLC; 2016.)

Radiology and Diagnosis

The most common diagnostic procedures in radiology are routine x-ray exams. They require little patient preparation, although you may need to explain them and answer patients' questions to reduce anxiety. Here are the preparation procedures that must be followed:

- Typically, patients must remove outer clothing from the area to be x-rayed. A gown should be provided if necessary.
- No metal objects can be worn on any area of the body that will be exposed to x-rays.
- Patients must remove jewelry and clothing with zippers, snaps, or other metal details, including underwire bras.

After patient preparations are finished, the patient is assisted into the proper position for the specific examination. In some cases, the patient may be standing near an upright film holder. In other cases, the patient will be positioned on the x-ray examination table.

After all the x-rays have been taken, the patient may be asked to wait until the x-rays are processed. This usually takes <10 minutes. If the processed x-ray films aren't clear, repeat exposures may be needed. If the x-rays are digital images, there is usually no need for the patient to wait because the images can be checked immediately.

In states where medical assistant scope of practice includes performing x-rays, further training is required. It is beneficial for all medical assistants to understand the basic steps in performing an x-ray. It may be necessary to answer initial questions from patients regarding the procedure.

Here are the general steps involved in a routine x-ray exam:

1. The film cassette is placed into the table or upright holder. A lead marker may be included to indicate which side of the patient (right or left) is being examined.
2. The patient is placed into the exact position for the specific radiograph.
3. The x-ray tube is moved to a specific distance from the film and body part.
4. Lead shields are positioned to protect the patient from radiation.
5. In the control booth, the radiographer sets the machine for the specific exposure.
6. Final instructions are given to the patient. Patients need to remain perfectly still during the exposure. The patient must hold the breath during certain x-ray positions. Remind the patient that he or she can breathe again once the x-ray has been taken.
7. The exposure is made.
8. If a different view is needed, a new film is placed in the film holder and the steps are repeated.

It is also necessary to understand the preparation of the patient for routine x-ray exams. Table 20-2 lists the preparation necessary for x-raying various body areas.

Case Questions

 Ms. Barber, the patient in the case study, will have an ECG performed; however, the physician also asked the medical assistant to schedule the patient for a chest x-ray. The patient is concerned that she may be having a heart attack and states that she does not see the need for an x-ray and asks the medical assistant if it is absolutely necessary to have the chest x-ray. If you were the medical assistant in this scenario, how would you explain the need for a chest x-ray? If the patient asks what the physician is looking for, what would you tell her?

Contrast Medium Examinations

Internal organs, like those within the abdomen, don't visualize very well on x-ray films. Many structures within the abdomen have similar absorption rates for radiation. In addition, some organs lie behind others in the abdominal cavity. These factors can make it difficult to see the different structures clearly in a two-dimensional x-ray.

In these cases, a contrast medium often is used to help differentiate between body structures. A **contrast medium** is a substance that temporarily changes the absorption rate of a particular structure to highlight a specific organ. Contrast media are introduced into the body in several ways. Here are some common ones:

- By mouth
- Intravenously
- Through a catheter

Table 20-2	Patient Preparation for Routine X-Ray Exams	
Region	**Areas to Which Preparation Applies**	**Patient Preparation**
Trunk	Chest, ribs, sternum, shoulder, scapula, clavicle, abdomen, hip, pelvis, as well as the sternoclavicular, acromioclavicular, and sacroiliac joints	Disrobing of the area and removing jewelry or clothing that might obscure parts of interest
Extremities	Fingers, thumb, hand, wrist, forearm, elbow, humerus, toes, foot, os calcis, ankle, lower leg, knee, patella, femur	Removing jewelry or clothing that might obscure parts of interest
Spine	Cervical, thoracic, or lumbar spine; sacrum, coccyx	Disrobing of the appropriate area
Head	Skull, sinuses, nasal bones, facial bones and orbits, optic foramen, mandible, temporomandibular joints, mastoid and petrous portion, and zygomatic arch	Removing eyewear, prosthetic eyes, removable dental appliances, earrings, hairpins, and hairpieces

The method used depends on the type of medium and the area of the body being examined. For example, a patient having an excretory urography will have the contrast medium injected. The anatomical structure of each kidney is evaluated as the medium passes through the urinary tract. The use of the contrast medium allows examination of each structure and its function.

Barium Studies

A patient with gastrointestinal (**GI**) symptoms may undergo barium studies to assist the physician in diagnosis. These are x-ray exams performed after parts of the patient's GI tract have been highlighted by a contrast medium called barium sulfate. The two most common barium studies are the upper GI examination and the barium enema. Figure 20-4 is an x-ray of the large intestine filled with barium.

- In an upper GI exam, the patient drinks the contrast medium. Then a series of x-rays follows the barium down the patient's esophagus, into the stomach, and into the small intestine. The barium enables the radiologist to examine the x-rays for abnormalities in each organ.
- In a barium enema, the contrast medium is injected through the rectum into the patient's large intestine, or colon. This highlights the organ when the patient's lower abdomen is x-rayed.

Barium studies are becoming less common than in the past. They have been replaced by a technology called endoscopy. Physicians now use a scope to visualize, biopsy, and even take pictures inside the esophagus, stomach, and large intestine.

Iodine—Contrast Medium

Some patients are allergic to contrast media that contain iodine. Always ask if they have an iodine allergy or if they're allergic to shellfish, which also contain iodine.

Iodine compounds are used in many areas of the body, including the kidneys and blood vessels. They're also used for some **CT** scans (computerized tomography).

Patients who have an intestinal perforation may be given an iodinated contrast medium instead of barium. That's because barium would be more troublesome to the patient if it leaked into the peritoneum (the lining of the abdominal cavity).

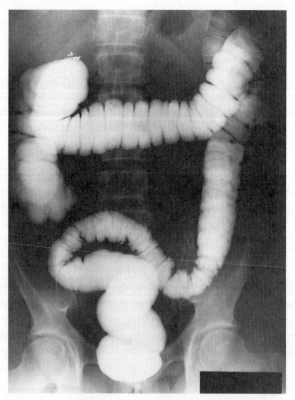

Figure 20-4   Barium-filled large intestine. (Reprinted from Kronenberger J, Ledbetter J. *Jones & Bartlett Learning's Comprehensive Medical Assisting.* 5th ed. Burlington, MA: Jones & Bartlett Learning, LLC; 2016.)

Scheduling X-Rays and Contrast Examinations

Most radiography procedures can be performed in any order, depending on what's convenient. However, some procedures must follow specific sequences. Here are some examples.

Gallbladder Exams

A patient with gallbladder symptoms may go through a series of tests. They begin with a simple, noninvasive oral cholecystogram. This is an x-ray of the gallbladder after the patient drinks a contrast medium. More complex procedures are performed later, such as an operative cholangiogram—an x-ray of the bile ducts after a contrast medium is injected during a surgical procedure.

Gastrointestinal Exams

If an endoscopic study of the upper gastrointestinal tract is ordered in addition to barium studies, the endoscopy is usually scheduled before any procedure involving barium. That way, the barium will not obstruct or interfere with the visualization of internal structures.

If an upper GI and a barium enema are ordered, the upper GI is usually scheduled first. But if results are needed quickly, the order is reversed. That's because barium from the small intestine will leave the body through the colon—and the second test can't be done as long as barium from the first test is in the organ to be examined.

Other Radiographic Diagnostic Procedures

Along with routine x-rays and contrast exams, several other procedures are used to visualize body structures for the purpose of diagnosis. These procedures include the following:

- Fluoroscopy
- Computed tomography
- Sonography
- Magnetic resonance imaging
- Nuclear medicine

Fluoroscopy

Fluoroscopy uses a continuous beam of x-rays to observe movement within the body. The image is in "real time" and is displayed on a monitor so the body part and its functioning can be seen in detail. The process may be highlighted by a contrast medium—for example, barium moving through the digestive system. Iodine compounds injected into the bloodstream allow the beating of the heart or blood flow through specific blood vessels to be examined.

Fluoroscopy also is used as an aid in treatment. Some ways it can help are in

- Reducing (setting) fractures
- Implanting devices such as pacemakers
- Inserting feeding tubes and other tubes into a patient's body

Computed Tomography

Computed tomography (**CT**) is a procedure that feeds x-rays from a tube circling the patient into a computer. All structures in each x-ray are blurred out except those desired. The computer analyzes these x-rays to create a series of cross-sectional "slices" of an organ or the body. Some CT machines can create three-dimensional images, so organs can be viewed from all angles. CT scans may be done with or without a contrast medium. Figure 20-5 is a CT scanner machine.

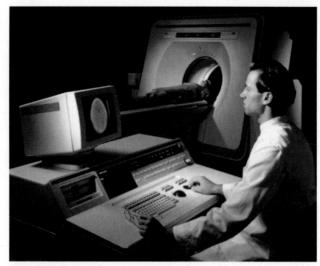

Figure 20-5 A CT scanner. (Reprinted from Kronenberger J, Ledbetter J. *Jones & Bartlett Learning's Comprehensive Medical Assisting.* 5th ed. Burlington, MA: Jones & Bartlett Learning, LLC; 2016.)

Sonography

Sonography, or **ultrasound**, uses high-frequency sound waves, instead of x-rays, to create images of the body, usually with the help of a computer. These images may be still or real-time, moving images. Sonography is often used to study heart function, abdominal structures, and pelvic structures. It's also commonly used in prenatal testing to visualize the developing fetus. Many obstetricians schedule at least one sonogram before the fourth month of pregnancy. Figure 20-6 shows a sonogram.

Magnetic Resonance Imaging

Magnetic resonance imaging (**MRI**) is a combination of high-intensity magnetic fields, radio waves, and computer analysis used to create cross-sectional images of the body. Like ultrasound, MRI doesn't use x-rays. The image depends on the chemical makeup of the body. MRI is used commonly for studying the central nervous system, joint structures, and a variety of other studies. Some MRI studies require contrast media.

During the MRI, the patient is enclosed for a long period of time in a machine that makes knocking and whirring noises. Some facilities use open MRI, which does not make a patient feel as claustrophobic as a closed MRI. Patients with a fear of enclosed places may require a mild sedative before a closed MRI. Figure 20-7 is an open MRI machine.

Nuclear Medicine

In nuclear medicine, the body is injected with small amounts of radionuclides, materials that emit radiation. The radionuclides are designed to concentrate in specific areas of the body for short periods of time. Special computer cameras detect the radiation and create an image. This method often is used to examine the thyroid, brain, lungs, liver, spleen, kidney, bone, and breast. These examinations are commonly called scans.

PET scans and **SPECT** scans are two sophisticated types of nuclear medicine studies.

- Positron emission tomography (PET) uses specialized equipment to produce detailed sectional images of physiological processes in the body.
- Single photon emission computed tomography (SPECT) produces sectional images of the body as detectors move around the patient.

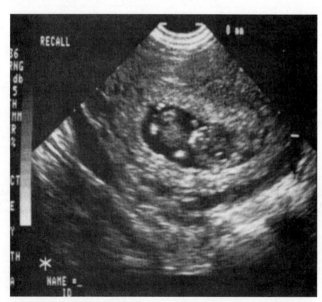

Figure 20-6 A sonogram. (Reprinted from Kronenberger J, Ledbetter J. *Jones & Bartlett Learning's Comprehensive Medical Assisting.* 5th ed. Burlington, MA: Jones & Bartlett Learning, LLC; 2016.)

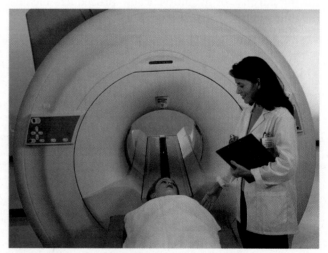

Figure 20-7 An open MRI. (Reprinted from Kronenberger J, Ledbetter J. *Jones & Bartlett Learning's Comprehensive Medical Assisting.* 5th ed. Burlington, MA: Jones & Bartlett Learning, LLC; 2016.)

Both procedures are useful in the early detection of physiological and cellular abnormalities, such as those associated with cancer.

Teleradiology

Teleradiology is the electronic transmission of radiological images, such as x-rays and CTs, from one location to another. Many institutions use a picture archiving and communication system (**PACS**) in which computers store and transmit images. Images can be transmitted using standard telephone lines, satellite connections, or local area networks (LANs).

Teleradiology has led to improved patient care. Physicians working on difficult cases can send images and information to specialists in other locations. This allows them to obtain expert opinions in a short period of time. For example, rural physicians may use teleradiology to send images taken in their office to a radiologist in a distant location for interpretation and consultation.

Radiology and Treatment

Radiological techniques are used to treat cancer and other conditions. Here are some examples of how radiology helps in treating some specific conditions. For many patients, these techniques are so effective, there's no need for surgery. In some cases, they may be lifesaving.

- Percutaneous transluminal coronary angioplasty (**PTCA**) is also known as balloon angioplasty. In this technique, the lumen of a coronary artery is enlarged using a balloon-tipped catheter. Guided by fluoroscopy, the catheter is placed at the point of partial occlusion (blockage) or stenosis (narrowing) of the artery. The balloon is then inflated, compressing the plaque against the sides of the artery. After the balloon is deflated, the catheter is removed. The diameter of the artery remains larger, improving blood flow.
- Laser angioplasty uses laser beams to remove deposits in vessels with the aid of fluoroscopy.
- Vascular stents are plastic or wire tubes inserted into a constricted or narrowed area of a blood vessel. The stent provides support and keeps the vessel open. Fluoroscopy is used to guide the placement of the stent.
- Embolization is a technique for artificially stopping active bleeding from a blood vessel. It also may be used to reduce blood flow to a diseased area or organ.

Radiation Therapy

For many years, radiation therapy has been a major force in the fight against cancer. In radiation therapy, high-energy radiation is used to destroy cancer cells. Because the radiation is so intense, it also may destroy adjacent normal cells. Treatments must be planned carefully and precisely by a radiologist, taking into account the following:

- The amount of radiation
- The frequency to be used
- The number of exposures during a given period of time

The area of the body to be exposed to radiation must be defined exactly so each treatment is identical. The patient is placed in a position described in the treatment plan, and an exact amount of radiation is directed at the treatment site by a technician. Usually, the patient has little to do but lie still.

The technician may make a small mark on the body to indicate exactly where the radiation should be directed. This helps the technician make sure that the radiation is put in the same spot every time.

Side Effects of Radiation

Most patients have some side effects from radiation therapy. Once the treatment plan is completed, most of the side effects disappear. Side effects may include

- Hair loss
- Weight loss
- Loss of appetite
- Skin changes
- Digestive system disturbances

The Medical Assistant's Role

As a clinical medical assistant, you're in an ideal position to help reduce patient anxiety over radiology procedures. You can do this by

- Giving patients information about procedures they don't understand
- Making patients feel comfortable enough to ask questions
- Answering questions using terms patients can understand

You also may have responsibilities that directly involve you with the procedures. These responsibilities may include the following:

- Assisting with examinations
- Handling, processing, and storing film
- Scheduling appointments
- Providing patient education

Educating Patients

Being sensitive to patients' feelings is one of the greatest talents you can possess. It should be an important part of every medical professional's training and personality.

Patients often must undergo procedures they don't understand. The technical aspects of radiology can make understanding its procedures especially difficult. Sometimes, patients feel they don't know enough even to ask the right questions.

One of the areas that the medical assistant can assist the radiology patient is explaining what to do after the procedure so the patient does not experience any distress. For example, a barium enema can lead to constipation if a patient does not drink enough fluids after the test.

As a medical assistant, you can affect patients' emotional response to a radiology procedure by explaining what to expect. Use everyday language, not technical medical terms. Keep your explanations simple, and leave the details to the physician. Here are some important topics you should cover:

- What preparations are needed prior to the procedure
- What to expect during the procedure
- What to do after the procedure

Assisting with Radiological Procedures

There are several ways you may be required to assist with radiological examinations:

- Telling the patient what clothing to remove or assisting with clothing removal as needed.
- Helping the patient take the position for the procedure. Emphasize the importance of remaining still and following instructions for breathing.
- Performing specific procedures, such as bone or chest radiography, as permitted by your state's laws and your education and training.
- Placing film in an automatic processor and reloading new film into the cassette.
- Distributing or filing radiographs and reports appropriately.

Handling and Storing Film

Automated processing machines are used to develop most x-ray film. This helps eliminate human error and simplifies the process. Processing machines usually can produce a developed image in <2 minutes.

Processors differ, according to their manufacturers. You need to be proficient in the operation of your facility's equipment.

No matter how your office develops x-ray film, here are some general tips for handling and storing it:

- Protect unexposed film from moisture, heat, and light by storing it in a cool, dry place. A lead-lined box is the best storage device.
- Open exposed or unexposed film packets in a darkroom, using only the darkroom light for illumination. The film must be placed in a cassette before using it in any areas outside the darkroom. Intensifying screens in the cassette are used to reduce the amount of exposure required.
- Store exposed film in special sleeves or envelopes of the right size. Be sure the film has been labeled with the date and the patient's name.

Transfer of Study Information

Any radiographic images obtained on site for use by the physician become part of the patient's medical record. Digital images can be saved in a computer file or on a compact disc (CD).

However, in many cases, a physician sends a patient to another office for x-rays or other diagnostic tests. Radiological films belong to the site where the study was performed. The physician or radiologist who examines the films generally writes a summary report of the examination findings. This report is sent to the referring physician. You may need to obtain the patient's permission to have the summary of findings sent to the office physician.

For a short-term referral, the physician who examines the films usually returns the films to the referring physician. When a patient needs a copy of their reports because they changed physicians, they may request the information after submitting a written request. The patient also may obtain copies of the actual x-rays. You may be responsible for filling these requests.

MAMMOGRAPHY

Mammography, or x-ray examination of the breast, is used as a screening tool for breast cancer. Each breast is compressed in a special device to even the thickness and allow the best diagnostic image. Using the mammogram as a guide, the physician can do a needle biopsy to withdraw small amounts of cells from suspicious areas for study under a microscope. Mammography thus makes it possible to detect breast cancer in a minimally invasive way.

The American Cancer Society has developed specific guidelines for mammography. By age 40, women should have a screening mammogram. Women who have no symptoms (such as palpable breast masses or masses shown on previous mammograms) should have mammograms on the following schedule:

- For ages 40 to 49, routine screening every 1 to 2 years
- For ages 50 and over, routine screening every year

Figure 20-8 is a mammography machine.

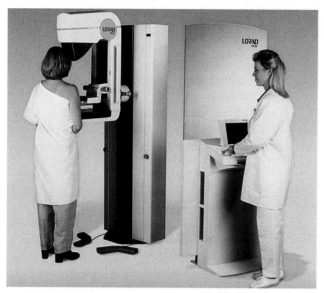

Figure 20-8 Mammography machine. (Reprinted from Kronenberger J, Ledbetter J. *Jones & Bartlett Learning's Comprehensive Medical Assisting.* 5th ed. Burlington, MA: Jones & Bartlett Learning, LLC; 2016.)

Cultural Connection

According to HHS, the federal Department of Health and Human Services, in the United States, heart disease is one of the leading causes of death for adults of all races. African American men are 30% more likely to die from heart disease than non-Hispanic white men. African American adults, both men and women, are 40% more likely to have high blood pressure and are less likely to have their high blood pressure under control. High blood pressure is a significant finding in most patients with heart disease. Years ago, men of all races were more likely to have heart disease than women. Now heart disease is the leading cause of death for American women.

DIAGNOSING CARDIOVASCULAR DISORDERS

Cardiovascular disease is a major cause of illness and death. A **cardiologist** is a physician who specializes in disorders of the heart. Many patients with chronic cardiac conditions are referred to the cardiology office for treatment and follow-up. However, some of these patients are seen in family practice or internal medical offices. You need to understand the common tests and procedures that are ordered for the diagnosis and treatment of cardiac patients.

Testing for cardiovascular disorders may be either invasive or noninvasive.

- Invasive techniques require entering the body by using a tube, needle, or other device.
- Noninvasive techniques don't involve entering the body or breaking the skin.

Depending on the patient's symptoms, testing may be basic and can be done easily during the general physical examination by auscultating the heart and chest.

The physician usually begins the cardiovascular examination with a review of the patient's history and the reason for the visit. She reviews the patient's vital signs and medications, noting any allergies to medications and other substances. The physician also inspects the patient to evaluate

- The general appearance
- The circulation and any swelling of extremities
- The color of the skin
- Any distention of the jugular vein (a large vein on each side of the neck that drains blood to the heart)

Palpation is used to evaluate the efficiency of the circulatory pathways and peripheral pulses. Using a stethoscope, the physician auscultates the sounds made as blood flows through the heart and the heart valves open and close. This allows the physician to detect abnormal heart sounds such as bruits or **murmurs** (abnormal sounds made as blood moves through the heart valves).

Common Cardiovascular Tests

After an initial exam, the physician may order additional tests that can be performed in the medical office, including chest radiography and electrocardiogram (ECG). Their results may reveal a need for further testing using more sophisticated procedures.

Some of these tests may take place outside the medical office. For example, invasive procedures are performed at an outpatient surgical center or hospital. Table 20-3 shows common invasive and noninvasive cardiovascular tests.

The Electrocardiogram

One of the most valuable diagnostic tools for evaluating the heart is the electrocardiogram (**ECG**). All muscle movements produce electrical impulses. The ECG picks up the electrical signals made by the heart muscle and records them on a graph. This test is often part of a routine physical exam. It's also performed as needed for a patient with chest discomfort or other signs and symptoms of possible cardiac problems.

ECGs help the physician in diagnosing

- Ischemia (insufficient blood flow)
- Delays in impulse conduction
- Hypertrophy of the cardiac chambers
- Arrhythmias (irregular heartbeats)

Table 20-4 summarizes the kinds of arrhythmias ECGs can detect. ECGs are not used to detect disorders

Table 20-3	Common Cardiovascular Tests	
Cardiac Test	**Description**	**Uses**
Chest radiography (noninvasive)	Diagnostic tool using high-energy waves	Detect and follow cardiovascular or other diseases
Electrocardiogram (ECG) (noninvasive)	Graph of electrical activity of the heart from various angles	Obtain a baseline or assess an acute situation
Holter monitor (noninvasive)	Continuous monitor of heart rhythm via portable device worn for an extended period during daily activities	Detect symptoms of rhythm disturbances not shown on ECG or during physical examination
Stress test (noninvasive)	ECG of heart rhythm during exercise on graded treadmill or stationary bicycle	Help diagnose patients with known or suspected heart problems
Echocardiogram (noninvasive)	Ultrasound of heart using sound waves generated by a transducer	Diagnose suspected or known valvular disease, severity of heart failure, or cardiomyopathy (weakness of heart muscle)
Cardiac catheterization (invasive)	Insertion of a catheter into the heart	Diagnose or determine severity of heart disease or atherosclerosis
Coronary arteriography (invasive)	Injection of contrast medium into coronary arteries (after cardiac catheterization) to see, via a monitor, any obstruction of arteries	Assess heart disease and damage after myocardial infarction, MI (death of the heart muscle)

Table 20-4	Arrhythmias	
Type of Arrhythmia	**Indications and Symptoms**	**Possible Causes and Consequences**
Sinus tachycardia	Abnormally rapid heartbeat (100–180 bpm) resulting in decreased ventricular filling and low blood pressure	Dehydration, extreme anxiety, heart failure, or hemorrhage; can also result from intense exercise
Sinus bradycardia	Abnormally slow heartbeat (<60 bpm), but with a normal rhythm	Can result from myocardial infarction or certain medications (such as digoxin); is also often seen in well-conditioned athletes
Paroxysmal atrial tachycardia (**PAT**)	Sudden, temporary onset of a heartbeat of 180–250 bpm; often accompanied by patient weakness and the feeling of a pounding or fluttering in the chest	Extreme anxiety or stress, excessive stimulants (such as nicotine or caffeine); also can have no known cause
Premature atrial contraction (**PAC**)	An electrical impulse starts in the heart before the next expected beat; patient may complain of feeling an "extra" or "skipped" beat	Thyroid disease, heart disease, central nervous system imbalances, stress, or excessive use of stimulants
Premature ventricular contraction (**PVC**)	Ventricles contract before the next expected beat; patient may complain of feeling an "extra" or "skipped" beat; can be more serious than PAC	Electrolyte imbalances, caffeine or other stimulants, anxiety, or stress; may also be a sign of pulmonary disease or an injured or diseased heart
Ventricular tachycardia (V tach)	Heart rate exceeds 100 bpm with 3 or more PVCs per minute; results in decreased cardiac output; patient may complain of pressure and the feeling that the heart is "beating out of my chest"	Similar to causes of PVCs; the longer V tach lasts, the more serious it is because cardiac output drops and the blood supply to organs is decreased; unchecked V tach can lead to V fib
Ventricular fibrillation (V fib)	Ventricles begin twitching, making the heart's pumping action ineffective and stopping the circulation of blood	The most serious of all arrhythmias; death will result if not immediately treated with CPR, a defibrillator, or cardiac drugs

in the heart's anatomy, such as those that may produce heart murmurs.

During the ECG, you may be responsible for explaining the procedure to the patient. The patient will lie on her back on the examining table, with her arms, chest, and lower legs accessible. (While patients are waiting, and after the electrodes are placed, you will offer female patients a drape to cover the chest area.) Electrodes are applied to the patient's arms, legs, and chest. These electrodes measure the electrical impulses of the heart. There are 10 electrodes. Combinations of these electrodes measure the heart's electrical activity in 12 different ways, called leads. The ECG machine converts the electrical impulses from each lead into markings on special graph paper.

The ECG tracing is printed on graph paper that is either red or black with a white coating that is sensitive to heat. Graph lines are printed over the white coating and appear as small blocks. Thicker lines outline every five small blocks. On standard ECG paper, each small block is 1 mm square. The large blocks are 5 mm long on each side. Each small square is 1 × 1 mm in size. Every fifth line is marked with a darker line to make a cube of 5 × 5 mm.

Some ECG machines contain a stylus that heats and melts the white coating. This exposes the background beneath to record the movement of the stylus as electrical impulses are detected. In newer ECG machines, the stylus uses ink to mark the ECG paper.

Each small horizontal line on the paper represents 0.04 seconds of time. (One large block therefore represents 0.2 seconds and five large blocks measure 1 second of time.) Each small vertical line represents 0.1 mV of electricity. After the heart's electrical activity is traced on the paper, the physician can read the graph to determine the patient's heart rate and the time required for the electrical impulses to spread through the heart.

Figure 20-9 shows a segment of ECG graph paper with the measurements.

Placing the Electrodes

A standard system of electrode placement records the electrical activity of the heart. Each lead records the heart's electrical activity from a different angle. The recordings these leads make on the graph paper give the physician a fairly complete "view" of the entire heart.

Wires from the ECG machine attach to the 10 electrodes. Four wires are labeled and color-coded for attachment to electrodes on the limbs. Six electrodes are placed on the anterior chest wall.

- One limb electrode is placed on each arm and leg. You should use muscular areas such as the calves, outer thighs, and the arm above the elbow. The electrodes should not be placed on bony areas. The right leg electrode is the grounding lead. It helps reduce electrical interference and keeps the average voltage for the patient the same as that of the machine. The other limb wires are attached to electrodes on the patient's left leg, right arm, and left arm.
- The chest electrodes must be placed in exact locations for an accurate ECG recording.

The skin where the electrodes are applied must be clean and dry. Body oils, lotions, and sweat must be removed with an alcohol wipe. Body hair generally can be separated by hand to make sure the electrodes make good contact with the skin. However, patients who are extremely hairy may need to have areas on which electrodes are placed shaved or trimmed. Electrodes also cannot be placed on open wounds, bandages, or skin that has recently healed. In such cases, place the electrode as close to the proper site as possible and inform the physician when this occurs.

What Electrocardiogram Leads Measure

Different combinations of the electrodes provide 12 different leads to show the electrical activity of the heart. There are three main types of leads:

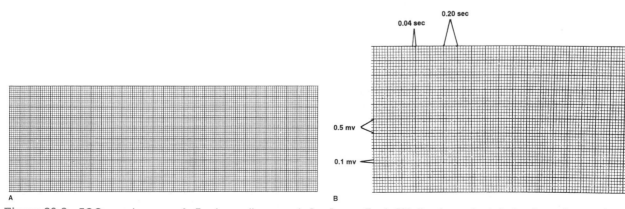

Figure 20-9 ECG graph paper. **A.** Each small square is 1 × 1 mm. Each fifth line is marked darker to make a cube of 5 × 5 mm (actual size). **B.** Horizontally, the graph paper represents time in seconds. Each small square represents 0.04 seconds, and each large square represents 0.2 seconds. Five large squares = 1 second (5 × 0.2). (Reprinted from Kronenberger J, Ledbetter J. *Jones & Bartlett Learning's Comprehensive Medical Assisting.* 5th ed. Burlington, MA: Jones & Bartlett Learning, LLC; 2016.)

- Standard bipolar leads. These leads measure electrical activity picked up from two-limb electrodes. The standard bipolar leads allow a frontal view of the heart's electrical activity from side to side. Roman numerals are used to describe these leads, which are known as leads I, II, and III.
- Augmented unipolar leads. These leads result from a combination of the impulses measured from all three-limb electrodes—RA, LA, and LL. (Remember that RL is the ground lead.) They allow visualization of the heart from a frontal view, top to bottom. They're called leads aVR, aVL, and aVF.
- Unipolar precordial leads. These leads measure electrical impulses picked up from the chest electrodes. Each lead measures the electrical activity from a specific part of the heart. The chest leads are referred to using numbers from 1 to 6—for example, V_1, V_2, and so on.

Electrocardiography Abbreviations

Like many other diagnostic tests, there's a special vocabulary associated with the ECG. It's important for you to become familiar with the common abbreviations used in performing ECGs.

- RA—right arm electrode
- LA—left arm electrode
- LL—left leg electrode
- RL—right leg electrode
- V_1–V_6—chest electrodes and leads (each number stands for a different position on the chest)
- aVR—augmented voltage right arm
- aVL—augmented voltage left arm
- aVF—augmented voltage left leg

Table 20-5 provides information about each lead and what it measures.

Electrocardiogram Chest Leads Attachment

If the chest ECG electrodes are not attached in the right places, the ECG leads may not provide an accurate tracing of the heart's electrical activity. The more you practice, the easier it will be to remember where to place the leads. But while you are learning, it might be helpful to take notes to review before working with a patient. Write the abbreviations for the chest leads on the left side of a 3 × 5 index card. Next to each one, write the location on the body.

V_1 fourth intercostal (between the ribs) space at right margin of sternum

V_2 fourth intercostal space at left margin of sternum

V_3 midway between V_2 and V_4

V_4 fifth intercostal space at junction of left midclavicular line

V_5 horizontal level of V_4 at left anterior axillary line

V_6 horizontal level of V_4 and V_5 at midaxillary line

Table 20-5	Lead Types and What They Measure	
Lead Type	**Lead**	**What's Measured**
Standard bipolar leads	Lead I	Electrical activity between LA and RA
	Lead II	Electrical activity between LL and RA
	Lead III	Electrical activity between LL and LA
Augmented unipolar leads	aVR	The electrical activity from LA + LL directed to RA
	aVL	The electrical activity from RA + LL directed to LA
	aVF	The electrical activity from RA + LA directed to LL
Unipolar precordial leads (chest leads)	V_1	The electrical activity from electrode V_1
	V_2	The electrical activity from electrode V_2
	V_3	The electrical activity from electrode V_3
	V_4	The electrical activity from electrode V_4
	V_5	The electrical activity from electrode V_5
	V_6	The electrical activity from electrode V_6

Study Skill

One way to remember the placement of the chest leads is to draw a diagram of the chest and put a mark at each of the six lead locations. Draw details like the ribs and sternum so that you have a clear understanding of the exact location of each lead. Write out the location of each chest lead. This tip will assist you when you are trying to learn anatomy also.

Interpreting the Electrocardiogram

It's not your responsibility to give patients ECG results. But you should still know how to basically interpret an ECG. During the ECG procedure, the graph of electrical activity from each lead is printed on the ECG paper. The paper speed on the machine is set at 25 mm/s. This allows the electrical impulses, recorded as waves on the ECG paper, to be measured. The blocks on the paper are used as a reference (each small block is 0.04 seconds). Each lead is marked clearly on the ECG paper as it is printed. In some cases, specific codes are printed on the paper to identify the wave from each lead.

Table 20-6 shows the standard codes for ECG leads.

Table 20-6 Coding ECG Leads

Lead	Code	Lead	Code
I	.	V_1	-.
II	..	V_2	-..
III	...	V_3	-...
aVR	-	V_4	-....
aVL	–	V_5	-.....
aVF	—	V_6	-......

If the ECG is performed correctly, the physician will be able to examine the wave forms that occur at different parts of the cardiac cycle, the pattern of events in the heart from the beginning of one heart beat to the beginning of the next. Several wave forms are examined. They include the following:

- P wave—This impulse measures the contraction of the atria, or upper chambers of the heart, at the beginning of the cardiac cycle, as the heart begins the process of pumping blood.
- P–R interval—This part of the wave form shows the electrical activity of the atria as they pump out blood.
- R wave—This measures the electrical activity through the left ventricle of the heart.
- QRS complex—The QRS segment of the wave form records the electrical activity of the ventricles (the lower, pumping chambers of the heart) as they pump out blood to the body.
- S–T segment—This represents the time period between the end of the contraction of the ventricles and the beginning of the period (T wave) when the ventricles are resting.
- T wave—This wave shows the resting period of the heart before the next cardiac cycle begins.
- U wave—This small "extra" wave is sometimes seen after the T wave in someone whose heart has a slow recovery time because he has a low potassium level or some other metabolic problem.

Figure 20-10 demonstrates the cardiac cycle waves, segments, and intervals.

The Electrocardiogram: What Is the Physician Looking For?

When interpreting the ECG, the physician takes into consideration the following:

- Heart rate, or how fast the heart is beating
- Heart rhythm, the regularity of cardiac cycles and intervals
- Axis, or the position of the heart and the direction of electrical movement through the heart
- Hypertrophy, enlarged size of the heart

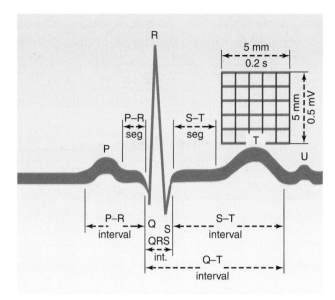

Figure 20-10 The cardiac cycle waves, segments, and intervals. (Reprinted from Cohen BJ. *Medical Terminology: An Illustrated Guide.* Burlington, MA: Jones & Bartlett Learning, LLC; 2003, with permission.)

- Ischemia, a decrease in blood supply to an area of the heart
- Infarction, the death of heart muscle resulting in a loss of blood flow to that area of the heart resulting in loss of function

Rhythm Strip

Sometimes, the physician requests a **rhythm strip** to provide more information for a particular problem. This is a long strip recording the heart activity for a certain lead or combination of leads. Most ECG machines have a button that automatically records the 12 view in the 12-lead ECG. However, for some machines, you may need to use the manual mode to obtain a rhythm strip. See Figure 20-11.

Getting a Good Electrocardiogram

You are responsible for obtaining good quality ECG tracings and avoiding artifacts. An **artifact** is an abnormal signal that doesn't represent the electrical activity of the heart during the cardiac cycle. Artifacts can result from

- Movement of the patient
- Mechanical problems with the ECG machine
- Improper technique
- Loose electrodes
- Broken cables or wires
- 60-Cycle (AC) interference

Table 20-7 describes three types of artifacts, what they look like, and how to prevent them.

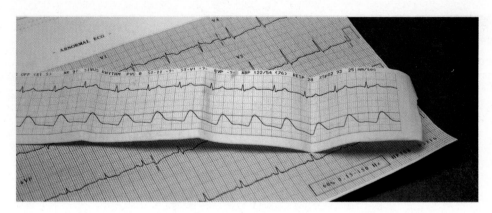

Figure 20-11 Rhythm strip. (Image from Shutterstock.)

Table 20-7	Types of Artifacts		
Artifact	**Possible Cause**	**How to Prevent Problems**	**Example of Appearance**
Wandering baseline	Electrodes too tight or too loose; tension on electrodes	Apply electrodes properly; drape wires over patient.	**WANDERING BASELINE**
	Electrodes dirty or corroded; gel used when applying electrodes to the patient has dried out	Clean and reapply electrodes or apply new electrodes.	
	Machine is picking up patient's breathing movements	Reposition and reapply electrode.	**SOMATIC MUSCLE TREMOR**
	Poor skin preparation; skin has oil, lotion, or excessive hair.	Repeat skin preparation and reapply electrodes.	
Somatic muscle tremor	Patient cannot remain still because of tremors.	Reassure patient; explain procedure and stress the need to keep still; patients with tremors or disease may be unable to stay motionless.	
Alternating current interference	Improperly grounded ECG machine	Check cables to ensure machine is grounded properly before beginning test.	**AC INTERFERENCE**
	Electrical interference in room	Move patient or unplug appliances in immediate area.	
	Dangling lead wires	Arrange wires along contours of patient's body.	

Wandering baseline, somatic muscle tremor, and alternating current (AC) interference. (Reprinted from Kronenberger J, Ledbetter J. *Jones & Bartlett Learning's Comprehensive Medical Assisting.* 5th ed. Burlington, MA: Jones & Bartlett Learning, LLC; 2016.)

Many patients may be anxious about having an electrocardiogram performed especially if they have never had one done before. They may be concerned because they don't understand the technology involved in the procedure. The term electrocardiogram brings to mind the word electricity. Some patients might actually believe that electricity will be emitted from the machine into their body. You can simply reassure the patient that no electricity will be put into their body. The ECG machine is designed to pick up the electrical activity generated by the patient's heart. Do not use medical language that the patient may not understand. Be simple in your explanation. Tell the patient that the record of the electrical signals from the heart provides information that gives the physician a good picture of how the heart is working.

As you talk, make sure your own body language shows you are listening and attentive to your patient's concerns. If the patient still refuses the procedure, tell the physician. The physician may be able to provide a convincing explanation for why it's necessary.

Electrode Maintenance

Most ECG machines have a patient cable that allows the use of disposable sensors. A clip at the end of each lead wire is attached to a sensor. When the ECG is completed, the sensors are discarded. If your ECG machine uses reusable electrodes, you need to thoroughly clean the metal electrodes and rubber straps with each use.

Holter Monitor

A Holter monitor is a portable ECG device that can be worn comfortably for long periods of time without interfering with daily activities. In many cases, an ECG that records the electrical activity of the heart for a brief moment in the medical office doesn't reveal cardiac problems. The Holter monitor is especially useful in diagnosing intermittent cardiac arrhythmias and dysfunctions because it records the electrical activity of the heart over periods of 24 hours or more. The Holter monitor is named after physicist Norman J. Holter, who invented telemetric cardiac monitoring in 1949. Clinical use started in the early 1960s. Figure 20-12 shows an example of a Holter monitor that a patient would have applied and wear for a designated period of time to record the heart's activity throughout the day and night.

The Holter monitor has two different settings:

- Continuous recording—The monitor can be set to record throughout the time the patient is wearing the monitor.

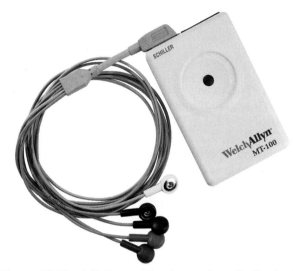

Figure 20-12 A Holter monitor. (Image from Shutterstock.)

- Incident recording—The monitor may be set to record only when the patient presses a button called the incident or event button. Patients press the button when they feel symptoms.

When instructing the patient on using a Holter monitor, make sure to explain what to do in case of problems. A flashing light on the monitor indicates a lead is loose, or an electrode has lost contact. If the patient notices right away, the patient can press on the electrodes to try to reestablish contact. You need to remind the patient to call the medical office right away if any problems are noticed.

Case Question

The ECG and chest x-ray that the patient, Ms. Barber, had didn't reveal any significant abnormalities so the physician is requesting that the patient have a Holter monitor test performed. The medical assistant is applying the electrodes and explaining the test to the patient. She asks what the reason is for this test since her ECG was normal. What would you tell her?

The Holter Diary

When the patient wears a Holter monitor, he or she must keep a diary of daily activities. Patients who press a button when they feel symptoms must record the event or activity that was occurring at the time of the symptoms. All types of activities and the times they took place should be recorded, including

- Working quietly at a desk
- Driving a car
- Eating a meal
- Watching television
- Sleeping

- Elimination
- Sexual activity
- Laughter
- Anger

The physician will interpret the ECG tracing recorded by the Holter monitor and compare these findings to the activities recorded in the diary. This helps to determine what activities, if any, precipitate cardiac arrhythmias.

To ensure an accurate test, tell patients to avoid using electrical devices, such as electric razors or toothbrushes, while wearing the monitor. Emphasize that they also should keep the electrodes dry and in contact with their skin at all times. Patients never should move an electrode or bathe, shower, or swim while wearing the monitor.

Other Cardiac Diagnostic Tests

Physicians often don't rely on one specific test to diagnose problems. They may need to gather information about heart function by looking at the results of several different tests. Many tests for diagnosing cardiovascular conditions typically are performed outside the medical office.

You've already read about x-rays and how they can provide information about the structures of internal body organs. This includes the heart. Other cardiac tests include

- Cardiac stress test
- Echocardiography
- Cardiac catheterization and coronary arteriography

Cardiac Stress Test

The physician orders a cardiac stress test to measure the response of the cardiac muscle to increased demands for oxygen. The patient is attached to an ECG monitor for constant tracing while performing physical activity. The heart is usually tested with the patient walking on a treadmill. The rate or angle of the walk or run is increased periodically during the test. The stress test also may be performed with the patient pedaling a stationary bicycle. The patient's blood pressure is monitored before, during, and after the test.

Echocardiography

Echocardiography uses sound waves to provide an image of the patient's heart. A small device called a transducer generates the sound waves. The waves pass through the cardiac chambers, walls, and valves and are transmitted back to a monitor for interpretation.

The **echocardiogram**, or image of the heart created by the sound waves, helps the physician diagnose valve disease and other defects in the heart. Echocardiograms also help in the diagnosis of

- The severity of heart disease
- The severity of cardiomyopathy
- Injuries to the heart in patients with trauma

Only the most specialized cardiac medical offices have the equipment and personnel (ultrasonographer) to obtain an echocardiogram. In most instances, your role will be to schedule an outpatient procedure and give the patient any instructions required by the facility. Usually, no patient preparations are needed for the echocardiogram.

Cardiac Catheterization

Cardiac catheterization is a common invasive procedure used to diagnose or treat conditions affecting circulation in the coronary arteries. It involves the insertion of a flexible tube called a catheter into a blood vessel in either the arm or the groin. The physician gently guides the tube toward the heart. It may be performed on patients with various cardiac symptoms, including

- Shortness of breath
- Angina
- Dizziness
- Palpitations
- Fluttering in the chest
- Rapid heartbeat

This procedure typically is used to determine the severity or cause of the cardiac problem. It is not performed in the medical office. However, you may be responsible for scheduling a cardiac catheterization at a local outpatient facility or hospital. You also will need to give the patient any instructions required by the facility.

If the procedure is for treatment, it must be done at an inpatient facility that has immediate access to open heart surgical equipment and personnel in the event of an emergency.

Coronary Arteriography

This procedure typically is performed after cardiac catheterization. Once the catheter is in place, a contrast medium is injected to reveal the heart's chambers, valves, great vessels, and coronary arteries on a monitor. If atherosclerotic plaques are found, an angioplasty may be performed or scheduled for later.

 # RESPIRATORY DISORDERS

The respiratory system works closely with the cardiovascular system to deliver oxygen to every cell in the body. The upper airways, bronchi (two main passages that move air into the lungs), alveoli, and other respiratory structures come into contact with air from the environment. In healthy individuals, body defense mechanisms protect the body from airborne disease and illness. However, disease can occur when the body is overwhelmed by cigarette smoke, air pollution, allergens, infectious organisms, or other irritants.

Respiratory disorders often are grouped according to their location in the body.

- Disorders of the upper respiratory tract involve the structures of the upper respiratory tract, including the nose, throat, and larynx. Common respiratory disorders are caused by infectious microorganisms or allergies. Examples include acute rhinitis, sinusitis, and tonsillitis.
- Lower respiratory tract disorders may be acute or chronic. Acute diseases of the lower respiratory tract include bronchitis and pneumonia. Examples of chronic diseases are asthma, chronic bronchitis, and emphysema, which are often grouped together as **COPD**, Chronic Obstructive Pulmonary Disease.

Figure 20-13 shows the upper and lower respiratory system.

 # RESPIRATORY TESTING

Many patients with respiratory conditions are seen in family practice medical offices. You need to understand some of the common tests and procedures required for diagnosing and treating respiratory conditions.

The traditional examination of the chest consists of inspection, palpation, percussion, and auscultation. During this examination, the patient must be sitting up. All clothing should be removed from the waist up. The patient should be given a gown and draped appropriately.

If the examination reveals any abnormalities or suspicious findings, such as crackling or wheezing sounds in the lungs, the physician may order additional respiratory tests. Two common respiratory tests performed in the medical office are

- Pulmonary function tests
- Oximetry

Pulmonary Function Tests

Pulmonary function tests are procedures for analyzing how well the patient moves air in and out of the lungs. A **spirometer** is a device used to measure the amount of air that is breathed in or out. The patient breathes into a

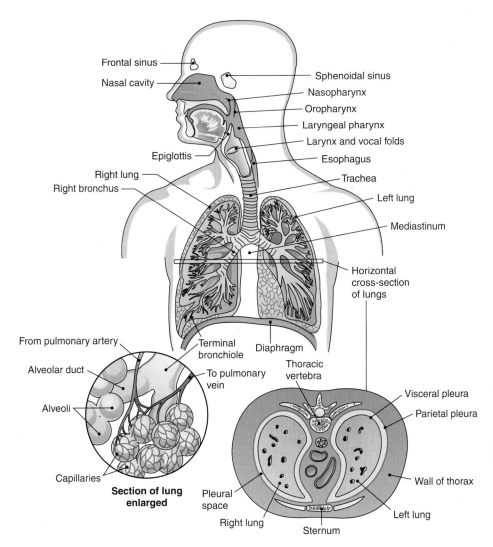

Frontal sinus
Nasal cavity
Sphenoidal sinus
Nasopharynx
Oropharynx
Laryngeal pharynx
Larynx and vocal folds
Epiglottis
Esophagus
Right lung
Trachea
Right bronchus
Left lung
Mediastinum
Horizontal cross-section of lungs
From pulmonary artery
Terminal bronchiole
Diaphragm
Alveolar duct
Thoracic vertebra
To pulmonary vein
Alveoli
Visceral pleura
Parietal pleura
Capillaries
Section of lung enlarged
Pleural space
Wall of thorax
Right lung
Left lung
Sternum

Figure 20-13 The respiratory system. (Reprinted from Cohen FJ. *Memmler's The Human Body in Health and Disease.* 11th ed. Burlington, MA: Jones & Bartlett Learning, LLC; 2009, with permission.)

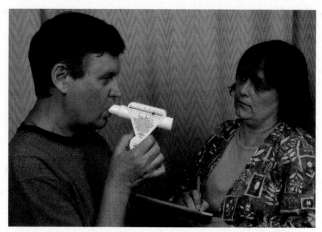

Figure 20-14 The peak flowmeter. (Reprinted from Kronenberger J, Ledbetter J. *Jones & Bartlett Learning's Comprehensive Medical Assisting*. 5th ed. Burlington, MA: Jones & Bartlett Learning, LLC; 2016.)

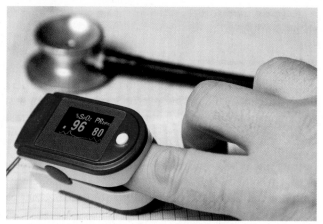

Figure 20-15 A pulse oximeter. (Image from Shutterstock.)

mouthpiece. Figure 20-14 shows a patient using a peak flowmeter, which will determine the amount of air moving into and out of the lungs.

During the test, you may ask the patient to perform different breathing maneuvers. The patient's airflow is measured and the results are compared with predicted values for the patient's height, weight, gender, age, and race. With this information, the physician can assess whether the patient has mild, moderate, or severe obstructive or restrictive disease. Two measurements may be obtained during the test:

- Tidal volume is the amount of air inhaled or exhaled with each normal breath. Although the human lungs can hold a large capacity of air, only a small amount of the total lung capacity is used during normal breathing.
- Forced expiration volume is the amount of air that can be exhaled forcefully after filling the lungs to capacity. The patient is asked to take a deep breath until the lungs are full and then to exhale as hard and completely as possible.

Oximetry

Many medical offices may have a pulse oximeter. This is a device that quickly and painlessly determines how much oxygen is in a patient's capillary blood cells. A sensor cable is attached to the nail bed of the patient's finger. The patient's pulse rate and oxygen saturation level are noted on a digital display on the small oximeter unit. See the picture of a pulse oximeter in Figure 20-15.

A pulse oximeter reading should be obtained as a baseline for patients with chronic respiratory conditions and for those with respiratory signs and symptoms, such as **dyspnea**, shortness of breath (**SOB**), or wheezing. The results should be recorded as a percentage.

- Saturation level readings above 95% are considered normal.
- Patients with chronic conditions, such as emphysema, may have readings of 90% or higher.
- Readings lower than 90% should be reported to the physician immediately.

Other Respiratory Tests

The physician may need information from more sophisticated or invasive respiratory tests to make a diagnosis and plan treatment. These tests typically are not performed in a medical office. However, you should be familiar with them in case patients ask questions about tests ordered by the physician.

Bronchoscopy

This endoscopic procedure involves inserting a lighted scope into the trachea and bronchi for direct visualization. This is considered an invasive procedure and requires the patient's written consent. Usually, it's performed in an outpatient surgical setting. You may have to schedule this procedure for patients.

Bronchoscopy is used for many diagnostic purposes, including

- Obtaining sputum specimens
- Obtaining tissue for biopsy
- Visually assessing airways

It also may be used therapeutically to clear out mucus plugs or remove a foreign body.

Blood Gases

Arterial blood gas (**ABG**) determination involves drawing a small amount of blood from a patient's artery. The levels of pH and dissolved oxygen and carbon dioxide in the blood are measured. The results can help show whether the lungs are functioning properly to exchange gases.

Drawing blood from an artery requires special training. It isn't done routinely in the medical office. However, you may be required to schedule a patient for an arterial puncture at a laboratory or hospital. You also may need to record the results, which usually are phoned in to the medical office.

Patient Education

Peak Flow for Patients

Patients with asthma may need to use a device called a peak flowmeter, which determines the amount of air moving into and out of the lungs. On days when the patient has no symptoms of asthma, breathing is tested at home using a peak flowmeter and the results are recorded on a chart or diary. This record helps the physician plan treatment for the condition.

You may be responsible for teaching patients how to use a peak flowmeter. You can follow these steps:

1. Wash your hands and gather the equipment. Explain to the patient how to read and reset the gauge after each reading. The peak flowmeter should be held upright.
2. Tell the patient to put the flowmeter's mouthpiece in the mouth. The patient's lips should be closed to form a tight seal around the mouthpiece, without biting down.
3. Ask the patient to take a deep breath and blow hard into the mouthpiece. Be sure to remind the patient not to block the back of the flowmeter, because this will interfere with the movement of the gauge.
4. Show the patient how to measure the airflow by noting the level where the sliding gauge stopped after blowing into the flowmeter.
5. Demonstrate how to set the gauge to zero.
6. Instruct the patient to perform the procedure three times consecutively, in the morning and at night. The highest of the three readings should be recorded on a form. Recording readings on a form also allows the patient to follow his or her progress based on medication therapy or exposure to allergens.
7. Show the patient how to clean the mouthpiece. It must be washed in soapy water and rinsed without immersing the flowmeter in the water. Disposable mouthpieces are also available to use with the device.

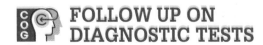

FOLLOW UP ON DIAGNOSTIC TESTS

Once diagnostic tests are completed, the testing facility or laboratory will send a report to the medical office. These reports provide important information for patient care and diagnosis. The office may receive reports for many different kinds of diagnostic tests.

- Pulmonary tests
- Cardiac tests
- Radiographic procedures
- Blood work
- Specimen testing

Reports usually are received through the electronic transmission to the EMR, courier services, or by fax machine. The medical assistant is responsible to review or screen the reports and provide them to the physician.

- Critical results may need to be reported to the physician right away. Follow the policies in your medical office for notifying the physician of abnormal or urgent results.
- Less urgent results may be placed in a specific location for later review by the physician.

When providing test results for the physician to review, make sure they're accompanied by the patient's medical record. The physician may need to refer to the patient's chart when interpreting the results. The EMR system may utilize a flagging system to alert the physician that a new report is pending review. If paper reports are received, never file paperwork in a patient's medical record until the physician has reviewed and signed it indicating he has reviewed it.

If a patient is coming in for a follow-up appointment based on the testing, it's your responsibility to check to make sure your office has received the results of all the diagnostic tests the physician has ordered. In some cases, you may need to call other medical facilities or hospital record facilities to obtain the test results before the patient's visit. The physician needs to have all the test results to diagnose and treat the patient properly.

After the physician has reviewed the test results, they may be filed in the patient's medical record. Check to see if any additional tests, follow-up procedures, or appointments are required. Depending on office policies, you may be required to notify the patient of test results by phone or through the mail. Always protect patient confidentiality.

Procedure 20-1 Performing a 12-Lead Electrocardiogram

Equipment: ECG machine, patient gown, antiseptic wipes, and electrodes.

1. Wash your hands and assemble the equipment. Greet and identify the patient and explain the procedure. Suggest that the patient use the restroom if necessary.

2. Turn on the machine. Make sure the patient cable is connected and working well.

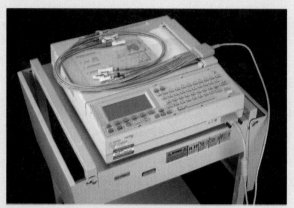

(Reprinted from Kronenberger J, Ledbetter J. *Jones & Bartlett Learning's Comprehensive Medical Assisting.* 5th ed. Burlington, MA: Jones & Bartlett Learning, LLC; 2016.)

3. Enter the appropriate data into the machine, including the patient's name or identification number, age, gender, height, weight, blood pressure, and medications.

4. Ask the patient to disrobe above the waist and provide a gown for privacy. Female patients also should be instructed to remove any nylons or tights. Pants do not have to be removed if they can be pulled up to expose the lower legs for attaching leads.

5. Assist the patient into a comfortable supine position, providing pillows as needed for comfort. Patients in cardiac or respiratory distress may also be placed in a semi-Fowler's or seated position. Drape the patient for privacy. It's important for the patient to feel comfortable. Uncomfortable patients may move during the test, resulting in artifacts on the ECG.

6. You need to prepare the patient's skin by wiping away skin oil and lotions with antiseptic wipes. Shave any hair that will interfere with good contact between the skin and the electrodes.

7. Apply the electrodes against the fleshy, muscular parts of the upper arms and lower legs, following the manufacturer's directions. Make sure the electrodes are snug against the skin, for a proper reading. In case of amputation or an otherwise inaccessible limb, you can place the electrode on the uppermost part of the existing extremity or on the anterior shoulder (upper extremity) and groin (lower extremity).

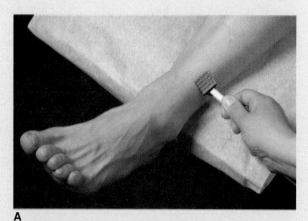

A

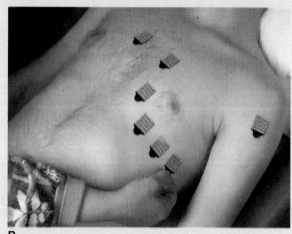

B

(Reprinted from Kronenberger J, Ledbetter J. *Jones & Bartlett Learning's Comprehensive Medical Assisting.* 5th ed. Burlington, MA: Jones & Bartlett Learning, LLC; 2016.)

8. Connect the lead wires securely according to the color-coded notations on the connectors (RA, LA, RL, LL, V_1–V_6). Untangle the wires before applying them to prevent electrical artifacts. Each lead should lie smoothly along the contours of the patient's body. You should double-check the placement of the leads. If the leads are placed improperly, the procedure may have to be repeated.

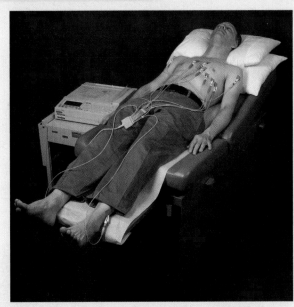

(Reprinted from Kronenberger J, Ledbetter J. *Jones & Bartlett Learning's Comprehensive Medical Assisting.* 5th ed. Burlington, MA: Jones & Bartlett Learning, LLC; 2016.)

It documents the accuracy of the machine and provides a reference point.

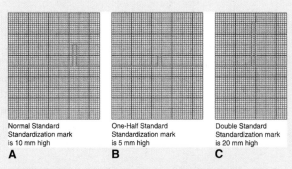

(Reprinted from Kronenberger J, Ledbetter J. *Jones & Bartlett Learning's Comprehensive Medical Assisting.* 5th ed. Burlington, MA: Jones & Bartlett Learning, LLC; 2016.)

9. Check the sensitivity, or gain, and paper speed settings on the ECG machine before running the test. Set the sensitivity or gain to 1 and the paper speed to 25 mm/s. These settings are necessary to obtain an accurate ECG and should not be changed without a direct order from the physician. If changes are made, you must note these on the final ECG tracing.

10. To start the tracing, press the automatic button on the ECG machine. The machine will move automatically from one lead to the next. If the physician wants a rhythm strip only, use the manual mode of operation and select the lead.

11. When the tracing is printed, you should check for artifacts and a standardization mark. When the sensitivity is set at 1, the standardization mark will be 2 small squares wide and 10 small squares high.

12. If the tracing quality is good, turn off the machine. Remove and discard the electrodes. Slowly assist the patient into a sitting position. Some patients become dizzy after lying supine. You can help with dressing if needed.

13. If a single-channel machine was used (each lead is printed on a single roll of paper, one lead at a time), carefully roll the ECG strip. Do not use clips to secure the roll. Folding or applying clips may make marks on the surface, which can obscure the reading. This ECG must be mounted on a special form or 8 × 11-inch paper before going into the patient's medical record. Follow the policies in your medical office.

14. Record the procedure in the patient's medical record.

15. Place the ECG tracing and the patient's medical record on the physician's desk, or give it directly to the physician, as instructed.

Procedure 20-2   Applying a Holter Monitor

Equipment: Holter monitor, incident diary, antiseptic wipes, patient gown, and electrodes.

1. Wash your hands and gather the equipment. Greet and identify the patient.

2. Explain the procedure, including how to use and care for the Holter monitor. You'll need to remind the patient of the need to carry out all normal activities for the duration of the test. A normal routine is necessary to allow the physician to identify areas of concern.

3. Explain the purpose of the incident diary. Emphasize the need to carry it at all times during the test. Ask the patient to remove all clothing from the waist up and to put on the gown. The patient must be exposed for placement of the electrodes. Drape patient appropriately for privacy.

4. With the patient seated, prepare the skin for electrode attachment. Be sensitive to patient privacy. Shave the skin only if necessary, and cleanse with antiseptic wipes. Clean skin will help the electrodes adhere properly.

5. Expose the adhesive backing of the electrodes. Follow the manufacturer's directions to attach each one firmly. Apply the electrodes at the specified sites:

    A. Right manubrium border

    B. Left manubrium border

    C. Right sternal border at fifth rib

    D. Fifth rib space at the left anterior axillary line

    E. Fifth rib space at the right anterior axillary line as a ground lead

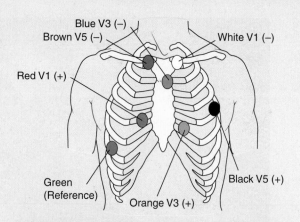

A

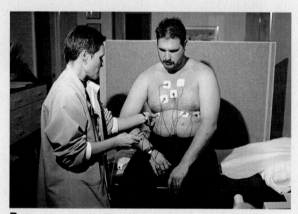

B

(Reprinted from Kronenberger J, Ledbetter J. *Jones & Bartlett Learning's Comprehensive Medical Assisting.* 5th ed. Burlington, MA: Jones & Bartlett Learning, LLC; 2016.)

6. Check the security of the attachments.

7. Position electrode connectors down toward the patient's feet. Attach the lead wires and secure them with adhesive tape. Putting tape over the connections helps to make sure the leads don't work loose.

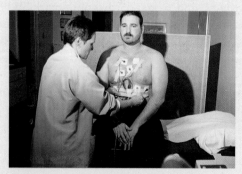

(Reprinted from Kronenberger J, Ledbetter J. *Jones & Bartlett Learning's Comprehensive Medical Assisting.* 5th ed. Burlington, MA: Jones & Bartlett Learning, LLC; 2016.)

Procedure 20-2 Applying a Holter Monitor (*continued*)

8. Connect the cable and run a baseline ECG by hooking the Holter monitor to the ECG machine with the proper cable hookup. You need to make sure the Holter monitor is working properly.

9. Assist the patient in dressing carefully, with the cable extending through the garment opening. You want to prevent any pulling or straining on the connectors or wires.

10. Plug the cable into the recorder and mark the diary. If needed, explain the purpose of the diary to the patient again. Give instructions for a return appointment to evaluate the recording and the diary.

11. Record the procedure in the patient's medical record.

Procedure 20-3 Performing a Pulmonary Function Test

Equipment: Pulmonary function test machine, calibration syringe, patient mouthpiece, and nose clip.

1. Wash your hands and assemble the equipment. Greet and identify the patient and explain the procedure.

2. Turn the pulmonary function test machine on. If necessary, calibrate the spirometer using the calibration syringe, according to the manufacturer's directions. The spirometer must be calibrated daily to ensure accurate results. Record the calibration in the appropriate log book, following office policy.

3. With the machine on and calibrated, attach the appropriate cable, tubing, and mouthpiece according to the type of machine being used. One cable is plugged into an electrical outlet and another is connected to the spirometer and the patient's mouthpiece.

4. Using the keyboard on the machine, enter the patient's name or identification number, age, weight, height, sex, race, and smoking history. The spirometer automatically takes these parameters into consideration when providing results.

5. Ask the patient to remove any clothing that may restrict the chest from expanding. Show the patient how to apply the nose clip to stop air from being expelled through the nose during the test.

6. Ask the patient to stand, breathe in deeply, and blow into the mouthpiece as hard as possible. The machine will indicate when the patient should stop blowing. The indicator may be a buzz, beep, or visual signal you can use to instruct the patient. Make sure a chair is available, and watch the patient carefully for signs of dizziness or imbalance.

7. During the procedure, coach the patient as necessary to obtain each reading. Many patients feel

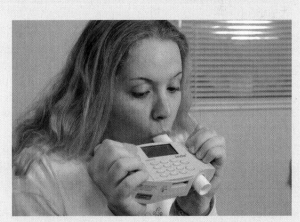

(Reprinted from Kronenberger J, Ledbetter J. *Jones & Bartlett Learning's Comprehensive Medical Assisting.* 5th ed. Burlington, MA: Jones & Bartlett Learning, LLC; 2016.)

they have exhaled all air from the lungs when the machine is instructing them to continue. The machine will indicate whether the reading is adequate. Three repetitions usually are required to obtain the patient's best result. Allow the patient to rest between them if necessary.

8. After printing the results, properly care for the equipment. Dispose of the mouthpiece in the biohazard container.

9. Wash your hands and document the procedure. Place the printed results in the patient's medical record.

Preparing for Externship

Your externship assignment may be at a medical facility where they perform procedures that are not included in the scope of practice for medical assistants in your state. These procedures may include x-ray and imaging exams. Even though you are not allowed to perform these exams, you might be able to observe the x-ray technician performing these exams. Ask about the opportunity to observe as many tests and exams possible. This will provide you the insight about the procedure, which will better prepare you to explain it to a patient when you have to schedule that exam in the future. Observing and asking questions is the best way to expand your medical knowledge.

Chapter Recap

- Radiology is a medical specialty that involves different imaging techniques to diagnose and treat diseases. These techniques include radiographs (x-rays), fluoroscopy, sonography (ultrasound), computed tomography (CT scans), magnetic resonance imaging (MRI), and nuclear medicine techniques. Radiologists interpret the images and send a report to the medical office.

- To produce a radiograph (commonly referred to as an x-ray), a beam of x-rays passes through the patient to record an image on radiographic film. Radiolucent tissues allow the x-rays to pass through and appear as black on the film. Radiopaque tissues are dense and absorb the x-rays, showing up as white on an x-ray.

- In some states, medical assistants are permitted to take and process simple x-ray images of the bones or chest. In other states, only licensed radiographers may take and process x-rays.

- Medical assistants who work in facilities where radiographs are performed may need to help prepare patients. Preparation includes removing any metal objects, including jewelry and clothing with metal fasteners.

- For some radiological procedures, contrast media are used to make it easier to differentiate body structures. A contrast medium may be introduced into the body by mouth, intravenously, or through a catheter.

- The medical assistant has a key role in educating patients about radiological examinations. Patients need information about what to expect during the procedure, what preparations they need to make, and what to do after the procedure.

- Diagnostic tests for cardiac disorders may be invasive or noninvasive. Some noninvasive tests are performed in the medical office, such as the electrocardiogram (ECG).

- The 12-lead electrocardiogram machine picks up electrical signals from the heart and records them on a graph. Sometimes, it is performed as part of a routine physician examination. It also can be used in the diagnosis of heart problems such as arrhythmias and ischemia. Placement of the electrodes is important for providing an accurate ECG tracing.

- Medical assistants are responsible for obtaining an accurate ECG. It's important to avoid artifacts that do not represent the electrical activity of the heart. Common factors that can produce artifacts are movement of the patient, mechanical problems with the ECG machine, and improper technique.

- The Holter monitor is a small, portable ECG worn by patients for a long period of time. It is useful in diagnosing intermittent cardiac arrhythmias and dysfunctions. While wearing the Holter monitor, the patient must keep a diary of all activities.

- Many cardiac procedures are not performed in the medical office. Some of these procedures are the stress test, echocardiography, cardiac catheterization, and coronary arteriography.

- The basic examination for respiratory disorders includes inspection, palpation, percussion, and auscultation. If the examination reveals abnormalities, the physician may order additional tests, such as pulmonary function tests, oximetry, bronchoscopy, or an arterial blood gas.

- When the results of diagnostic tests are received in the medical office, the medical assistant screens them to determine if they require immediate attention. The medical assistant attaches the test results to the patient's medical record for review by the physician.

- After the physician has reviewed the test results, the medical assistant places them in the patient's medical record. The medical assistant may be required to inform patients of test results.

Online Resources for Students

Student Resources available on the text's online site include:

- Audio Glossaries
- Animations
- Competency Evaluation Forms

- Videos
- Anatomy & Physiology Module with Heart and Lung Sounds
- Weblinks
- Worksheets

Exercises and Activities

Certification Preparation Questions

1. The specialist who interprets visual images is called a:

   a. radiologist.
   b. radiographer.
   c. radiography.
   d. radiogram.
   e. radiograph.

2. The term radiolucent describes:

   a. an x-ray that is computerized.
   b. a substance that allows x-rays to pass through them.
   c. a dense substance that absorbs radiation.
   d. a substance that does not allow x-rays to pass through them.
   e. a two-dimensional image.

3. The position used where the patient is standing erect facing the x-ray film is:

   a. AP.
   b. RPO.
   c. PA.
   d. LPO.
   e. RAO.

4. Which of the follow would not be a safety procedure to protect patients during x-ray procedures?

   a. Applying the ALARA principle
   b. Limiting the area exposed to radiation
   c. Confirming pregnant status of females
   d. Taking numerous x-rays to ensure a quality one
   e. Shielding the gonads

5. A cholangiogram would be useful to visualize the:

   a. coronary vessels of the heart.
   b. ureters and the renal pelvis of the kidneys.
   c. lower colon including the sigmoid area.
   d. gastrointestinal system.
   e. bile ducts of the gallbladder.

6. Which of these is an invasive test?

   a. Coronary arteriography
   b. Echocardiogram
   c. Chest radiography
   d. Holter monitor
   e. Electrocardiography

7. Which of these is associated with PVC?

   a. A feeling of fluttering in the chest.
   b. The heart ventricles contract prematurely.
   c. A sudden onset of heartbeat over 100 bpm.
   d. The ventricles begin to twitch.
   e. An abnormal slow heartbeat <60 bpm

8. A characteristic of ECG paper is:

   a. five large blocks measure 10 seconds.
   b. each horizontal line represents 1 second.
   c. each vertical line represents 1 mV of electricity.
   d. each small square is 1 × 1 mm.
   e. the large blocks are 10 × 10 mm.

9. aVR measures the electrical activity from:

   a. LA + LL directed to RA.
   b. RA + LL directed to LA.
   c. RA + LA directed to LL.
   d. electrical activity between LA + RA.
   e. electrical activity between LL + RA.

10. The amount of air inhaled and exhaled with each normal breath is referred to as:

   a. vial inspired amount.
   b. limited capacity.
   c. total lung capacity.
   d. forced exhaled volume.
   e. tidal volume.

CareTracker Connection

 HARRIS Ordering Laboratory and Diagnostic
CareTracker Tests

CareTracker Activities Related to This Chapter

- Case Study 11: Ordering Stat Labs and Copying the Referring Provider
- Case Study 13: Recalling and Recording Patient Results

NOTE: *Case Studies 11 and 13 have prerequisite cases (in addition to Cases 1 to 10 and 12), which must be completed first. See Case Studies 11 and 12 on the-Point for the list of prerequisites.*

Although some illnesses can be diagnosed on the basis of the patient's symptoms and a physical examination, many others require further testing to determine the cause and to guide the treatment of the condition. This testing typically consists of laboratory tests, such as a blood panel or urine analysis, and diagnostic imaging,

such as an x-ray or computed tomography scan. It is the medical assistant's job to enter orders for such tests into the practice's system. CareTracker allows you to easily perform these tasks using its Order application.

Tasks discussed in this chapter that can be performed in CareTracker include the following:

- Ordering laboratory and diagnostic tests
- Documenting the performance of diagnostic tests during the office visit
- Documenting the results of diagnostic tests in the patient's medical record

Many of these tasks are discussed in CareTracker Connection features in other chapters. A task we'll consider here is ordering a laboratory test.

To place an order with a patient in context, you would open the patient's Medical Record module and click on the ⚕ icon at the top of the screen, and a new Order window will appear.

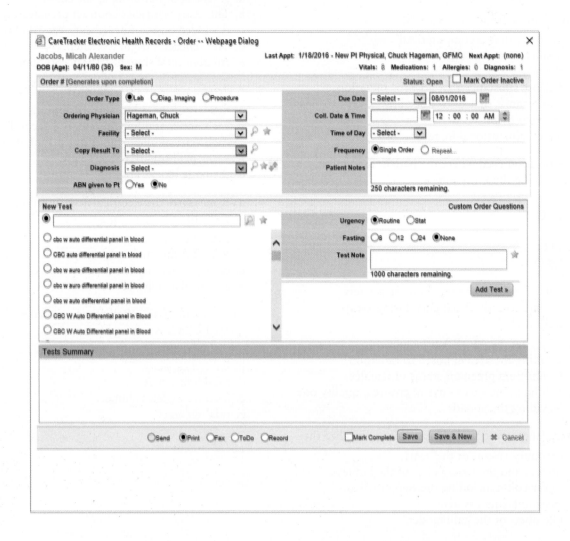

You would then select "Lab" as the Order Type and enter the ordering physician, laboratory facility desired, date due, collection date, collection time, order frequency, notes, and related diagnosis. Next, you would search for the laboratory test being ordered (such as "Hemoglobin A1c") by typing its name in the New Test search field and clicking on the Search icon. A list of related tests will appear, as shown below.

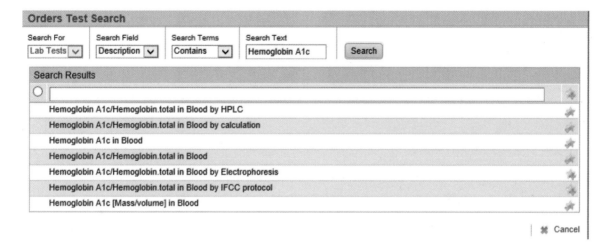

You would select the test desired (such as "*Hemoglobin A1c/Hemoglobin.total in Blood by calculation*"), select the urgency and fasting time associated with the test, and click on the Add Test button. The completed laboratory order would appear as below.

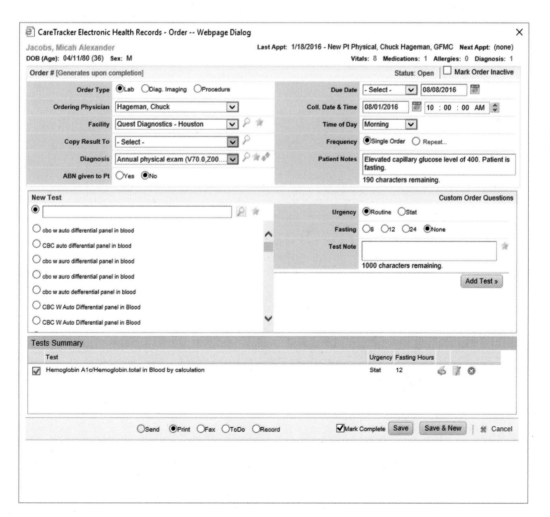

You would then click Save to complete the order.

21 | Patient Education

Chapter Objectives

- List the five main steps in a teaching plan.
- Describe four different teaching strategies.
- List five conditions necessary for learning.
- Summarize Maslow's hierarchy of needs and explain how to use it.
- Identify three factors that can promote learning.
- Provide instruction for health maintenance and disease prevention.
- Discuss four obstacles that can interfere with patient learning.
- Identify some considerations for adapting teaching materials to meet the needs of specific patients.
- Instruct individuals according to their needs.
- Identify community resources.

- List the recommended annual screenings for maintaining good health.
- List and describe the main food groups in the food groups system.
- Explain how to modify a basic diet to treat a medical condition.
- Define range-of-motion exercises and explain why they're used.
- Explain what to teach patients about herbal supplements.
- Identify different stressors associated with illness or disease.
- Describe three relaxation techniques for managing stress.
- Explain the role of the medical assistant in educating patients about substance abuse.

CAAHEP & ABHES Competencies

CAAHEP

- Instruct and prepare a patient for a procedure or a treatment.
- Instruct a patient according to patient's special dietary needs.
- Use feedback techniques to obtain patient information including reflection, restatement, and clarification.
- Use medical terminology correctly and pronounced accurately to communicate information to providers and patients.
- Coach patients regarding office policies, health maintenance, disease prevention, and treatment plan.

- Coach patients appropriately considering cultural diversity, developmental life state, and communication barriers.
- Develop a current list of community resources related to patients' health care needs.
- Facilitate referrals to community resources in the role of a patient navigator.

ABHES

- Teach self-examination, disease management and health promotion.
- Identify community resources and Complementary and Alternative Medicine practices (CAM).

Chapter Terms

Assessment	Implementation	Learning objectives	Rationalization
Denial	Learning goal	Noncompliance	Repression

Abbreviations

AA	CDC	OCD	USDA
AAP	FDA	ROM	USP
ADHD			

Case Study

Henry's mother is accompanying her 6-year-old son to the medical office for follow-up training on insulin injections. Henry has been receiving insulin injections from his mother and the school nurse; however, the physician is requesting that Henry should start to learn how to do this himself.

Patient education is an important part of a clinical medical assistant's job. Educating patients involves more than telling them what medications to take or which behaviors they need to change. To educate patients effectively, you need to:

- Help them adjust to and accept their illness or condition
- Involve them in gaining knowledge that will change their attitudes or behaviors
- Provide them with positive reinforcement, or encouragement

THE PROCESS OF PATIENT EDUCATION

Effective patient education involves five basic steps:

- Assessment
- Planning
- Implementation
- Evaluation
- Documentation

Together, these five steps form a teaching plan. The plan may be written as the process is occurring, or it may be documented after the teaching has taken place. It is important to always consider how your actions and responses will affect the patient. You must treat each patient fairly and without prejudice.

Assessment

Assessment is a process that involves gathering information about a patient's abilities and needs. Before you begin this first step, you need to review your own attitudes. This means being aware of your personal feelings about the patient and the materials to be taught. At times, you may be uncomfortable with the situation, the material, or the patient. However, as an educator, you must set aside your feelings, beliefs, and experiences. For example, you may be asked to instruct a patient about something you personally oppose. Your job is to teach objectively to the best of your ability and without making any judgments or opinions.

You can get the information necessary for assessment from a variety of sources. The best source is the patient's medical record. It includes all the information about current diagnoses, treatments, medications, past medical history, and other documentation. Most medical records have a problem list on the inside cover. This can give you

Case Question

If you were the medical assistant doing the training, what kind of questions do you think Henry will ask that you should be prepared to answer?

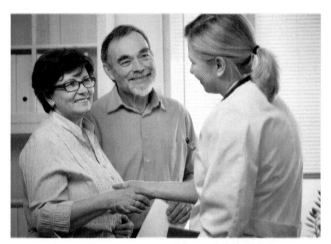

Figure 21-1 Female patient with her husband for support during training session with medical assistant. (Image from Shutterstock.com.)

a snapshot of the patient and may save you time. Other sources of information might be

- The physician
- The patient's family members
- The patient's significant other, if any
- Other members of the health care team

Remember that if you talk to family or friends when doing a teaching assessment, be extra careful not to violate the patient's privacy. Don't share any medical information. Figure 21-1 is a wife with her husband. She will be receiving health education from the medical assistant.

Making a Good Assessment

In doing a good assessment, here are some of the things you should consider:

- The patient's current health care needs
- The patient's past medical and surgical conditions
- The patient's current understanding and acceptance of her health problems and status
- The patient's need for additional information
- Factors that may hinder the patient's learning

Planning the Education

In planning, you use the information gathered during the assessment phase to decide how to approach the patient's instruction. Try to involve the patient in this part of the process if you can. Work with the patient to establish goals and objectives.

- The **learning goal** is what the patient should achieve at the end of the program. This might be knowledge, an action or behavior, or even an attitude toward something. Whatever it is, the learning goal is the desired outcome of your teaching.

- **Learning objectives** are tasks to help reach the goal that will be performed at different points in the program. The learning objectives must be specific to each patient. They also must be measurable. That way, you will be able to determine whether the patient has successfully completed them.

Case Question

If a patient must learn to limit his fluid intake, which of these two objectives would better allow you to measure the patient's progress in reaching the learning goal?

- The patient understands why he should limit his fluid intake.
- The patient is able to prepare a schedule for daily fluid intake and explain why it's important that he limits his fluids.

The second objective is better because it requires the patient to demonstrate that he understands.

Having patients prepare their own schedules also gets them involved in their own health care. It lets them create schedules to fit their lifestyles. This will be likely to increase a patient's compliance, or how well the patient follows the physician's recommendations.

Implementation

After you and the patient agree on goals and objectives, you begin to put them into practice. **Implementation** is the process used to perform the actual teaching. The implementing stage may occur once or several times over a longer period. The length of the teaching process depends on the following:

- The patient's disease process
- The patient's ability to understand
- The patient's access to resources

For example, teaching a patient about diabetes probably will require several sessions. The first session may focus on what diabetes is. Later teachings might include topics such as diet, foot care, glucose monitoring, and insulin injection.

Teaching Methods

You'll probably use one or more of these methods in the teaching process. Choose teaching methods that will best help that particular patient understand and remember the learning. The subject to be taught also will influence which of these methods you choose. Each teaching session is usually carried out in several steps. You should

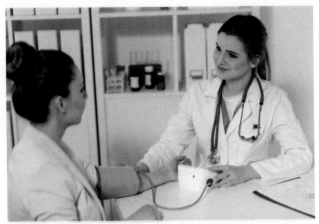

Figure 21-2 Medical assistant demonstrating the use of a digital blood pressure unit for home use. (Image from Shutterstock.com.)

use more than one method. Figure 21-2 is a medical assistant demonstrating how to use a digital blood pressure device that the patient will use at home.

Lecture and Demonstration

Lecture and demonstration are both good ways to present basic information to the patient. However, no patient participation is involved. Participation helps patients remember the information.

Role-Playing and Demonstration

During role-playing and demonstration, the patient watches you perform a medical procedure. Then the patient performs it in a return demonstration. Active participation will help the patient remember the information.

Discussion

A discussion is a two-way exchange of information. It works well when teaching patients about lifestyle changes. This method isn't as useful for teaching about medical procedures. This method does allow the patient to ask questions throughout the discussion.

Audiovisual Presentation

DVDs, videos, and CDs often can be taken home. Patients and family members can then review the material as needed. This provides reinforcement of your teaching. This type of material also provides auditory and visual stimulation.

Printed Material and Programmed Instructions

When you give a patient printed instructions or other material, you need to make sure the patient understands it. Discuss the information with the patient to clarify points. Encourage the patient to ask questions. Print materials are able to be presented in the language that the patient and family best understand. For example,

even if the family speaks English, they may actually understand print materials better in Spanish.

Teaching Aids

Patients also can benefit from the use of teaching aids. Booklets, DVDs, and CDs provide handy references for patients to use at home as a means for reinforcement of the training. Here are some aids you might find useful:

- Drawings
- Charts and posters
- Graphs
- Pamphlets and booklets
- Videos and DVDs
- Audiocassettes and CDs
- Mannequins or models

Evaluation

After you've taught a patient, you need to determine if your teaching was effective. The process of finding this out is called evaluation. It begins by asking some basic open-ended questions, those that don't require just a yes or no answer.

- How is the patient progressing?
- How well did the teaching plan work?
- What kind of changes does the plan need, if any?

Contact with patients in the medical office is limited. So part of the evaluation process might have to be done by patients at home. If you can't schedule office visits for direct observation of patients, they'll be responsible for phoning in and reporting their status. When you speak to these patients on the phone, you need to find out if the patient can do the task you taught or if the patient is having trouble with the task. The evaluation process is ongoing and you can expect to update and modify your teaching plan from time to time.

If the patient mentions any concerns, or seems unclear about the instructions, try to resolve the problems over the phone. However, you may need to schedule an office appointment.

During the evaluation, you may discover **noncompliance**. This is the patient's inability or refusal to follow a prescribed order. When you discover noncompliance, your first step is to find out why. The patient may have misunderstood the instructions. In some cases, the noncompliance is because the patient simply refuses to follow them. In either case, you need to notify the physician.

Documentation

All teachings must be documented in the patient's chart. Table 21-1 shows what kinds of information a teaching note should contain.

Table 21-1	Documenting Patient Education
Things to Be Documented	**Example**
Date and time of teaching	06/03/2015 4:15 PM
What information was taught	Diabetes foot care was discussed. It consisted of the proper method for toenail cutting and the need for regular examination by a podiatrist.
How the information was taught	ADA (American Diabetes Association) foot care video was shown to the patient.
Evaluation of the teaching	Patient verbalized the need to make an appointment with a podiatrist.
Any additional teaching planned	Patient will return on 6/10/2015 to the office with his wife for glucose monitoring instructions.

Your signature implies that you did the teaching. If another staff member helped with the education, clearly note that in the patient's chart. Also include the names of any interpreters, if used, who were involved in the education sessions.

Documenting patient education is important for phone conversations too. You might write, "Spoke with patient by phone today; he said he is testing his blood sugar every morning without problem."

 ## CONDITIONS NEEDED FOR PATIENT EDUCATION

Patients will have a hard time learning new information and skills if the conditions aren't right. Here are some of the things that are necessary:

- A patient's perceived need to learn and readiness to learn
- An appropriate environment
- The right equipment
- A knowledgeable teacher
- *Different* ways to teach the information

Why Learn?

Learning isn't likely to occur unless a patient perceives, or sees, a need to learn. Suppose you're planning to teach a patient with hypertension about low-sodium diets to help manage high blood pressure. However, the patient doesn't feel his hypertension is a problem. Because he hasn't accepted the need for teaching, he isn't motivated to learn the diet. Before you begin teaching this patient, three things must occur.

- The patient must accept that hypertension needs to be managed.
- The patient has to accept that there's a relationship between high sodium intake and hypertension.
- The patient needs to be willing to make a dietary change.

Maslow's Hierarchy of Needs

Basic human needs must be met before people can focus on higher needs, such as taking personal responsibility for their health. A psychiatrist named Abraham Maslow viewed human needs as being like a pyramid. Basic needs are at the bottom or foundation of the pyramid, while higher needs are at the top. The patient makes upward progress as different levels of needs are met. If the patient reaches the highest level, she has reached a state of health and well-being. A patient can move up and down the pyramid depending on her situation. Figure 21-3 is an image of the Maslow Hierarchy of Needs pyramid.

Physiological Needs

At the base of Maslow's pyramid are basic needs like water, food, rest, and comfort. Until these needs are met, the patient can't begin the process of meeting higher

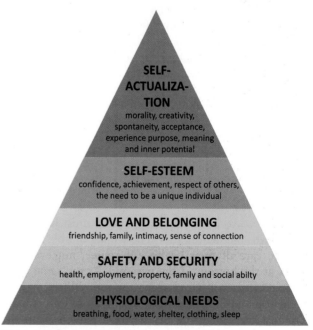

Figure 21-3 Maslow Hierarchy of Needs Pyramid. (Image from Shutterstock.com.)

needs. Everyone has a different level of tolerance and expectation for basic needs. For example, one person might expect to have his food in three meals with drinks and dessert. Another may skip lunch regularly to attend work meetings.

Safety and Security

These needs include a safe environment and freedom from fear and anxiety. Patients can be affected by fear and anxiety because of their medical conditions. Some people who are diagnosed with cancer may be so frightened that they're unable to think of anything but dying. Patients who have experienced trauma or disaster may place the need to feel safe above all other needs.

Belonging and Affection

The need for love and belonging is essential for feeling connected and important to others. A sense of love and belonging can be an important motivation for patients to try to regain good health.

Esteem and Self-Respect

These needs involve our need to feel self-worth. We can develop esteem ourselves, or it can come from those who admire us. If others value us, or we value ourselves, we are more likely to strive to maintain good health. Patients who lack self-esteem are less likely to accept education that targets improving their health. They aren't likely to have much motivation to learn.

Self-Actualization

A person at the top of the pyramid has satisfied all the lower level needs. This person feels responsible and in control of his or her own life. Self-actualized patients will work eagerly to control their state of wellness by following medical teaching and orders. They even may help others achieve wellness. Not all patients will reach this level. But patients who have reached it will be ready to learn health care skills. They will work to regain good health and maintain it. They also will follow guidelines to prevent possible medical problems in the future.

Using Maslow's Hierarchy of Needs

How can you use Maslow's hierarchy of needs to help in teaching patients?

You need to be aware that patients must have their basic needs met before they'll be willing or able to learn to take care of their health. Of course, not everyone starts at the bottom of the pyramid. At the same time, some patients will never reach the top. Others may be at the top and slide backward as a result of unfortunate circumstances. Figuring out where a patient is on the pyramid will help you decide what type of education is appropriate, if any.

- If a patient isn't meeting basic needs, you should help in arranging for him to get those needs met before beginning teaching.
- Patients who are in the middle levels may be able to focus and learn certain skills, but they may not be ready for complex teachings. In this case, you should involve family or significant others in the teaching process, if possible.

The Teaching Environment

You need to teach in an environment that will promote learning. For example, it's not appropriate to teach patients in a hallway, a waiting room, or any other high-traffic area. The room where you teach should meet the following criteria.

- Good lighting
- Quiet
- Private
- Free of distractions

Patients learn best when they feel relaxed. For example, it wouldn't be worthwhile to teach a patient who is on the examination table with her feet in the stirrups. Little learning will take place until she's more comfortable. First, remove her from the stirrups and have the patient get dressed. Then invite her to sit in a chair. If the patient had a procedure done in the room and bloody dressings or suture equipment is still present, clean the area and then return for teaching. Try to make the patient as comfortable as possible.

Teaching with Equipment

Often, you'll need to teach patients to perform a psychomotor skill. A psychomotor skill requires the patient to perform a physical task. Some examples of psychomotor skills are as follows:

- Crutch walking
- Glucose monitoring
- Eye drop instillation
- Dressing changes

In order to teach the skill, you need to have the equipment on hand and ready to use. If possible, the equipment should be from the patient's home or be an exact copy of what the patient will use.

Using Different Strategies

For patient education to be effective, you should use several techniques or approaches. The more techniques you use, the more the patient will learn and remember. People learn in three different ways, by seeing, hearing and touching. Your teaching should involve at least two of these three senses. When there are different ways to learn the material, patients are more motivated to learn. They also will learn more information.

Here's an example. Suppose you were teaching a patient about the dangers of smoking. Which method would be the most effective?

1. Giving the patient a pamphlet that explains the dangers of smoking, along with statistical data.
2. Showing a patient photos comparing a smoker's and a nonsmoker's lung, explaining what happens to the lungs when the patient smokes, and giving the patient pamphlets about smoking cessation programs.

The teaching in the second approach will be more effective. The patient sees the photos and hears your explanations about the dangers of smoking. He also receives a brochure with practical hands-on information he can refer to later.

When using the various strategies, take into consideration special situations that will need to be incorporated in the learning. These include the following:

- Family or significant others may need to be present if the information is complex, or if it requires their help. Family members are essential if the patient is confused or unreliable.
- Patients should be wearing any sensory devices they need (e.g., glasses, hearing aids, etc.).
- Some patients may require a qualified interpreter.

OBSTACLES TO PATIENT EDUCATION

Even when you have the right conditions for learning, some factors can get in the way of the process. You need to recognize these factors and be able to intervene, if appropriate. In some cases, your teaching may be delayed. Also, you may need to adjust your teaching plan. Some of the factors that can interfere with patient learning are

- Illness and pain
- The patient's age
- The patient's educational background
- Any physical impairments

Existing Illness and Pain

The type of illness patients have will play a key role in their ability and willingness to learn. In general, patients with acute, short-term illnesses will be motivated to learn a skill that will speed up healing. Some illnesses include colds and viruses as well as orthopedic injuries such as uncomplicated fractures and sprains.

However, many illnesses have symptoms and complications that may make learning more difficult. Untreated or persistent pain can affect the healing process and affect the patient's quality of life. Table 21-2 shows several kinds of illness or conditions that will negatively affect learning.

Patient's Age

You need to consider the age of the patient when deciding on the amount and type of education you can do. Children need to be educated at an age-appropriate level. For example, it wouldn't be appropriate to teach a 2-year-old how to assemble an asthma nebulizer. You would need to teach that to the parent or caregiver. However, it would be appropriate to explain to the child that the nebulizer is not a toy and that it contains medication. It's important to focus on safety issues when teaching small children and their parents.

Table 21-2	Medical Conditions That Affect Patient Education
Condition	**Examples**
Illness that results in moderate to severe pain	Neuropathies, bone cancer, kidney stones, recent surgical procedures
Illness with poor prognosis or limited rehabilitation potential	Progressive neurological disorders, certain cancers, traumatic events
Illness with weakness or general malaise as a primary symptom	Gastrointestinal disorders that cause vomiting or diarrhea, anemia, Lyme disease, recent blood transfusions
Illness that impairs the patient's mental health or cognitive abilities	Brain tumors, Alzheimer disease, substance abuse, psychiatric disorders
More than one chronic illness	Diabetes with cardiac, renal, or integumentary (relating to skin, hair, and nails) complications
Illness that results in respiratory distress or difficulty breathing	Chronic obstructive pulmonary disease, pneumonias, lung cancer, asthma

Children

Children mature at different rates. You need to assess what information a specific child can handle and what information should not be shared with the child. To do this, talk to the child's parents first, to gather information about the child's developmental stage.

Here's an example. A 7-year-old child has just been diagnosed with diabetes. He needs to know the signs and symptoms of low blood sugar and how to treat it. But the child may not be ready to learn about the long-term complications of the disease, such as blindness or renal failure. You need only to teach the child that the disease must be well controlled to prevent future problems. You don't want to provide so much information that the child becomes fearful. Figure 21-4 is a medical assistant talking with a child about the child's illness. The medical assistant needs to initially establish a good relationship with the child.

Adults

The challenge in teaching adults is that they often have many responsibilities and obligations. These may relate to children, spouses, or aging parents. Social or work obligations also limit their free time. As a result, adults may be less willing to learn or have little time to learn something new. Your teaching may have to occur in short sessions over long periods of time.

Older Patients

Elderly patients may be challenging to teach for several reasons, including

- Confusion
- Lack of interest

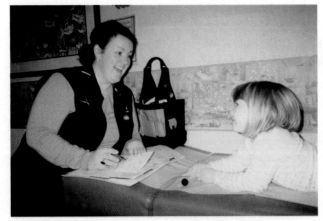

Figure 21-4 Medical assistant establishing rapport with the child. (Reprinted from Kronenberger J, Ledbetter J. *Jones & Bartlett Learning's Comprehensive Medical Assisting.* 5th ed. Burlington, MA: Jones & Bartlett Learning, LLC; 2016.)

- Overall poor health
- Sensory deficits

But remember never to stereotype any of your patients. Some older patients can be the most attentive and curious learners.

Educational Background

On most assessment forms, patients are asked to fill out the level of education they've obtained. This information can help you determine their ability to understand written information. You need to be careful in making this assessment, however. Education level may not guarantee how well the patient can read. You'll need to use tact and diplomacy to evaluate the situation.

Also keep in mind that patients who have an educational background in health care may need the same attention and teaching as other patients. Don't assume you can skip teaching a skill just because your patient is a nurse or a physician. Her specialty may be in an unrelated area.

Physical Impairments and Other Factors

For patients with physical impairments, some types of learning may be difficult. For example, patients with severe arthritis in their hands may have difficulty performing certain psychomotor skills, such as giving themselves insulin. For patients with physical impairments, an occupational therapist is the best resource to assist you. Speak to the physician to obtain the proper referrals.

Along with physical impairments, other factors may hinder your efforts to teach patients.

- A patient's culture may guide which teaching methods you use.
- Patients with financial troubles may feel distracted and have a difficult time focusing on your instruction. This applies to any patients under a good deal of stress.

It's important for you to assess the patient's readiness to learn and to try to remove any obstacles that may be present.

PATIENT TEACHING PLANS

Medical assistants usually are given only a small amount of time for patient teaching. Often, you may find yourself needing to teach without a written plan. To make sure the teaching process follows a logical order, develop a general plan in your mind. Following the steps you learned earlier in the chapter—assessing, planning, implementing, evaluating, and documenting—will help you do this.

Elements of a Teaching Plan

No matter what the design, all teaching plans need these elements:

- Learning goal—this is a description of what the patient should learn from your teaching.
- Material to be covered—this should include all the major topics you will teach.
- Learning objectives—these are the steps or procedures the patient needs to understand or demonstrate to meet the learning goal.
- Evaluation—you need to describe how you will measure the patient's progress.
- Comments—the plan should include a place for remarks about circumstances that may be preventing the patient from reaching the learning objectives. It also includes how the patient is meeting the objectives and revisions to the teaching plan.

Adapting Teaching Material

A huge amount of material is available for patient education. Although the physician or office may provide much of the material you use, you may be responsible for selecting some teaching aids. Here are several things to consider when choosing this material:

- The material should be clear and easy to read with an appealing appearance.
- Make sure the information in commercial materials is accurate, truthful, and current.
- Be sure the information in any outside source you use agrees with your office's policies and procedures.

A good rule of thumb is to use commercial material only from nationally recognized organizations or government agencies.

Creating a Teaching Plan

You may be asked to instruct a patient about a specific topic or subject; however, there is no teaching plan or outline available on a topic. So how do you meet the needs of the patient? You get your creative juices flowing and create a dynamic teaching plan. Chances are that you will need to use the plan with other patients so when you get a great plan, it will be there ready for the next time you need something on that topic. Start your teaching plan design by reviewing available resources and teaching aids. Then, adapt the information to

benefit your patient. Here are some important things to remember when developing teaching material.

- Include the objective of the information.
- Personalize the information so the patient will want to learn.
- Make sure the information is clear and well-organized.
- Use lists and outlines, which are easier to read and remember than paragraphs.
- Avoid medical jargon (terminology and phrases) as much as possible.
- Focus on the key points.
- Select appropriate printing type or font.
- Use diagrams that are simple to understand and well labeled.
- Include the names and telephone numbers of people or organizations whom patients can contact for further information and to answer questions.
- Recommend various Web sites or books that provide appropriate and accurate information.

After patients have used the material, ask for feedback from the patients about the usefulness of the information and how it might be improved. If materials and a teaching plan are not effective, you are not meeting the goal or objective for the patient.

 ## TEACHING SPECIFIC HEALTH CARE TOPICS

The medical assistant's role in patient education varies greatly. The topics you will teach can depend not only on the patient, but also on your medical office and the physician's wishes. Some of the topics medical assistants teach about include

- Preventive medicine
- Medications
- Nutrition
- Exercise
- Alternative medicine
- Stress management
- Smoking cessation
- Substance abuse
- Diseases, such as hypertension and diabetes

Preventive Medicine

Preventive medicine is the branch of medicine that's concerned with promoting health and preventing disease, the key to living a long, healthy life. As a medical assistant, you have two important roles in preventive medicine:

- Promoting preventive screenings
- Teaching safety tips to prevent injury

Many hospitals, clinics, and public health departments offer free preventive screenings for patients. Your office should keep a list of which free screenings are available in the local community.

In addition to free screenings, physicians also recommend that their patients have

- Regular physical examinations for all age groups
- Annual flu and regular pneumonia vaccinations
- Adult immunizations for tetanus, influenza, and hepatitis A and B
- Childhood immunizations
- Regular dental checkups
- Regular blood pressure checkups
- Monthly breast self-examinations for women
- Mammograms on a regular basis for certain groups of women
- Papanicolaou (Pap) tests for women
- Bone density tests for women
- Monthly testicular self-examinations for men
- Prostate-specific antigen (PSA) blood tests for all men, along with the need for regular digital rectal examinations

The Centers for Disease Control (**CDC**) and the National Institutes for Health publish recommended screenings and examinations that most physicians suggest for their patients.

Teaching Safety Tips

Another large part of preventive medicine is teaching safety tips. Preventable injury is the leading cause of death in people between the ages of 1 and 21. In addition, about 25% of children will require at least one emergency room visit for treatment of a preventable accident during childhood. Preventable injuries and deaths can arise from

- Bicycle and car accidents
- Poisoning
- Fires
- Choking
- Falls
- Drowning
- Firearms
- Lawn mowers
- Toys (broken or defective)

The American Academy of Pediatrics (**AAP**) offers injury prevention tips for parents and health care providers. The AAP Web site offers valuable teaching tips for parents and child care providers. They also have educational materials that can be downloaded or mailed to physicians' offices for distribution to patients.

Patient Education

Many injuries result from slips and falls that may have been avoided. These accidents may result in strains, sprains, and fractures. Offer these tips to older patients and others who are at high risk for falls.

- Encourage patients to remove all scatter and throw rugs in their home. Use double-sided rug tape to keep area rugs in place.
- Remind patients to keep hallways free from clutter.
- Good lighting should be available in all rooms and hallways of the home.
- Patients should avoid steps and have only one floor living, if possible.
- Encourage patients to store frequently used items on low shelves and cabinets so they don't need a step stool to get to these items.
- Ensure that patients have well-soled shoes or sneakers. Advise patients to avoid slippers with soft soles. Advise female patients to avoid wearing shoes with heels.
- Instruct patients to place nonskid surfaces in bathtubs and to use a shower chair.
- Installing handrails or grab bars in bathtubs, hallways, and stairwells will provide a higher level of safety for the patient.
- Encourage patients to have smoke detectors installed and remind them to change the batteries twice a year.
- Advise patients taking medications that lower their blood pressure to stand up slowly and get their balance before they begin to walk.
- Recommend that patients have regular eye examinations and have their glasses adjusted as needed.
- Patients should prepare their living space for emergency situations like power outages and severe storms.

Medications

With new medications available all the time, patient education becomes even more essential. Some medication information comes in package inserts. If this isn't available, the patient may not understand the importance of the medication therapy. This could lead to noncompliance, drug interactions, or other serious side effects. You may be responsible for gathering the information needed and preparing teaching materials for patients. Your teaching will help prevent complications.

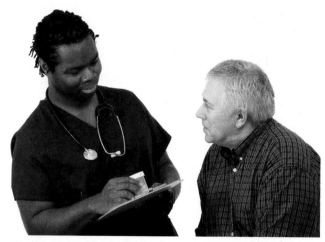

Figure 21-5 Medical assistant explaining a new medication to a senior patient. (Image from Shutterstock.com.)

Figure 21-5 is a medical assistant explaining the new medication to a senior patient.

When preparing a teaching tool about medication therapy, you need to consider factors such as the patient's financial abilities, social or cultural demands, physical disabilities, and age. Be sure to include the following information in any teaching:

- Medication name (generic or brand)
- Dosage to be taken
- Route of administration
- What the medication is for
- Why the medication must be taken as prescribed
- Possible changes in bodily functions (e.g., colored urine)
- Possible side effects
- Other medications (including over-the-counter ones and natural supplements) that might interfere with the action of this medication
- Foods, liquids, and any medications to be avoided
- Activities to be avoided
- A phone number to call for any questions or concerns

For patients taking many medications, scheduling can be a prime concern. For example, the patient may be taking several types of medications at different times of the day or week. Evaluate the patient's daily routine to see how a medication schedule will affect his lifestyle. Some questions you might ask the patient are as follows:

- How late do you sleep each morning?
- What time do you go to bed?
- When do you usually eat?

Once you've collected information about the patient's lifestyle, you can create a scheduling tool. This will help remind your patient what medications to take when.

Pillboxes also can help remind patients to take their medications. Pillboxes are plastic containers prelabeled with the days of the week and times. They're sold in most pharmacies. You may need to instruct the patient on how to fill the pillbox.

Nutrition

Nutrition is the study of what people eat and how the body uses food to maintain and repair itself. Proper nutrition is important for everyone, not just people who are ill. Here is some basic information you can teach all patients.

- There are no "quick fixes" for losing weight.
- Moderation is the key to proper nutrition. It's not necessary to totally eliminate favorites like ice cream, candy, or chips.
- A well-balanced meal should have a rainbow of colors.
- Daily salt intake should be limited, avoiding prepared foods that have higher sodium.
- Eat three balanced meals a day.
- Avoid eating at least 2 hours before going to bed.
- Drink plenty of water. Avoid ingesting large amounts of soda or caffeine.

The Food Guide

Materials are available to help you instruct patients about healthy eating. The U.S. Department of Agriculture (**USDA**) has developed a basic food group system and a Food Guide Pyramid. The USDA system organizes foods into five main groups, plus an extra category for oils.

- Grains—foods made from wheat, rice, oats, cornmeal, barley, or other grains (cereals, pasta, bread, tortillas).
- Vegetables—raw or cooked vegetables or 100% vegetable juice.
- Fruits—raw or cooked fruits or 100% fruit juice.
- Milk and milk products—milk fluids (including flavored milks) and products made from milk, such as cheese or yogurt.
- Meats and beans—often called proteins, include different kinds of meats as well as poultry, fish, eggs, nuts, seeds, and legumes.
- Oils—fats that are liquid at room temperature. This group includes oils that are used for cooking, such as canola oil or corn oil, as well as oils used for flavorings (e.g., sesame oil). The group also includes foods that are naturally high in oils, such as olives, nuts, avocados, and some fish.

Table 21-3 is information that can be used to teach patients about how to incorporate the food groups into their diet.

Figure 21-6 is a chart explaining the anatomy of the MyPyramid established by the USDA.

Table 21-3 Teaching Tips for Food Group Categories

Food Group	What to Teach Patients
Grains	• At least half of the grains eaten each day should be whole grains. • Eat three or more ounces of whole grain products per day. Look for whole before the word grain on the ingredient list. • Avoid croissants, biscuits, sweet rolls, and pastries. • The best cereals are oat, bran, and whole grain cereal. Avoid frosted or sweet cereals.
Milk	• Use skim or 1% milk. Avoid creams and buttermilks. • Eat low-fat cheeses, such as 1% cottage cheese. • Choose low-fat or nonfat yogurt.
Fruits	• Eat a variety of fruits each day. Canned, frozen, and dried fruits are all acceptable. • When choosing canned fruits, look for fruits canned in water or fruit juice instead of syrup. • Avoid drinking too many fruit juices. Fruit juices should be less than half of the total fruit intake.
Vegetables	• Choose a variety of vegetables each day. Try to eat vegetables from different groups (dark green, orange, starchy vegetables, legumes, other vegetables) several times a week. • Fresh, frozen, or canned vegetables all count. Low-salt or no-salt versions of canned vegetables are best.
Meats and Beans	• Choose low-fat or lean meats and poultry. Use USDA-select grade beef, and avoid beef with large amounts of marbling (fat). • Limit bacon to small serving sizes and limit its frequency. • Use preparation methods that don't add fat, such as roasting, broiling, or grilling. • Fish should be fresh. Cook unbreaded and avoid sauces. Good fish choices are salmon, trout, and herring.
Oils	• Limit solid fats like butter, shortening, stick margarine, and lard. • Choose low-fat snacks such as air-popped popcorn, pretzels, and rice cakes to avoid saturated or trans fats. • Use low-fat versions of salad dressings and mayonnaise.

Anatomy of MyPyramid

One size doesn't fit all
USDA's new MyPyramid symbolizes a personalized approach to healthy eating and physical activity. The symbol has been designed to be simple. It has been developed to remind consumers to make healthy food choices and to be active every day. The different parts of the symbol are described below.

Activity
Activity is represented by the steps and the person climbing them, as a reminder of the importance of daily physical activity.

Moderation
Moderation is represented by the narrowing of each food group from bottom to top. The wider base stands for foods with little or no solid fats or added sugars. These should be selected more often. The narrower top area stands for foods containing more added sugars and solid fats. The more active you are, the more of these foods can fit into your diet.

Personalization
Personalization is shown by the person on the steps, the slogan, and the URL. Find the kinds and amounts of food to eat each day at MyPyramid.gov.

Proportionality
Proportionality is shown by the different widths of the food group bands. The widths suggest how much food a person should choose from each group. The widths are just a general guide, not exact proportions. Check the Web site for how much is right for you.

Variety
Variety is symbolized by the 6 color bands representing the 5 food groups of the Pyramid and oils. This illustrates that foods from all groups are needed each day for good health.

Gradual Improvement
Gradual improvement is encouraged by the slogan. It suggests that individuals can benefit from taking small steps to improve their diet and lifestyle each day.

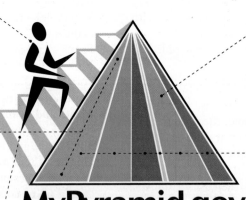

MyPyramid.gov
STEPS TO A HEALTHIER YOU

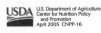 U.S. Department of Agriculture
Center for Nutrition Policy and Promotion
April 2005 CNPP-16

USDA is an equal opportunity provider and employer.

GRAINS VEGETABLES FRUITS OILS MILK MEAT & BEANS

Figure 21-6 Anatomy of MyPyramid. (Reprinted from Kronenberger J, Ledbetter J. *Jones & Bartlett Learning's Comprehensive Medical Assisting.* 5th ed. Burlington, MA: Jones & Bartlett Learning, LLC; 2016.)

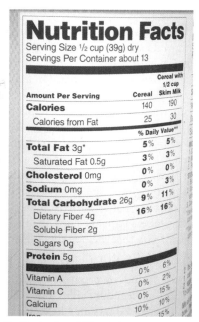

Figure 21-7   Typical nutrition label on packaged food product. (Image from Shutterstock.com.)

General Dietary Guidelines

The USDA and the U.S. Department of Health and Human Services developed a food guide and food pyramid as well as general guidelines for improving diet. Here are some of the key recommendations.

- Choose a variety of foods from the five basic food groups.
- Maintain a healthy weight by balancing the food you eat with physical activity.
- Keep your diet low in saturated fats and keep trans fats as low as possible.
- Choose a diet with plenty of vegetables, fruits, and whole grain products.
- Prepare and choose foods with little salt or added sugar.
- Drink alcoholic beverages in moderation.

Food Labels

When teaching patients about nutrition, you need to encourage them to read the labels on food containers. These labels provide several important pieces of information:

- The nutritional value of the product
- The specific ingredients that were used
- What additives are in the food

All information on food labels is based on the portion or serving size. Remind patients that if they eat double the portion, they need to double the nutritional facts. The serving size is at the top of the label. Below the serving size is the number of servings per container. For certain foods, it's easy to determine the serving size. The label may say two cookies or one slice of bread. In other cases, it may be more difficult. Generally, serving sizes are listed as measured in grams. Figure 21-7 is an example of a nutrition label on packaged food product.

When teaching about the nutritional facts on a label, you should point out the key information on the label that patients should look for.

Dietary Portion Control

Teach your patients these simple rules for measuring.

- 50 g of cheese is about the size of two thumbs.
- 50 to 100 g of meat is about the size of the palm of an adult's hand.
- One cup of raw greens or salad is about the size of a fist.

Figure 21-8 is a reminder to have patients use appropriate measuring devices for accuracy in portion control.

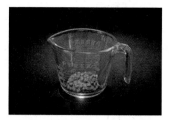

Figure 21-8   Measuring cup for accurate serving size. (Reprinted from Kronenberger J, Ledbetter J. *Jones & Bartlett Learning's Comprehensive Medical Assisting.* 5th ed. Burlington, MA: Jones & Bartlett Learning, LLC; 2016.)

Daily Fat Intake

Total fat is the first nutritional fact on the food label. It lists the total grams of fat in one serving.

The average diet consists of 2,000 calories per day. Each gram of fat contains 9 calories. On a 2,000-calorie diet, the maximum grams of fat per day should be <65, with <20 g of saturated fat. Teach patients to add their total grams of fat per day.

The label also will list a percentage number. The percentage refers to what percent of allowed fat is contained in one serving. However, most patients will find it easier to add up the total grams of fat they eat instead. Different kinds of fat also are listed under the total fat heading on the label. Patients need to understand the different types of fats that include the following:

- Unsaturated fats are the best choices for healthy eating. They are found in products made from plant sources, including vegetable oils, seeds, and nuts, and some fish. Unsaturated fats may be called monounsaturated (canola, olive, and peanut oils) or polyunsaturated (sunflower, corn, soybean oil) on food labels. Both types of unsaturated fats can reduce the risk of heart disease.
- Saturated fats typically are found in products that are solid at room temperature. They are found in meat, seafood, egg yolks, and dairy products made with whole milk. They are also found in products made with coconut, coconut oil, or palm oil. Saturated fats raise the levels of LDL ("bad" cholesterol) in the blood.
- Trans fats are created when hydrogen is added to vegetable oil during a food-manufacturing process. The ingredient lists on food products list them as hydrogenated or partially hydrogenated fats and oils. Trans fats are found in baked goods like crackers, cookies, and other snack foods, as well as in shortening and some margarine. Like saturated fats, diets with high levels of trans fats increase the risk of cardiovascular disease.

Daily Carbohydrate Intake

Carbohydrates are the sugars and starches found in many foods. They are converted to simple sugars in the body to provide energy for body cells. Any portion of sugar the body doesn't use is stored as fat.

The nutrition label tells how many carbohydrates are in each serving. Each gram of carbohydrates contains 4 calories. Based on a 2,000-calorie diet, the total carbohydrates per day should not exceed 300 g. Patients should add their total carbohydrate intake for 24 hours. It's essential that patients learn to count carbohydrates if they have diabetes.

Carbohydrates also include fiber (also called roughage). Fiber is the parts of fruits and vegetables that can't be digested. It helps digestion by stimulating

peristalsis—muscle contractions that push food through the digestive tract. It also helps lower blood cholesterol levels (LDL).

Daily Intake of Sodium, Cholesterol, and Protein

Amounts for these nutrients are also listed on food labels. Patients with special diets can use this information to determine how much of a particular nutrient they're eating. Amounts are listed in grams per serving, as well as by the percentage of the nutrient in an average 2,000-calorie diet. Each gram of protein contains 4 calories.

Large fast food chains will have this information available at each of their stores. You should encourage your patients to ask for and read this information.

Daily Vitamin and Mineral Intake

Food labels also list percentages for vitamins and minerals. These percentages show how much of the daily recommended amount of a vitamin or mineral is contained in a serving. Recommended amounts are different for each vitamin and mineral. Food labels are not required to show all the vitamins and minerals in the food.

Healthy Food Preparation

After discussing healthy foods, provide some information about healthy food preparation. Give patients these tips for preparing healthy foods:

- Broil, bake, roast, or grill meats instead of frying them.
- Trim the fat from beef.
- Use a cooking rack so fat drips away from the meat.
- Remove the skin from chicken. Use caution with raw chicken. Wash hands and cutting surfaces immediately.
- Homemade soup or gravy should be chilled after cooking. When chilled, skim the fat off the top and reheat to use.
- Use unsaturated oils (canola, corn, sunflower). Use nonstick spray when possible. Avoid saturated oils (butter, lard).

Other Dietary Considerations

As with any patient teaching, you need to consider several factors before sending a patient home with a pre-printed diet form. Some factors that influence how well a patient complies with dietary changes are

- Age
- Culture
- Religion
- Geographic background
- Social and financial circumstances

Some patients may have questions about vegetarian diets. Vegetarian diets typically have low levels of saturated fat and high levels of fiber and vitamins. There are three types of vegetarian diets:

- Lacto-ovovegetarian means that a diet of vegetables is supplemented with milk, eggs, and cheese.
- Lactovegetarian means the diet is supplemented only with milk and cheese.
- Pure vegetarian means that the diet is only vegetables and excludes all foods of animal origin.

Modifying Diets for Medical Conditions

Diets that limit or balance the intake of specific nutrients are used to treat some diseases. Some examples are listed in Table 21-4.

Other patients may require special diets to help treat an illness or disease. The patient's normal diet is assessed and then modified. A specific nutrient may need to be limited through careful diet planning. Figure 21-9 shows the use of computer technology to provide training on nutrition. It is very interactive and the patients can participate from their home.

Exercise

Exercise can be any activity that uses muscles to help maintain fitness. If done in moderation, there are several reasons why it benefits the body:

- Maintains healthy body weight
- Increases circulation
- Strengthens the heart and lungs
- Increases muscle tone
- Keeps bones strong
- Decreases stress and helps patients manage depression
- Helps patients sleep better

All patients should get some form of exercise on a regular basis. Patients who are under age 35 and in good health usually don't need medical clearance before starting a routine exercise program. However, a physician consultation is recommended for patients aged 35 or

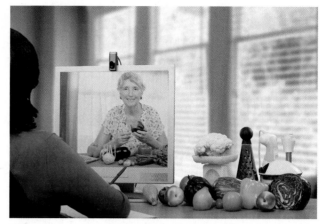

Figure 21-9 Computer technology used to deliver nutrition training to a patient in their home. (Image from Shutterstock.com.)

older who have not been active in several years. Patients with known medical disorders also should check with the physician before exercising including pregnant patients who should consult their obstetrician before beginning an exercise program. These disorders include the following:

- Hypertension
- Cardiovascular problems
- Family history of strokes

Range-of-Motion Exercises

If patients are unable to perform exercises without assistance, it may be necessary to instruct them or their family members on range-of-motion (**ROM**) exercises. In these exercises, the patient moves the affected limb or joint through all of the movements that the joint is capable of making, until resistance is met.

In most cases, ROM exercises are ordered by the physician to prevent further loss of motion or disfigurement after a musculoskeletal injury, surgery, or neurological damage. ROM exercises are performed several times a day on each involved joint.

Table 21-4	Special Diets for Medical Conditions	
Type of Diet	**Description**	**Disease or Condition**
Bland diet	Foods that contain irritating chemicals (peppers, spices, caffeine) or bulky fiber are eliminated.	Gastrointestinal disorders
Diabetic diet	Food intake is controlled to keep blood glucose levels under control. Foods are grouped according to protein, carbohydrates, and fats.	Diabetes mellitus types 1 and 2
Elimination diet	Specific foods are limited (e.g., milk, eggs, wheat).	Food allergies
Low-sodium diet	Foods that are high in sodium are eliminated (e.g., avoid processed foods and canned vegetables with added salt).	Hypertension (high blood pressure)

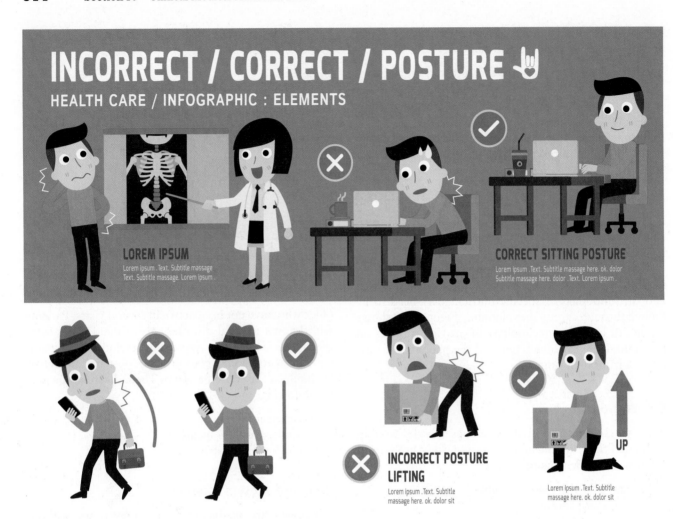

Figure 21-10 Printed materials used as a visual aid to teach patients proper lifting techniques. (Image from Shutterstock.com.)

Some patients are unable to perform any exercise on the affected area. In that case, passive ROM is performed. This requires someone else to exercise the limb or joint for the patient. ROM exercises help promote blood circulation and improve muscle tone. If they're not performed as ordered, the patient may not be able to regain use of the affected area.

Patients with a major loss of motor skills often will be referred to physical therapy or occupational therapy for intense ROM teachings. In these cases, your role will be to assess their compliance in going to their therapy appointments and to provide positive reinforcement. Figure 21-10 is an example of a picture brochure demonstrating proper lifting techniques. Patients with back problems are at a higher risk of injury due to improper lifting technique. This is a great visual tool to use when doing patient education.

Alternative Medicine

Alternative medicine is health care practices that are used instead of standard medical treatments. Some ancient remedies that were once dismissed by Western medicine have proven to be beneficial in some circumstances. There are many kinds of alternative medicine. Let's look at four of the most common therapies.

Acupuncture

Acupuncture is one of the oldest forms of Chinese medicine. It's based on the principle that there are 2,000 acupuncture points in the human body. These points are connected throughout the body by 12 pathways called meridians. When the meridians are triggered, they conduct energy, or qi (pronounced "chee") in the body. The trigger comes in the form of very thin needles that are inserted at certain acupuncture points. When a meridian is stimulated, it prompts the brain to release certain chemicals and hormones.

Acupuncture is used to treat many conditions. Here are some of the more common ones:

- Addictions, such as smoking
- Fibromyalgia
- Osteoarthritis
- Asthma
- Chronic back pain

Acupuncture is also sometimes used to treat children with attention deficit hyperactivity disorder (**ADHD**). About 40 states require that acupuncturists be licensed to practice. Training and licensing requirements vary by state.

Acupressure

Acupressure is similar to acupuncture, but it does not use needles. The practitioner applies pressure to the meridians through direct touch. Acupressure has several uses:

* To treat nausea and vomiting associated with chemotherapy
* To ease chronic pain
* To boost the immune system

Hypnosis

On television, hypnosis is portrayed as a magical method for reaching the inner workings of the brain. However, when conducted properly, there are some health care benefits. Here are some of its most common uses:

* In weight loss programs
* Treating obsessive–compulsive disorder (**OCD**)
* For smoking cessation

Yoga

Yoga is useful for relieving stress and improving flexibility. It involves a mix of physical exercises, posture, breathing exercises, and meditation. There are many types or forms of yoga.

Herbal Supplements

Many people think of herbal supplements as "natural" and, therefore, safe. However, the Food and Drug Administration (**FDA**) does not regulate herbal supplements and similar substances. Patients need to understand that there has been no formal government testing or approval of these substances. Without testing, many aspects of herbal supplement use are unclear, including:

* What are appropriate dosages?
* What side effects may exist?
* What potential interactions with other substances may exist?
* What are the possible benefits of these supplements?

There's also no guarantee that what the label claims is in the bottle is actually in there.

The quality and purity of herbal supplements can vary greatly, depending on the manufacturer. Patients who wish to use herbal supplements should buy only those that are stamped on the label with a U.S. Pharmacopeia bar code. This bar code means that the manufacturing site has met certain standards. However, it does not mean that the supplement has been tested for health care benefits.

The use of some herbal supplements has evolved through folklore, various cultures, or clinical research. In some cases, the supplement may involve an element of the placebo effect. The placebo effect is the power of believing that something will make you better when there's no chemical action from the substance that creates a medical benefit.

Some common herbal supplements and their reported benefits are as follows:

* Echinacea—treatment of colds; stimulates immune system, attacks viruses
* Garlic—treatment of colds; diuretic; prevention of cardiac diseases
* Ginkgo—increased blood flow to the brain; treatment of Alzheimer disease
* Ginseng—mood elevator; antihypertensive
* Glucosamine—treats arthritis symptoms; improves joint mobility

Patient Education

Medical assistants are frequently asked to ensure that patients understand how to safely use herbal supplements. Here are a few general teaching tips on herbal supplements:

* Emphasize that it's important for patients to always tell the physician or other health care provider about any herbal supplements they're taking.
* Tell patients that just because it is a natural product, it does not mean it is safe to use. For example, all mushrooms are natural, but some are very poisonous.
* Teach patients to look for the **USP** (United States Pharmacopeia) label as well as the expiration date of the product.
* Advise patients not to depend on health store clerks for information about supplements. They should speak to physicians or pharmacists.
* Caution patients not to trust advertisements that use words like magical or breakthrough or that claim to detoxify the whole body.
* Emphasize that patients need to check with the physician about taking herbal supplements at least 2 weeks prior to surgery. Tell them they also must advise the surgeon what supplements they've been taking, how much, and for how long. Some supplements can increase bleeding time.
* Warn diabetic patients that many supplements will interfere with blood sugar levels.
* Parents should avoid giving herbal supplements to their children unless approved by a physician.
* Pregnant or breast-feeding patients need to consult with a pharmacist or physician before taking any supplements.

Stress Management

When people are affected by illness or injury, they often experience stress. Stress is a state of physiological and/or psychological strain that may disturb normal functioning. It can result from forces such as fear, anger, anxiety, crisis, or joy. When the body is healthy, it can handle stress more easily. But when dealing with an illness or injury, a patient may face:

- Physical pain
- The inability to perform self-care
- Treatments, procedures, and possible hospitalization
- Changes in self-image and roles in life
- Loss of control and independence
- Changes in relationships with family and friends

If patients are able to deal with stress factors, then they may be more likely to adjust to lifestyle changes. Patients with chronic conditions may need more time to adjust than those with acute illnesses. Also, some patients may not be capable of coping with stress on their own, even with the help of teaching by medical office staff. These patients may need professional counseling.

Positive and Negative Stress

Two types of stress affect all of us—positive stress and negative stress. Positive stress motivates us to work efficiently and to perform to the best of our abilities. Examples of positive stress include

- Working on a challenging new job or project
- Getting married
- Giving a speech or performance

Many people work best under positive stress. When faced with this kind of stress, our brain releases chemicals that increase our heart rate and breathing capacity. Our body releases stored glucose that gives us an energy boost.

Once a stressful situation is over, we must take time to relax, to prepare for the next one. Positive stress can become negative stress if relaxation techniques aren't part of our daily routine. Negative stress is the inability to relax after a stressful encounter. Left unchecked, it can lead to physical responses such as

- Headache
- Nausea and diarrhea
- Sweating palms
- Insomnia
- Malaise
- Rapid heart rate

If stress is not relieved, patients will progress to higher anxiety levels. It will require all their energy and attention to focus on the problem at hand. Most mental and physical activity will be directed at relief of the stress. Patients try to avoid the ultimate anxiety level known as panic—a sudden, overwhelming state of anxiety or terror. Long-term physical effects of unrelieved stress include increases in

- Blood pressure
- Glucose levels
- Metabolism
- Intraocular pressure

Stress also can lead to exhaustion and unrelieved stress is associated with an increased risk of heart attack, stroke, diabetes, certain cancers, and immune system failure.

Dealing with Stress

Most people have developed methods for reducing the effects of intense stress. These methods are referred to as coping skills. Usually, we have no conscious control of them. They're a psychological defense against unpleasant situations. Here are some common coping skills.

- **Repression** means the mind blocks uncomfortable or distressing ideas from conscious awareness.
- **Denial** is when a person rejects a fact that's painful or difficult to accept.
- **Rationalization** is the process of finding excuses for thoughts or feelings that would otherwise be hard to accept.

Stress Coping Skills

There are several coping skills you can teach to patients suffering from psychological effects of negative stress. Applying these skills may help them manage their stress.

- Encourage patients to try to reduce stressors (things that cause stress), but make it clear that it's not possible to remove all stressors. Caution them that trying to make everything perfect adds its own stress.
- Encourage patients to organize and limit their activities as needed.
- Try to lessen patients' fear of failure so they just do the best they can.
- Encourage patients to talk to someone when they're feeling anxious or stressed. Talking about their problems allows them to "let off steam."
- Encourage patients to utilize relaxation techniques to help them regain control over their stressors.

Relaxation Techniques

There are several relaxation techniques that patients might use. To find what works best for them, they must first consider how much time they have and what type of relaxation they need. Three different types of relaxation techniques are

- Breathing techniques
- Visualization
- Physical exercise

Breathing Techniques

Breathing exercises can be done anywhere. Most people are shallow breathers and need to be instructed on deep-breathing techniques. Deep breathing can get the oxygen flowing through the body at a faster rate. It sometimes can relieve boredom, tension, and stress.

Follow these steps for instructing patients to use deep breathing exercises:

1. Tell the patient to sit up straight and place the hands on the stomach.
2. Instruct the patient to take a deep breath through the nose. The patient should keep breathing in as the hands are pushed away by the stomach. This may feel awkward, because most people try to pull their stomach in when they breathe deeply.
3. Tell the patient to hold the breath for a few seconds.
4. Instruct the patient to exhale through pursed lips. The hands will be pulled in.

 VISUALIZATION

This relaxation technique involves allowing the imagination to run free and focus on positive and relaxing situations. It's similar to "daydreaming." It can help the patient feel removed from a stressful situation and help the mind to relax.

Instruct the patient to find a quiet place, close the eyes, and visualize a soothing scene. Remind the patient that it's important to choose appropriate times for this daydreaming technique.

Physical Exercise

As you read earlier in the chapter, exercise has many health benefits. Another important benefit of exercise is that it relieves tension and anxiety. Most people who exercise regularly say that it helps them relax and rest better at night.

The key to using exercise to manage stress is to find the type of exercise that is right for the individual. Here are some tips to teach your patients.

- The vigorous activity in recreational sports such as squash or tennis can help the body cope with stress.
- Even a brisk 20-minute walk every day can help relieve tension and stress.
- If possible, break up the workday by exercising for a short period of time every 90 minutes.

Exercises at work can include stretching, walking up and down stairs, or a short walk outside. A 10-minute break can help relax a person's mind and reduce tension.

Substance Abuse

Substance abuse is the excessive use of and dependency on drugs. Some abused substances are legal (e.g., alcohol and nicotine), whereas others are illegal (e.g., marijuana and cocaine). Patients affected by commonly abused substances usually work with trained specialists or counselors.

Substance abuse can have serious effects on patients' health. It's important that you give them information about substance abuse if they ask for it. This information may come from various national organizations. You also should have information available about any local organizations or groups that may help these patients.

A patient with a substance abuse problem may need detoxification before counseling. Detoxification is the process of clearing drugs out of the patient's body. Factors that affect the detoxification process include

- The type of substance that's been abused
- The length of time the patient has abused the substance
- The patient's overall level of health
- Any physical or mental effects that result from the body's withdrawal from the substance

In some cases, detoxification may require hospitalization.

The most important role of the medical assistant in educating patients about any type of substance abuse is to be supportive.

- Provide positive reinforcements as appropriate.
- Offer services to patients for cessation programs.
- Never condemn a patient for not seeking help. Always be nonjudgmental.

Smoking Cessation

Nicotine is highly addictive, whether it's ingested by smoking or chewing. This drug reaches the brain in 6 seconds. It damages blood vessels, decreases heart strength, and is associated with many cancers. Patients who try to stop smoking experience withdrawal symptoms, such as

- Anxiety
- Progressive restlessness
- Irritability
- Sleep disturbances

Many different methods are used to try to stop smoking. Some programs have the patient stop gradually. Others try a total, abrupt stoppage. There are research data to support both methods.

Here are some suggestions to help patients stop smoking:

- Find local smoking cessation support groups. Provide phone numbers and contact names of these groups to your patients.
- If you don't have a local group, the American Heart Association, American Lung Association, or American Cancer Society may help.

- Discuss with the physician the options of prescribing various patches, gums, or other interventions for the patient. Some products have side effects and the physician may choose not to order them. The decision may be based on the patient's age or other medical illnesses.

Alcohol

Alcohol is chemically classified as a mind-altering substance because it contains ethanol. Ethanol depresses the action of the central nervous system and affects motor coordination, speech, and vision.

Many people use alcohol in moderation. However, in large amounts, alcohol can affect respiration and heart rate. There are also several long-term effects of alcohol use or abuse:

- Liver failure
- Various types of cancer
- Strokes
- Nutritional deficiencies

The leading organization for treating alcoholism is Alcoholics Anonymous (**AA**). Patients complete a 12-step program during recovery. Recovering alcoholics provide many of its support services. AA has many chapters and support services for patients and patient families. There are also special services for teenage alcoholics.

Recovering alcoholics should avoid over-the-counter and prescription medications that contain alcohol. This is a common ingredient in many cough and cold medicines.

Illegal Drugs

Many people assume that users of illegal drugs have criminal tendencies or come from a certain type of background. However, drug abuse affects a wide range of people from different cultures and with different social experiences. The abuse of prescription drugs or the use of illegal drugs can have long-term effects on brain function. It's important to understand drug abuse so you can work to help prevent it.

Drug abuse can affect several areas of an individual's life.

- Personality changes might include mood swings, depression, or frequent lying. Some individuals may become verbally or physically abusive.
- Changes in physical appearance may be noticeable. Some examples are neglecting personal hygiene, changes in sleeping behavior or activity level, and changes in weight.
- Changes in social activity may include withdrawal from family and friends, dropping social connections, or a loss of interest in school and work.

There are also other effects related to the type of drug being abused.

Marijuana

Marijuana and hashish have many effects on the brain and body. Here are just a few:

- Impaired short-term memory
- Impaired comprehension
- Reduced ability to perform tasks requiring concentration or coordination
- Increased heart rate and appetite

Long-term users may develop psychological dependence. Because these drugs are inhaled as unfiltered smoke, users take in more cancer-causing agents and do more damage to the respiratory system than with regular filtered tobacco smoke.

Cocaine and Crack

These drugs stimulate the central nervous system and are extremely addictive. Crack cocaine is particularly dangerous. This pure form of cocaine is usually smoked and absorbed rapidly into the bloodstream. It can cause sudden death. The use of cocaine can cause psychological and physical dependency. There are many side effects, such as

- Dilated pupils
- Increased pulse rate
- Elevated blood pressure
- Insomnia
- Loss of appetite
- Paranoia
- Seizures

Cocaine also can cause death by disrupting the brain's control of the heart and respiration.

Amphetamines

Amphetamines and other stimulants boost the central nervous system and have similar effects as cocaine. Some stimulants are legally prescribed to treat medical conditions, such as depression or ADHD. However, when they are abused or used illegally, these drugs can be addictive and dangerous. They cause increased heart rate and blood pressure. Symptoms of stimulant use include dizziness, sleeplessness, and anxiety. Amphetamine use causes

- Psychosis
- Hallucinations
- Paranoia
- Physical collapse (in extreme cases)

The long-term effects of these substances are hypertension, heart disease, stroke, and renal and liver failure.

Depressants

Depressants and barbiturates are sometimes referred to as "downers." That's because they may calm nerves, relax muscles, and have a tranquilizing effect. Chemically, they depress the action of the central nervous system. Use of these substances can cause physical and psychological dependence. Depressants are especially dangerous when taken with alcohol. Some depressants are prescribed to treat medical conditions. However, illegal use or abuse of these drugs can have serious effects, such as respiratory depression, coma, and even death. Withdrawal from them can lead to

- Restlessness
- Insomnia
- Convulsions
- Death

Hallucinogens

There are many different types of hallucinogens. These substances interrupt the brain's messages that control thinking and the processing of sensory experiences. They affect individuals by causing them to hallucinate—to hear, see, or feel things that aren't really there. Here are some examples of hallucinogens:

- Lysergic acid diethylamide (LSD)
- Phencyclidine (PCP or "angel dust")
- Mescaline
- Peyote

Large doses of hallucinogens can produce seizures, coma, and heart and lung failure. Chronic users complain of memory problems and speech difficulties for up to a year after they stop using the drugs.

One effect of hallucinogens is that they stop the brain's pain sensors. Users can hurt themselves and not even know it.

Narcotics

Narcotics are addictive drugs that relieve pain by preventing pain messages from being sent to the brain. They include natural substances derived from the opium poppy as well as synthetic substances designed to have similar effects. Narcotics may be prescribed to ease pain, to suppress coughing, or to produce anesthesia. Some examples are codeine and morphine. There are regulations for prescribing narcotics (controlled substances) because they are addictive and highly susceptible to abuse. Some narcotics are illegal substances, such as heroin. Others are commonly prescribed drugs.

Narcotics have many effects on the body. Here are some of the common ones:

- Feelings of euphoria
- Drowsiness
- Fluctuations in blood pressure
- Fluctuations in pulse

An overdose of narcotics can lead to seizures, coma, cardiac arrest, and death.

Many substances of abuse can harm a fetus; some examples include fetal alcohol syndrome and cocaine

dependency in babies. Teach all pregnant women about the dangers of these substances to their unborn children.

USING INTERNET RESOURCES FOR PATIENT EDUCATION

When you're teaching patients, you'll need to find reliable information to use. Also, patients may want to use the Internet to search for information on their own. It's important to be knowledgeable about Web sites that will provide solid information based on facts and research. Look for Web sites with extensions such as .org, .gov, or .edu. Avoid personal or commercial Web sites (e.g., .com). Table 21-5 lists some Web sites you can use to search for more information.

Study Tip

Summarizing lecture or reading materials will help you when you review your materials at a later time. When you hear your instructor say that there are three items related to a subject or topic summarize and write down the three using a number for each one. Too many students get "bogged" down when listening to a lecture or reading a chapter and lose interest in the topic. When you organize the information into numbered lists, it will help you in your exam review.

Table 21-5	Internet Resources for Patient Education	
Organization	**Web Site**
Alcoholics Anonymous	www.aa.org
American Academy of Pediatrics	www.aap.org
American Cancer Society	www.cancer.org
American Heart Association	www.heart.org
American Lung Association	www.lung.org
Food and Drug Administration	www.fda.gov
Food and Nutrition Information Center	https://fnic.nal.usda.gov/
National Center for Complementary and Alternative Medicine	https://nccih.nih.gov/
National Institute of Drug Abuse	www.drugabuse.gov
U.S. Department of Agriculture (MyPyramid)	www.mypyramid.gov

Procedure 21-1   Implementing Individualized Teaching

1. Gather your supplies, including the patient's medical record and physician's orders. Read the physician's orders. Clarify any questions you have before you begin.

2. Identify factors that may get in the way of the teaching or learning process.

3. Consult resources for the specific topic you are teaching the patient.

4. Create a set of instructions you can give to the patient. This may involve adapting existing instructions from resources in your medical office. If your teaching involves equipment, include instructions on how to maintain it.

5. After you have prepared your materials, greet and identify the patient. If necessary, involve the patient's parent or legal guardian.

6. Explain the procedure to the patient in a logical, step by step manner.

7. Show the patient how to perform the procedure.

8. Ask the patient to return the demonstration. Provide feedback and positive reinforcement to the patient.

9. Ask questions to check whether the patient has understood the information. You also can use questions to determine whether the patient is compliant.

10. Provide the patient with the prepared instructions and any other materials such as pamphlets, DVDs, or CDs.

11. Document your teaching in the patient's medical record using a formal teaching plan.

Teaching Plan: 32-year-old female with Iron Deficiency Anemia
Patient Learning Goal: Increase patient's knowledge of Iron Deficiency Anemia, its complications and treatments
Material to be Covered: Description of disorder, complications, diet, medications, procedures

Learning Objectives Comments	Teaching Methods/Tools	Procedure Explained/Demonstrated Date/Initial	PT Demonstrated/ Objectives Met Date/Initial
1. Patient describes what happens when body's demand for oxygen is not met. a. oxygen and hgb concentration decrease b. signs/symptoms of anemia c. anemia occurs only after body stores of iron are depleted	Instruction		
2. Patient describes complications caused by decrease of oxygen concentration a. chronic fatigue b. dyspnea c. inability to concentrate, think d. decrease in tissue repair e. increase of infection f. increase in heart rate	Instruction		
3. Patient discusses importance of diet in prevention of iron deficiency anemia a. including iron-rich foods in diet (beef, poultry, green vegetables) b. including foods that contain ascorbic acid to assist in absorbing iron in body (fruits) c. importance of limiting large meals if fatigued; stress importance of several small meals	Instruction/Video: "Your Diet: Why It Is Important"		
4. Patient describes prescribed medication, its purpose, dosage, route, and side effects	Instruction/Pamphlet: *Taking Your Iron Supplements*		
5. Patient aware of importance of follow-up appointments for evaluation of prescribed plan of treatment	Instruction/Appointment slip with next scheduled appointment		

Teaching Plan. (Reprinted from Kronenberger J, Ledbetter J. *Jones & Bartlett Learning's Comprehensive Medical Assisting.* 5th ed. Burlington, MA: Jones & Bartlett Learning, LLC; 2016.)

Procedure 21-2 | Identifying and Using Community Resources

1. Determine what types of resources will be most useful for the patients in your medical office. These may include support groups and/or services for:
   - Patients with serious and fatal diseases (e.g., cancer, multiple sclerosis)
   - Patients suffering from abuse
   - Patients who are ill or elderly and need assistance
   - Patients with limited financial resources
   - Patients who are hearing impaired or sight impaired
   - Patients with mental disabilities
   - Patients with chronic diseases

2. Compile a contact list of resources you can use to find out about community services. Your list may include:
   - Social service departments at hospitals
   - Local public health departments
   - Nursing home associations
   - Local charities and church organizations
   - Community services in the phone book
   - Web sites

3. Contact the resources to determine what services they offer. Create a list of services available. Include addresses, e-mail addresses, Web sites (if available), and phone numbers. Store this master list on your office computer.

4. When needed, use this master list to create a list of services specific to your patient's needs. Answer any questions your patient may have about the services available.

5. Offer to make contact with the service for your patient. However, some patients may prefer to do this for themselves. Be sensitive to your patient's wishes.

6. Document in your patient's chart that you provided the information.

Preparing for Externship

You are actually providing patient education each time you answer a patient's question. During your externship, be very careful to refer patient questions to the staff unless you have been authorized to provide specific information. Medical assistants need to be aware that offering advice to a patient may be a form practicing medicine. Most patients may not understand that you are a student and inexperienced. You should listen very carefully to the other medical assistants when they encounter questions from the patients. See how they handle the patient's questions.

Chapter Recap

- Medical assistants have an important role in patient education. They teach patients information about health care and disease prevention. They also help patients to accept their illnesses and provide support and encouragement.
- Effective patient education requires a teaching plan. Five main steps in the teaching plan are assessment, planning, implementation, evaluation, and documentation.
- Medical assistants use different strategies to implement the teaching plan. Some of these are lectures, demonstrations, role-playing, discussion, audiovisual presentations, and printed materials. Teaching aids such as diagrams, charts, or audiocassettes are useful.
- All teaching must be documented in the patient's medical record. Documentation must include the date and time of teaching, how the information was taught, and an evaluation of the teaching.
- Before they can learn new information, patients need to be motivated or realize they need to learn. Basic needs must be met before patients will be ready to learn health care skills.

- Factors that may be obstacles to learning are existing illness and/or pain, age, educational background, and physical impairments. The medical assistant should try to remove any obstacles to learning.

- Medical assistants often teach preventative medicine. They focus on promoting preventive screenings and teaching safety tips to prevent injury. Teaching patients about medications helps to prevent noncompliance and to avoid drug interactions or other serious side effects.

- Food labels can provide patients with nutritional information. Medical assistants may teach patients to look for the serving size when assessing the nutrients in a food product. Patients with specific medical conditions may need special diets.

- All patients should participate in some form of exercise on a regular basis. If patients are not able to exercise without assistance, range-of-motion exercises may be necessary.

- Alternative medicines may be useful for treating some medical conditions. Four therapies that have proven effective are acupuncture, acupressure, hypnosis, and yoga.

- Herbal supplements are not regulated by the Food and Drug Administration. Medical assistants need to assess whether patients are using herbal supplements, how long they have been using them, and any reported benefits. This information should be reported to the physician.

- Illness or disease often can lead to stress as patients experience changes in lifestyle, relationships, and anxiety associated with medical procedures. Medical assistants may teach patients about relaxation techniques to cope with stress. Three main relaxation techniques are controlled breathing, visualization, and physical exercise.

- Substance abuse can have serious health effects. Medical assistants provide patients with information from national organizations and may help patients find community resources if they ask for them. The most important role of the medical assistant is to be supportive.

Online Resources for Students

Student Resources available on the text's online site include:

- Audio Glossaries
- Animations
- Competency Evaluation Forms
- Videos
- Anatomy & Physiology Module with Heart and Lung Sounds
- Weblinks
- Worksheets

Exercises and Activities

Certification Preparation Questions

1. Which of these is not one of the five basic steps to effective patient education?
   a. Assessment
   b. Planning
   c. Documentation
   d. Follow-up
   e. Implementation

2. Tasks that are designed to help the patient reach the goal of the education program are referred to as:
   a. key elements.
   b. learning objectives.
   c. techniques of learning.
   d. styles of learning.
   e. measurable items.

3. Which of these training tools would be most effective with a patient who has vision impairment?
   a. Illustrations and drawings
   b. Charts and posters
   c. Videos and DVDs
   d. Audiocassettes and CDs
   e. Pamphlets and booklets

4. Which of these would not be recommended for patients who are at a greater risk for falls?
   a. Keep hallways free from clutter.
   b. Wear sneakers and shoes with no high heels.
   c. Use stairs whenever possible as a means of exercise.
   d. Store items frequently used on low shelves for easy access.
   e. Install handrails in the bathtub.

5. A patient who wishes to quit smoking should be told that he or she may experience these withdrawal symptoms except:

   a. muscle pain.
   b. anxiety.
   c. progressive restlessness.
   d. irritability.
   e. sleep disturbances.

6. Which of the following is not critical to discuss with the patient when you are teaching about a new medication therapy?

   a. The dosage to be taken
   b. The route of administration
   c. The cost of the drug
   d. The purpose for the medication
   e. Possible side effects

7. Which of these would not be a factor that would not need to be considered when the medical assistant is developing the patient's training plan?

   a. The patient's illness and pain
   b. The patient's age
   c. The patient's insurance company
   d. Any physical limitations the patient has
   e. The patient's educational background

8. The term used to describe a patient's inability or refusal to follow a prescribed order is:

   a. difficult.
   b. assertive.
   c. noncompliant.
   d. arrogant.
   e. irritable.

9. Which of these foods would provide the greatest amount of daily protein in the diet?

   a. Vegetables
   b. Grains
   c. Meat
   d. Oils
   e. Fruits

10. The term used for the process of performing the actual patient teaching is:

   a. evaluation.
   b. planning.
   c. implementation.
   d. questioning.
   e. documenting.

22 Medical Office Emergencies and Emergency Preparedness

Chapter Objectives

- Identify duties that may be required of a medical assistant during an emergency.
- List the key elements for a medical office emergency action plan.
- List signs that may indicate an emergency.
- Describe the general steps to take after identifying an emergency.
- Discuss the steps involved in the primary assessment of a patient in an emergency.
- Compare the two methods for opening an airway and explain when each is used.
- Describe the steps involved in cardiopulmonary resuscitation (CPR).
- Describe the purpose and use of the automatic external defibrillator (AED).
- Describe the signs, symptoms, and treatment of shock.
- Explain how to control severe bleeding from a wound.
- Explain how to classify burn injuries and how to assess the extent of a burn using the rule of nines.
- Explain the difference between sprains, strains, fractures, and dislocations and the emergency treatment for each condition.

- Identify the early symptoms of heart attack.
- Explain the signs of seizure and how to manage a seizure patient.
- Identify the signs and symptoms of an anaphylactic reaction.
- List the information needed before calling a poison control center.
- Contrast hyperthermia and hypothermia and list the dangers of each condition.
- Discuss the difference between a psychiatric emergency and an emotional crisis.
- Describe the steps in managing a patient who has fainted.
- Explain how to control a nosebleed.
- Identify unusual patterns of illness or patient behavior that could suggest bioterrorism.
- Explain the use of heat and cold in emergency treatments and identify adverse reactions to watch for.
- Describe the steps to follow for weather-related emergencies.
- Discuss the importance of preparedness in a catastrophic emergency.

CAAHEP & ABHES Competencies

CAAHEP

- Identify safety techniques used in responding to accidental exposure to blood, other body fluids, and chemicals.
- Discuss fire safety issues in the office or clinic.
- Describe fundamental principles for evacuation of a health care setting.

- Identify critical elements of an emergency plan for response to a natural disaster or other emergency.

ABHES

- Recognize and respond to medical office emergencies.

Chapter Terms

Abrasion	Dehydration	Hypothermia	Rule of Nines
Allergen	Diaphoresis	Hypovolemic shock	Seizures
Amputation	Ecchymosis	Immobilized	Septic shock
Anaphylactic shock	Edema	Infarction	Shock
Anaphylaxis	Epistaxis	Ischemia	Sprain
Avulsion	Hematoma	Luxation	Strain
Bioterrorism	Hemorrhage	Melena	Subluxation
Cardiogenic shock	Hemorrhagic shock	Neurogenic shock	Syncope
Contusion	Hyperthermia	Pressure points	Vasodilation
Defibrillation	Hyperventilation	Rescue breathing	

Abbreviations

AAPCC	CAB	LOC	RICE
AED	CPR	MI	SOB
BSA	EMS	PASS	

Case Study

Robert McNeil, a 40-year-old new patient, reported to the office for a well exam and medical clearance to participate in a Triathlon. When Bella, the medical assistant, was taking another patient from the waiting room, she noticed that Mr. McNeil appeared to be short of breath and diaphoretic. She placed her patient in a room, apologized briefly and explained she would return. She returned to the waiting room for Mr. McNeil. Bella notified another medical assistant that she had a potential emergency and asked that MA to notify the physician. As Bella and Mr. McNeil entered an exam room, he stated he didn't feel right. At that moment, with Bella walking behind and slightly to the side of him, Robert began to fall to the ground. Bella braced Mr. McNeil against her body and used her body to lower him safely to the ground. She immediately called for an AED and 9-1-1.

A medical emergency can happen anytime, anywhere, and to anyone. The outcome of any emergency hinges on the actions of those in the area. Proper planning and training will aid in the promptness and accuracy of your response. In this chapter, you'll learn about different types of emergencies that may occur in the medical office and how to handle them effectively.

EMERGENCY CARE IN THE MEDICAL OFFICE

Emergency medical care is immediate care given to persons who are sick or injured. Proper emergency care can sometimes mean the difference between:

- Temporary disability versus permanent disability
- Rapid recovery versus a long recovery
- Life versus death

Emergencies are classified as major and minor. In cases of major emergencies, treat the patient until help arrives to handle the situation and transport the patient to a hospital emergency room. For minor emergencies, treat the patient and send him home with instructions for follow-up care.

Steps for Handling Medical Emergencies

Providing proper care and treatment in medical emergencies is dependent on the following steps:

1. Correctly identify the emergency.
2. Deliver basic first aid.
3. If needed, provide temporary help or basic life support until an emergency response team arrives.

As a medical assistant, you are a valuable member of the team when medical emergencies occur. Some of the duties you may be called upon to perform include:

- Providing basic life support or assisting in life support procedures.
- Providing or assisting in basic first aid and other treatments.
- Contacting emergency rescue help and providing information about the situation when they arrive.
- Documenting emergency treatment delivered by medical office personnel.
- Calming the patient's relatives, other patients in the office, and any other bystanders during the emergency.

THE EMERGENCY ACTION PLAN

Every medical office should have an emergency action plan. The plan should include the:

- Local emergency rescue service phone number, if not 9-1-1
- Location of the nearest hospital emergency department, name and address
- Phone number of the local or regional poison control center
- Location and list of contents of the emergency medical kit or crash cart

- Procedures for various emergencies
- List of office personnel who are trained in CPR

You should be able to find the emergency action plan in the procedure manual for your medical office. Read it carefully so you know your office's protocol for handling emergencies.

Medical assistants need to be trained and certified to perform cardiopulmonary resuscitation (**CPR**). This technique temporarily circulates blood through the body when the heart has stopped. You also should know how to clear a person's airway when an object is blocking it. The American Association of Medical Assistants requires that certified medical assistants show proof of current CPR certification in order to certify or renew their CMA credential.

Providing emergency care requires you to coordinate many different events. Emergencies become complicated by added factors. Here are just a few examples:

- Panicky family members
- Arrival of emergency personnel
- Language barriers

You need to stay calm and focused, no matter what happens. You also need to perform your work competently, professionally, and within your scope of practice and state guidelines.

Additional Emergency Training and Certification

Although this chapter provides an overview of handling medical office emergencies, it is not a substitute for comprehensive training in emergency care. Your office may provide you with such training, as well as training in its own policies and procedures for handling emergencies. Other training may be available from the following organizations:

- American Red Cross
- American Heart Association
- American Health and Safety Institute
- National Safety Council

Emergency Medical Kit/Crash Kit

Proper equipment and supplies must be ready and easily accessible in the event of a medical emergency. The equipment and supplies in a medical office may vary with the medical specialty. However, emergency equipment and supplies are usually standard in all medical facilities. The equipment and supplies are stored in a place where all staff members can get to them. Replace items used during an emergency as soon as possible. In addition, a staff member should check the emergency kit or crash cart regularly to make sure all necessary items are present and that no items have passed their expiration dates.

Items in the Emergency Medical Kit/Crash Cart

Standard supplies for an emergency medical kit include the following:

- Activated charcoal
- Adhesive strip bandages, assorted sizes
- Adhesive tape, 1- and 2-inch rolls
- Alcohol (70%)
- Alcohol wipes
- Antimicrobial skin ointment
- Chemical ice pack
- Cotton balls
- Cotton swabs
- Disposable gloves
- Elastic bandages, 2- and 3-inch widths
- Gauze pads, 2-by-2-inch and 4-by-4-inch widths
- Rolls of self-adhesive gauze, 2- and 4-inch widths
- Safety pins, various sizes
- Scissors
- Syrup of ipecac
- Thermometer
- Triangular bandage
- Tweezers

In addition to these supplies, the following equipment should be available:

- Blood pressure cuff (pediatric and adult)
- Stethoscope
- Bag–valve–mask device with assorted size masks
- Flashlight or penlight
- Portable oxygen tank with regulator
- Suction unit and catheters
- Automatic external defibrillator (**AED**)

If possible, the following additional equipment also could be included:

- Various sizes of endotracheal tubes
- Laryngoscope handle and various sizes of blades
- Intravenous supplies (catheters, administration set tubing, assorted solutions)
- Emergency drugs (atropine, epinephrine, sodium bicarbonate)

Case Question

 Emergencies occur without warning. Mr. McNeil, the case study patient, was coming into the office for a physical and release to compete in a triathlon. He actually ended up as the victim of an emergency. Bella, the medical assistant, was able to identify the emergency immediately thanks to her training. What training or knowledge was required in order for Bella to handle this type of emergency?

Recognizing an Emergency

You may rarely see some types of emergencies in your medical office; however, you should still be aware of the signs. Here are some signs that can indicate an emergency:

- Fainting or loss of consciousness (**LOC**)
- Difficulty breathing or shortness of breath (**SOB**)
- Chest pain
- Choking
- Coughing up or vomiting blood
- Persistent vomiting
- Continuous bleeding or large wound
- Change in mental status (confusion, unusual behavior)
- Ingestion of a poisonous substance
- Head or spine injury
- Sudden injury, such as burns, smoke inhalation, a motor vehicle accident, or near drowning
- **Diaphoresis** (profuse sweating)

You should be able to recognize when an emergency exists and notify emergency medical services (**EMS**) when it is life threatening or could become life threatening.

Case Question

 Recall that Bella called for an AED and 9-1-1 immediately after Robert lost consciousness. Bella noticed Mr. McNeil's symptoms and identified them as an emergency. Her prompt actions resulted in Mr. McNeil receiving CPR with AED immediately. Being able to identify the signs of an emergency is critical to the patient's care. If Bella had not reacted so quickly in this situation, what might have happened to Mr. McNeil?

Steps to Follow in a Medical Emergency

In an emergency, the victim is always your first priority. Once you've identified the emergency, here are the general steps to follow:

1. Provide immediate care to the patient, including CPR if necessary.
2. While you're providing emergency care, direct another staff member to notify the physician.
3. Continue to provide first aid, or assist the physician in providing first aid, as the physician assesses the patient. Direct another staff member to notify EMS unless the physician tells you to do so.
4. When EMS arrives, assist EMS workers as necessary. Let them examine the patient and take over emergency care.

The staff member who calls EMS must be able to describe the emergency to the communications operator. This will tell the operator what level of emergency personnel and rescue equipment to send.

Documenting the Emergency

Once other medical staff members have taken over the emergency, you should turn to documenting the events. EMS personnel will need several pieces of information when they arrive:

- The patient's symptoms and duration
- The nature of the emergency
- Any treatment already provided and duration
- The patient's age
- Medications the patient is currently taking
- Allergies

Record this information in the patient's health record. Record events in chronological order as they occurred or as treatment was performed. In some cases, the emergency may involve visitors or staff. Document the treatment of these persons also. Most facilities complete report forms available in their electronic health record (EHR) system. These forms contain a format to insure that all information is time-lined and recorded. Additional items that will need to be documented include the following:

- Basic identification, including the person's name, age, address, and an emergency contact if known
- The chief complaint, if known
- Times of events, beginning with recognition of the emergency, management techniques, and changes in the person's condition

- The person's vital signs
- Specific emergency management performed in the office. Some examples might be CPR, bandaging, splinting, or any medications given by the office before, during, and after the emergency
- Observations of the patient's condition, such as slurred speech, lethargy, or confusion
- Any medical history, allergies, or current medications, if known

 EMERGENCY ASSESSMENT

During an emergency, you have two immediate goals:

- Identify and correct any life-threatening problems
- Provide necessary care

Meeting these goals requires an emergency assessment of the patient. There are three main steps to an emergency assessment. Manage each step effectively before proceeding to the next one.

- Primary assessment
- Secondary assessment
- Physical examination

You'll need to survey the scene quickly to identify any hazards to the patient (as well as yourself) and any clues to the patient's condition.

- Don't assume the obvious injuries are the only ones. Less noticeable or internal injuries also may have occurred.
- Look for the causes of the injury. They may provide a clue to the extent of the physical damage.

The Primary Assessment

When you reach the patient, do a quick check to assess the situation. The primary assessment is usually completed in <45 seconds. The purpose is to identify and correct any life-threatening problems. Immediately assess:

- Responsiveness—Is the patient conscious or unconscious? In some emergencies, the patient may be conscious and able to respond to your voice. If the patient is unconscious, try to wake him or her. Speak and touch the patient's shoulder. If there's no response, activate EMS.
- Circulation—In adults and children, you evaluate circulation by checking the carotid pulse. For infants, you need to use the brachial pulse. If no pulse is found, you must begin cardiopulmonary resuscitation (CPR) immediately. Starting with compressions then airway and respiration or breathing (**CAB**). If a pulse is present, move on to assess airway and respiration, noting the rate and quality.

- Airway—Open the patient's airway using the head tilt/chin lift (no suspected neck or spinal injury) or jaw thrust (suspected neck or spinal injury).
- Respiration—Once you've opened the airway, evaluate the patient's breathing. For an unconscious patient, look at the patient's chest to see if it's rising and falling. Listen for breathing sounds and feel for air moving out of the patient's mouth or nose. If the patient isn't breathing but has a pulse, start artificial respiration or **rescue breathing** immediately. If there is no pulse, initiate CPR, give two breaths and continue with CPR.

When performing CPR, check the patient's pulse frequently. Evaluate perfusion, or blood flow through the tissues, by checking the temperature and moisture of the skin. While assessing circulation, you also should check for any **hemorrhage**, the excessive flow of blood. Control any bleeding quickly.

Once you're sure the patient's heart is beating, you should recheck the patient's breathing. Respirations that are too fast, too slow, or irregular will require medical intervention. Immediate intervention for these conditions may include the following:

- Breathing into a mask or paper bag to treat **hyperventilation** (respirations that are too fast)
- Administering oxygen as directed by the physician

Assessing and Opening the Airway

There are two ways to assess the airway. The patient's condition will determine which one you'll use:

- For an unconscious patient, you normally assess the airway using the head-tilt/chin-lift technique. Figure 22-1 demonstrates the head-tile/chin-lift technique.
- Unconscious patients who may have neck injuries should have the airway opened using the jaw thrust technique. Figure 22-2 shows the jaw thrust technique used to open an airway.

An unconscious patient who is supine may have a partial or total airway obstruction, if the tongue has fallen back into the oropharynx. This would produce either snoring respirations or a total airway obstruction. In either case, you will need to open the patient's airway to allow for adequate respirations. The Table 22-1 explains both techniques for opening airways.

Obstructive Airway

The way to help a patient with a blocked airway will depend on the patient's condition. For a conscious patient, first ask, "Are you choking?" If the patient can speak or cough, the obstruction isn't complete. The patient can breathe. Observe the patient closely, and assist as needed. The patient may be able to remove the

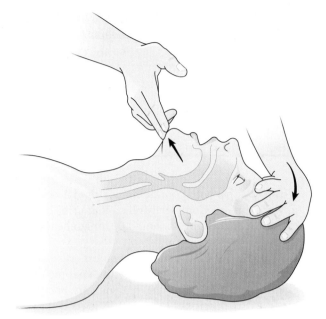

Figure 22-1 The head-tilt/chin-lift technique for opening the airway. The head is tilted backward with one hand while the fingers of the other hand lift the chin forward. (Reprinted from Kronenberger J, Ledbetter J. *Jones & Bartlett Learning's Comprehensive Medical Assisting.* 5th ed. Burlington, MA: Jones & Bartlett Learning, LLC; 2016.)

obstruction without help. Don't perform abdominal thrusts, as this may cause injury to the patient.

For a conscious patient who can't speak or cough:

1. Ask for permission to help the patient.
2. Stand behind the patient, slightly to the side. Wrap your arms around the patient's waist.
3. Stand behind the patient. Wrap your arms around the patient's waist.
4. Make a fist with your nondominant hand. Place the thumb side against the patient's abdomen approximately two fingers above the navel.

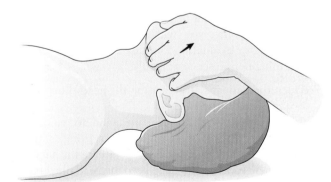

Figure 22-2 The jaw thrust technique for opening the airway. The hands are placed on either side of the head. The fingers of both hands grasp behind the angle of the jaw, bringing it up. (Reprinted from Kronenberger J, Ledbetter J. *Jones & Bartlett Learning's Comprehensive Medical Assisting.* 5th ed. Burlington, MA: Jones & Bartlett Learning, LLC; 2016.)

Table 22-1	Opening a Patient's Airway	
Patient's Situation	**Airway-Opening**	**Description of Technique**
Patient is unconscious and unresponsive.	Head tilt/chin lift	Tilt the head backward with one hand on the forehead. Lift the chin forward with the fingers of the other hand.
Patient is unconscious and may have neck injuries.	Jaw thrust technique	Place your hands on either side of the patient's head. Grasp behind the angle of the jaw with your fingers on both sides, and gently bring the jaw up.

5. Grasp your fist with your dominant hand. Give quick upward thrusts. Completely relax your arms between each thrust. Each thrust should be forceful enough to dislodge the obstruction.
6. Repeat the thrusts until the object is expelled. Several thrusts may be necessary to expel the object. Continue thrusts until the patient can breathe or becomes unconscious.
7. If you cannot reach your arms around the patient's waist or if the patient is pregnant, place your arms round their chest and perform chest thrusts.

If the patient becomes unconscious (if patient is unconscious when you arrive on scene follow protocol for CPR):

1. Activate EMS then begin CPR, starting with chest compression.
2. Following compressions, open airway and check for obstruction. If seen, remove it otherwise give two breaths.
3. Continue with CPR be sure to check for objects prior to breaths. Do not blind sweep. Only sweep if the object is visible.

Rescue Breathing

In your primary assessment, you'll determine whether the patient is breathing or not. If the patient has a pulse but isn't breathing, you will need to perform rescue breathing. After evaluating for pulse and respiration and determining the presence of a pulse you will:

1. Open the patient's airway using the head tilt/chin lift or jaw thrust.
2. With the airway open, use one hand to pinch the patient's nostrils shut. This stops air from escaping through the patient's nose. Rest the heel of the hand on the patient's forehead to help keep the head tilted back.
3. If available, place a one-way CPR valve or bag–valve–mask over the patient's mouth. This prevents transmission of disease. If not using a breathing mask, be sure to seal your mouth over the patient's mouth while blowing to prevent the air from escaping.
4. Turn your head to the side. Listen and watch for signs of breathing. If there are no signs of breathing,

deliver two breaths (each lasting about 1 second). Watch for chest rise. Use caution so that breaths are not too forceful as it will cause gastric distension and can promote vomiting.
5. If the patient's lungs don't inflate, the airway may be obstructed. Reposition the patient's head and give two additional breaths.
6. Check for signs of breathing and check the patient's pulse.
   ○ If the patient is still not breathing but has a pulse, give one slow breath every 5 seconds (adults and children) or one breath every 3 seconds for infants. Continue with breaths for 2 minutes and then check pulse and respiration. Repeat until the patient begins breathing, EMS arrives, someone with equal or greater training takes over, or you are too exhausted to continue.
   ○ If at any point the patient has no pulse, initiate CPR.

Cardiopulmonary Resuscitation

Cardiopulmonary resuscitation keeps the patient's blood circulating until the patient can receive appropriate medical care. The two main components of CPR are chest compressions and respirations.

Begin CPR anytime there is an absence of pulse. Once you have determined the patient is nonresponsive activate EMS, call 9-1-1 or your emergency team and begin CPR steps (for a single rescuer):

1. CPR begins with chest compression. Place your hand in the center of the chest, the lower half of the sternum.
2. Place the palm of the other hand on top of the hand on the chest and lace your fingers together.
3. Position yourself so your upper body is perpendicular to the patient's chest. Lock your elbows. Press straight down compressing the chest about 2 inches or 5 cm on adults and children.
4. Push hard and fast, allowing the chest to completely recoil between compressions.
5. After 30 compressions, give 2 breaths.
6. Compression rate will be 100 to 120 beats per minute.
7. Continue CPR until EMS arrives, or a pulse is palpated. Stop if you are too exhausted or the patient is breathing and has a heartbeat, or if the scene becomes unsafe.

Be sure to document the procedure as soon as you can. Here is an example of typical charting of the incident:

10/14/20xx 10:30 A.M. Pt. arrived complaining of chest pain. Skin diaphoretic, color pale. Pulse 125 and regular, BP 88/54 (L.). Collapsed in exam room, Dr. Barton notified. Pulse and respirations absent, CPR started. EMS notified. Signature: S. Pencil, CMA

10/14/20xx 10:40 A.M. CPR continued per EMS. Pt. transported to General Hospital. Signature: S. Pencil, CMA

CPR for Infants and Children

The CPR procedure for infants and children is slightly different from the procedure for adults. Here are the steps to follow:

1. Check for responsiveness. For children, gently tap shoulder and call to the child. For infants, flick the bottom of the foot.
2. If the patient is unresponsive, another person should notify EMS, or if you are alone, and the incident was unwitnessed, provide one full cycle of care and then activate EMS. If you are alone and witnessed the attack, notify EMS first and then begin CPR.
3. Place the infant or child on her back on a flat surface.
4. Assess for breathing and pulse. If not breathing with pulse, begin rescue breathing.
   ○ For children, pinch the nostrils and breathe into the mouth. If available, use a one-way CPR valve.
   ○ For infants, use your mouth to cover the mouth and nose. If available, use an infant one-way CPR valve mask.
5. Checking for a pulse.
   ○ For children, check the carotid pulse as you would for an adult.
   ○ For infants, check the brachial pulse.
   ○ As you palpate for a pulse, assess for signs of breathing.
   ○ If you feel a pulse and there are no signs of breathing, continue rescue breathing.
   ○ For children, give one breath every 3 to 5 seconds.
   ○ For infants, give one breath every 3 to 5 seconds.
6. If there's no pulse, begin chest compressions.
   ○ For children, place your hand in the same position as for adults. Use one hand or two hands to compress to approximately one-third the depth of the chest or 2 inches (5 cm). Give compressions at a rate of at least 100 to 120 beats per minute.
   ○ For infants, use two fingers to compress the middle of the chest just below the nipples. Compress to approximately one-third the depth of the chest or 1.5 inches or 4 cm. The rate of compressions should be about 100 to 120 beats per minute.

7. Give 2 breaths for every 30 compressions if you're delivering CPR on your own. If there are two rescuers attempting CPR on a child or an infant, give 2 breaths for every 15 compressions.
8. Continue CPR until EMS or advanced life support providers arrive or until the patient begins to move.

Defibrillation

Some medical offices may have an automatic external defibrillator (AED) as part of the emergency medical kit. **Defibrillation** is the process of using electric shock to restore normal heart rhythm. If your office or facility has an AED, take time to review its use prior to an emergency. Figure 22-3 is an AED used as soon as it is available. It aids in cardioversion.

How to Use an AED

In cases when a pulse is absent, use an AED as soon as it is available. Follow these steps for using the AED:

1. Turn on the AED and follow prompts.
2. While another rescuer performs CPR, remove, cut, or tear the patient's shirt. Prepare the chest for electrodes.
   ○ Remove medication patches and quickly wipe away any medication that may interfere with placement of the electrodes.
   ○ Make sure the chest is dry so the electrodes will have good contact.
   ○ Make sure the patient is not in water or is dried off.
   ○ Make sure the patient is not on any metal.

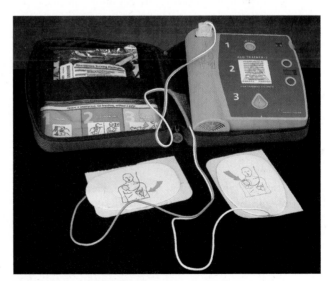

Figure 22-3 The AED is used to defibrillate a life-threatening heart rhythm. (Reprinted from Kronenberger J, Ledbetter J. *Jones & Bartlett Learning's Comprehensive Medical Assisting.* 5th ed. Burlington, MA: Jones & Bartlett Learning, LLC; 2016.)

3. The other rescuer should continue CPR while you remove the sticky paper backing and press electrodes onto chest.
   - Place the first electrode on the upper right chest.
   - Place the second electrode on the lower left chest.
4. Once electrodes are properly placed, plug in the pad connector and advise the other rescuer to stop CPR. The AED will analyze the heart rhythm. Don't touch the patient or perform CPR. Make sure the patient is not moving or in a moving vehicle. Follow instructions on the device.
   - If no shock is indicated, the AED will instruct you to restart CPR. Immediately restart CPR beginning with compressions.
   - If the AED indicates that shock is advised, make sure no one is touching the patient or the examination table. Shout, "Clear." Deliver the shock by pressing the button on the AED.
5. After delivering a shock, begin CPR immediately, starting with chest compressions. Check the victim's rhythm after giving about five cycles of CPR (about 2 minutes).
6. Continue the process until the EMS team arrives.

As with any procedure, defibrillation must be documented.

Secondary Assessment

By the end of the primary assessment, you will have checked and corrected the patient's airway, breathing, and circulation. Once this is done, and if EMS or other help has not yet arrived, you'll need to perform the secondary assessment. The secondary assessment involves asking the patient questions to get more information and doing a more thorough physical evaluation to find less obvious problems. When you evaluate the patient, you'll be assessing four things:

- General appearance
- Level of consciousness
- Vital signs
- Skin

General Appearance

The patient's skin color and moisture, facial expression, posture, motor activity, speech, and state of alertness are all clues to the patient's mental and physical condition. Check for a medical bracelet or necklace. Medicine bottles in a pocket or purse also can give you useful information.

Level of Consciousness

After examining the patient's general appearance, you may have a good indication of his level of consciousness.

Many conditions can alter a patient's level of consciousness, such as:

- A decrease in oxygen to the cells of the brain
- Neurological damage from a cerebrovascular accident (CVA or "stroke")
- Intracranial swelling

Vital Signs

The third part of the secondary assessment is taking vital signs, including pulse, respiratory rates, and blood pressure. It's also important to remember to check the patient's temperature. Temperature assessment is essential for:

- Patients who have altered skin temperature
- Patients who have been exposed to extreme environmental conditions
- Patients with a history of infection, chill, or fever
- Children with seizures

Skin

You'll have already noted the temperature and moisture of the skin during the primary assessment. A more thorough look is performed in the secondary assessment. Skin is normally dry and somewhat warm. Moist, cool skin may indicate poor blood flow to the tissues and likely, shock. The color of the skin provides information about circulation near the surface of the body and the oxygenation of tissues. Table 22-2 lists various abnormal skin colors and their causes.

Physical Examination

After performing the primary and secondary assessments, the patient should be examined from head to toe. The physician usually performs this examination, but you should be prepared to assist. It's important for you to keep providing reassurance to the patient.

Head and Neck

If a cervical spine injury is suspected, the patient's spine must be **immobilized** (unable to move) immediately. Also, avoid moving the neck when the head is examined. The head examination should include:

- Inspecting the face for **edema** (swelling due to fluid accumulation), **ecchymosis** (bruising), bleeding, and drainage from the nose and ears
- Examining the mouth for loose teeth and dentures
- Inspecting the eyes with a flashlight or penlight

Checking the pupils of the eyes can show the condition and severity of a neurological injury. This can help to assess patients with altered consciousness. The pupils should be checked for:

Table 22-2	Abnormal Skin Colors and Their Causes	
Skin Color	**Possible Causes**	**Possible Conditions**
Pink	Vasodilation Increased blood flow	Heat illness Hot environment Exertion Fever Alcohol consumption
White, pale	Decreased blood flow Decreased red blood cells Vasoconstriction	Shock Fainting Anemia Cold exposure
Blue	Inadequate oxygenation	Airway obstruction Congestive heart failure Chronic bronchitis
Yellow	Increased bilirubin (a waste product formed by the liver when breaking down red blood cells) Retention of urinary elements	Liver disease Renal disease

- Equality in size
- Dilation bilaterally in darkness or in dim light
- Rapid constriction to light in both eyes
- Equal reaction to light

To evaluate the pupils, you or the physician must shade the eyes from the light. A small flashlight or penlight is held 6 to 8 inches from each eye. A conscious patient should not look directly into the light. If you perform the examination, you should report the findings to the physician.

Cervical Fractures

The degree of injury to the patient depends on which cervical vertebrae are fractured. There are seven cervical vertebrae in the neck:

- C-1—Fractures to the first cervical vertebra are often fatal. They must be treated immediately and aggressively by EMS before the patient is transported to the hospital.
- C-2 and C-3—Fractures to the second and third cervical vertebrae often result in permanent or long-term respiratory dependency.
- C-4 to C-7—Fractures of the fourth to seventh cervical vertebrae usually result in different levels of paralysis and motor impairment.

If you think a patient has a cervical or spinal fracture, keep the patient still and call for EMS. Don't move the patient unless the patient is in immediate danger.

Chest, Back, and Abdomen

You may have examined the chest somewhat when you checked for respirations. You may need to remove clothing from the chest for a more thorough examination. Patients who should have a more thorough examination include patients with trauma, abnormal vital signs, and with cardiac or respiratory complaints.

A distended abdomen may indicate hemorrhage in the abdominal cavity. Palpation of the chest and back may also reveal possible fractures.

The abdomen of all patients is examined and inspected for scars, bruises, and masses. This examination is particularly important for patients with:

- Gastrointestinal symptoms
- Vaginal bleeding
- Vomiting
- **Melena** (blood in the stool)

Arms and Legs

Examination of the arms and legs is the last step in the head-to-toe survey. Arms and legs should be inspected for swelling, deformity, and tenderness. Also, any tremors in the hands should be noted. The neurological status of the arms and legs is checked by assessing:

- Muscle strength—in the upper extremities, it is checked by having the patient squeeze both the examiner's hands at the same time. Leg strength is assessed by having the patient push each foot against the examiner's hand, again at the same time.
- Range of motion—ensure that all limbs move in their full motion.
- Sensation—assessed by using a safety pin or other tool on the arms and legs to determine the patient's response to pain.

The examiner must compare both sides and note any weakness or decreased sensation in one side compared to the other. While the physician normally performs these tests, you should be prepared to assist as needed.

TYPES OF EMERGENCIES

Many different kinds of emergencies could need handling in a medical office. Although the physician or EMS probably will provide most of the emergency treatment, you may need to assist or care for the patient until help arrives. Knowing about the different types of emergencies you could encounter will prepare you for what to expect.

Shock

Shock is a lack of oxygen to individual cells of the body, including the brain. It results from a decrease in blood pressure. The reasons for this decrease can vary; the body reacts to any type of shock in much the same way:

- Strength of heart contractions increases.
- Heart rate increases.
- Blood vessels constrict (narrow in diameter) throughout the body.

As shock progresses, the body has more difficulty trying to adjust. Eventually, tissues and organs have such severe damage that the shock becomes irreversible, causing death.

Signs and symptoms of shock are as follows:

- Low blood pressure
- Restlessness or signs of fear
- Thirst
- Nausea
- Cool, clammy skin
- Pale skin with cyanosis (bluish color) at the lips and earlobes
- Rapid and weak pulse

Types of Shock

There are several types of shock, each with a different set of causes:

1. **Hypovolemic shock**—caused by loss of blood or other body fluids. If the cause is blood loss, it is called **hemorrhagic shock**. **Dehydration** (excessive water loss) caused by diarrhea, vomiting, or heavy sweating also can lead to hypovolemic shock.
2. **Cardiogenic shock**—an extreme form of heart failure. It occurs when the heart's left ventricle is so impaired it can't pump adequate blood to body tissues. This type of shock may follow the death of cardiac tissue during a myocardial infarction (**MI**), a heart attack.
3. **Neurogenic shock**—caused by a dysfunction of the nervous system following an injury to the spinal cord. After a spinal cord injury, the nervous system loses control of the diameter of the blood vessels, resulting in **vasodilation**. Once the blood vessels are dilated,

there is not enough blood in the general circulation. Blood pressure falls and shock occurs.
4. **Anaphylactic shock**—an acute general allergic reaction. It occurs within minutes or hours after the body has been exposed to an offending foreign substance. You must observe patients carefully for this type of shock after giving medications and during allergy testing.
5. **Septic shock**—caused by a general infection of the bloodstream. It may be associated with an infection such as pneumonia or meningitis. It also may occur without any apparent source of infection, especially in infants and children. The patient appears seriously ill. Initially, a fever is present, but the body temperature falls. This fall in temperature is a clinical sign suggesting sepsis.

Managing Patients in Shock

Shock can occur following many types of medical crisis or trauma. After doing primary and secondary assessments, you'll need to care for the patient. Here's a list of guidelines for managing a patient in shock:

1. Maintain an open airway and adequate breathing.
2. Control any bleeding.
3. Administer oxygen as directed by the physician.
4. Immobilize the patient if spinal injuries may be present.
5. Splint any fractures.
6. Prevent loss of body heat by covering the patient with a blanket, especially if the patient is cold.
7. If the patient's blood pressure is low, elevate his or her feet and legs.
8. Do not let the patient move unnecessarily.
9. Do not let the patient eat, drink, or smoke.
10. Be sure that someone stays with the patient at all times. The patient should not be unattended.
11. Call EMS to transport the patient to the hospital as soon as possible.

Implied Consent in Emergency Situations

In some emergencies, patients aren't able to give informed consent. For example, if the patient is unconscious, it's not possible to obtain her consent.

If treatment can be delayed without putting the patient in danger, the physician should obtain consent first. Conscious patients have the right to make choices about their emergency care.

If the patient is not competent or is unable to give consent, a surrogate may be asked to give it. A surrogate is a person authorized to make decisions on the patient's behalf. However, if no surrogate can be found and the patient's life is at stake, the physician can provide emergency treatment without informed consent.

Soft Tissue Injuries and Bleeding

Soft tissue injuries involve the skin and/or the muscles underlying the skin. An open injury to these tissues is referred to as an open wound.

When a blunt object strikes the body, it may crush the tissue beneath the skin. Although the skin doesn't always break, severe damage to the tissues and blood vessels may cause bleeding within a confined area. This is a closed wound.

Closed Wounds

There are three main types of closed wounds:

- **Contusion** is a collection of blood under the skin or in damaged tissue. The site may swell immediately, or 24 to 48 hours later. As blood gathers in the area, a characteristic black and blue mark called ecchymosis, or a bruise, can be seen.
- **Hematoma** is a blood clot that forms at the injury site. This often occurs when large areas of tissue are damaged. When a large bone is fractured, as much as a liter of blood can be lost in the soft tissue.
- **Crush injuries** are usually caused by extreme external forces that crush both tissue and bone. Even though the skin remains intact, the organs underneath may be severely damaged.

No matter what type of swelling occurs in a closed wound, the treatment is the same. You need to apply ice to the area to reduce and prevent more swelling.

Open Wounds

In an open wound, the skin is broken. This exposes the patient to external hemorrhage and wound contamination. You need to follow standard precautions to protect yourself against disease transmission and to protect the patient from further contamination. There are several kinds of open wounds. Some are more serious than others and each presents its own set of problems. Table 22-3 lists and describes the common types of open wounds.

Figure 22-4 is an example of a laceration, a type of open wound. Depending upon the depth of the laceration, suturing may be needed.

Some types of open wounds require special treatment. For amputations, you need to control the bleeding. However, you also need to preserve the severed part for possible reattachment later. Here are the steps for preserving a severed body part:

- Place the severed part in a plastic bag.
- Place this bag in a second plastic bag. This will provide added protection against moisture loss from the severed part.
- Place both sealed bags in a container of ice or ice water. Don't use dry ice.

Wounds with impaled objects also require special attention. Do not remove the impaled object and immobilize the body area impaled. Movement of the impaled object might cause more damage to the wound and underlying tissue. Place gauze pads around the object and stabilize. The immobilized, impaled object can be removed carefully after the patient is transported to the hospital.

Table 22-3	Types of Open Wounds	
Type of Wound	**Description**	**Examples/Causes**
Abrasion	The least serious open wound; it's basically a scratch on the skin's surface. All abrasions are painful because they affect nerve endings.	Scrapes
Laceration	Results from snagging or tearing of tissue, leaving jagged edges; skin may be partly or completely torn away.	Wound caused by broken bottle or piece of jagged metal
Major arterial laceration	Sharp or jagged instrument cuts the wall of a blood vessel; it may result in shock or death if bleeding is not controlled.	Same causes as lacerations
Puncture wound	Results from penetration of skin by sharp, narrow object; it also can be caused by high-speed penetrating objects, such as bullets.	Wound caused by knife, nail, or ice pick
Impaled object wound	Like a puncture wound; however, the object that caused the injury remains in the wound.	Wound with steel rod, stick, or glass
Avulsion	A wound with a flap of skin torn loose; the flap may remain hanging or tear off altogether. This wound usually bleeds profusely.	Wounds caused by machinery, lawn mowers, or power tools
Amputation	This is a wound caused by a force that is strong enough to rip away or crush limbs from the body.	Wounds caused in industrial or automobile accidents

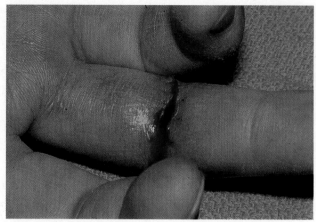

Figure 22-4 An open wound; laceration. (Reprinted from Kronenberger J, Ledbetter J. *Jones & Bartlett Learning's Comprehensive Medical Assisting.* 5th ed. Burlington, MA: Jones & Bartlett Learning, LLC; 2016.)

Managing Soft Tissue Injuries and Bleeding

Open wounds often involve bleeding. Here are some essential steps for controlling bleeding:

- Have the patient lie down to reduce the risk of fainting.
- Raise the body part above the level of the heart, if possible.
- Apply direct pressure to the wound by using a clean gauze pad and holding it firmly on the wound.
- If blood soaks through the gauze pad, place another pad on top. Keep applying pressure.
- Don't remove a pad that is soaked with blood. You could disrupt the process of blood clotting.
- If bleeding stops, secure the gauze pads with a bandage.

Controlling Severe Bleeding

Elevation and pressure to the wound alone may not stop severe bleeding. You also may need to apply direct pressure to an artery. **Pressure points** are specific places where you can press an artery against a bone. This will slow the flow of blood.

Here are some tips for using pressure points:

- Apply pressure to the artery at a point between the wound and the heart. Continue to apply direct pressure to the wound.
- Check if bleeding has stopped by slowly removing your fingers from the pressure point. However, keep direct pressure on the wound.
- Once the bleeding has stopped, don't continue to apply pressure to the artery.
- Only use pressure points if direct pressure doesn't stop the bleeding. Body tissues can be damaged without sufficient blood flow.

Figure 22-5 shows some wounds that require the use of applied pressure.

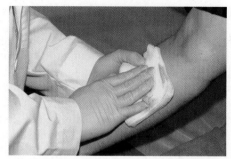

Figure 22-5 Applying direct pressure to a wound. (Reprinted from Kronenberger J, Ledbetter J. *Jones & Bartlett Learning's Comprehensive Medical Assisting.* 5th ed. Burlington, MA: Jones & Bartlett Learning, LLC; 2016.)

Burns

Burn injuries come from four main sources:

- Thermal burns (heat burns) are caused by contact with hot liquids, solids, superheated gases, or flame.
- Electrical burns are caused by contact with low- or high-voltage electricity. Lightning injuries are also considered electrical burns.
- Chemical burns result when wet or dry corrosive substances come into contact with the skin or mucous membranes. The amount of injury with a chemical burn depends on the amount and concentration of the substance and how long it's in contact with the skin.
- Radiation burns are similar to thermal burns. They can result from overexposure to ultraviolet light or from any extreme exposure to radiation.

Burn injuries are classified according to their depth and the layers of tissue affected. The depth of the burn depends on three factors:

- Agent causing the burn
- Temperature
- Length of time exposed

Classifying Burn Injuries

There are four classifications of burn injuries:

- First-degree burn or superficial burn
- Second-degree burn or partial-thickness burn
- Third-degree burn or full-thickness burn
- Fourth-degree burn

Figure 22-6 is an example of the redness and blisters that are signs of a second-degree burn.

Table 22-4 lists the four types of burns and their characteristics.

Body Surface Area and Burns

To treat burn patients, you need to assess how much of the body surface area (**BSA**) has been injured. The most

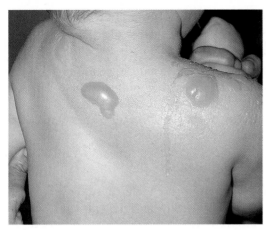

Figure 22-6 Partial-thickness burns. Toddler with second-degree burn caused by scalding. (Reprinted from Hatfield NT. *Broadribb's Introductory Pediatric Nursing.* Philadelphia, PA: Lippincott Williams & Wilkins; 2006.)

common method for doing this is the **Rule of Nines**. This method uses percentages to calculate the total surface area of specific sections of the body.

Adult Burns

In an adult, 9% of the skin is estimated to cover the head. Another 9% covers each arm, including front and back. Twice as much, or 18%, of the total skin area

covers the front of the trunk. Another 18% of the skin area covers the back of the trunk, and 18% covers each lower extremity (including front and back). The area around the genitals, or the perineum, is 1% of the total body surface area.

Pediatric Burns

In infants and children, the percentages are the same as for adults, with two exceptions. The head is 18% of the total skin area, and the lower extremities are each 13.5%.

Figure 22-7 shows figures of the Rule of Nines and how it is used to calculate the percent of burned area of the body.

Managing a Burn Patient

If you need to provide emergency treatment to a patient with burns, you can follow these guidelines. You should handle minor burns and major burns differently.

For minor burns that are second degree and not larger than 3 inches in diameter, you should follow the following steps:

1. Cool the burn by holding the burned area under cool running water for about 5 minutes. If this is not possible, use cold compresses. You should never put ice on a burn.
2. Cover the burn with sterile gauze. Do not wrap the gauze too tightly.

Table 22-4	Characteristics of Burns According to Depth				
Burn Depth	**Causes**	**Skin Layers Involved**	**Symptoms**	**Wound Appearance**	**Recovery Course**
First degree or superficial	Sunburn and low-intensity flash	Epidermis	Tingling, hyperesthesia (abnormal sensitivity to touch), and pain soothed by cooling	Reddened; blanches (or turns white) with pressure; little or no edema	Complete recovery within a week; some peeling
Second degree or partial thickness	Scalds and flash flame	Epidermis and dermis	Pain, hyperesthesia, and sensitivity to cold air	Blistered, mottled red base; broken epidermis; weeping surface; edema	Recovery in 2–3 weeks; some scarring, depigmentation; infections may convert to third degree
Third degree or full thickness	Flame, long exposure to hot liquids, and electric current	Epidermis, dermis, and sometimes subcutaneous tissue	Pain-free; shock; hematuria (blood cells in urine); possible entrance and exit wounds if electrical	Dry, pale, white, leathery, or charred; broken skin with fat exposed; edema	May require escharotomy (incisions made through dead tissue to relieve pressure) and skin grafting; scarring; loss of function; loss of digits or extremity possible
Fourth degree	Prolonged contact with flame, high-voltage electrical injury	Epidermis, dermis, subcutaneous tissue, muscle tissue, and potentially bone	Pain-free; shock	Possibly black and depressed; exposed bones and ligaments	Skin grafting usually needed; scarring; loss of function; loss of digits or extremity possible; recovery time depends on severity.

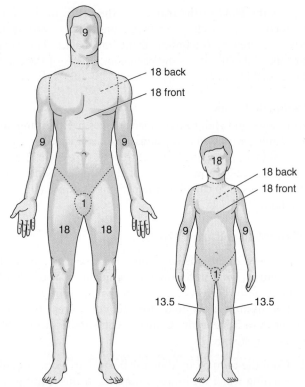

Figure 22-7 The rule of nines. (Reprinted from Kronenberger J, Ledbetter J. *Jones & Bartlett Learning's Comprehensive Medical Assisting.* 5th ed. Burlington, MA: Jones & Bartlett Learning, LLC; 2016.)

For major burns, here are the steps you should follow:

1. Eliminate the source of the burn, if necessary. Be sure that the patient is not in contact with any smoldering materials or heat.
2. Have someone notify the physician and call EMS.
3. Assess the patient's airway, breathing, and circulation. Begin CPR if necessary.
4. Cover the area of the burn using a sterile bandage or sheet.
5. Administer oxygen as instructed by the physician.
6. Treat the patient for shock and accompanying low blood pressure.
7. Assist with necessary procedures for transporting the patient to the hospital.

Musculoskeletal Injuries

Injuries to muscles, bones, and joints are some of the most common problems you'll encounter. These injuries vary widely in their seriousness. Some injuries are simple, such as a fractured finger while others may be life threatening, such as an open fracture to the femur, which can cause severe bleeding.

Injuries to muscles, tendons, and ligaments occur when a joint or muscle is torn or stretched beyond its normal limits. Fractures and dislocations usually result from external forces. However, they also can arise from diseases and bone degeneration.

Here are the major types of musculoskeletal injuries:

- **Strain**—an injury to a muscle and its supporting tendons
- **Sprain**—an injury to a joint capsule and its supporting ligaments
- **Dislocation**—bones of the joint are not in place
- **Fracture**—a broken bone

Sprains and Strains

Strains and sprains both can cause the affected site to be unstable. If a ligament is torn, it can't stabilize the joint properly. Common symptoms of strains include pain, limited motion, inflammation, and muscle spasm or weakness. Symptoms associated with sprains are also pain and inflammation as well as bruising, loss of ability to move the joint, and redness around the affected area.

You can help reduce these symptoms by following **RICE** therapy:

- R—rest by reducing physical activity and keeping your weight off the injured area for 48 hours.
- I—ice the area for approximately 20 minutes about four to eight times a day.
- C—compression of the injury by a wrap or special cast or boot can help reduce swelling.
- E—elevation above heart level can reduce swelling.

Figure 22-8 demonstrates a variety of splints used to immobilize sprains, strains, and dislocations.

Dislocations

A dislocation, or **luxation**, occurs when the end of a bone becomes displaced from its normal position in a joint. Dislocations may be caused from sudden impact to the joint in a fall, a blow, or other trauma. Common sites of dislocation are as follows:

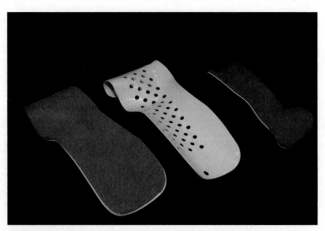

Figure 22-8 Types of splints. (Reprinted from Kronenberger J, Ledbetter J. *Jones & Bartlett Learning's Comprehensive Medical Assisting.* 5th ed. Burlington, MA: Jones & Bartlett Learning, LLC; 2016.)

- Shoulders
- Elbows
- Fingers
- Hips
- Ankles

Sometimes, a bone is pulled out of its socket, but all structures in the joint, such as ligaments and tendons, keep their proper relationships. This is referred to as a partial dislocation, or **subluxation**. Patients who have a dislocation or partial dislocation may have several symptoms, including:

- Pain
- Pressure
- Limited movement
- Deformity
- Numbness or loss of pulse in the affected extremity

Usually dislocations are treated by realigning the bones and immobilizing the joint. The patient may require a program of exercises to strengthen the supporting muscles.

Fractures

A fracture is a break or disruption in a bone. Fractures often are caused by falls or other trauma. Other causes may be disease, tumors, and unusual stresses on a bone. Symptoms of fractures include the following:

- Pain
- Swelling
- Lack of movement or unusual movement
- Bruising
- Deformity of the body part
- Exposure of the bone through the skin
- Numbness

Here are some types of fractures you might see as emergencies in a medical office:

- Simple or closed—a type of fracture that doesn't protrude through the skin.
- Compound or open—the broken end of a bone protrudes through the skin. Infection is a major concern.
- Greenstick—a type of fracture that is common in children. It is a partial or incomplete break. Only one side of a bone is broken.
- Compression—a type of fracture where the damage results from applying a strong force against both ends of the bone. It often results from falls. Vertebrae are susceptible to compression fractures.
- Pathological—fractures that result from disease processes are called pathological. Some diseases that may cause fractures are osteoporosis (brittle bones), Paget disease (a skeletal disease noted by bowing of the long bones), bone cysts, tumors, or cancer.

Managing Musculoskeletal Injuries

It can be difficult in some emergencies to tell whether an injury is a strain, sprain, dislocation, or fracture. In most cases, it's best to treat the area as a fracture. This means you'll need to immobilize the joint above and below the injury site. Doing this helps the patient by:

- Preventing further injury to soft tissues, blood vessels, and nerves
- Relieving pain by stopping motion at the site

Ice should be applied to the injured area as soon as possible. You should not apply the ice directly to the skin; instead, wrap the ice in a towel to avoid burning the skin. Ice will reduce the swelling that commonly occurs with this type of injury.

Types of Splints

A splint is any device used to immobilize a sprain, strain, fracture, or dislocated limb. Splinting material may be soft or rigid. Almost any object that will provide stability will do in an emergency. However, there are several types of commercial splints:

- Traction
- Air
- Wire ladder
- Padded board

Applying a Splint

With any type of splint, you need to check the injured extremity for signs of impaired circulation. Here are some tips to insure proper circulation:

- Observe the extremity's skin color and the nail beds of the hand or foot. A pale or cyanotic color indicates that circulation is blocked.
- Locate a pulse in an artery away from the affected extremity. A weak or absent pulse indicates decreased circulation to the area.
- Watch for increased swelling of the extremity. While this may not indicate that the circulation is impaired, the swelling itself may reduce circulation.
- If the circulation is impaired with the splint in place, loosen or remove it immediately. Without adequate blood flow, tissue **ischemia** (decrease in oxygen) and **infarction** (death of tissue) may occur.

Slings

If the injured body part is an arm, a sling will help to immobilize the limb as well. A sling usually is applied after the arm has been splinted. If available, you can use a canvas triangular arm sling, or a triangular bandage. A sling also could be improvised from a large piece of cloth, such as a pillowcase or clothing.

Here are some key points when applying an arm sling:

1. Position the injured limb across the patient's upper body. The hand should be at slightly less than a 90-degree angle. The fingers should be higher than the elbow. This helps to reduce swelling in the hand and fingers.
2. Place the triangle across the patient's upper body and under the injured arm.
   - The upper corner of the triangle is placed at the shoulder on the uninjured side of the body. Extend the corner across the nape of the neck.
   - The middle corner is placed under the elbow of the injured arm.
   - The third corner should be pointing at the foot on the uninjured side.
3. Bring up the third corner to meet the upper corner at the side of the neck.
4. Tie or use safety pins to secure the two corners together at the side of the neck. Never knot the sling at the back of the neck. It's uncomfortable for the patient.
5. Secure the elbow by fitting any extra fabric neatly around the injured limb and pinning.
6. Check the patient's comfort and the circulation to the distal part of the extremity.

Patient Education

Crutches are often prescribed for conditions when the patient can't bear weight on one foot or leg. They may be wooden or aluminium. Medical assistants are frequently responsible for teaching patients how to use them safely. Here are some techniques that aid in teaching patients how to properly use crutches:

A. Moving to a Standing Position
   1. Move both crutches to the hand on the affected side.
   2. Slide to the edge of the chair.
   3. Push down on the chair with the arm on the unaffected side and stand up.
   4. Rest on crutches until you get your balance.
B. Moving to a Sitting Position
   1. Back up to the chair until its edge is against the back of the legs.
   2. Move both crutches to the hand on the affected side.
   3. Reach back for the chair with the hand on the unaffected side.
   4. Lower yourself slowly into the chair.
C. Walking with Crutches
   1. Move both crutches forward. The unaffected leg should bear your weight.
   2. Support your weight on the hand grips of the crutches as you bring the unaffected leg forward.
   3. Insure that your armpits do not rest on the crutches or bear weight.
D. Walking up Stairs
   1. Hold on to the handrail and hold both crutches under the opposite arm. If there is no handrail to grasp, keep a crutch under each arm for balance.
   2. Stand close to the bottom step.
   3. Support the body's weight on your hands on the crutches. Step up to the first step with the unaffected leg. Remember that the good leg always goes up first.
   4. Push down on the crutches, and then step up with the weaker leg.
   5. Get your balance before attempting the next step.
E. Walking Down Stairs
   1. Stand close to the edge of the top step.
   2. Bend from the hips and knees to adjust to the height of the step below you. Don't lean forward! That can cause you to fall.
   3. Carefully lower the crutches and the affected leg to the next step.
   4. Then lower the unaffected leg to the lower step.
   5. Get your balance before you attempt the next step.

Other Crutch Gaits

Not all patients will be able to put weight on one leg. There are other types of crutch gaits that you should be familiar with.

- Four-point gait—used for patients who can put some weight on each foot. It is a slow gait, but one that provides stability and maximum support. The patient starts with the right foot and then advances the left crutch. Next the patient advances the left foot and then the right crutch. Once the patient is back to the beginning stance, the sequence starts again.
- Two-point gait—faster than the four-point gait, but it requires more stability and offers less support. The sequence starts with moving the right foot and left crutch and then the left foot and right crutch. This is repeated again once more until back to the beginning position.
- Three-point gait—requires good balance and good arm strength to support body weight. While it is a faster gait, it is not for everyone. The patient moves both crutches and the weaker leg forward at the same time. Then the stronger leg is moved forward while the arms support the body weight.

- Swing-to gait—requires good arm and upper body strength and a bit of practice, too. To begin, the patient lifts both feet and swings forward, landing the feet next to the crutches. Then he advances both crutches and repeats the same swinging move.
- Swing-through gait—similar to the swing-to gait. However, the main difference is that the body lands past the crutches during the swing movement. This is the fastest of all of the gaits.

Cardiovascular Emergencies

Cardiovascular disease accounts for nearly a million deaths each year in the United States. The most common problem is coronary artery disease. As coronary artery disease progresses, less and less oxygen can get to the heart. This leads to tissue ischemia and eventual infarction of the cardiac tissue.

About two-thirds of sudden deaths from coronary artery disease occur out of the hospital. Most occur within 2 hours after symptoms begin. The early symptoms of myocardial infarction, or heart attack, include the following:

- Chest pain not relieved by rest
- Complaint of pressure in the chest or upper back
- Nausea or indigestion
- Chest pain that radiates up into the neck and jaw or down one arm
- Anxiety
- Shortness of breath
- Cold sweats
- Paleness

Early treatment can prevent many deaths related to heart attacks. This treatment may include basic life support, early defibrillation, and advanced life support.

If CPR is started right away and the patient is quickly and successfully defibrillated, chances of survival improve greatly. If the patient has no pulse and you suspect a heart attack is the cause, the AED should be used as soon as possible, if one is available.

Neurological Emergencies

Seizures are caused by abnormal electrical activity in the brain. During a seizure, several different behaviors can occur. Here are some typical examples:

- Erratic muscle movements
- Strange sensations
- Complete loss of consciousness

A seizure is not a disease. It's a symptom of another disorder. Epilepsy, head injury, and drug toxicity are potential causes of seizures.

Assessing Seizure Patients

It's important to review the patient's history when assessing a seizure patient. The review should include the following:

- Information about previous seizure disorders
- Frequency of the seizures, if they've happened before
- Medications the patient is taking
- History of head trauma
- History of alcohol or drug abuse
- History of recent fever
- Presence of neck stiffness (as seen in meningitis)
- History of heart disease, diabetes, or stroke

Managing Seizure Patients

In managing a patient having a seizure, your first priority is to assess the patient's responsiveness, airway, breathing, and circulation. In some types of seizures, the patient loses consciousness.

During a seizure, the body's muscles will contract tightly, including the muscles of the face. Because of this, it's important that you don't try to put any object in the patient's mouth. If you try to force an object between the teeth to prevent the patient from biting his or her tongue, you may injure yourself or the patient.

Patients often vomit during a seizure and lose bowel and bladder control. You need to clear and maintain the patient's airway. You should never give the patient any food or water. Assisting the patient into the recovery position (on one side) will help secretions such as blood or vomit drain from the mouth. You also may remove secretions from the mouth using a suction machine, if one is available.

After gaining control of the airway, the most important thing you can do for a patient during a seizure is to protect the patient from injury. Don't hold the patient down at any time. Move the patient only if you are in a dangerous place such as the top of a flight of stairs. Move items that could hurt the patient away from the area. If possible, you should put something soft under the patient's head to prevent injury. If the patient lost consciousness and fell at the beginning of the seizure, you will need to protect the neck and cervical spine until the spine can be immobilized.

Allergic Reactions

An **allergen** is a substance that causes a person to have an allergic reaction. This general reaction occurs after the body has been exposed to a substance to which it's sensitive. Common types of allergens include drugs, insect venom, pollen, and certain foods. Allergens can enter the body in several ways. The most common ones are injection, inhalation, and absorption through the skin or mucous membranes

In some cases, a person may have symptoms within seconds after exposure to the allergen. In other cases, the reaction is delayed for several hours. It's important to ask patients about their allergies at every visit since new allergies can develop at any time. Enter any allergies into the patient record.

Signs and Symptoms

Always check the patient's medical record and ask about allergies before administering any medications in the office. This is critical to preventing reactions in patients with known allergies.

Repeated exposures to a substance that produces a simple allergic reaction eventually may lead to anaphylaxis. An anaphylactic reaction is much more severe than an ordinary allergic reaction.

You should know the signs and symptoms of allergic reactions and watch for them in your patients. A key rule to remember is that the sooner the symptoms occur after the exposure, the more severe the reaction is likely to be. Be observant and ready to treat any patient who shows any of these early symptoms:

- Severe itching
- Feeling of warmth
- Tightness in the throat or chest
- Rash

If these conditions are left untreated, and the situation worsens, anaphylaxis could be the result.

Allergy Injections

Patients with moderate to severe allergy symptoms often receive frequent injections of specific allergens. These can reduce the symptoms associated with certain allergies.

After an injection, the patient should be monitored closely for anaphylaxis. The patient should not be permitted to leave the office for a prescribed amount of time, usually 20 to 30 minutes after the injection. When documenting an injection, you should always note the condition of the patient at discharge.

Anaphylaxis

Anaphylaxis occurs when the body's immune system recognizes a substance to which the person is extremely allergic. Most of the emergencies that result from allergic reactions are due to anaphylaxis. Anaphylactic reactions can lead to airway obstruction, cardiovascular collapse, shock, and even death.

The main cause of death in anaphylactic reactions is swelling of the tissues in the airway, leading to airway obstruction. You need to observe a patient having an allergic reaction closely for any signs of airway involvement. You should watch for:

- Wheezing
- Shortness of breath
- Coughing
- Choking
- Feelings of tightness in the neck and throat

Along with these signs of airway involvement, patients with severe allergic reactions may experience:

- Tachycardia
- Hypotension
- Pale skin
- Dryness of the mouth
- Diaphoresis (profuse sweating)
- Other signs of shock

Managing Allergic and Anaphylactic Reactions

Patient care will depend on the severity of the allergic reaction. Some allergic reactions are mild, without respiratory problems or signs of shock. These can be managed by administering oxygen or medications, such as antihistamines, to relieve symptoms (as directed by the physician). If respiratory involvement occurs without signs of shock, the physician may order epinephrine to be given subcutaneously.

The patient with a severe anaphylactic reaction who is in shock needs more aggressive treatment. This treatment will include additional medications, an intravenous line, and monitoring of the patient's cardiac rhythm and other vital signs.

Treating Anaphylactic Reactions

The main goal in treating a patient who's having an anaphylactic reaction is to restore respiratory and circulatory function. The following steps should be followed:

- Don't leave the patient alone. Have another staff member call the physician immediately and bring the emergency kit or crash cart, including oxygen. Another staff member also should call EMS.
- Help the patient into a semi-Fowler position.
- Assess the patient's respiratory and circulatory status by obtaining blood pressure, pulse, and respiratory rates.
- Observe the patient's skin color and warmth.
- If the patient complains of being cold or is shivering, cover her with a blanket.
- Administer oxygen and other medications as ordered.
- Document vital signs and any medications and treatments.
- Communicate relevant information to the EMS personnel, including copies of the patient's progress notes or medication record as needed.

Poisoning

There are many substances in the home and workplace that lead to poisoning. Some examples are medications, both over-the-counter and prescription, and household and industrial chemicals.

Most toxic exposures occur in the home. Almost half of these occur in children ages one to three. Household chemicals often have a pleasant odor and color. This may make them appealing to young children if not stored properly.

About 90% of reported poisonings are accidental. Intentional exposure usually involves adolescents and adults who are abusing these substances. They tend to have a higher death rate. Your office's emergency action procedures should include directions on how and when to contact poison control.

The Poison Control Center

The American Association of Poison Control Centers (**AAPCC**) has established standards and regional poison control centers throughout the country. Physicians, nurses, and pharmacists are on the staff at these centers. The poison control center is a valuable resource. The phone number should be posted near all phones in the medical office.

The professionals at the poison control center will help in several ways:

- Evaluation a potential or known toxic exposure
- Instruction on steps to take, including when to use of syrup of ipecac to induce vomiting
- Check on the patient's progress by follow-up telephone calls

Managing Poisoning Emergencies

Few toxic substances have specific antidotes or remedies to control or stop the effect of the poison. So managing a poisoning emergency involves treating the signs and symptoms and assessing the organ systems involved.

The patient may arrive at the medical office after the poisoning. More commonly, the patient or caregiver phones the office requesting information. In either case, you need to obtain the following information before calling a poison control center:

- Nature of the poisoning (ingested, inhaled, skin exposure)
- Age and weight of the patient
- Name of the substance
- Estimate of the amount of substance involved
- When the exposure occurred
- Patient's present signs and symptoms

Once the poison control center is notified, and instructions provided, you must be prepared to treat the patient as directed. Also, notify EMS to transport the patient to the hospital, if needed.

Heat- and Cold-Related Emergencies

Life depends on the body's ability to control its core temperature within a range of several degrees. Measured rectally, this core temperature is about 99.6°F (37.6°C). The peripheral temperature is usually lower (98.6°F orally). However, several conditions can disrupt the normal temperature-regulating mechanisms of the body. These conditions are grouped under two main categories.

- **Hyperthermia** is a general condition of excessive body heat.
- **Hypothermia** is an abnormally low body temperature.

Another cold-related condition that may require emergency care is frostbite.

Managing Hyperthermia

Correct management of hyperthermia depends on assessing its type. The three main types of hyperthermia are heat cramps, heat exhaustion, and heat stroke.

Heat Cramps

Heat cramps are muscle cramps that follow a period of heavy exertion and profuse sweating in a hot environment. Sweat is mainly water, but it also contains sodium, a key electrolyte needed for muscle function. An electrolyte is a substance found in the body that includes dissolved minerals such as potassium, sodium, and calcium. Heavy sweating will result in a sodium deficit. This will impair muscle function and cause cramps. A patient with heat cramps often complains of cramping in the calves of the legs and in the abdomen; however, cramping also may occur in the hands, arms, and feet. Mental status and blood pressure usually remain normal, although an increased pulse rate is common.

Patient Education

Teaching patients to recognize the signs and symptoms of heat- and cold-related illness will help prevent serious issues. Encourage patients to drink an electrolyte solution and plenty of water before and during physical activities on a hot day. They should drink water every 20 minutes during outdoor exercise.

Heat Exhaustion

Physical exertion in a hot environment without adequate fluid replacement can result in heat exhaustion. Heat cramps may or may not occur before this stage is reached. Body temperature usually remains normal or slightly above normal. Patients have central nervous symptoms, such as:

- Headache
- Fatigue
- Dizziness
- *Syncope* (fainting)

Typically, the skin will be moist and the pulse rate will be high. However, skin color, blood pressure, and respiratory rate will vary with the degree to which the body is able to hold off the distress. A patient in the late stage of heat exhaustion will have pale skin, low blood pressure, and rapid respirations.

A person with heat exhaustion does not usually need to see a physician unless the conditions worsen. Tell patients that the first step in managing heat exhaustion is to get out of the heat and get inside or to a shady location. The person should lie down with her legs elevated. She should also drink cool water or a sports drink with electrolytes.

The person must be monitored so the condition doesn't become more serious and turn into heatstroke. If there is a fever > 102°F, fainting, confusion, or seizures, the patient must seek emergency medical assistance immediately.

Heat Stroke

Heat stroke is a true emergency. In heat stroke, the body is no longer able to compensate for the rapid rise in body temperature (>105°F). This can lead to brain damage or death. Patients with heat stroke can deteriorate quickly into coma. Many patients have seizures. Here are the signs and symptoms of heat stroke:

- Skin is classically hot, flushed, and dry with the absence of sweating.
- Vital signs are elevated at first, but may drop and cardiac arrest may follow.
- Patient may be confused, irritable, or unconscious.

To manage heat stroke, you need to cool the patient's body. Alert the physician. Then, follow office policy for the management of hyperthermia and heat stroke. You should include these steps:

1. Move the patient to a cool area.
2. Remove clothing that may be holding in the heat.
3. Place a wet sheet on the body or cool wet cloths on these key surface areas, where the ability to cool its blood is greatest:
   - Scalp
   - Neck
   - Axilla (armpits)
   - Groin
4. Administer oxygen as directed by the physician and apply a cardiac monitor.
5. Notify EMS for transporting the patient to the hospital.

Hypothermia

The body can tolerate a drop in core temperature of 3°F to 4°F without loss of normal body function. However, further drops due to internal metabolic factors and significant heat loss to the environment can lead to hypothermia. Hypothermia may result from very cold air or immersion in cold water. These are common signs and symptoms:

- Cool, pale skin
- Lethargy and mental confusion
- Shallow, slow respirations
- Slow, faint pulse rate

There are several steps involved in managing a patient with hypothermia. You should contact EMS so the patient can be taken to a hospital emergency room. Until the ambulance arrives, manage the patient by handling gently, remove wet clothing and cover the patient to prevent further cooling. You should not massage or rub the patient's skin. And do not apply any direct heat. Wrapping the patient in a blanket is enough until he gets to the hospital.

If there's evidence of rewarming (warm skin, no shivering, and respirations approaching normal), and if the patient is alert and able to swallow, give warm fluids by mouth. Avoid drinks that constrict peripheral blood vessels, such as coffee, tea, or other drinks containing caffeine. Fluids that cause dilation of the blood vessels, such as alcohol, should also be avoided. Warm beverages with sugar, such as hot chocolate, can be given to begin replacement of fuel the body needs to restore normal heat production.

Frostbite

The greatest risk of frostbite occurs in windy, subfreezing weather. Body parts with a high ratio of surface area to tissue mass are the most vulnerable to frostbite. These areas include the fingers, toes, ears, and nose. Larger areas of the extremities are also vulnerable during profound cooling. The main factors that determine the extent of the frostbite are the type of contact and the duration of contact.

For example, touching cold fabric is not as dangerous as coming into contact with cold metal, especially if the skin is wet or damp.

Superficial frostbite can be managed by warming the affected part with another body surface. For example, placing an ungloved hand over the nose and ears can provide the necessary warmth. For more severe cases of frostbite, rapid rewarming is necessary.

Behavioral and Psychiatric Emergencies

Psychological distress may be mild, moderate, or severe. The type and amount of intervention necessary depends on the degree of intensity. It's important for you to know the difference between a psychiatric emergency and an emotional crisis.

- Psychiatric emergency—any situation in which the patient's moods, thoughts, or actions are so disordered or disturbed that harm or death may result for the patient or others if there is no intervention.
- Emotional crisis—is a situation with much less intensity. It may be distressing to the patient. But it is not likely to end in danger, harm, or death. However, an emotional crisis can't be neglected. That's because it may turn into a full psychiatric emergency.

Like a medical emergency, a behavioral emergency can be very serious. Urgent situations usually require some form of professional intervention including transfer to a hospital.

Study Skill

There's so much to remember in dealing with emergencies that it may seem overwhelming. Here's a study tip that may help. Make a summary chart that shows what to do in different situations.

On the left, list the different types of emergency situations that might occur, such as fracture, frostbite, heat emergencies, shock, poison, etc. On the right, list the key steps you need to follow.

Making the chart will help you organize and remember the information. Drill yourself on the steps by covering up the right side of the chart. Look at the heading you made on the left, and see if you can remember what you need to do.

OTHER URGENT SITUATIONS

As a medical assistant, you may encounter other situations that can lead to emergencies if first aid is not delivered promptly or if complications arise. In the medical office, the physician is usually available to treat these situations. However, it's important for you to know what to do in case the physician isn't available or so you can provide assistance.

Fainting

Syncope, or fainting, is a sudden loss of consciousness due to insufficient oxygen or blood to the brain. Sometimes, fainting occurs without any warning signs. In other cases, one or more of these warning signs may be present:

- Abnormally pale appearance
- Feelings of dizziness
- Nausea
- Numbness or heaviness in extremities

Most fainting episodes last less than a couple of minutes. The main danger to the patient is from injuries that may occur as a result of falling when losing consciousness.

If a patient shows signs of fainting, ask the patient to lower his or her head to increase the blood supply to the brain. You also may decide to ask the patient to lie down to avoid a potential fall. For a patient who has fainted, follow these steps:

1. Check the patient's airway and perform rescue breathing or CPR if necessary. Check the patient's vital signs.
2. Notify the physician of the patient's condition.
3. Loosen tight clothing. Cover the patient with a blanket for warmth.
4. Elevate the patient's feet above the level of the heart. This may help to relieve symptoms of fainting. But don't move the patient's legs if there is any chance of head or neck injuries or if the patient has heart problems.
5. Monitor vital signs.
6. Once the patient has recovered, slowly assist the patient into sitting position. Don't leave the patient alone until he has recovered.

The fainting episode should be documented in the patient's medical record, along with any care or treatment provided.

If the patient doesn't recover consciousness quickly or has other symptoms that may be life threatening (such as chest pain, loss of speech, or visual disturbances), it may be necessary to call EMS.

In rare cases, fainting may be a sign of a serious medical problem, such as heart disease or stroke. It also can be a complication of diabetes (low blood sugar) or medication use. Patients who don't regain consciousness may have slipped into a coma.

Asthma Attacks

Patients with asthma sometimes may experience an acute attack. The symptoms of an asthma attack are as follows:

- Wheezing
- Coughing
- Tightness in the chest
- Shortness of breath

Patients often become frightened during an attack, because they're concerned about getting enough air. In managing an asthma attack, there are some key steps to follow:

1. Notify the physician that the patient is having breathing difficulties.
2. Assess the patient's airway, breathing, and circulation.
3. If the patient has an asthma inhaler, help the patient get out the device and use it, if necessary. Provide reassurance to keep the patient calm.
4. Administer asthma treatments with a nebulizer or medications to open up the patient's bronchi, as directed by the physician.

Fever

Fever is a sign that the body is working to fight infection. The discomfort associated with a fever can usually be managed with acetaminophen or aspirin. However, a fever > 105°F (40°C) can lead to irreversible brain damage.

If a patient has an abnormally high temperature, you must provide treatment right away.

1. Check the patient's responsiveness and other vital signs.
2. Notify the physician of the patient's condition.
3. Cool the patient by placing cool, damp towels on the axilla and groin.
4. Watch the patient carefully for signs of seizure, especially if the patient is a child.
5. Continue to monitor vital signs.

Eye Injuries

Injuries to the eye can be painful or irritating. Types of eye injuries include the following:

- Burns to the eye
- Foreign objects in the eye
- Chemicals in the eye
- Cuts or punctures of the eye or eyelid
- Blows to the eye

Here are some tips for managing eye injuries:

- Have the patient wait for the physician in a darkened room. Patients with eye injuries are often sensitive to light.
- Remind the patient not to rub or touch the eye. An ophthalmic topical anesthetic may be applied to relieve pain or irritation, as directed by the physician.
- If there is swelling or contusion, apply cold, wet compresses.
- Don't try to remove any foreign object from the eye.

If the injury is a result of a foreign object or substance, the physician may order eye irrigations. See Procedure 22-1 for steps to perform eye irrigation.

Ear Emergencies

Ear emergencies may involve the outer, middle, or inner ear. They have many different causes. For example, young children sometimes stick objects in their ears. Excessive buildup of cerumen (earwax) also can cause problems.

Some signs and symptoms of ear emergencies include the following:

- Dizziness
- Loss of hearing
- Nausea and vomiting
- Earache
- Bleeding or discharge from the ear
- Swelling or redness
- An object visible in the ear

A common treatment for removing debris or foreign objects from the ear is irrigation.

Impacted wax can impair hearing, cause discomfort or even pain, and result in possible injury to the ear. Sometimes, before beginning the irrigation, medication is instilled into the ear to soften the wax or relieve pain. Procedure 22-2 provides steps in performing ear irrigation.

Nosebleeds

Nosebleeds, or **epistaxis**, can occur as a result of injury to the membranes in the nose. They also may result from another disease process, such as hypertension or cancer.

Most nosebleeds are not serious. They can be managed by following these steps:

1. Have the patient sit upright, with his or her head tilted slightly forward. This helps prevent nasal drainage down the throat, which can lead to nausea.
2. Compress the nostril (nares) against the septum using ice or a cold, wet compress. The nostril should remain compressed for 5 to 10 minutes.
3. Remind the patient to sit still. The patient should not blow their nose until the physician advises that it's okay to do so.

If a nosebleed continues for more than 10 minutes after treatment begins, it's considered severe. The patient may need to be transported to the hospital or the physician may perform additional treatment. Some additional treatments you may need to assist with are inserting nasal packing material, inflating a balloon catheter in the nose, or cautery treatment to seal off blood vessels.

Disaster Emergencies

Your training and knowledge about medical emergencies may be useful in situations where large numbers of people are injured. Examples of such situations are as follows:

- Natural disasters such as tornados, floods, fires, hurricanes, or earthquakes
- Terrorist acts, including acts of bioterrorism

Natural Disasters

In a natural disaster, medical personnel often are summoned to treat a wide range of emergency conditions. Some of the injuries you might have to deal with in a natural disaster include shock, muscular and soft tissue injuries, musculoskeletal injuries, and burns.

You can prepare yourself for a disaster situation by becoming familiar with standard protocols for responding to disasters. Here are some general tips for managing victims during or after a natural disaster:

- Make sure the scene is safe. You may need to wait for the scene to be secured by proper authorities (police, fire, civil defense) before you evaluate the patient.

- Practice standard precautions when caring for wounds. After some natural disasters, it may be difficult to find running water. If water is not available, use an alcohol-based product to wash your hands.
- Watch carefully for the presence of other injuries that may not be obvious.
- Obtain a history from the patient, and perform a head-to-toe examination to rule out other injuries.

Acts of Terrorism

In an act of **bioterrorism**, toxic substances or biological agents are deliberately released to harm people in the community. Several substances have been identified as possible weapons:

- Anthrax
- Smallpox
- Plague
- Tularemia
- Botulism

There's an additional risk of tetanus for both victims and responders in a disaster. Tetanus is a nervous system disorder caused by bacteria that can enter the body through punctures and other cuts and wounds. As a medical assistant, it is important to issue your tetanus vaccine up to date.

If bioterrorism occurs, medical offices will provide an important resource for health care. They are likely to be one of the places where unusual patterns of illness or behavior are first noticed. You should be alert to any unusual patterns. Here are some important events to watch for and alert the physician:

- An unexpected number of patients with a particular illness
- Clusters of patients arriving from the same location
- Clusters of patients with the same disease arriving within a short period of time
- An unusual age distribution for a disease
- A disease with an unusual exposure route
- A disease that occurs outside its normal transmission season
- Disease that has an unusual pattern of resistance
- An unusual strain of a disease

EMERGENCIES PREPAREDNESS

The best way to prepare for an emergency is to plan ahead and expect the unexpected. Floor plans with emergency escape routes should be posted in every office and examination room. Escape routes should be color coded to indicate the primary, secondary, etc. Additionally, exits should be well lit with battery backup lighting.

Risk of Fire

In most areas, the fire marshal will perform a yearly inspection to insure that all exit signs are lit and that the battery backup system is in working order. The fire marshal will also check your sprinkler system and smoke alarm. Despite the fire marshal's yearly visit, you should schedule monthly checks to insure everything is in working order. In the event of a fire, a plan should be in place for exiting patients. This plan should include who will be responsible for patients in the different areas of your office. Quarterly drills should be performed, without patient involvement, to insure everyone remembers their responsibilities. Time should be spent reviewing the results of the drill as well as discussing any modifications that might need to occur.

Fire Extinguisher

Every employee should know where fire extinguishers are located and how to properly use them. Fire extinguisher will need to be check and maintained a minimum of yearly. Anytime an extinguisher is used, it will have to be recharged or replaced. Housing units for your extinguisher should have easy access. At the first sign of fire, smelling of unexplained smoke or seeing smoke, call 9-1-1.

Use of a Fire Extinguisher

When using a fire extinguisher remember to **PASS**—Pull, Aim, Squeeze Sweep. The steps are as follows:

1. Pull the pin and hold the extinguisher with the nozzle pointing away from you.
2. Aim at the base of the fire.
3. Squeeze the level slowly and evenly.
4. Sweep from side to side.

Be sure you know your escape route in the event you can't contain the fire. Be mindful of time and smoke. Remember you will be inhaling smoke while you are working to put out the fire.

WEATHER EMERGENCIES

There may be times that your office and patients are at risk from weather-related events. Your emergency plan should detail any possible weather-related emergency that could occur in your area. You should be familiar with the plans and where the safest places for patients and staff. Your plan should include precautions for loss of electricity resulting in loss of heating or cooling, as well as how to treat any injuries. Your office should have a battery-operated emergency or weather radio. Be sure that you stock up-to-date batteries so that you can stay informed. Additionally, stocking some provisions like water and food would be advisable.

Procedure 22-1 | Performing Eye Irrigation

In this procedure, sterile solution is used to wash out the eye. The steps for performing eye irrigation are as follows:

Equipment: Unpowdered gloves, irrigation solution (warmed to body temperature), emesis basin, sterile irrigation syringe, and tissues.

1. Wash your hands and put on gloves (unpowdered) for infection control and assemble equipment.

2. Check the label for the solution three times, as you would for other medications. Make sure the solution label states it is for ophthalmic use.

3. Have the patient lie down with the affected eye down or sit with the head tilted so the affected eye is lower than the other eye. This helps to prevent contamination of the unaffected eye.

4. Drape the patient to protect the patient's clothing.

5. Place an emesis basin against the upper cheek near the eye. You may ask the patient to hold it.

6. Use clean gauze to wipe the eye from the inner canthus outward. This removes any debris from the lashes that might wash into the eye.

7. Separate the patient's eyelids with the thumb and forefinger of your nondominant hand. Hold the syringe in your dominant hand. To steady the syringe, you may rest it lightly on the bridge of the patient's nose.

8. Keep the tip of the syringe about 1 inch from the eye. Gently irrigate from the inner to the outer canthus. Use gentle pressure. Don't touch the eye.

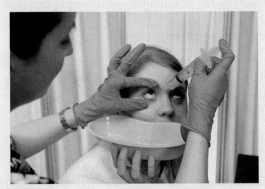

(Reprinted from Kronenberger J, Ledbetter J. *Jones & Bartlett Learning's Comprehensive Medical Assisting.* 5th ed. Burlington, MA: Jones & Bartlett Learning, LLC; 2016.)

9. Use tissues to wipe away any excess solution from the patient's face.

10. Assist the patient to a sitting position and remove the drape.

11. Document the procedure in the patient's medical record.

Procedure 22-2 | Performing Ear Irrigation

Ear irrigation is not a sterile procedure, but you must wash your hands and apply gloves prior to performing the irrigation.

Equipment: Otoscope, irrigation solution (warmed to body temperature), waterproof barrier or towel, emesis basin, irrigating syringe, and gauze.

1. Wash hands and assemble equipment.

2. First examine the ear by straightening the auditory canal. For an adult's ear, gently pull the ear up and back. In children, gently pull the ear slightly down and back. Then view the ear with an otoscope to locate the foreign matter or cerumen.

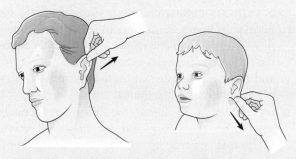

(Reprinted from Kronenberger J, Ledbetter J. *Jones & Bartlett Learning's Comprehensive Medical Assisting.* 5th ed. Burlington, MA: Jones & Bartlett Learning, LLC; 2016.)

3. Drape the patient with a waterproof barrier or towel.

4. Tilt the patient's head toward the affected side.

5. Place an emesis basin under the patient's ear.

6. Fill an irrigating syringe or turn on an irrigating device. Make sure the solution is warmed to body temperature to prevent further discomfort or issues for the patient.

7. With your nondominant hand, straighten the ear canal (as described above). With your dominant hand, place the tip of the syringe in the ear opening (auditory meatus). Direct the flow of the solution up toward the roof of the canal.

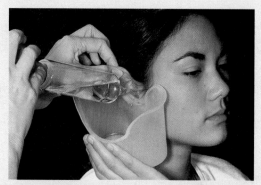

(Reprinted from Kronenberger J, Ledbetter J. *Jones & Bartlett Learning's Comprehensive Medical Assisting.* 5th ed. Burlington, MA: Jones & Bartlett Learning, LLC; 2016.)

8. Continue irrigating for the prescribed period or until the debris or cerumen is removed.

9. Dry the patient's external ear with gauze. Have the patient sit for a while with the affected ear down. This allows the solution to drain.

10. Inspect the ear with the otoscope to see if the debris or cerumen has been removed. If the patient is experiencing any pain during this procedure stop and inform the physician.

11. Document the procedure in the patient's medical record.

Preparing for Externship

Your externship will provide you with hands-on experience and the opportunity to apply the skills you learned in the classroom. Each night, record the activities of your day. Then, near the end of your externship, compile a list of the skills and duties you performed and add them to your resume. Remember, externship is a great time to start actively searching and applying for positions. Of course, you should never do this while at your externship site. Use your time off to job search, even if you think your site is a hiring site. It's always nice to have options.

Chapter Recap

- Emergencies in the medical office may involve staff, patients in the office, or patients who arrive seeking emergency treatment. For major emergencies, the patient is helped until EMS arrives. For minor emergencies, the patient is treated and sent home with follow-up instructions.

- Every medical office should have an emergency action plan and a crash cart or kit with emergency medical supplies and equipment. All staff should know where to locate the emergency supplies and equipment, including an AED. Emergency numbers should be displayed by all telephones. It's also important that staff be familiar with signs and symptoms that can indicate an emergency.

- In any emergency, there are three steps to follow: identify and treat any life-threatening problems, including rescue breathing or CPR; gather information by asking the patient questions and assessing general appearance, level of consciousness, vital signs, and skin; perform a physical examination for a head-to-toe assessment to identify problems not immediately known.

- Patient reassurance is a critical aspect of emergency care. Patients may be panicky, confused, or in pain. The medical assistant needs to remain calm and focus on the patient.

- All emergency care must be documented. Documentation should include the patient's symptoms, the nature of the emergency, and any treatment performed. Events should be recorded in chronological order.

- Major emergencies that may require immediate treatment include shock, soft tissue and musculoskeletal injuries, cardiovascular injuries, neurological injuries, severe allergic reactions, poisoning, and cold- and heat-related emergencies. Each of these has its own set of signs, symptoms, and procedures for management.

- Injuries to bones, muscles, and joints vary widely in their severity. In an emergency, it can be difficult to tell the difference between sprains, strains, dislocations, and fractures. In most cases, the injured area should be immobilized using splints.

- It's important to know the difference between a psychiatric emergency and an emotional crisis. A psychiatric emergency is life threatening for the patient or others without immediate intervention. An emotional crisis is not likely to result in danger or harm.

- Some of the minor emergencies medical assistants may need to deal with are fainting, asthma attacks, severe diarrhea or vomiting, high fevers, eye injuries, ear emergencies, or nosebleeds.

- Training and knowledge about medical emergencies may be useful in natural disasters or if acts of terrorism occur. Medical assistants need to be familiar with standard protocols for emergencies.

- Heat and cold are used to treat many different kinds of major and minor emergencies. Common treatments include compresses, soaks, hot packs or hot water bottles, and cold packs or ice bags.

- All office personnel should be know the locations of fire extinguishers and their proper use.

Online Resources for Students

Student Resources available on the text's online site include:

- Audio Glossaries
- Animations
- Competency Evaluation Forms
- Videos
- Anatomy & Physiology Module with Heart and Lung Sounds
- Weblinks
- Worksheets

Exercises and Activities

Certification Preparation Questions

1. When using a fire extinguisher utilize the _____ method.
   a. AIM
   b. PASS
   c. PULL
   d. FIRE
   e. PAS

2. When you apply heat to an area and vasoconstriction occurs this represents an example of:
   a. recoil.
   b. hot packs.
   c. rebounds.
   d. compresses.
   e. soaks.

3. When the end of a bone is displaced from its normal position in a joint, this is referred to as:
   a. closed fracture.
   b. greenstick fracture.
   c. luxation.
   d. subluxation.
   e. compound fracture.

4. A skeletal disease noted by bowing of the long bones is an example of a:
   a. pathological fracture.
   b. open fracture.
   c. closed fracture.
   d. compound fracture.
   e. greenstick fracture.

5. When performing CPR, the compression/ ventilation ratio for 2-person child CPR is:
   a. 30:2.
   b. 30:1.
   c. 15:2.
   d. 15:1.
   e. 5:2.

6. When performing CPR, you should use the AED:
   a. after performing CPR for 2 minutes.
   b. after performing five cycles of CPR.
   c. immediately upon arrival.
   d. after completing 10 cycles of CPR.
   e. following 5 minutes of CPR.

7. When performing ear irrigation the solution should be:
   a. room temperature.
   b. body temperature.
   c. 115°F.
   d. 50°F.
   e. 130°F.

8. A hematoma is a:
   a. collection of blood under the skin or in damaged tissues.
   b. blood clot that forms at the injury site.
   c. black and blue marks.
   d. scratch on the skin's surface.
   e. flap of skin torn loose.

9. Yellow discoloration of skin is an indication of:
   a. shock.
   b. anemia.
   c. congestive heart failure.
   d. liver disease.
   e. fever.

10. Skin that is pink is an indicator of:
    a. alcohol consumption.
    b. cold exposure.
    c. airway obstruction.
    d. renal disease.
    e. liver disease.

Section V

Clinical Laboratory

23 Medical Assistant Role in the Clinical Laboratory

Chapter Objectives

- List the reasons for laboratory tests.
- Describe the medical assistant's role in the lab.
- Identify the kinds of labs where medical assistants work and describe what these labs do.
- List the various positions in a lab and the duties of each.
- Name each type of lab department and explain what it does.
- List the common equipment used in most small labs and the purpose of each.
- Identify the types of hazards encountered in a lab and summarize how to manage them.
- Recognize safety signs, symbols, and labels.
- Explain how OSHA makes labs safer.
- List the safe behaviors employees should practice in the lab.
- Identify the information included on Safety Data Sheets (SDS) and the purpose of these sheets in a health care setting.
- Identify CLIA and explain how it affects lab operations.
- Describe how quality control affects lab operations.

CAAHEP & ABHES Competencies

CAAHEP

- Identify safety signs, symbols, and labels.
- Identify safety techniques that can be used in responding to accidental exposure to blood, other body fluids, needle sticks, and chemicals.
- Describe the purpose of Safety Data Sheets (SDS) in a health care setting.
- Discuss protocols for disposal of biological chemical materials.
- Identify principles of body mechanics and ergonomics.
- Demonstrate proper use of eyewash equipment and sharps disposal containers.

ABHES

- Comply with federal, state, and local health laws and regulations as they relate to health care settings.
- Practice quality control.
- Dispose of biohazardous materials.

Chapter Terms

Aerosol	Cytology	Normal values	Quality control
Anticoagulant	Graduated	Phlebotomists	Reagents
Blood-borne pathogens	Histology	Plasma	Safety data sheets
Caustic	Microorganisms	Quality assurance	Serum
Centrifuge			

Abbreviations

CLIA	NFPA	PPE	QA
CMS	POC	PPM	QC
COC	POCT	OSHA	SDS
FDA	POL		

Case Study

Sheila, the medical assistant for Dr. Lawrence, just received laboratory results from the reference laboratory for a patient who is anxiously awaiting the findings of a blood test to determine if she is positive for hepatitis or HIV. The good news is that the results are negative for both of these tests. When the patient calls the office to get the results, Sheila explains that she cannot release the results. She reminds him that the physician requested that he return to the office to review the results and discuss the next steps to deter-mine what condition is causing his symptoms. As the medical assistant is talking on the phone with the patient to schedule the appointment, the patient again asks Sheila if the results were positive or negative. Sheila answers by saying "you have nothing to worry about." The patient then asks, "Does that mean that the tests were negative?" Again, the medical assistant tells the patient "you have nothing to worry about." The patient responds by saying, "I'll take that as a negative, thank you so much."

Laboratories test a person's blood, urine, and other body fluids and tissues to help identify diseases and disorders. This chapter presents information about the different types of laboratories where a medical assistant might work. Also, you will find information about how to use a microscope and other laboratory equipment, as well as how to work safely in the laboratory.

LABORATORIES AND WHAT THEY DO

Laboratories have established **normal values**, which refer to the acceptable ranges for laboratory test results. The patient's test values are compared to these normal test values. Using the laboratory results, the health care provider assesses the health of a particular organ or determines if a patient's medication dosage is correct.

The most common laboratory testing purpose is to:

- Diagnose disease
- Determine the progress of a disease or its response to treatment
- Perform legal blood tests, such as for work-related drug testing or alcohol levels of drivers

Case Questions

 Did the medical assistant properly handle the patient's question? What would you have said to the patient?

Some other common tests provide information to assist the health care provider to:

- Monitor a patient's medication and treatment
- Find the levels of key substances in the body
- Determine the cause of an infection
- Establish a baseline value
- Prevent disease

Laboratories and the Medical Assistant

As a medical assistant, you'll have many types of responsibilities to both your patients and your physician, or employer. Your role in lab testing will be vital because such tests provide some of the most powerful diagnostic tools available.

You'll need to tell patients how to collect their own specimens, or samples, such as stool or urine. This is to be sure they provide quality specimens—those that are reliable and free from contamination.

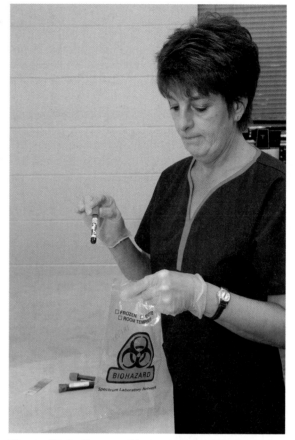

Figure 23-1 Transport bags are used to maintain the integrity of the specimen and to protect those who are responsible for handling the specimen from possible contact with hazardous bodily fluids and substances. (Reprinted from Kronenberger J, Ledbetter J. *Jones & Bartlett Learning's Comprehensive Medical Assisting.* 5th ed. Burlington, MA: Jones & Bartlett Learning, LLC; 2016.)

Cultural Connection

When communicating with patients and their family members who do not use or understand English as their first language, it is necessary to take care when discussing laboratory testing. There are very specific requirements for specimen collection and preparation prior to the collection. Try to speak slower, not louder. Use appropriate gestures and facial expression to emphasize critical points. Ask patients to repeat their understanding of instructions. Avoid technical, uncommon, or complicated terms and words. Organize your thoughts and don't muddy the waters with unnecessary chatter or lengthy explanations. Keep it as simple as possible.

- Supplies and instruments
- Policies and procedures
- Equipment maintenance

The medical assistant may be in charge of ordering lab supplies and choosing **reagents**, the substance used to produce a test reaction. Biohazard safety and waste disposal are two critical areas that all health care professionals need to understand and apply every day.

Types of Laboratories

Medical assistants may work with various types of laboratories. These include reference labs, hospital labs, and physician office labs (**POLs**). Depending on the size of the lab, reference and hospital labs typically perform hundreds of specialized tests each day. The POL may only do a few types of tests on a limited number of patients.

Some of the more common lab tests are ones you will perform right in the physician's office where you work. At other times, you'll need to arrange to transport specimens to an off-site lab. Figure 23-1 shows a medical assistant packaging a specimen for transport to a reference lab. The specimen transport bag needs to be strong and fluid resistant to contain the contents if the specimen were to break or leak inside.

One of the most important duties in the medical setting or laboratory is keeping records using a **quality assurance** (**QA**) program. Among other things, QA helps ensure good patient care. A good QA program includes **quality control** (**QC**) processes. These help ensure accuracy in testing by monitoring things like:

Reference Laboratories

A reference lab, also known as a referral laboratory, is a large facility resembling a factory. Some operate 24 hours a day with different shifts of employees completing many tests each day. The reference lab receives specimens from many different facilities, such as doctors' offices, hospitals, and clinics, and rarely sees patients directly.

The reference lab completes tests in bulk "runs" or "batches." This method allows testing of multiple patient specimens at a time. Patient results entered into a computer are reported to the health care providers, who discuss the results with their patients.

Specimens sent to a reference lab are delivered by these methods:

- Special courier
- US mail
- Ground delivery service
- Air delivery service

Hospital Laboratories

A hospital lab located in or close to a hospital serves hospitalized patients. The hospital lab personnel include the following:

- **Phlebotomists**—Obtain blood specimens from patients
- Lab assistants—Collect and process specimens
- Lab technicians and medical technologists—Perform most of the specimen testing
- Administrative assistants or receptionists—Process patients and manage the laboratory records

The medical assistant's role might be to perform the administrative duties, assist the laboratory technicians, or perform phlebotomy. The laboratory job description may include a variety of these functions.

Physician Office Labs

A common type of lab is the POL, or physician office laboratory. Most POLs only do waived or moderately difficult tests. If qualified lab technicians are available, more difficult or complex tests are performed in a POL. The federal government regulates the kinds of tests performed by a physician office lab. In general, the POL conducts only two kinds of tests:

- Tests done on semiautomated machines
- Tests done with self-contained test kits

The instructions in test kits are the best source of information on how to conduct those tests safely and accurately. So are the instructions inside packages of reagents for test machines and QC instructions for the machines themselves. Information from these sources, combined with the POL's routine procedures, provide written instructions for each test it performs.

The most common tests done in a POL include the following:

- Urinalysis
- Blood cell counts
- Hemoglobin and hematocrit
- Blood glucose
- Cholesterol levels

Pregnancy tests and quick screening tests, such as for mononucleosis or strep throat, also may be done in a POL. The medical assistant in a POL will work under the physician's supervision and may have duties that include the following:

- Collecting samples
- Performing tests
- Managing QC
- Maintaining lab instruments
- Maintaining records
- Reporting results to the health care provider

Point of Care Tests

Point of Care (**POC**) or Point of Care Tests (**POCT**) include those lab tests performed at the location where the patient is cared for. POC tests are typically performed on handheld devices that are easily transported to the patient. POCT are utilized in the hospital setting at the patient's bedside, in the physician's office, in the patient's home, and even in some pharmacies. Just because the devices are small and simple to use does not mean that these tests can be performed by anyone. There are minimum education and training requirements to qualify a health care professional to perform these tests. It is critical to follow the manufacturer's instructions to ensure reliable results.

Laboratory Forms

There are two primary documents used in the processing of specimens and reporting the results. The laboratory requisition form is used to accompany a specimen to the lab, and the laboratory results form is used to document the results.

Laboratory Requisition Form

The requisition form is necessary to accompany specimens to the off-site laboratory so that the lab will know the patient and physician information and the tests requested. The medical assistant will complete the form with the necessary data and place the form in the transport vehicle (bag) to send it to the lab. Figure 23-2 is an example of a simple requisition that accompanies the specimen to the lab. Requisition forms are customized by each lab with much more information including the CPT codes and patient insurance information.

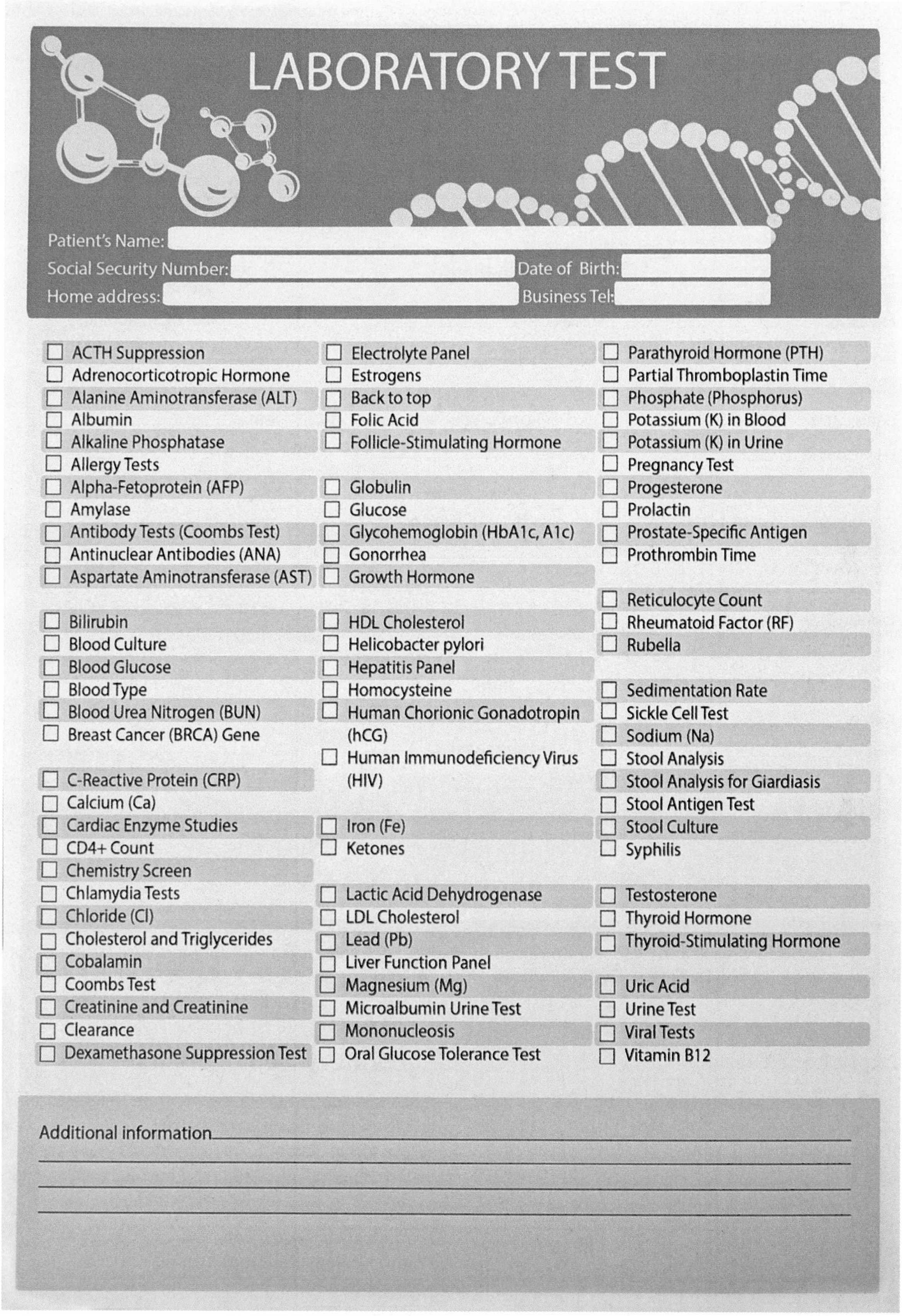

LABORATORY TEST

Patient's Name:

Social Security Number: Date of Birth:

Home address: Business Tel:

- ☐ ACTH Suppression
- ☐ Adrenocorticotropic Hormone
- ☐ Alanine Aminotransferase (ALT)
- ☐ Albumin
- ☐ Alkaline Phosphatase
- ☐ Allergy Tests
- ☐ Alpha-Fetoprotein (AFP)
- ☐ Amylase
- ☐ Antibody Tests (Coombs Test)
- ☐ Antinuclear Antibodies (ANA)
- ☐ Aspartate Aminotransferase (AST)

- ☐ Bilirubin
- ☐ Blood Culture
- ☐ Blood Glucose
- ☐ Blood Type
- ☐ Blood Urea Nitrogen (BUN)
- ☐ Breast Cancer (BRCA) Gene

- ☐ C-Reactive Protein (CRP)
- ☐ Calcium (Ca)
- ☐ Cardiac Enzyme Studies
- ☐ CD4+ Count
- ☐ Chemistry Screen
- ☐ Chlamydia Tests
- ☐ Chloride (Cl)
- ☐ Cholesterol and Triglycerides
- ☐ Cobalamin
- ☐ Coombs Test
- ☐ Creatinine and Creatinine
- ☐ Clearance
- ☐ Dexamethasone Suppression Test

- ☐ Electrolyte Panel
- ☐ Estrogens
- ☐ Back to top
- ☐ Folic Acid
- ☐ Follicle-Stimulating Hormone

- ☐ Globulin
- ☐ Glucose
- ☐ Glycohemoglobin (HbA1c, A1c)
- ☐ Gonorrhea
- ☐ Growth Hormone

- ☐ HDL Cholesterol
- ☐ Helicobacter pylori
- ☐ Hepatitis Panel
- ☐ Homocysteine
- ☐ Human Chorionic Gonadotropin (hCG)
- ☐ Human Immunodeficiency Virus (HIV)

- ☐ Iron (Fe)
- ☐ Ketones

- ☐ Lactic Acid Dehydrogenase
- ☐ LDL Cholesterol
- ☐ Lead (Pb)
- ☐ Liver Function Panel
- ☐ Magnesium (Mg)
- ☐ Microalbumin Urine Test
- ☐ Mononucleosis
- ☐ Oral Glucose Tolerance Test

- ☐ Parathyroid Hormone (PTH)
- ☐ Partial Thromboplastin Time
- ☐ Phosphate (Phosphorus)
- ☐ Potassium (K) in Blood
- ☐ Potassium (K) in Urine
- ☐ Pregnancy Test
- ☐ Progesterone
- ☐ Prolactin
- ☐ Prostate-Specific Antigen
- ☐ Prothrombin Time

- ☐ Reticulocyte Count
- ☐ Rheumatoid Factor (RF)
- ☐ Rubella

- ☐ Sedimentation Rate
- ☐ Sickle Cell Test
- ☐ Sodium (Na)
- ☐ Stool Analysis
- ☐ Stool Analysis for Giardiasis
- ☐ Stool Antigen Test
- ☐ Stool Culture
- ☐ Syphilis

- ☐ Testosterone
- ☐ Thyroid Hormone
- ☐ Thyroid-Stimulating Hormone

- ☐ Uric Acid
- ☐ Urine Test
- ☐ Viral Tests
- ☐ Vitamin B12

Additional information _____

_____

_____

_____

Figure 23-2 Laboratory requisition forms are completed and accompany the specimens to the laboratory. (Image from Shutterstock.com.)

Third Street
PHYSICIAN'S OFFICE, INC.

123 Main Street
Baltimore, MD 21201

Time Order Received:

Time Collected:

Time Reported:

Doctor:

Date:

LABORATORY

Patient Name

Chart No.

URINALYSIS

PHYSICAL

Color _____

Clarity_____

CHEMICAL

Leuk. Esterase _____

Nitrite _____

Urobilinogen _____

Protein _____

pH _____

Specific Gravity _____

Blood _____

Bilirubin _____

Ketones _____

Glucose _____

PREGNANCY

Urine HCG _____

Serum HCG _____

PROTHROMBIN TIME

Seconds _____

INR _____

SEDIMENTATION RATE

_____ Males 0–10

_____ Females 0–20

GLUCOSE

_____ 80–110 mg/dL

MONO

_____ NEG

STREP SCREEN

_____ NEG

PROVIDER PERFORMED MICROSCOPY

URINE MICROSCOPIC

Epis _____

WBCs_____

RBCs _____

Bacteria _____

Mucus _____

Amorphous _____

Other _____

KOH

_____

_____

WET PREP

_____

_____

_____

_____

_____

Performed by: _____

Figure 23-3   Laboratory result form with reference values provided for various tests. (Reprinted from Kronenberger J, Ledbetter J. *Jones & Bartlett Learning's Comprehensive Medical Assisting.* 5th ed. Burlington, MA: Jones & Bartlett Learning, LLC; 2016.)

Laboratory Result Form

The result form documents the findings or results of the test performed. Reference and hospital labs use a form that has normal values or ranges printed on the form. The physician can easily see the patients' results compared against the normal range. The form typically highlights or flags any abnormal value that falls outside the range being either too high or too low. Figure 23-3 is an example of a simple laboratory result form that a Physician's Office Laboratory might use to formally report the results of the waived and moderate complexity tests that would be performed in that type of setting.

Laboratory Departments

POLs may have only one department. Reference and hospital labs perform such a wide variety of tests that they need special departments to manage these. Here are the basic departments usually found in a hospital or reference lab.

- Hematology department
- Clinical chemistry department
- Immunology department
- Microbiology department
- Pathology department
- Immunohematology department, may also be called "blood bank"

As you think about the types of laboratories and the various departments, it would probably be helpful to contact a local reference or hospital laboratory near you to see if the lab will allow you to take a tour of the lab and possibly talk with some of the lab employees. When a medical facility knows that you are a student studying to work in the health care industry, they are usually willing to help you understand the concepts of the lab. Visualizing the laboratory and the departments will give you a better appreciation for the work accomplished in a lab.

Hematology

The hematology department tests the blood for various types of cells and how many of each type are present. Common tests include the following:

- Complete blood count (CBC)
- White blood cell count (WBC)
- Platelet count
- Hemoglobin and hematocrit (H & H)
- Differential count
- Erythrocyte sedimentation rate (ESR, sed rate)
- Reticulocyte count

Coagulation studies, performed in the hematology department, indicate how well the body responds to damaged blood vessels. The most common tests are as follows:

- Prothrombin time (PT)
- Partial prothrombin time (PPT)
- Fibrinogen
- Bleeding time

These tests also check levels of **anticoagulant** medicines, such as heparin and Coumadin. Anticoagulant medicines prevent blood clotting in conditions caused by clot formation and blocked blood vessels. These conditions include heart attacks, strokes, pulmonary embolisms, and some types of phlebitis.

Clinical Chemistry

The clinical chemistry department measures chemical substances in the blood. Examples include the following:

- Hormones and enzymes
- Medicines and drugs
- Sugars, proteins, and fats
- Waste products

The most common chemistry tests performed in a small lab are as follows:

- Glucose
- Cholesterol
- Blood urea nitrogen (BUN)
- Electrolytes

Toxicology is often a separate part of a chemistry department. Toxicology testing involves measuring levels of both medical drugs and illegal drugs in a person's blood.

Immunohematology

The immunohematology department, sometimes referred to as the blood bank, operates in hospitals and blood donor centers. This department performs blood typing to ensure the stored blood products are safe for patient transfusions. When the blood is required for transfusion, a crossmatch is performed to further ensure that the blood is compatible with the recipient's blood.

Immunology

Immunology is sometimes called serology. This department performs tests for specific diseases based on the reactions of antibodies to foreign substances in the body. Immunology tests are used to detect HIV, mononucleosis, syphilis, and other diseases.

Microbiology

The microbiology department identifies **microorganisms** that cause disease and identifies the drugs that will combat them most effectively. Microorganisms are living organisms that are only visible with a microscope. The specialties within the microbiology department include the following:

- Bacteriology, or the study of bacteria
- Virology, or the study of viruses
- Mycology, or the study of fungi and yeasts
- Parasitology, or the study of parasites (e.g., certain protozoa and worms)

The Pathology Department

The pathology department studies specimens from:

- Aspirations—Fluids or gases suctioned from a body cavity
- Biopsies—Living tissue surgically removed for examination
- Autopsies—Examinations of dead bodies
- Surgically removed organs

Pathology departments usually have histology and cytology sections. In larger labs, however, histology and cytology may be departments of their own.

Histology is the study of tissue. Tissue samples are prepared and studied under a microscope to show if disease is present. Biopsies and frozen specimens that need immediate results are examined in this department.

Cytology is the study of cells. Individual cells in body fluids and other types of specimens are studied under a microscope to find things like cancer or other disease. The most common cytology test is the Papanicolaou (Pap) test. This test evaluates cells from a woman's cervix to determine the presence of cancerous cells.

Cytogenetics is a special form of cytology that examines the genetic information contained in the cells found in tissue, blood, or other body fluids. The cells are examined for DNA deficiencies related to disease.

Laboratory Personnel

The various lab departments employ many people to carry out their duties. Most positions require specific education or training. Table 23-1 summarizes the personnel found in laboratories.

Laboratory Equipment

There are many types of lab equipment, but even if you do not use the equipment, you need to be familiar with a few of them. Here are the types of basic equipment with which you should be familiar:

- Microscope
- Centrifuge
- Chemistry analyzer
- Incubator
- Glassware
- Lab refrigerator or freezer
- Automated cell counter

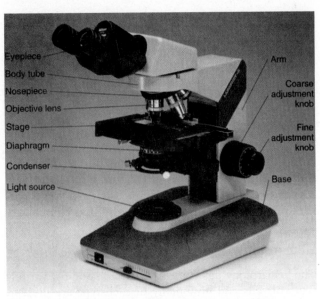

Figure 23-4   Binocular microscope. (Image from Shutterstock.com.)

Microscopes

A microscope is the instrument used to identify cells and microorganisms in specimens. The microscope most commonly used in a POL is a compound microscope. It has two lenses to magnify the objects on the microscope slide. A strong light helps you see the object better. Figure 23-4 is a binocular microscope showing the various components.

Table 23-1   Laboratory Personnel

Position	Function
Pathologist	A physician who studies disease, usually serves as the manager of the technical functions of the laboratory
Chief Technologists or Laboratory Manager	A person who supervises the laboratories' day-to-day operations
Certified Medical Technologist	A specially trained, 4-year education, and nationally certified medical technologist; performs all levels of laboratory tests according to CLIA rules
Medical Laboratory Technician	Has completed 1 year of college and 1 year of clinical training; performs lab tests but is not a supervisor
Medical Assistant	Has a high school diploma or equivalent and has completed a medical assistant program; may collect and process specimens and perform waived laboratory procedures
Laboratory Assistant	Has a high school diploma or equivalent and has completed an occupational or on-the-job training program; collects and processes specimens and may perform some tests
Phlebotomist	Is trained to draw blood and process specimens; have additional duties that are more involved; may be called medical or laboratory assistant
Histologist	A person trained to process and evaluate tissue samples, such as biopsies
Cytologist	A person professionally trained to look for abnormal changes in tissue and blood cells, under a microscope
Specimen processor or accessioner	A person who is specially trained to accept shipments of specimens and prepare them for testing; labels and numbers the specimens and enters the specimen data into a computer

Here are the basic parts of a compound microscope.

- The frame is the main part of the microscope. It holds the arm and the base.
- The eyepiece or ocular at the top of the microscope is what you look through. Binocular microscopes have two eyepieces. This causes less eyestrain.
- The adjustment knobs are used to bring the object you're looking at into focus. There is a coarse and fine adjuster knob.
- The stage is the flat surface that holds the slide you are studying. The stage has clips or guides to control the slide's movement.
- The condenser focuses the light onto the slide. The lower the position of the condenser, the less light is available. The higher the position, the brighter the light will be.
- The diaphragm is part of the condenser. It acts like the iris in your eye, in that its opening can be adjusted to allow for more or less light. The more highly magnified the slide is, the greater the need for light.
- The light source is housed in the microscope's base.

Microscopes are delicate, expensive instruments. Proper care in handling and storing them ensures that they stay in good working order. Although a medical assistant will not be performing microscopic exams, you should understand some rules to follow when storing a microscope.

- Turn off the light source and rotate the nosepiece until the lowest-power lens faces the stage.
- Cover the microscope when not in use.
- Keep the microscope in a location where it cannot be damaged.
- Make sure it's away from any source of vibration, such as a centrifuge.

The medical assistant may be responsible for caring for the microscope. Here are some tips for cleaning the microscope in your lab.

- Wash your hands before handling the microscope.
- Assemble cleaning supplies and always use both hands to carry the microscope, one hand on the base and the other on the arm of the microscope.
- Clean the ocular areas using lens paper and cleaner. Don't use gauze or tissue, as these may scratch the glass. Don't touch the glass with your fingers.
- Start with the eyepiece—or ocular—and work down to the lenses near the base. Clean each piece of glass. Change lens paper often, once it appears dirty. The cleanest area of a microscope is usually the eyepiece and the dirtiest is the highest-power lens.
- Use a clean lens paper to wipe each ocular area again to make sure no dirt or cleaner remains. Residue from dirt or cleaner will distort images viewed through the microscope.

- All other areas of the microscope such as the stage, the base, and the knobs can be cleaned using a mild soap solution and gauze. Clean them regularly to avoid buildup of oil and dirt.
- Cover the microscope at the end of the day.

Centrifuge

A **centrifuge** is a machine that separates liquids into their different parts. It does this by using centrifugal force, or spinning that exerts force outward. This action separates the heavy and light parts of the liquid. This is similar to the spin cycle of a washing machine. Figure 23-5 is an example of a centrifuged blood specimen. Notice the layers of blood that have separated into the plasma on top, the thin, buffy coat in the middle, and the heavier, packed red blood cells on the bottom.

When a blood specimen is processed in a centrifuge:

- The heavier part of the blood, the red blood cells, go to the bottom of the tube.
- A middle layer, known as the buffy coat, forms. This layer contains the white blood cells and platelets.
- The topmost layer of separated blood is either plasma or serum. If the specimen was allowed to clot (in a red tube top), its top layer is called serum.

Serum and plasma are straw colored and look identical. However, there are chemical differences. **Plasma** is the liquid part of the blood with the clotting agents. It is collected in an anticoagulated tube (lavender, blue, gray, or yellow tube top). **Serum** is the liquid part of the blood with the clotting agents removed. A red top tube is used

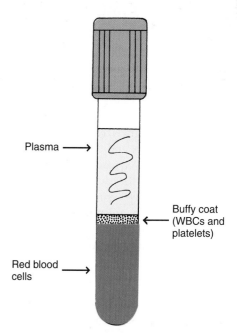

Plasma →

Buffy coat (WBCs and platelets)

Red blood cells →

Figure 23-5 Centrifuged blood specimens; clear plasma on top, thin buffy coat of WBCs and platelets and RBCs on the bottom. (Image from Shutterstock.com.)

for collection when serum is needed. This tube allows the blood to clot before centrifuging the specimen.

When working with a centrifuge, safety practices must be applied including:

- Spinning an even number of tubes to keep balance during the process. An unbalanced centrifuge may "walk" along the counter and fall off the edge. When only one tube needs processing, balance the centrifuge with a tube of equal size filled with water equal to the amount of blood.
- Have the same level of liquid in all the tubes and tightly cap each one.
- Lock the lid before starting the centrifuge.
- Wait until the centrifuge has stopped spinning before opening it and never use your hand to try to stop the machine.
- Perform regular cleaning and maintenance following manufacturer's instructions.

A microhematocrit machine is a special type of centrifuge used to perform a hematocrit test. The hematocrit is the amount of packed red blood cells compared to the total volume of the sample. This test represents the percentage of red blood cells in whole blood.

The hematocrit test requires a special test tube called a capillary tube. This is a very small tube used for collecting and testing tiny blood samples. The tube is filled with blood, sealed on one end with clay, and placed in the centrifuge with the sealed end to the outside.

Chemistry Analyzers

Chemistry analyzers are machines used to run multiple tests on a sample. Complex analyzers can perform 30 or more tests and are operated by computer.

Some analyzers are handheld so are small and manageable. They're simple to use and don't require a large sample. Best of all, they can give results within minutes. A computer shows the results on a digital screen or it can provide a printout of the results.

POLs use benchtop analyzers when they conduct a variety of chemistry tests and do a lot of testing. Some of these machines use wet reagent systems. A separate reagent pack is required for each type of test.

Other chemistry analyzers use dry reagent technology. All the test reagents are put on a special strip or card, which is put into the machine. Then a drop of blood or serum is added to the strip with a special pipet.

Glassware

Glassware includes glass and sometimes plastic. Plastic is great because it does not break easily like glass and it is disposable. The medical assistant will probably not use these items to perform the tests they will be doing; however, if you are working in a major laboratory, you need to understand the items you may see or be asked to clean and take care of. Here are some examples of the glassware or plasticware you might use in the lab.

- Beaker—A container with a wide opening for mixing or heating liquids.
- Flask—A container with a narrow opening and round base for holding or moving liquids.
- Glass slides–Slides and coverslips hold a specimen for viewing under a microscope. They are disposable.
- Graduated cylinder—A container used for measuring liquids. **Graduated** means it's marked with divisions—usually in milliliters (mL) for exact measurements.
- Petri dish or plate—A shallow, covered dish filled with a substance that grows microbes in a specimen (culture).
- Pipet or Pipette—Is used to move or measure small amounts of liquid. Mechanical pipettes come in either fixed or variable sizes and have replaceable tips.
- Test tube—A cylinder-shaped container that's open at one end and round or pointed at the other. It's used to hold lab specimens. Evacuated blood tubes are an example of a type of test tube.

Other Lab Equipment

Other equipment that you may see used in a laboratory include the following:

- Incubator—Used to keep microbiology specimens at a certain temperature (usually about 95°F to 99°F or 35°C to 37°C). You'll notice that this is close to body temperature. Some bacteria and other microbes must be this warm to grow and reproduce. Lab employees should keep a daily log that records the incubator's temperature.
- Refrigerators and freezers—Used to store reagents, kits, and specimens. Like the incubator, keeping the temperature constant is vital. The temperature is monitored and recorded daily. Storing food or beverages in a lab refrigerator is a danger to your health and violates OSHA regulations. Specimens stored in the refrigerator or freezer may contain diseases that could be transferred to your food.
- Automated cell counter—Used to analyze blood specimens for white and red blood cell counts plus hematocrit, hemoglobin levels, and platelet counts. Many counters perform calculations (called indices) and a basic white blood cell differential. Using a cell counter requires special training from a qualified person.

LAB SAFETY

People who work in a lab must pay special attention to safety. Every specimen should be treated as if it's hazardous. To avoid injury to yourself or others, you also should be aware of the three basic types of hazards in a lab that include physical, chemical, and biological hazards. Everyone in your workplace should be aware of how to handle each type of hazard. Written policies and procedures for lab safety are designed to keep risks to a minimum.

Physical Hazards

Physical hazards include fires, broken glass, or spills that could cause someone to slip and fall.

If a fire breaks out, all employees should know where the fire extinguishers are located. You also must know how to use the extinguisher. It's equally important to know all the escape routes out of the lab.

With so much equipment in the average lab, the risk from electrical fires is especially high. Follow these precautions to help avoid electrical fires.

- Avoid using extension cords.
- Do not overload electrical outlets.
- Always unplug equipment before servicing or repairing it.

Chemical Hazards

Chemical hazards involve substances that create fumes or could hurt you by coming into contact with your eyes or skin. Other chemical hazards arise from chemicals that could catch fire or explode.

All chemicals have a **safety data sheet** (**SDS**) available from the product vendor. Each SDS gives the manufacturer's instructions for how to store, handle, and dispose of the chemical or substance. The SDS also contains information about:

- The risk involved using this chemical
- How to prevent exposure to the chemical
- How to treat or manage a situation when there is exposure to the chemical

Safety data sheets are stored in a binder in the lab. You can quickly look up the safety procedures when needed in an emergency. The binder also should contain the lab's own rules and procedures for handling hazardous chemicals.

To reduce chemical hazards, read each bottle or container label for storage information. Failure to read this storage information can result in:

- Damage to the chemical
- Release of fumes that could be dangerous and should have been vented
- Placing two chemicals next to each other that could result in a reaction between the two stored reagents

Biological Hazards

The laboratory binder should include rules and procedures for the handling of test specimens as well. Nearly all types of specimens are capable of passing on disease if they contain microbes that cause the disease. Most of the biological hazards in a lab relate to possible exposure to these microbes.

Lab accidents and careless procedures could result in dangerous exposures. Some of the worst are exposure to the microbes that cause diseases such as:

- HIV/AIDS
- Hepatitis
- Tuberculosis

In some cases, you may be testing for such diseases. At other times, you'll be handling specimens from patients that have infectious diseases, although no one may suspect it.

To reduce the risks from biological hazards, the Occupational Safety and Health Administration (**OSHA**) requires the use of personal protective equipment (**PPE**) in the lab.

The National Fire Protection Association

The National Fire Protection Association (**NFPA**) has a labeling system to identify the risks from various hazardous chemicals. This system uses a diamond-shaped symbol divided into four sections, each with a different color.

- Blue means health hazard.
- Red means fire hazard.
- Yellow means reactive hazard, such as an explosion.
- White is left blank unless there's a specific hazard, such as radiation, or a reaction if a substance comes into contact with water.

A number from zero (little or no danger) to four (great danger) appears in each color section. This number rates the seriousness of that type of hazard. The ratings will depend on what chemicals are used and stored in the area.

Hazardous materials posters should be displayed in all lab areas, in places where they're easy to see. You should know the NFPA system well enough to understand what each poster means. Figure 23-6 is an example of the hazardous material rating system.

Occupational Safety and Health Administration Requirements

The Occupational Safety and Health Administration (OSHA) is a federal government agency that protects the health and safety of all workers. Following OSHA standards will reduce, eliminate, or prevent hazards and accidents in the workplace. Two very important OSHA standards that apply to medical labs are the:

- Occupational Exposure to Blood-borne Pathogens Standard
- Hazardous Communication (HazCom) Standard

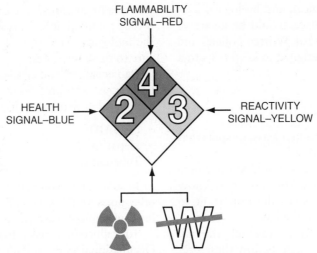

Identification of Health Hazard Color Code: **BLUE**		Identification of Flammability Color Code: **RED**		Identification of Reactivity (Stability) Color Code: **YELLOW**	
	Type of possible injury		Susceptibility of materials to burning		Susceptibility to release of energy
SIGNAL		**SIGNAL**		**SIGNAL**	
4	Materials that on very short exposure could cause death or major residual injury even though prompt medical treatment was given.	4	Materials that will rapidly or completely vaporize at atmospheric pressure and normal ambient temperature, or that are readily dispersed in air and that will burn readily.	4	Materials that in themselves are readily capable of detonation or of explosive decomposition or reaction at normal temperatures and pressures.
3	Materials that on short exposure could cause serious temporary or residual injury even though prompt medical treatment was given.	3	Liquids and solids that can be ignited under almost all ambient temperature conditions.	3	Materials that in themselves are capable of detonation or explosive reaction but require a strong initiating source or that must be heated under confinement before initiation or that react explosively with water.
2	Materials that on intense or continued exposure could cause temporary incapacitation or possible residual injury unless prompt medical treatment is given.	2	Materials that must be moderately heated or exposed to relatively high ambient temperatures before ignition can occur.	2	Materials that in themselves are normally unstable and readily undergo violent chemical change but do not detonate. Also materials that may react violently with water or that may form potentially explosive mixtures with water.
1	Materials that on exposure would cause irritation but only minor residual injury even if no treatment is given.	1	Materials that must be preheated before ignition can occur.	1	Materials that in themselves are normally stable, but that can become unstable at elevated temperatures and pressures or that may react with water with some release of energy, but not violently.
0	Materials that on exposure under fire conditions would offer no hazard beyond that of ordinary combustible material.	0	Materials that will not burn.	0	Materials that in themselves are normally stable, even under fire exposure conditions, and that are not reactive with water.

Figure 23-6   Hazardous material rating chart. (Reprinted with permission from McCall R. *Phlebotomy Essentials.* Burlington, MA: Jones & Bartlett Learning, LLC; 2007.)

If your lab is not following OSHA rules, the health of you and your coworkers could be in danger. OSHA fines the lab for all violations and requires corrective action. After initial fines, OSHA inspectors revisit the lab to ensure the violations are corrected. If the lab failed to correct its problems, or continued to have other violations, it could even lose its license.

Blood-borne Pathogens Standard

OSHA requires training of all lab personnel to protect themselves from contact with **blood-borne pathogens.** These are dangerous organisms than can exist in the blood of an infected person. The standard also applies to all other body fluids and secretions.

Working in a laboratory carries the risk of exposure to such pathogens. If accidentally punctured by a needle, or if any body fluid splashes into your eyes, nose, mouth, or other opening in your skin, you could be at risk.

One of the most vital protections your employer must provide is immunization for you against hepatitis B virus and other blood-borne pathogens. Employers are required to provide the immunizations at no cost to the employee within 10 days of assignment to lab duties or specimen collection.

OSHA also requires all medical employers to train their staff about the dangers of blood-borne pathogens. Safety manuals must be available to guide you and other employees in the lab.

OSHA also requires medical employers to provide workers with personal protective equipment (**PPE**). This reduces your chance of coming into contact with materials that might be hazardous. This is a list of PPE items you might need:

- Latex or vinyl disposable gloves (do not use latex products if allergic to latex)
- Gown, lab coat, or apron
- Face shield, goggles, or glasses with side shields
- Face mask
- Shoe covers

PPE should fit the level of hazard resulting from exposure. For example, when drawing blood or assisting with the collection of tissue samples, you should wear disposable gloves. If you might encounter splashes or splatters, or an **aerosol** (particles suspended in gas or air), cover and protect your eyes, face, and even your shoes.

HazCom Standard

The HazCom Standard requires that all hazardous materials have a visible manufacturer's label. The label must include the following information:

- A warning, such as "DANGER"
- A statement of the specific hazard, such as "FLAMMABLE"
- Precautions to follow to avoid exposure
- First aid measures to take if exposed to the materials

In addition, manufacturers must provide a safety data sheet for their products. The SDS must include guidelines for safe storage, information about fire risk, and exposure precautions.

The standard requires employers to have written guidelines for handling each hazardous material in the workplace. This information should include the manufacturer's SDS.

All this information should be available in a binder in the lab. You should review the SDSs regularly to keep safety precautions and first aid procedures fresh in your mind.

It's Up To You

A medical laboratory can be a safe place to work—or it can be a not-so-safe place. Your daily behaviors and those of your coworkers will help determine which kind of place your lab will be. Here are some tips for making the lab a safe place to work for you and the people around you.

Personal Behaviors

Daily routine activities can affect lab safety. Here are some important guidelines for the lab.

- Never eat, drink, or smoke in the lab area.
- Never touch your face, mouth, or eyes with pens, pencils, or any other items used in the lab (including your gloves).
- Don't apply makeup or insert contact lenses in the lab.
- Wear glasses instead of contact lenses when working around chemicals that produce fumes.

Protect Yourself

Here are some precautions you should take to lessen your risk of exposure to lab hazards.

- Wear gloves whenever there is a possibility of contact with blood, body fluids, secretions, excretions, broken skin, or mucous membranes.
- Wash your hands frequently. Always wash your hands before and after gloving, and before leaving the work site.
- Wear appropriate PPE when splatters, splashes, spills, or aerosols are a possibility. Use a splatter guard or splash shield whenever these risks exist.
- When opening a container, hold its mouth or opening away from you and others to avoid aerosols, splashes, and spills.
- When removing a stopper, hold the opening away, use gauze around the cap, and twist gently. Avoid glove contact with the specimen since you may contaminate the specimen and you will have specimen residue on your gloves, depositing it in other areas of the workspace that you touch.
- Avoid spills by pouring carefully. Pour at eye level if possible, but never too close to your face.

Protect Your Coworkers

Some of your work practices in the lab will make it a safer place to be. The following practices will protect both you and your coworkers.

- Store all chemicals according to the manufacturer's instructions. Most chemicals that are **caustic** (corrosive or abrasive) are stored below waist level typically under sinks.

- Discard any container with a label that you cannot read clearly.
- Label all specimen containers with biohazard labels and never store chemicals in unlabelled containers.
- Tightly replace lids on all containers immediately after use.
- Clean reusable glassware and other containers with recommended disinfectant or soap. Dry them thoroughly before using them again. Wear gloves when washing and drying.
- Disinfect all lab surfaces when you're finished using them and at the end of each day. Use a 10% bleach solution (nine parts water: one part bleach) or an appropriate disinfectant.
- Never allow clutter to accumulate.
- Dispose of needles and broken glass in sharps containers. Use biohazard containers to discard all other contaminated materials.

Be Informed and Prepared

Here are some other tips for preventing lab accidents and for being prepared in case one occurs.

- Read equipment manuals and know how to operate the equipment safely. Don't use damaged electrical equipment.
- Keep fire extinguishers close at hand. Many chemicals can catch fire and burn.
- Know the location and operation of all safety equipment, such as fire extinguishers, safety showers, and eyewash stations. Use an eyewash station by turning on the water and lowering your face into the stream. Flush your eyes with the water until they are clear.
- Immediately report any biohazard exposure or work-related injury to your supervisor.

Cleaning Up Spills

Use proper procedures for removing chemical or biological spills. If the spill is chemical, follow the manufacturer's instructions on the SDS. Commercial kits are available for such cleanups.

If the spill is biological, follow this procedure:

1. Put on gloves.
2. Cover the area with disposable material, such as paper towels, to soak up the spill. Discard the towels in a biohazard container.
3. Flood the area with disinfecting solution. Let the solution remain for 10 to 15 minutes.
4. Wipe up the solution and discard all waste in a biohazard container.

Incident Reports

Complete an incident report whenever any kind of accident occurs in a medical office. Of course, any exposure to a chemical or biological hazard should result in such a report. Other situations requiring an incident report is when

- An employee, patient, or visitor is accidentally stuck by a contaminated needle.
- A medication error takes place.
- Blood is drawn from the wrong patient.

CLINICAL LABORATORY IMPROVEMENT AMENDMENTS

Congress passed the Clinical Laboratory Improvement Amendments (**CLIA**) to improve the quality of medical testing in the United States. CLIA standards apply to all medical labs, from the largest reference labs to the smallest physician office laboratory (POL). States also create their own rules for labs. These rules can be more strict than CLIA standards, but not less strict.

Two US government agencies oversee the CLIA program. They are the Centers for Medicare and Medicaid Services (**CMS**) and the Food and Drug Administration (**FDA**). CMS regulates the labs that conduct the tests. The FDA assigns each test to one of three categories, based on its level of difficulty.

- Waived tests—The easiest to conduct and interpret. Many are simple enough for patients to do at home. Many POLs perform only waived tests. Medical assistants may perform all waived tests.
- Moderate-complexity tests—POLs must become CMS certified to perform these tests. The difficulty of these tests requires lab workers to have more training. Most of this testing is done in reference or hospital labs.
- High-complexity tests—Requires high levels of training to conduct and interpret; rarely performed in POLs.

CLIA has identified some moderate-complexity tests that involve using procedures called provider-performed microscopy (**PPM**). POLs must have a special certificate from CMS to perform these procedures. Only the following persons can perform PPM procedures:

- Physician
- Dentist
- Medical technologist
- Nurse practitioner (under a physician's direct supervision)
- Nurse midwife (under a physician's direct supervision)
- Physician assistant (under a physician's direct supervision)

Table 23-2	Typical Laboratory Tests and Level of Testing	
Waived	**Moderate Complexity**	**High Complexity**
Dipstick urinalysis or reagent tablets	Urine and throat cultures	Advanced cell studies (cytogenetics)
Fecal occult blood packets	Automated testing for cholesterol, high-density lipoproteins, and triglycerides	Cytology (such as Pap smears)
Ovulation testing in packets with color comparison charts	Gram staining	Histocompatibility
Urine pregnancy test kits using color comparison charts	Microscopic urinalysis	Histopathology
Manual erythrocyte sedimentation rate tests	Automated hematology with or without differential and no histogram	Manual cell counts
Manual copper sulfate hemoglobin tests	Manual white blood cell count differentials without identification of atypical cells	
Centrifuged microhematocrits	Automated coagulation tests that do not require intervention during analysis	
Blood glucose tests	Automated chemistry tests	
Flu kits and some rapid strep test kits	Automated urinalysis tests	

The PPM category includes the following microscopic examination tests:

- Direct wet-mount preparations testing for bacteria, fungi, parasites, and cell properties
- Potassium hydroxide preparations
- Pinworm tests
- Fern tests for amniotic fluid
- Postintercourse exams of vaginal or cervical mucous
- Urine sedimentation exams
- Nasal smear granulocytes
- Fecal leukocytes
- Semen analysis

Table 23-2 is a list of the typical lab tests that CLIA has assigned to the various categories that include waived, moderate complexity, and high complexity.

 LABORATORY STANDARDS

Each year, the CMS or the FDA may conduct unannounced visits to inspect labs that do moderate- or high-complexity tests. The inspectors show up without warning to ensure that the lab meets CLIA standards. They pay special attention to patient test management and quality control (QC).

Here are some things inspectors look for in judging patient test management:

- Written standards of patient care and employee conduct
- Clear policies and procedures for preparing patients and handling specimens

- A system to ensure that specimens are kept and identified properly for testing
- Written procedures for performing tests, evaluating their safety and reliability, and handling questionable results
- A system to ensure that results are accurately recorded and reported

Quality Control (QC)

A good QC, program covers every part of the lab's performance. This includes making sure it measures up to required standards in the following areas:

- Specimen collection and processing
- Testing and reporting results
- Reagents and equipment
- Actual test performance
- Personnel qualifications

Written procedures must exist to ensure that QC standards for monitoring test quality, accuracy, and reliability are in place.

Control Samples

Control samples are specimens provided by manufacturers. The outcome of tests is predictable since the contents of a control sample have a known value.

Good QC procedures require testing control samples each time a new reagent kit is opened. This ensures that the kit's materials are performing correctly. If the test results don't fall within the range given in the kit's package insert, the kit can't be used. Control samples are tested each time the test is run on patient specimens to check on the accuracy of the patients' results. If the results on the control sample aren't in the range given in the test kit's package insert, the patient results can't be reported. If the control sample test results fall outside the required range, here are the steps you should take.

1. Check the expiration dates of the reagent and control sample.
2. If the reagent has been prepared by mixing it with a liquid, check the mixture's accuracy and its expiration date.
3. Check that the testing equipment is clean and functioning accurately.
4. If these steps are completed and the control sample is not providing reliable results, remix the reagent or open a new reagent or control sample and test the control sample again.

Management of Reagents

Reagents are chemicals that produce a reaction. They each have a manufacturer's lot number and expiration date. You'll need to record these in your lab's QC log, as well as the dates the reagent was received and opened. If there's anything wrong with the reagent, the lot number and the dates can help the manufacturer identify the problem.

Instrument Calibration

Handle and operate all lab instruments according to manufacturer's standards. Follow the recommended schedule for maintenance of their equipment. In the QC log, record all maintenance or repairs to equipment.

There are three components of instrument calibration.

- *Reportable range* is the range of tests an analyzer, instrument, or procedure is capable of producing results.
- *Calibration* is setting the calculation points for the instrument by processing solutions of known values within the reportable range of the instrument. The solutions may or may not resemble clinical specimens. They may be measured quantities, a substance or standardized serum, or aqueous-based solutions. If a machine's calibration is correct, and the control sample results fall within its reportable range, patient's tests run on the machine will be correct.
- *Quality control specimens* are specimens that resemble clinical specimens. They have values that cover the calibrated range of the instrument. They may not exceed the upper or lower limits of the calibrated range. There are usually three levels—lower, middle, and upper. QC specimens are selected to cover the expected range of patient results found in both healthy and sick patients. The controls have expected values and the instrument matches these results plus

or minus a small preset amount. The amount is the *standard deviation*.

After you run the required controls for a procedure and they are all within acceptable ranges, you can report patient results with confidence. If they are not within acceptable ranges, the procedures and instruments must be evaluated. You must make the necessary changes and have acceptable QC results before you can rerun the tests and give the results to patients.

Quality Control Log

A lab must keep a QC log to show compliance with CLIA testing requirements. The log is kept as a book or on the computer. It must include a record of each control sample and standard test. Figure 23-7 is an example of a QC log sheet used to document testing controls.

Here's what these entries must contain:

- The date and time of the test
- The results expected
- The results obtained
- The action taken for correction, if necessary

Your office must keep test records for 2 years. Records on maintenance of equipment and supplies are also kept in the QC log.

Quality Assurance

QC programs also must contain written policies and procedures to make sure lab employees meet the standards required by CLIA. Labs must keep a record of this information and make it available for inspection. The employer can help the lab employees meet the standards by:

- Determining each employee's educational background
- Providing opportunities for continuing education and training
- Conducting proficiency testing and use other methods to evaluate employees' competence

Proficiency Testing

Besides inspections, another way of finding out if a lab and its employees are competent is proficiency testing. Labs doing tests for patients covered by Medicare must participate in three proficiency tests each year. They must also agree to at least one on-site inspection. Here's how the proficiency program works.

- The lab receives specimens from an outside testing agency.
- The lab tests the specimens using the same methods it does for patient tests.
- The lab mails the results to the testing agency.
- The testing agency reviews the results and evaluates the lab's performance.

QUALITATIVE QC LOG SHEET FOR _____
RECORD LOT NUMBER IF DIFFERENT FROM LAST LOT NUMBER.

TEST DATE	KIT LOT	POSITIVE CONTROL LOT #	NEGATIVE CONTROL LOT #	POSITIVE CONTROL RESULT	NEGATIVE CONTROL RESULT	OK TO USE?	IF NO, CORRECTIVE ACTION	INITIALS

Figure 23-7   QC Log. (Reprinted from Kronenberger J, Ledbetter J. *Jones & Bartlett Learning's Comprehensive Medical Assisting.* 5th ed. Burlington, MA: Jones & Bartlett Learning, LLC; 2016.)

Patient Education

The medical assistant will be collecting specimens from patients. It is important to educate the patient on the collection process to ensure the best quality specimen. Before collecting a patient's specimen, provide the patient with the following information:

- The name of the test (such as a blood cell count test)
- The type of specimen the patient needed for the test (such as blood, urine, or stool)
- The purpose of the test
- What kind of preparation the patient needs to do (such as fasting or following a certain diet)
- How long it will take to get results back from the lab
- How the patient will be informed of the results

Proper preparation is especially important. In testing for diabetes for example, if the patient doesn't prepare properly, the test results may be wrong. Do not use language that the patient cannot understand such as "we are testing to see if you have hyperglycemia." Simply say high blood sugar.

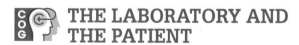

THE LABORATORY AND THE PATIENT

Of course we need to consider the patient when collecting specimens and performing laboratory testing. The medical assistant needs to understand the chain of custody of the specimen to maintain the integrity and protect the patient's privacy with test results.

Chain of Custody

When you work in a lab, you may be in charge of collecting specimens for drug or other testing done for legal purposes. Chain of custody (**COC**) is a process that accounts for a specimen at all times. Each person who handles the specimen until the testing is complete signs the COC form. This procedure documents that the specimen is genuine and that no one has tampered with it. The chain of custody process is required when determining blood alcohol levels in situations involving vehicle accidents. Urine drug testing is a preemployment requirement of many employers. Procedure 23-1 outlines the steps in urine collection while maintaining the chain of custody.

Packaging Specimens for Reference Labs

The medical assistant will frequently be responsible for processing the specimens sent out of the office to a reference laboratory. Carefully package these specimens to prevent damage that can occur due to:

- Rough handling
- Very high or low temperatures
- Pressure changes

Use only containers that meet federal regulations for transporting biohazardous materials. These containers are designed to protect the specimens and are leak proof. The special containers used to send specimens to a lab protect both the contents and those who handle the package. The results of tests sent off-site are usually ready in 24 to 48 hours.

Test Results and Patient Privacy

As a medical assistant, you have access to sensitive laboratory test results, such as:

- Human immunodeficiency virus (HIV)
- Pregnancy
- Illegal drugs
- Sexually transmitted infections or diseases (STI, STD)

You have a responsibility to keep the results of these tests, or any test results, from persons who are unauthorized to review or see the results. Only the physician and the patient are entitled to the results. The only exception is when laws require reporting certain results to protect public health and safety. However, deciding when to do this is not your responsibility. Always follow the protocols established by your medical facility for the disclosure of test results.

Procedure 23-1 — Maintaining the Chain of Custody for Urine Collection

Supplies required to maintain the chain of custody (COC) when collecting urine include a tamper-proof collection container and transport bag, chain of custody forms, and patient's picture ID. The steps for collection are as follows:

1. Obtain a picture ID and have the subject empty his pockets before collecting the specimen.

2. Turn off the water supply in the restroom used for collection. Add dye to toilet water to prevent the subject from using it as the specimen.

3. Ask the patient to wash their hands prior to the collection to ensure there is no soap residue that would affect the specimen quality.

4. Record the collection of the specimen and the name of the witness, if there was one present during the collection.

5. Record the specimen's temperature (90.5°F to 99.8°F is acceptable). The minimum volume collected should be 35 mL.

6. Have the subject and the collector sign the COC form, with the date and time of collection.

7. Sign and attach tamper seals to each side of the container, going across the lid.

8. Put the specimen and COC form in a tamper-proof bag.

9. Seal the bag for transport to the testing facility department.

Preparing for Externship

During your Externship, it is critical that you apply the safety measures that you learned in the classroom. Unfortunately, even some health care professionals do not always follow the OSHA standards when performing patient care. As a reminder, when you are caring for patients, you must assume that everyone has a potentially dangerous and communicable disease or condition, regardless of age. You are required to use personal protective equipment when performing invasive procedures and handling blood and body fluids. If you have any cuts on your hands, keep the area bandaged and change it when it becomes wet. Also, remember to wash your hands frequently and maintain good grooming of your fingernails.

Chapter Recap

- Medical assistants play an important role in the process of performing certain lab tests, which are critical to diagnosing, preventing, and treating medical conditions and diseases.
- Large hospital labs and reference labs have specialized departments that perform complicated tests. Most physician office laboratories perform tests that are less complex.
- Microscopes, centrifuges, and chemical analyzers are basic equipment for lab tests. To ensure the accuracy of test results, they must be handled gently, operated correctly, and kept in good repair.
- Machines, chemicals, and testing specimens in a lab can make it a hazardous place to work. Reduce possible dangers by following safe practices for the operation, storing, and handling of these items.
- OSHA rules set lab safety standards and procedures. CLIA standards regulate tests and testing methods. Failure to meet either set of requirements can have serious consequences.
- Good QC practices are basic to lab operations. These include careful control over reagents, test instruments, and test methods. They are also necessary for meeting CLIA requirements.

Online Resources for Students

Student Resources available on the text's online site include:
- Audio Glossaries
- Animations
- Competency Evaluation Forms
- Videos
- Anatomy & Physiology Module with Heart and Lung Sounds
- Weblinks
- Worksheets

Exercises and Activities

Certification Preparation Questions

1. Which of these statements best describes the types of laboratories?
   a. Reference laboratories primarily perform point of care testing.
   b. Physician's office laboratories specialize in performing high-complexity tests.
   c. Hospital laboratories usually perform point of care testing.
   d. Physician's office laboratories perform waived tests.
   e. Point of care testing includes many moderate complexity tests.

2. Which department performs a CBC?
   a. Serology
   b. Immunology
   c. Hematology
   d. Pathology
   e. Cytology

3. The purpose of an SDS is to:
   a. track the use of reagents for testing.
   b. log the quality controls when performing tests.
   c. provide information about substances and chemicals.
   d. notify the laboratory when to perform equipment maintenance.
   e. track the chain of custody of a specimen.

4. Which two government agencies oversee the CLIA program?
   a. CMS and COC
   b. FDA and CMS
   c. POL and POCT
   d. NFPA and FDA
   e. COC and POC

5. The person specifically trained to process and evaluate tissue samples, such as biopsies is a:
   a. cytologist.
   b. phlebotomist.
   c. medical technologist.
   d. histologist.
   e. medical laboratory technician.

6. The equipment that separates liquids into their different parts is a/an:
   a. incubator.
   b. centrifuge.
   c. autoclave.
   d. analyzer.
   e. POC device.

7. Coagulation studies determine the effectiveness of:
   a. antibiotics.
   b. diuretics.
   c. hormones.
   d. anticoagulants.
   e. enzymes.

8. Which of these tests is not performed in the hematology department?
   a. CBC
   b. BUN
   c. ESR
   d. H & H
   e. WBC

9. The part of the microscope that holds the slide is the:
   a. condenser.
   b. adjuster knob.
   c. diaphragm.
   d. ocular.
   e. stage.

10. Which of these is not a reason to perform laboratory testing?
    a. Monitor a patient's medication and treatment.
    b. Find the levels of key substances in the body.
    c. Determine the cause of an infection.
    d. Satisfy a patient's insurance deduction.
    e. Establish a baseline value.

Internet Resources

For additional information regarding CLIA rules, visit the Centers for Medicare and Medicaid Services web site at www.cms.hhs.gov/CLIA/.

24 Hematology

Chapter Objectives

- List the components of blood.
- Explain the functions of the three types of blood cells.
- Describe the role of the hematology lab.
- Identify the leukocytes normally seen in the blood and explain their functions.
- List the different tests in a complete blood count.
- Specify the normal ranges for each test in a complete blood count.
- Understand process for preparing a peripheral blood smear.
- Describe the structure of red blood cells and explain the tests that are performed on the cells.
- Describe the various types of anemia and the cause of each.
- Understand the process for performing a manual microhematocrit determination.
- Perform a manual hemoglobin determination.
- Understand process for determining erythrocyte sedimentation rate using the Westergren method.
- Explain the functions of platelets.
- Explain the process of how blood clots form in the body and describe the tests that measure the ability to form clots.

CAAHEP & ABHES Competencies

CAAHEP

- Identify CLIA-waived tests associated with common diseases.
- Instruct and prepare a patient for a procedure or a treatment.
- Perform a quality control measure.
- Obtain specimens and perform CLIA-waived hematology test.
- Define basic units of measurement in the metric system.
- Analyze health care results as reported in graphs and tables.
- Reassure a patient of the accuracy of the test results.
- Differentiate between normal and abnormal test results.

ABHES

- Practice quality control.
- Perform selected CLIA-waived tests that assist with diagnosis and treatment.
- Perform CLIA-waived hematology testing.

Chapter Terms

Anemia	Hematology	Leukemia	Neutrophilia
Anisocytosis	Hematopoiesis	Leukocytosis	Poikilocytosis
Erythropoietin	Hemoglobin	Leukopenia	Thrombocytopenia
Hematocrit	Hemostasis	Neutropenia	Thrombocytosis

Abbreviations

CBC	Hgb	PT	WBC
CLIA	MCH	PTT	
ESR	MCHC	PT/INR	
HCT	MCV	RBC	

Case Study

Maria Stone, a 24-year-old patient, is seeing the physician for symptoms of fatigue and feeling cold all the time. She has not seen the physician since she had a high school sports physical 7 years ago. After the physician is finished talking with Maria, he asks the medical assistant to draw blood for a CBC and comprehensive metabolic panel. He also orders a routine urinalysis. As the medical assistant is drawing Maria's blood, the patient asks "Is this normal to do this much lab testing?" She also states "The doctor thinks I may just have a vitamin or iron deficiency so I think I will just go to the drug store and load up on vitamins."

 HEMATOLOGY

Hematology is the study of blood, blood-forming tissues, and blood diseases. In this chapter, you'll learn the vital role that blood plays in our overall health and how it is often used to perform important tests and diagnose illnesses. In addition to learning about blood tests used for diagnostic purposes, you'll also learn about coagulation tests used to monitor patients undergoing certain treatments. It may not always fall within your scope of practice as a medical assistant to perform certain tests or to analyze specimens. However, you'll need to be familiar with these tests and the techniques involved to prepare specimens that are usable to perform these tests.

 BLOOD BASICS

Blood is made of two parts, the liquid part and the formed elements. The liquid part is known as plasma and the formed elements are the cells. The three basic types of cells are as follows:

- Leukocytes, commonly called white blood cells or **WBCs**
- Erythrocytes, commonly called red blood cells or **RBCs**
- Thrombocytes, also known as platelets

Leukocytes

Leukocytes are the body's main line of defense against bacteria and viruses. There are two main kinds of leukocytes, granulocytes and nongranulocytes.

Nongranulocytes include the following:

Case Question

 How should the medical assistant respond to the patient's question and comments?

- Lymphocytes
- Monocytes

Granulocytes include the following:

- Neutrophils
- Eosinophils
- Basophils

Erythrocytes

Red blood cells, or erythrocytes, carry gases between the lungs and the body's tissues, mainly oxygen and carbon dioxide. Hemoglobin molecules, made of protein, are in each red blood cell. This allows the red blood cells to carry these gases to the body tissues and cells.

Thrombocytes

Platelets are not actual whole cells but are cell fragments. Their main function is to help stop bleeding by participating in the clot formation. The term thrombocyte literally means clotting cells.

How Blood Is Made

Blood cells form in the bone marrow. Most blood cells are made in the long bones, skull, pelvis, and sternum. Blood cells are also made in the liver, in the spleen, and in the yolk sac of a developing fetus.

Hematopoiesis is the process of blood cell production. Here's how it works. Young, immature cells in the bone marrow divide and differentiate. To differentiate means that cells take on different characteristics and begin to mature. These maturing cells become erythrocytes, leukocytes, and thrombocytes depending on what the body needs. Figure 24-1 is a very detailed chart showing the process of blood cell formation from the initial hematopoietic stem cell to the final mature cells.

This process is influenced by many factors such as specific hormones and certain nutrients that are required for cells to function properly. Once the cells reach maturity, they're released from the bone marrow and into the bloodstream.

 THE HEMATOLOGY LAB

The hematology lab analyzes blood cells, their quantities, and their characteristics to assist physicians to diagnose and manage many conditions. Some of the illnesses diagnosed in the hematology lab include the following:

- **Anemia**—condition resulting from reduced numbers of RBCs in the blood or from reductions in the amount of hemoglobin the RBCs contain.
- **Leukemia**—disease in which unusually high numbers of abnormal WBCs are produced.

- Infection—invasion of the blood and body tissues by bacteria and other microorganisms. (A microorganism is a living thing that can only be seen under a microscope.)

Hematology also includes the study of **hemostasis**, to control bleeding or stop flow of blood from the body. This is the body's ability to keep blood in a fluid state in the vessels. The hematology lab helps evaluate patients who have trouble forming blood clots, as well as those who form clots unexpectedly in their blood vessels.

As you work in the medical field you will encounter various units of measurement. Blood test results are reported using some of these measurements. The metric system measurements are used to express many of the laboratory findings. Table 24-1 explains the prefixes in the metric system and their meanings. For example, you can see that milli- means "one thousandth of." If something is a milliliter, you know it's one thousandth of a liter. In hematology, the measurements you'll see the most are the ones that are less than the number 1, for example, picogram.

Hematology Testing

Hematology testing does more than just help diagnose and treat problems with the blood cells. It's also useful in detecting and dealing with the following types of problems:

- Metabolic disorders—problems with the body's chemical and physical processes, such as growth and producing energy
- Nutritional disorders—problems with how food is used for nourishment and body repair
- Immunological disorders—problems resulting from bacteria, viruses, and other foreign substances in the body
- Neoplastic disorders—problems related to abnormal growth of tissue, such as tumors

Hematology Testing and the Medical Assistant Scope of Practice

The Clinical Laboratory Improvement Amendments (**CLIA**) was adopted to help regulate the functions and operations of medical laboratories. The amendments include personnel requirements to perform specific tests. The CLIA regulations allow medical assistants to perform waived tests and with additional training, some moderately complex tests have recently been approved. Overall, waived tests do not require a higher level education and training to perform highly complex tests. Hematology tests medical assistants currently can perform include the following:

- Erythrocyte sedimentation rate (not automated)
- Hematocrit (all spun microhematocrit procedures)

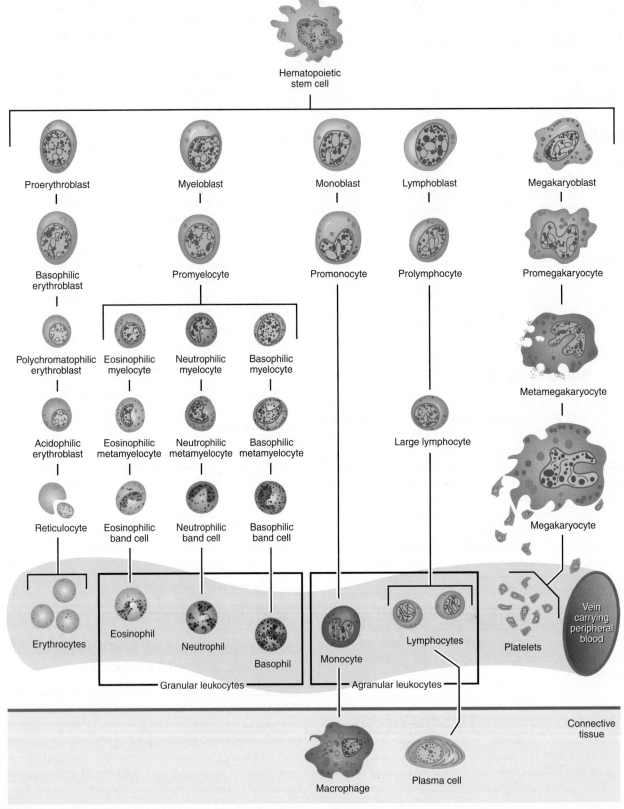

Figure 24-1 Stem cell. The development of red blood cells, leukocytes, macrophages, lymphocytes, and platelets. (Image from Shutterstock.)

Table 24-1   Prefixes of the Metric System

Decimal Multiples	Prefix	Symbol	Meaning
1,000,000,000,000	tera-	T	One trillion times
1,000,000,000	giga-	G	One billion times
1,000,000	mega-	M	One million times
1,000	kilo-	k	One thousand times
100	hector-	h	One hundred times
10	deka-	da	Ten times
1			One times
0.1	deci-	d	One tenth of
0.01	centi-	c	One hundredth of
0.001	milli-	m	One thousandth of
0.000001	micro-	mu	One millionth of
0.000000001	nano-	n	One billionth of
0.000000000001	pico-	p	One trillionth of
0.000000000000001	femto-	f	One quadrillionth of

- Hemoglobin (selected methods)
- Prothrombin time (selected methods)

The entire list of waived tests is updated regularly by the Centers for Medicare and Medicaid Services (CMS). As a medical assistant, you should know which tests you're allowed by law to perform.

Remember that even with waived tests, it's still possible to make a mistake. If test results are inaccurate, patients could go untreated or receive an improper diagnosis or treatment. In some cases, this could be disastrous.

To protect yourself and your employer against possible legal action, make sure you follow the proper procedures and the manufacturer's instructions for whatever test you are performing. Also, always stay within your scope of practice.

 COMPLETE BLOOD COUNT

The complete blood count (**CBC**) is one of the most frequently ordered lab tests. It consists of several related tests:

- WBC count and differential
- RBC count
- Hemoglobin (**Hgb**) determination

- Hematocrit (**Hct**) determination
- Mean cell volume (**MCV**)
- Mean corpuscular hemoglobin (**MCH**)
- Mean corpuscular hemoglobin concentration (**MCHC**)
- Platelet count

White Blood Cell Count and Differential

White blood cells (WBC), or leukocytes, are the body's main line of defense against bacteria and viruses. Different types of WBCs have different functions in the body. Some circulate in the bloodstream. Others work their way into the body's tissues and cavities to do their job.

Study Skill

When you study normal values for blood tests, it is easier if you understand the abbreviations used to express the quantity. For example, when you see "mm³," it means cubic millimeters. Imagine a small perfectly square box, or cube, that is 1 mm long by 1 mm wide by 1 mm tall.

The quantity of a blood cell count is thousands or millions of cells that are in the amount of blood that can fill that cube.

The normal WBC range is 4,500 to 11,000/mm³. A WBC count measures the white blood cells in the peripheral blood (blood circulating in the body). The differential reveals the types of WBCs and the quantity of each. It means that you are sorting the WBC in to their individual types. For example, there are many types of apples available at the grocery store; however, they are sorted according to type such as gala, red and yellow delicious, granny smith, etc. The five types of white blood cells in order of their abundance from greatest to smallest amount are as follows:

- Neutrophils
- Lymphocytes
- Monocytes
- Eosinophils
- Basophils

Figure 24-2A–H are microscopic images of the various white blood cells and red blood cells.

All types of WBCs are colorless but have specific identifying characteristics. The manual method to study them, involves putting a drop of blood on a microscope slide, spreading it into a thin layer and staining it. This way, the different kinds of WBCs can be seen under a microscope. Once a blood sample has been stained, 100 WBCs are counted and divided according to type. Then, the different types are reported as percentages. Most CBC tests that include a differential are performed on an automated cell counter in a laboratory. CLIA does now allow medical assistants to perform manual cell counts; however, some

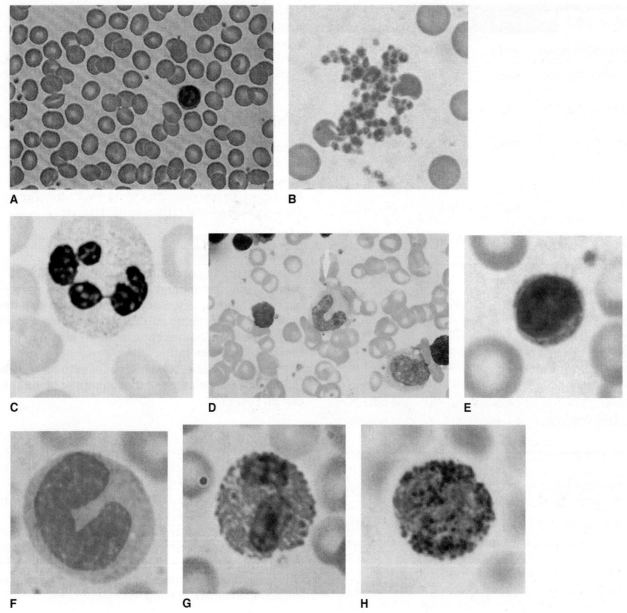

Figure 24-2 **A-H.** Blood smear and cells. (Reprinted from Kronenberger J, Ledbetter J. *Jones & Bartlett Learning's Comprehensive Medical Assisting.* 5th ed. Burlington, MA: Jones & Bartlett Learning, LLC; 2016.)

cell analyzers may have waived status, which would allow medical assistants to use those machines. The number of white blood cells can increase or decrease from specific conditions or diseases in the body. Terms used to describe these conditions are as follows:

- **Leukopenia**—a condition where there are too few WBCs in the body; factors that can decrease the number include the following:
  - Chemical toxicity
  - Poor nutrition
  - Chronic or overwhelming infection
  - Certain malignancies

- **Leukocytosis**—a condition when there are too many WBCs in the body; factors that can increase the number include the following:

- Infection
- Inflammatory condition
- Certain drugs
- Injury to tissue
- Certain malignancies

Neutrophils

Neutrophils are the most plentiful leukocytes and the primary granulocyte. Normally, 50% to 70% of white blood cells are neutrophils. The percentage of neutrophils is higher in patients who have bacterial infections. When the neutrophils are released from the bone marrow into the bloodstream, they circulate in the blood for about 7 hours, and then they move into the tissues where they can perform their function.

Neutrophils defend the body against bacteria by phagocytosis, or surrounding and digesting them. The bacteria are killed by digestive enzymes. An enzyme is a protein that starts a chemical reaction. Eventually, the digestive enzymes kill the neutrophil, too.

When a neutrophil is stained, it has a light pink cytoplasm. The nucleus is dark purple and usually has five or fewer segments. If a patient's neutrophils have more than five segments (hypersegmented), this condition can mean a vitamin B_{12} or folate deficiency. (Folate is an essential nutrient.)

A band (or stab) is a younger version of the neutrophil, not fully mature. Its appearance is much the same as a regular neutrophil, but the nucleus is not segmented. The normal percentage of bands is 0% to 5%. A higher percentage may indicate acute infections that require immediate attention. Terms used to describe the quantity of neutrophils include:

- **Neutrophilia**—an increase in the percentage of neutrophils that can be a sign of inflammation or bacterial infections, such as syphilis and tuberculosis
- **Neutropenia**—a low number of neutrophils that can result after an overwhelming infection, or after certain drugs have been given to a patient

Lymphocytes

Lymphocytes are the next most common leukocyte and they are also the smallest. A lymphocyte's purpose is to recognize that a foreign cell or particle is a threat to the body and then make antibodies to destroy it. These antibodies coat the foreign cell or particle, and then one of two things happens:

- The pathogen is destroyed by being surrounded and digested (the phagocytic system).
- A group of chemicals in the blood destroys the foreign cell or particle by puncturing holes in its membranes (the complement system).

The normal percentage of lymphocytes is 20% to 40%. The percentage increases in patients with viral infections, such as infectious mononucleosis.

Most lymphocytes live 4 to 7 days, although some can last for years. When lymphocytes are stained, they have a small, round, dark purple nucleus, and their cytoplasm is sky blue.

Monocytes

Monocytes are the third most common leukocyte with a normal percentage of 3% to 8% of the total WBCs. They are twice the size of nonreactive lymphocytes and slightly larger than neutrophils. The main purpose of monocytes is to digest foreign cells or particles—much like neutrophils—and to assist the lymphocytes in the destruction of foreign cells or particles by antibodies.

The shape of a monocyte's nucleus can vary. When a monocyte is stained, the cytoplasm is gray-blue and looks like ground glass.

Monocytes stay in the bloodstream for about 3 days and then move into body tissues.

Eosinophils and Basophils

Eosinophils are the fourth most common leukocyte with 0% to 6% of the total WBCs. Their function in the body is not completely understood. The nucleus of an eosinophil is divided into two segments, with large orange granules in the cytoplasm. The percentage of eosinophils is higher in patients with allergic reactions and parasitic infections.

Basophils are the least plentiful type of leukocyte. In fact, <1% of WBCs are basophils. The nucleus of a basophil is either two or three segments. When stained, very large dark blue-purple granules appear in the cytoplasm.

Table 24-2 is a recap of the types and characteristics of white blood cells.

Red Cell Count

Red blood cells (RBCs), or erythrocytes, transport gases between the lungs and the body tissues. They are shaped like disks that are concave on both sides and contain hemoglobin. Their special design allows them to easily change shape and pass through small capillaries. They exchange gases in the body tissues and lungs by:

- Releasing carbon dioxide, picked up at the tissues, as the blood moves through the capillary bed of the lungs; carbon dioxide is a by-product of metabolism
- Releasing oxygen, picked up in the lungs, into the tissues as it circulates to the organs

Red Blood Cell Production

RBCs are made in the bone marrow with all the other blood cells. The hormone **erythropoietin** is released from the kidneys and influences the production of RBCs. This is a reason why individuals with kidney problems may become anemic due to the malfunction of the kidney.

Erythropoietin stimulates the production of RBCs to increase blood oxygen levels. This process occurs when:

- Inadequate oxygen (hypoxia) is detected and erythropoietin travels to the bone marrow to increase RBC production.
- Anemia is corrected by increasing the production of RBCs releasing more into circulation.

Nutrition can also affect the quality and quantity of red blood cells (RBCs). Vitamin B_{12} and folic acid are

Table 24-2	Types and Characteristics of WBCs		

White Blood Cell	Percent of Normal WBC	Function	Nucleus Appearance
Segmented neutrophils (Segs)	50%–70%	Fight bacterial infections	Dark purple; 2–5 lobes
Neutrophilic band (Band)	0%–5%	An immature Seg; a young warrior that doesn't fight infections as well as a Seg	Dark purple; tube shaped, may be twisted and turned, but not pinched
Eosinophils (Eos)	0%–6%	Slightly increased in allergic reactions 10%–15%; markedly increased in parasitic infections, up to 40% of WBC	Dark purple; 2–3 lobes, usually obscured by orange granules
Basophils (Baso)	0%–1%	Granules contain histamine and heparin	Dark purple; 2–5 lobes, usually obscured by purple granules
Lymphocytes (Lymph)	20%–40%	Fight viral infections	Dark purple; normal RBCs are the same size as nucleus of lymph
Reactive lymphocytes	0%–5%	Usually B lymphocytes producing antibodies to fight infections	Nucleus not as dark as regular lymph; usually smooth consistency
Monocytes (Mono)	3%–8%	Clean up cell and microbe debris; the "garbage collector" after the battle	Lighter purple to blue; less dense

necessary to properly mature the RBCs. At first, RBCs have a nucleus. As they mature, the nucleus is pushed out. The color of their cytoplasm changes from blue to red. A mature RBC is a pale red biconcave (concave on both sides) disk that is able to squeeze through very small capillaries. The average RBC lives about 120 days.

Cultural Connection

Sickle cell disease describes a group of inherited red blood cell disorders. People with this disease have hemoglobin S in their red blood cells, which is an abnormal form of hemoglobin. People of African ancestry or identify as black make up the majority of people in the United States who have this disease. Statistics show that about 1 in 13 African American babies is born with the sickle cell trait. This means that they do not actually have the disease but carry the trait on their genes. Other ethnic groups that have a higher incidence of this disease are Hispanic, Middle Eastern, and Asian Indian. In the United States, there are approximately 100,000 who have sickle cell disease. For more information and statistics on sickle cell disease, visit the website for the National Institutes of Health at http://www.nhlbi.nih.gov/health/health-topics/topics/sca/atrisk.

Measuring Red Blood Cells

Measuring RBCs helps to detect anemia, which can be caused by:

- Decreased RBC production (iron deficiency anemia)
- Increased RBC destruction (hemolytic anemia)
- Blood loss (hemolytic anemia)
- Vitamin B_{12} deficiency (pernicious anemia)

Figure 24-3 shows the difference between various red blood cells including those that are microcytic, smaller than normal, and hypochromic, lighter color than normal.

Case Question

Maria Stone, the patient mentioned earlier in the chapter was diagnosed with vitamin B_{12} deficiency and will be started on a series of injections to increase her vitamin level. As the medical assistant is preparing to give the patient her first injection, Maria asks her why she is so cold all the time. How should the medical assistant respond to her?

The normal range of RBCs differs among men and women. For men, the normal range is 4.6 to 6.2 million/mm³. For women, the range is 4.2 to 5.4 million/mm³.

A report on the morphology, or appearance, of RBCs is included in a WBC differential count. The report comments on variations in the size (**anisocytosis**)

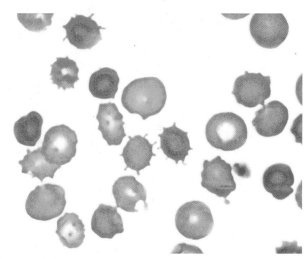

Figure 24-3 Microcytic, macrocytic, and hypochromic red blood cells in anemia. (Image from Shutterstock.)

and shape (**poikilocytosis**) of the RBCs. Table 24-3 describes some common RBC abnormalities and the conditions they may indicate.

Other less common RBC shapes include:

- Elliptocytes/ovalocytes—RBCs are distinctly oval in shape; liver impairment, anemias (especially thalassemia), and hemoglobin C disease (genetic blood disorder)
- Schistocytes—RBCs are fragmented; hereditary spherocytosis, hemolytic anemias, and burns

- Spherocytes—RBCs show no area of central paleness; artifact as blood dries and hyperosmolarity (a condition of increased numbers of dissolved substances in the plasma)
- Burr cells—RBCs have small, regular spicules (sharp points)

Hematocrit Testing

The percentage of RBCs in whole blood is called the **hematocrit**. For example, if a patient has a hematocrit of 40, it means that 40% of the patient's total blood volume is RBCs. The other 60% is plasma.

The purpose of the hematocrit test is to detect anemia. To get a hematocrit measurement, the blood is centrifuged to pack the RBCs into one area so a percentage can be read. A microhematocrit centrifuge doesn't actually calculate the hematocrit. Instead, it must be read on a chart, which is in the centrifuge or a separate reader card. Cell counting machines measure the RBC count and the mean cell volume (MCV) and then calculate the hematocrit from these two values using the formula for MCV. The normal hematocrit range for men is 45 to 52 and for women, 37 to 48.

Red Blood Cell Indices

Red blood cell indices are part of the complete blood count (CBC) test. They are used to help diagnose the

Table 24-3	Erythrocyte (Red Blood Cell) Abnormalities
Abnormality	**Associated Conditions**
Hypochromia—reduced hemoglobin in the RBCs; appear lighter with more area of central pallor	Anemias, especially iron deficiency and thalassemia, a hemolytic anemia
Hyperchromia—increased hemoglobin in RBCs; appear to have less or no area of central pallor	Megaloblastic anemia (characterized by large, dysfunctional RBCs), hereditary spherocytosis (condition in which nearly all the RBCs are spherocytes), and hemolysis, acute blood loss
Polychromia—some RBCs have a blue color	Iron deficiency anemia and thalassemia
Microcytosis—RBCs are smaller than usual	B_{12} and folate deficiencies and megaloblastic anemias
Macrocytosis—RBCs are larger than normal	Hereditary elliptocytosis (condition in which all or almost all of the RBCs are elliptical or oval in shape), iron deficiency anemia, myelofibrosis (disorder in which bone marrow tissue develops in abnormal sites), sickle cell anemia (hereditary anemia characterized by the presence of sickle-shaped RBCs), hereditary elliptocytosis (condition in which all or almost all of the RBCs are elliptical or oval in shape), iron deficiency anemia, myelofibrosis (disorder in which bone marrow tissue develops in abnormal sites), and sickle cell anemia (hereditary anemia characterized by the presence of sickle-shaped RBCs)
Target cells—RBCs resemble targets with light and dark rings	Hemolysis, burns, and intravascular coagulation (clot formation within the vessels)

cause of anemia. These indices include the MCV, MCH, and MCHC which are as follows:

- MCV—average red blood cell size
- MCH—the quantity of hemoglobin per red blood cell
- MCHC—the hemoglobin concentration (amount of hemoglobin) relative to the size of the cell

Knowing the MCV value helps to diagnose anemias such as those caused by the nutritional deficiencies that affect RBC production. Too little iron often results in microcytosis (when the MCV is below normal). This test finding, along with RBC counts, hematocrit and hemoglobin tests, and tests for forms of iron and related compounds, may lead to a diagnosis of iron deficiency anemia.

A deficiency of vitamin B_{12} or folic acid is often the cause of macrocytosis (when the MCV is above normal). This abnormality can also indicate anemia. In addition, liver disorders can raise the MCV.

Erythrocyte Sedimentation Rate

Erythrocyte sedimentation rate (**ESR** or sed rate) measures the rate at which RBCs settle out in a tube or column of blood. Anticoagulated blood is placed into a calibrated glass tube and is allowed to settle, undisturbed, for 1 hour. The ESR reading is determined by the number of millimeters the RBCs have fallen during the hour. The normal range for ESR in men is 0 to 10 mm/h. For women, it's 0 to 20 mm/h. A higher ESR value doesn't point to a specific disorder, but it does indicate inflammation or other conditions that indicate increased or altered proteins in the blood (e.g., rheumatoid arthritis). The ESR can also be higher in patients who are pregnant or who have an infection. The more quickly the RBCs fall in the tube, the greater the inflammation is in the patient.

Medical assistants are permitted to perform manual CLIA-waived ESR tests. Figure 24-4 shows the blood tube system used for ESR determination. This method of ESR testing requires a vial of EDTA-anticoagulated whole blood. Automated ESR tests are available but are not CLIA waived at this time. In an automated ESR, a centrifuge spins the sample for 3 minutes, forcing the RBCs to the end of the tube. About 100 measurements are taken during the process. The ESR is calculated from these measurements.

Measuring Hemoglobin

Hemoglobin is the part of the red blood cell that binds the gases it carries. There are millions of hemoglobin molecules in each RBC. Each hemoglobin molecule also contains four protein chains called globins. The most common globin chains are named alpha and beta. Newborns have some gamma (fetal) globin chains instead of alpha chains in their fetal hemoglobin. Fetal hemoglobin percentages should drop to <3% after 6 months. When there's a defect in those globin chains, patients have abnormal hemoglobins. For example, sickle cell anemia is one condition caused by abnormal hemoglobins.

Like RBCs in general, the normal range for hemoglobin differs among men and women. For men, the normal range is 13 to 18 g/dL (grams per deciliter) and for women, 12 to 16 g/dL. Anemia can be detected with a hemoglobin measurement—this shows the body's ability to oxygenate tissues. There are several CLIA-waived handheld devices that easily determine the hemoglobin using a single drop of blood either from a capillary finger puncture or from anticoagulated whole blood.

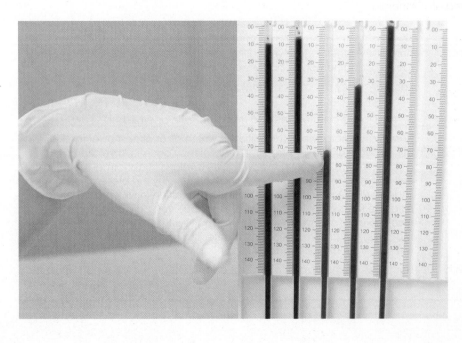

Figure 24-4 Erythrocyte sedimentation rate. (Image from Shutterstock.)

Platelet Count

Like other blood cells, platelets, also called thrombocytes, are made in the bone marrow. Platelets are not actually cells, but cell fragments. They can attach themselves to damaged endothelium (a layer of flattened cells that lines the inside of some body cavities). Platelets perform two important functions:

- Aid in sealing wounds and stopping bleeding until a clot can form.
- Help initiate the clotting factors to form a sturdier fibrin clot.

The normal number of platelets ranges from 150,000 to 450,000/mm³. Having too few platelets is called **thrombocytopenia**. This can be caused by a variety of conditions. Increased bleeding also can result when the number of platelets is decreased.

Having too many platelets is called **thrombocytosis**. This condition is often benign. It sometimes occurs after a splenectomy (removal of the spleen) or during an inflammatory disease. However, marked thrombocytosis (more than 1 million/mm³) may be associated with increased clotting, or even severe bleeding if the platelets aren't functioning properly. As the platelet count decreases, the risk of bleeding increases. Platelets are much smaller than RBCs. When stained, they are a light purplish blue. They have an irregular shape and no nucleus.

 COAGULATION TESTS

Coagulation tests measure the ability of whole blood to form a clot. When the body suffers a cut, proteins in the blood, called clotting factors, work together to form a clot. The process of clot formation and repair involves these steps:

- Vasoconstriction—the vein narrows to reduce blood loss.
- Platelet plug forms—platelets stick to the wound and form a plug to slow or stop the blood flow.
- Fibrin clot forms—the blood's clotting factors form a clot at the site of the wound.
- Clot lysis and vascular repair—as the body repairs the damage (the cut heals), another set of proteins slowly dissolves (lysis, break down) the clot.

The two most common tests for determining how well a fibrin clot can form are prothrombin time (**PT**) and partial thromboplastin time (**PTT**).

These tests are common when treating patients with clotting problems (including heart attacks, stroke, and pulmonary embolism). When treating these patients, the physician may start patients on two medications. Heparin is used for immediate inhibition of the formation of new clots and Coumadin, for the long-term inhibition of new clot formation.

Prothrombin Time

The prothrombin time (PT) is a test designed to measure clotting time. It is used to monitor Coumadin therapy. The normal PT range is 12 to 15 seconds; however, laboratories may have their own range of normal set by the analyzer used. The following factors may lengthen a patient's prothrombin time:

- Liver disease
- Vitamin K deficiency
- Coumadin (oral anticoagulant) therapy

When the PT starts to show abnormal results, it's a sign that the physician needs to adjust the heparin and Coumadin therapy. There are several point-of-care instruments that medical assistants can use in the medical office to determine PT times that are CLIA-waived coagulation testing devices. They measure the prothrombin time/international normalized ratio (**PT/INR**). Figure 24-5 demonstrates the blood sample required for a PT/INR used to perform PT/INR in a physician's office. This test requires only one drop of blood from a venipuncture or capillary specimen. A handheld device is used to complete the test.

Partial Thromboplastin Time

The partial thromboplastin time (PTT) is a two-stage test to determine clotting time. The normal range is 32 to 51 seconds, but like a PT test, a lab may set its own range based on instrumentation used to perform the test. PTT can be delayed when certain clotting factor deficiencies are present in the blood, especially ones that cause hemophilia (uncontrolled bleeding). Heparin (anticoagulant) therapy also prolongs the PTT. This is why the PTT test is often used to monitor heparin therapy.

Monitoring Anticoagulation Therapy

Patients need to understand the importance of PT and PTT monitoring when on heparin or Coumadin therapy. If a patient is on anticoagulation medication and does not come in for testing, the medical assistant should let the physician know. It is the physician's responsibility to decide whether a refill should be called in to the pharmacy. Try to contact the patient to find out why he didn't return for the blood work. Perhaps transportation is a problem. Many communities have programs where health care workers will draw patients' blood in their homes. The medical assistant can:

- Make sure the patient understands the purpose of the medication and why the blood tests are important to his health.
- Inform the patient about the dangers of self-dosing Coumadin. For example, he could experience excessive bleeding with an overdose and clotting with an underdose.

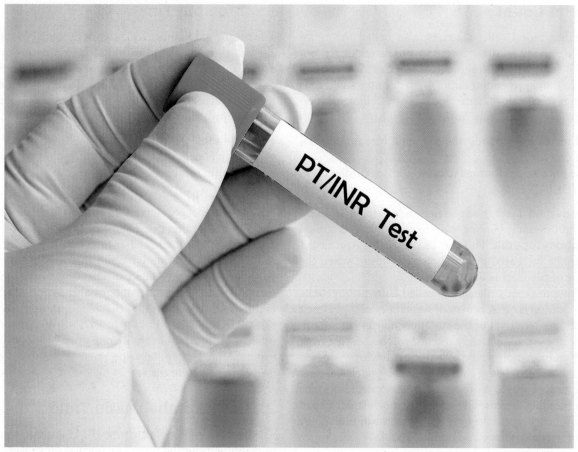

Figure 24-5   PT/INR testing requires whole blood from venipuncture or capillary puncture. (Image from Shutterstock.)

• Document all phone conversations with the patient, including the date, time, and message and record the patient's responses; try to quote his exact words when possible.

Patient Education

The medical assistant may be asked to educate patients with thrombocytopenia. Patients with low platelet counts may need instruction to help them understand their condition and the precautions they should take. Inform patients that if they bruise easily, any of these other signs could indicate thrombocytopenia:

• Prolonged bleeding from a cut
• Tiny red or purple spots on the skin (called petechiae)
• Black or bloody stool
• Brown or red urine
• Nose bleeds or bleeding gums
• Increased vaginal bleeding

   It is also critical to instruct patients with low platelet counts to take these precautions:

• Avoid aspirin or any medication that contains aspirin; if you aren't sure if a medication is safe, talk to the physician before taking it.
• Use a soft toothbrush. Brush gently and floss carefully.
• Use an electric shaver instead of a razor.
• Avoid foods that might irritate your digestive tract or make you constipated.
• Avoid clothing with tight-fitting elastic waist or wristbands.
• Always wear shoes.
• Avoid enemas, rectal thermometers, and suppositories. Women should avoid douches and tampons.
• Blow your nose gently.

   Advise patients with thrombocytopenia to ask the doctor if sexual intercourse is a safe activity. Also, tell them to call the office right away in the following situations:

• New bruising or petechiae
• Bleeding from your nose, mouth, or gums
• Blood in your urine or stool
• A headache that doesn't go away

Procedure 24-1 Making a Peripheral Blood Smear

Equipment: Clean glass slides with frosted ends, a pencil, a well-mixed whole blood specimen, and a transfer pipette.

Follow these steps to prepare a blood sample for microscopic examination:

1. Wash your hands.

2. Get your equipment ready.

3. Greet and identify the patient. Explain the procedure. Ask for and answer any questions.

4. Put on gloves, an impervious gown, and a face shield.

5. Perform a venipuncture to get an EDTA (lavender-top tube) blood specimen from your patient. A capillary puncture is also a method to obtain one drop of blood to place on the slide.

6. Label the slide with the patient's name or identification number on the frosted area using a pencil.

7. Hold the slide flat between the thumb and first finger on your nondominant hand. Place a drop of blood 1 cm from the frosting at one end of the slide. The slide also can be held on a flat surface and the smear made on the surface. Try both ways and see which is more comfortable and gets the best results.

8. Use your thumb and forefinger on your dominant hand to hold the second (spreader) slide against the surface of the first slide at a 30-degree angle.

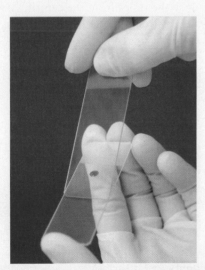

Preparing Blood Smear Slide Begin. (Reprinted from Kronenberger J, Ledbetter J. *Jones & Bartlett Learning's Comprehensive Medical Assisting*. 5th ed. Burlington, MA: Jones & Bartlett Learning, LLC; 2016.)

- The angle of the spreader slide may have to be greater for large or thin drops of blood.
- The angle of the spreader slide may have to be <30 degrees for small or thick drops.

Move the spreader slide back until it is touching the drop of blood. Allow the blood to spread under the edge for a fraction of a second. Then push the spreader slide at a medium speed toward the other end of the slide. Make sure the two slides are in contact the entire time.

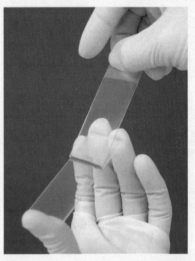

Preparing Blood Smear Slide Blood Drop Spread. (Reprinted from Kronenberger J, Ledbetter J. *Jones & Bartlett Learning's Comprehensive Medical Assisting*. 5th ed. Burlington, MA: Jones & Bartlett Learning, LLC; 2016.)

9. Allow the slide to air dry. (The photograph shows a properly prepared smear.)

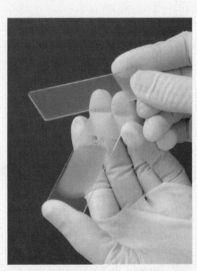

Prepared Blood Smear Slide Final. (Reprinted from Kronenberger J, Ledbetter J. *Jones & Bartlett Learning's Comprehensive Medical Assisting*. 5th ed. Burlington, MA: Jones & Bartlett Learning, LLC; 2016.)

Procedure 24-1   Making a Peripheral Blood Smear *(continued)*

10. Properly take care of or dispose of equipment and supplies. Clean your work area. Then, remove your gloves, gown, and face shield, and wash your hands.

Make sure you don't hesitate too long before pushing the spreader slide toward the other end of the slide. If you wait too long, platelets will collect along the edge of the spreader slide.

A thin film of blood is desired at the feathered end of the smear. After staining, a proper smear should have a significant area where the RBCs are close to each other, but not on top of each other. Too much blood on the slide will make the smear unusable.

Procedure 24-2   Performing a Manual Microhematocrit Determination

Equipment: Microcollection tubes, sealing clay, microhematocrit centrifuge with a reading device or a separate microhematocrit reading care, biohazard container and sharps container, lancet, gauze, sealing clay, and gloves.

1. Wash your hands and gather your supplies.

2. Apply PPE including gloves and if desired a lab gown and faceshield.

3. Use one of the following methods to draw blood into the capillary tube.

   A. Directly from a capillary puncture:

      - Touch the tip of the capillary tube to the blood at the puncture site and allow the tube to fill to three-quarters or the indicated mark.

      - For a finger stick, use heparinized capillary tubes.

      - Place your forefinger over the top of the capillary tube, wipe excess blood off its sides, and push its bottom into the sealing clay. (Make sure you push the end opposite to the end the blood was drawn in.) Use caution while sealing tubes as they can break and puncture gloves and skin if you use too much force.

      - Then, draw a second specimen in the same way. (The second tube is for a duplicate test as a part of quality control.)

   B. From a well-mixed EDTA tube of whole blood:

      - Touch the tip of the capillary tube to the blood in the EDTA tube and allow the capillary tube to fill three-quarters.

      - Place your forefinger over the top of the capillary tube, wipe excess blood off its sides, and push its bottom into the sealing clay. (Make sure you push the end opposite to the end the blood was drawn in.) Use caution while sealing tubes as they can break and puncture gloves and skin if you use too much force.

      - Draw a second specimen in the same way. (The second tube is for a duplicate test as a part of quality control.)

4. Place the tubes, with the clay-sealed end out, in the radial grooves of the microhematocrit centrifuge opposite each other. Put the lid on the grooved area and tighten by turning the knob clockwise. Close the lid. Spin the tubes for 5 minutes or as directed by the manufacturer of the machine.

5. Remove the tubes from the centrifuge and read the results. Instructions on how to do this are printed on the device.

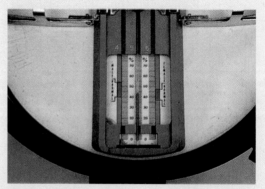

Hematocrit Centrifuge reader. (Reprinted from Kronenberger J, Ledbetter J. *Jones & Bartlett Learning's Comprehensive Medical Assisting.* 5th ed. Burlington, MA: Jones & Bartlett Learning, LLC; 2016.)

Procedure 24-2 Performing a Manual Microhematocrit Determination (*continued*)

Take the average of the two tube readings and report it as a percentage. (The figure shows the determinations of microhematocrit values. Results should be within 2% of each other. Results that have greater than a 2% variation are unreliable. A 3% difference is the equivalent of a patient losing about a pint of blood.)

Note how the results are displayed on this centrifuge-reading device.

6. Dispose of the microhematocrit tubes in a biohazard container. Properly take care of or dispose of other equipment and supplies. Clean your work area. Then, remove your gloves, gown, and face shield, and wash your hands.

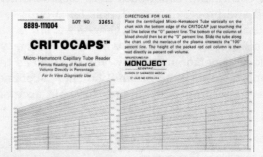

Hematocrit Reader Card. (Reprinted from Kronenberger J, Ledbetter J. *Jones & Bartlett Learning's Comprehensive Medical Assisting.* 5th ed. Burlington, MA: Jones & Bartlett Learning, LLC; 2016.)

Note: Some microhematocrit centrifuges have the scale printed in the machine at the radial grooves.

Procedure 24-3 Performing a Westergren Erythrocyte Sedimentation Rate

Equipment: Whole blood sample collected in EDTA (free of clots and <4 hours old), a Sediplast system vial pre-filled with 0.2 mL of 3.8% sodium citrate, an autozero calibrated Sediplast pipette, a sed rate rack, and a disposable transfer pipette.

Follow these steps to determine the ESR:

1. Wash your hands.

2. Get your equipment ready.

3. Put on gloves and personal protective equipment.

4. Remove the stopper on the prefilled vial. Using a transfer pipette, fill the vial to the bottom of the indicated fill line with 0.8 mL of blood to make the required 4:1 dilution. (The test can also be run with no dilution.)

Use a transfer pipette to fill the vial.

5. Replace the pierceable stopper and gently invert several times. This way, there will be a good mixture of blood and diluent.

6. Place the vial in its rack on a level surface. Carefully insert the pipette through the pierceable stopper using a rotating downward pressure until the pipette comes in contact with the bottom of the

vial. The pipette will autozero the blood and any excess will flow into the reservoir compartment.

Invert the vial to get a good mixture of blood and diluent.

Insert the pipette through the stopper.

7. Make sure the pipette makes firm contact with the bottom of the vial. Otherwise, you may get inaccurate test results.

8. Let the sample stand for exactly 1 hour and then read the numerical results of the erythrocyte sedimentation in millimeters. Make sure the test is set up on a surface that is free from vibration and away from anything that may cause a change in temperature (windows, refrigerators, motors, AC ducts). Most of these will cause an increase in sedimentation rate, but cold will cause a decrease.

It's essential that the pipette makes firm contact with the bottom of the vial.

9. Read the result at exactly 60 minutes and record the results.

10. Properly take care of or dispose of equipment and supplies. Clean your work area. Then remove your gloves and other PPE and wash your hands.

Preparing for Externship

Your externship experience may include drawing blood and processing specimens for submission to an outside laboratory. Even though the site assigns a preceptor or supervisor who will oversee your work, that person may allow you to do some tasks independently. When handling lab specimens, always use proper techniques to avoid accidental contact with the contents. You may observe some medical assistants who become complacent about doing their job. They lose focus and become careless in performing their tasks. This is typically when accidents happen. Always pay attention, listen carefully and follow directions. Do not take short cuts.

Chapter Recap

- There are three basic types of blood cells—erythrocytes, leukocytes, and thrombocytes.
- Blood tests can help diagnose anemias and infections.
- Medical assistants perform a variety of important duties in hematological testing.
- Several types of blood tests are CLIA waived, which means the medical assistant can perform these tests in a typical physician office setting.
- The most common hematological tests are the complete blood count (CBC), erythrocyte sedimentation rate (ESR or sed rate), and coagulation tests.

- Red blood cells (RBCs), or erythrocytes, transport gases (oxygen and carbon dioxide) between the lungs and the body tissues.
- The mean cell volume (MCV) measures the average size of the RBCs.
- The purpose of the mean corpuscular hemoglobin (MCH) and the mean corpuscular hemoglobin concentration (MCHC) is to show the relative hemoglobin concentration in a single RBC.
- Coagulation tests such as prothrombin time (PT) and partial thromboplastin time (PTT) help to determine the patient's ability to maintain hemostasis.

Online Resources for Students

Student Resources available on the text's online site include:
- Audio Glossaries
- Animations
- Competency Evaluation Forms

- Videos
- Anatomy & Physiology Module with Heart and Lung Sounds
- Weblinks
- Worksheets

Exercises and Activities

Certification Preparation Questions

1. Which of these cells is responsible for carrying gases to the body?
   a. Thrombocytes
   b. Erythrocytes
   c. Granulocytes
   d. Leukocytes
   e. Lymphocytes

2. Which of these is characteristic of the platelet?
   a. They have red granules when stained.
   b. They are biconcave.
   c. They are cell fragments.
   d. They have a segmented nucleus.
   e. They have blue granules when stained.

3. Which of these is a condition resulting from a reduced number of RBCs?

   a. Neutropenia
   b. Thrombocytopenia
   c. Leukemia
   d. Anemia
   e. Leukopenia

4. Which of these is not included in a CBC?

   a. WBC
   b. RBC
   c. Hgb
   d. HCT
   e. ESR

5. The normal range for WBC is:

   a. 12 to 16 g/dL.
   b. 10 to 20 mm/h.
   c. 45% to 52%.
   d. 4,500 to 11,000/mm^3.
   e. 4.6 to 6.2 million/mm^3.

6. Which of these readings would not constitute a diagnosis of thrombocytopenia?

   a. 160,000/mm^3
   b. 140,000/mm^3
   c. 100,000/mm^3
   d. 75,000/mm^3
   e. 50,000/mm^3

7. A patient's prothrombin time may be lengthened due to a deficiency of:

   a. vitamin A.
   b. vitamin B.
   c. vitamin C.
   d. vitamin D.
   e. vitamin K.

8. Which of these is most prevalent in a normal differential count?

   a. Basophil
   b. Eosinophil
   c. Lymphocyte
   d. Monocyte
   e. Neutrophil

9. Which of these blood tests would not be within the medical assistant's scope of practice?

   a. Spun microhematocrit
   b. White cell differential count
   c. Selected hemoglobin methods
   d. Selected prothrombin time methods
   e. Nonautomated erythrocyte sedimentation rate

10. Which of these blood cells increase in patients with allergic reactions and parasitic infections?

    a. Basophil
    b. Eosinophil
    c. Neutrophil
    d. Lymphocyte
    e. Monocyte

25 Phlebotomy

Chapter Objectives

- Identify the main methods of phlebotomy.
- Identify equipment and supplies used in routine venipuncture and skin puncture.
- Understand the proper use of venipuncture and skin puncture equipment.
- List the major evacuated tubes, their additives, color stoppers and the suggested order in which they are used for a venipuncture.

- Perform venipuncture and describe proper site selection and needle positioning.
- Perform skin puncture.
- Identify complications of venipuncture and skin puncture and how to prevent them.
- Explain how to handle exposure to blood-borne pathogens.

CAAHEP and ABHES Competencies

CAAHEP

- Perform venipuncture.
- Perform capillary puncture.
- Practice standard precautions.
- Select appropriate barrier/personal protective equipment (PPE) for potentially infectious situations.
- Display sensitivity to patient rights and feelings in collecting specimens.

- Explain the rationale for performance of a procedure to the patient.
- Show awareness of patients' concerns regarding their perceptions related to the procedure being performed.

ABHES

- Collect, label, and process specimens.
- Perform venipuncture.
- Perform capillary puncture.

Chapter Terms

Antecubital space
Anticoagulants
Antiseptics
Bevel

Capillaries
Gauge
Hematoma
Hemoconcentration

Hemolysis
Phlebotomy
Skin puncture
Syncope

Tourniquet
Vacuum
Venipuncture

Abbreviations

CLSI	HIV	OSHA	SST
EDTA	mL	PST	

Case Study

One of Dr. Alhambra's patients, Martha Williams, is in for a follow-up visit to evaluate her pernicious anemia. She developed this condition during her pregnancy and has been receiving B$_{12}$ injections twice a month for 3 months. Dr. Alhambra wants to see if the injections are helping her condition. He asks his medical assistant, Rebecca, to draw blood for a complete blood count. In the past, Kim, a different medical assistant in the office, has always drawn this patient's blood. As the medical assistant escorts Ms. Williams to the blood draw area, she says, "I hope you don't leave a huge bruise like the one I got when Kim did the draw."

Physicians often analyze a patient's blood to help them determine the state of the patient's health. Blood tests are a valuable tool used in the diagnosis of various diseases and conditions. Tests are used to detect infections, as well as diabetes, heart disease, and many other disorders.

As a medical assistant, you may be responsible for collecting blood in your office. To make sure that diagnostic tests are accurate, you must collect these specimens using established guidelines. Specimens must be handled, stored, and transported according to set protocols. A laboratory result is only as reliable as the specimen submitted for testing.

THE BASICS OF PHLEBOTOMY

The process of collecting blood is known as **phlebotomy**. The main methods for doing this are venipuncture and skin puncture.

- In **venipuncture**, you use a hollow needle to puncture a large blood vessel, a vein. Small amounts of blood are withdrawn through the needle and are tested on site or sent to a reference lab for testing.
- In **skin puncture**, you pierce the skin with a sharp object. This causes **capillaries** (small blood vessels in the skin) to bleed, producing a specimen for testing.

Basic Blood-Drawing Equipment

Both types of phlebotomy typically are performed at a blood-drawing station. This is a place that is specially equipped for drawing blood. See Figure 25-1 which is a typical drawing station complete with a phlebotomy chair and a supply station.

Venipuncture and skin puncture each have their own specialized equipment and methods. Basic equipment and supplies used for venipuncture and skin puncture that should be available in the station include the following:

- Table—It should be high enough to reach easily and large enough to hold a variety of supplies.
- Phlebotomy chair—This special chair has adjustable armrests and safety locks to prevent falls in case of fainting.
- Bed or reclining chair—This should be available for patients with a history of fainting or for taking blood from infants and small children.
- Gloves—The Centers for Disease Control and Prevention (CDC) and the Occupational Health and Safety Administration (**OSHA**) require wearing gloves when drawing blood. The gloves are disposable and nonsterile and usually are latex-free.
- Antiseptic—**Antiseptics** block the growth of bacteria. The most common one used in blood collection to cleanse the skin is 70% isopropyl alcohol.

Case Question

 What should Rebecca say to this patient? What could have caused the patient's huge bruise? As you read through this chapter, you will discover the proper technique used to do a venipuncture.

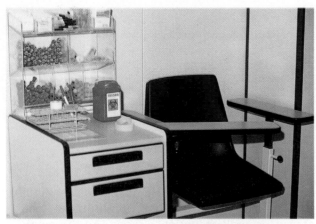

Figure 25-1 A well-stocked blood-drawing station. (Reprinted from Kronenberger J, Ledbetter J. *Jones & Bartlett Learning's Comprehensive Medical Assisting.* 5th ed. Burlington, MA: Jones & Bartlett Learning, LLC; 2016.)

- Gauze pads—Two-inch square gauze pads to hold pressure over the puncture site to stop the bleeding. Cotton balls leave fibers at the puncture site that would disrupt the clot formation when removed so are not used.
- Bandages—A small adhesive bandage to cover the puncture site once the bleeding has stopped.
- Sharps containers—Puncture-resistant containers used to dispose of needles and other sharp objects.

Venipuncture Equipment

There are several methods for collecting blood by venipuncture. In general, the following equipment is used.

- **Tourniquet**—A soft, flexible rubber strip that you wrap around the patient's arm to block the flow of blood in the veins. Using a tourniquet enlarges the veins, making them easier to find and puncture with a needle. Disposable tourniquets are available so a new one can be used for each patient. This practice will prevent bacteria from being transferred from one patient to another. If tourniquets are reused, they must be sanitized after each use.
- Needles—Used for drawing blood are hollow and coated with silicon so they will penetrate the skin smoothly. The **bevel** is the slanted end of the needle where the opening is located. Needles are sterile, used only one time, and disposed of in a sharps container. Needles should have a safety lock device that can be engaged immediately after the blood draw.
- Evacuated tubes—Containers that hold the blood as it is drawn and used to transport the blood to the lab or testing site. They are made of glass or plastic and range in size from 2 to 15 milliliters (**mL** or **ml**). A rubber stopper seals the end of the tube to protect the

vacuum inside. (A vacuum is a space from which the air has been removed, or "evacuated.")

Needle Gauges

Needles have different gauges. The **gauge** of a needle refers to the size of its opening, or lumen. The larger the gauge number, the smaller the opening of the needle. A 21- to 22-gauge needle is desirable for most blood collection. Choose a gauge that best fits the size and condition of the patient's vein. As you gain more experience with this process, you'll feel more confident choosing the needle size. However, there are a few factors to consider when considering the condition of a patient's vein and which needle to choose.

- Veins in infants and the elderly may collapse under the normal vacuum of a normal-size evacuated tube. The veins in infants and elderly patients may also be too small to accommodate a 20- or 21-gauge needle, so a smaller 23-gauge needle and smaller evacuated tube or syringe are used.
- Veins that are not straight are called tortuous veins. These veins may be easier to access with a 23-gauge needle.
- *Never* use a needle with a gauge larger than 23 to collect blood. The opening is too small. This will cause **hemolysis**, the rupture of the blood cells. The specimen that is hemolyzed is not able to be used for laboratory tests.

The Evacuated Tube System

The most commonly used venipuncture collection method is the evacuated tube system with an attached safety multisample needle and holder. A winged infusion set may also be used instead of a multisample needle. A syringe can also be attached to the winged infusion set to collect the specimen. The syringe-collected specimen is transferred into an evacuated tube for transport to the laboratory. Figure 25-2 includes images of the items that constitute an evacuated tube blood draw system.

The evacuated tube system has three parts:

- A multisample needle
- Various collection tubes
- A single-use plastic holder that attaches to the needle and holds the collection tubes

Using the evacuated tube system allows you to collect multiple tubes with a single venipuncture. It's a closed system. That means the patient's blood flows from the vein through the needle and into the collection tube without exposure to air.

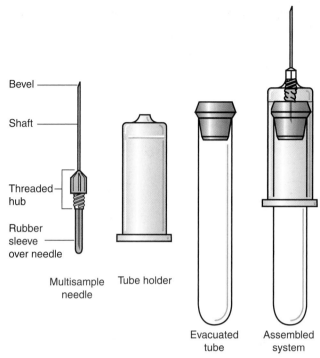

Figure 25-2 Traditional components of the evacuated tube system. (Reprinted from McCall R. *Phlebotomy Essentials.* Burlington, MA: Jones & Bartlett Learning, LLC; 2007, with permission.)

Choosing the Right Tube

The tube or tubes used in collecting the blood depends on several things including these.

- The size of the tube and amount of vacuum in the tube can vary depending on the patient's age, amount of blood needed, and the condition of the patient's veins. The vacuum in each tube causes it to automatically fill with the amount of blood needed for that test. Larger tubes have more vacuum and draw blood through the needle faster. The larger tube with greater vacuum may also allow a vein to collapse.
- The size of the tube also can depend on the amount of blood needed and whether serum or plasma is needed by the lab to perform the tests ordered.
- The tube stopper color selected depends on the tests the physician orders. In some cases, more than one tube of a given color may be required for the number of tests ordered.

Tube Additives

The tube stopper color indicates what additive the tube contains. An additive is a substance that is placed in the tube to affect the blood that is collected in it.

Laboratory tests require different types of blood specimens. Some tests require serum samples. For these, the blood is drawn into a tube that contains no additive or one that has a clot activator to speed the clotting of the blood. Other tests require whole blood, or plasma. For these tests, blood is drawn into a tube that contains an additive to prevent clotting.

The most common additives are:

- **Anticoagulants**—Prevent the blood from coagulating, or clotting
- Clotting activators—Accelerate the coagulation of the blood to the specimen allowing centrifuging sooner
- Thixotropic gel separator—Forms a physical barrier between the cellular portion of a blood and the serum or plasma portion after they have been separated by spinning the tube in a centrifuge

Table 25-1 provides information on the evacuated tube system and the color coding used to designate the various tubes with the additives. The table also provides information about how to properly mix the blood with the additive in each tube.

You must use a tube with the correct colored stopper and the correct additive for each test the physician orders. The test results can be altered if you don't select the proper tube for each test. If a medical facility uses an outside laboratory for testing blood, the lab will supply a directory of the tests performed, type of specimen, and tube required.

Case Study

Martha Williams needs to have blood drawn for a complete blood count. Review the information in Table 25-1 that discusses the evacuated tube color order of draw. This patient will need a lavender tube drawn for the complete blood count, a hematology test.

Case Question

 If this patient also needs a gray tube drawn for a glucose test, which tube would be drawn first? According to Table 25-1, why are the tubes drawn in this order?

The Syringe System

Syringes are made of glass or disposable plastic varying in volume from 1 to 50 mL. When you choose a syringe, make sure it's big enough to hold the amount of blood necessary to perform all the tests that have been ordered.

Table 25-1	Order of Draw, Stopper Color, and Rationale for Collection Order	
Order of Draw	**Tube Stopper Color**	**Rationale for Collection Order**
Blood cultures (sterile collections)	Yellow sodium polyanethole sulfonate (SPS) (or sterile media containers)	Minimizes chance of microbial contamination
Plain (nonadditive) tubes	Red (glass)	Used as a discard tube when drawing blood with winged infusion set Prevents contamination by additives in other tubes
Coagulation tubes	Light blue	Second or third position in order of draw prevents tissue thromboplastin contamination. Must be the first additive tube in the order because all other additive tubes affect coagulation tests
Serum separator gel tubes (**SST**)	Red and gray (marbleized) rubber; gold plastic	Prevents contamination by additive in other tubes Drawn after coagulation tests because silica particles activate clotting and affect coagulation tests; carryover of silica into subsequent tubes can be overridden by the anticoagulant in them.
Plasma separator gel tubes (**PST**)	Green and gray (marbleized) rubber; light green plastic	Contains heparin, which affects coagulation tests and interferes in collection of serum specimens Causes the least interference in tests other than coagulation tests
Heparin tubes	Green	Same as PST
Ethylenediaminetetraacetic acid (**EDTA**) tubes	Lavender	Causes more carryover problems than any other additive Elevates sodium and potassium levels Chelates and decreases calcium and iron levels Elevates prothrombin time and partial thromboplastin time results
Oxalate/fluoride tubes	Gray	Sodium fluoride and potassium oxalate elevate sodium and potassium levels, respectively. Drawn after hematology tubes because oxalate damages cell membranes and causes abnormal red blood cell morphology

Pulling on the plunger of a syringe creates a vacuum in the barrel. The vacuum created by pulling on the plunger while a needle is in the patient's vein fills the syringe with blood. Pull the plunger slowly and rest between pulls so the vein has time to refill with blood. A syringe with a needle attachment may be used or a syringe with a winged infusion set may also be used to collect the blood into the syringe. After collecting blood in the syringe, you must transfer the blood from the syringe into the evacuated tube for each test ordered. A blood transfer device is used to transfer the blood from the syringe to the evacuated tube. The use of this device will reduce the risk of transfer-related injuries while maintaining specimen integrity.

Winged Infusion Set

The winged infusion set, or the butterfly collection system, is used to collect blood from difficult or small veins.

Examples might be veins in the back of the hand or the veins of elderly patients or small children. This device consists of a beveled needle with wing-shaped plastic extensions. These extensions are connected to a 6- to 12-inch length of tubing. The winged infusion set is also known as a butterfly set because the plastic extensions attached to the needle resemble butterfly wings.

The butterfly system can be used with either a syringe or an evacuated tube system. A multiple sample Luer adapter is used to connect the needle to the tube system.

Figure 25-3 is an example of a winged infusion set attached to a syringe and to an evacuated tube holder.

Safety Device Needles

OSHA has many regulations to promote safety in the medical office and to prevent needlestick injuries and blood-borne pathogen hazards. OSHA requires that

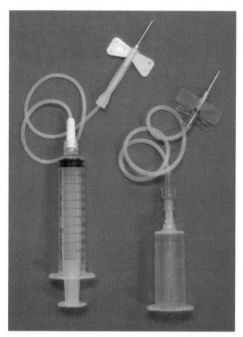

Figure 25-3　Winged infusion sets. (Reprinted from McCall R. *Phlebotomy Essentials.* Burlington, MA: Jones & Bartlett Learning, LLC; 2007, with permission.)

all needles have a safety feature to reduce the risk of exposure. These sharps with engineered sharps injury protection are nonneedles or needles with built-in safety features that prevent needlesticks. These safety features should be simple and require little training to use effectively. They should also be activated using a one-handed behind-the-needle technique.

Figure 25-4 shows the safety device on a multisample needle attached to a plastic tube holder or adapter.

Skin Puncture (Microcollection) Equipment

There are times when venipuncture may not be indicated to obtain blood. Here are some examples when a skin puncture is indicated.

- Only a few drops of blood are needed for the test.
- A small quantity of blood is required from patients with small volumes of blood, such as infants.
- Patients, such as those with extensive burns or scarring, may not have veins available for venipuncture.

In such cases, shallow punctures of the skin can be made, usually on the patient's fingers or heels, to obtain blood for testing. The equipment used to collect the specimen depends on the test being performed.

- Lancets—If drops of blood are needed for testing, you may use a sterile single-use disposable lancet to pierce the skin. Lancets are available in various sizes, which are designed to control depth of punctures, shallow or deeper. They also have safety features to reduce acci-

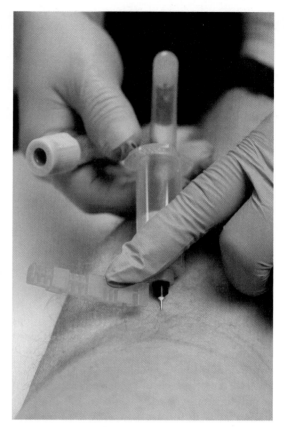

Figure 25-4　Safety device used to shield the needle after blood draw. (Image from Shutterstock.)

dental sharps injuries. Once the lancet is activated and the skin is punctured, the lancet automatically retracts into the holder so there is no risk of accidental puncture from the contaminated, sharp puncture device. Figure 25-5 is an example of a retractable, single-use lancet used for finger and heel capillary puncture.

- Microcollection containers—These containers consist of plastic tubes and color-coded stoppers that indicate the additive in the tube. The color coding is the same as the coding on the blood collection tubes used in

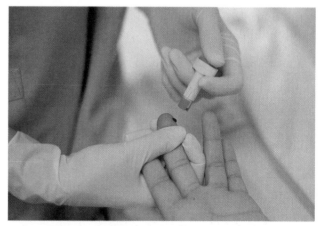

Figure 25-5　Retractable lancet used for capillary puncture of finger or heel. (Image from Shutterstock.)

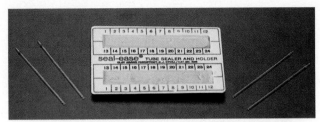

Figure 25-6 Microcollection tubes and clay sealant. (Reprinted from Kronenberger J, Ledbetter J. *Jones & Bartlett Learning's Comprehensive Medical Assisting.* 5th ed. Burlington, MA: Jones & Bartlett Learning, LLC; 2016.)

venipuncture. With a microcollection container, you can fill with blood to the proper measure, stopper the tube, then centrifuge, and store the blood in one container.

- Microcollection and microhematocrit tubes—These are small thin glass or plastic disposable tubes that fill by capillary action and hold 0.50 to 0.75 mL of blood. Blue-line hematocrit tubes are plain glass or plastic and will clot if used to do a fingerstick hematocrit. Red-line hematocrit tubes are coated with an anticoagulant and won't clot when used for blood collected directly from a finger or heel. Once filled, the microhematocrit tube is closed on one end with sealing clay. Figure 25-6 is a picture of microcollection tubes and clay sealant.

Filter Paper Test Requisitions

Another microcollection device is filter paper that is part of a test requisition. This special filter paper is used to test newborns for genetic defects, such as hypothyroidism and phenylketonuria. The filter paper is printed with circles that must be filled with blood.

To use the paper test:

1. Clean the bottom lateral surface of the infant's heel with alcohol and wipe dry with a sterile gauze pad or allow to air-dry.
2. Puncture the bottom lateral surface of the newborn's heel. Wipe away the first droplet with sterile gauze.
3. Allow a large blood droplet to form. Gently touch the circle on the filter paper against the droplet so it can be absorbed into the filter paper card.
4. Repeat, using a new droplet for each circle. Let the blood droplet soak through to the other side of the filter paper.
5. Allow the filter paper to air-dry in a horizontal position. Do *not* stack with other collection requisitions.

Warming Devices

Warmers increase blood flow before the skin is punctured. This is especially important for heel sticks. Heel-warming devices provide a temperature not exceeding 42°C or 105°F.

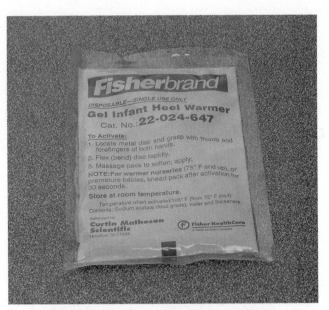

Figure 25-7 Infant heel warmer. (Reprinted from McCall R. *Phlebotomy Essentials.* Burlington, MA: Jones & Bartlett Learning, LLC; 2007, with permission.)

Heel warmers are typically used only on infants. They may also be used on any individual with poor circulation. As an alternative, you can fill a latex glove with warm water. Then, tie the opening in a knot. Figure 25-7 shows an example of an infant heel warmer.

PERFORMING PHLEBOTOMY

Some patients are anxious about having blood collected. Putting the patient at ease is part of the process. These are ways that the medical assistant can reassure the patient prior to performing a venipuncture.

- Introduce yourself and explain the procedure in simple terms.
- Talk quietly and speak in a pleasant manner.
- Be cheerful and confident.

Also make sure that you listen to the patient. Some patients know from prior experience having blood drawn where it is easiest to find an accessible vein.

Before the Procedure

There are several steps you must take before you begin the actual collection of blood. First, you must identify the patient to be sure that you are collecting blood from the right person. Ask the patient to state:

- Full name
- Date of birth
- Any other information to verify identity

Patient's Rights and Consent to Collect Blood

It's always important to respect the patient's rights. Even when the physician has ordered the collection of a blood sample, the patient must in some way give his consent to it. Rolling up his sleeve would be one way of showing consent. This is called implied consent because the action suggests or implies that he's willing to cooperate. It's better, however, to get a direct verbal consent, also known as expressed consent. Simply ask the patient, "Are you ready to begin?" before starting the procedure. If you go ahead without obtaining the patient's consent, and he objects, you could be charged with assault and battery.

Performing Venipuncture

Most often, you will use the forearm veins in the **antecubital space** (the inside of the elbow) for venipuncture. The three main veins in this area are:

- Median cubital—first choice
- Cephalic
- Basilic

Figure 25-8 shows the principal veins of the arm, including major antecubital veins. On this diagram, notice where the median nerve travels down the inner aspect of the upper arm and across the anterior elbow area. It is critical to avoid hitting a nerve when performing venipuncture. This is why it is so important to palpate a vein and be certain that you feel the elasticity of a vein beneath the surface. Do not enter blindly into unknown territory.

Applying a Tourniquet

As with any medical procedure, wash your hands and put on your gloves before applying the tourniquet. Here are the steps to follow:

1. When you're ready to apply the tourniquet, place it 3 to 4 inches above the site from which you plan to take blood.
2. Secure the tourniquet with a half-bow knot. Using this knot lets you rapidly release the tourniquet with just one hand. Rapid removal is important. If it stays in place longer than 1 minute, **hemoconcentration** of the blood will occur, or the pooling of blood components. This may cause inaccurate lab results.
3. Tie the tourniquet with the ends away from the puncture site so they will not contaminate or fall into the puncture field.
4. Apply the tourniquet tightly enough to slow venous blood flow without affecting arterial blood flow. You will learn by experience how tight to put on a tourniquet by observing what tightness gets the best results on different patients.

Right arm in anatomic position

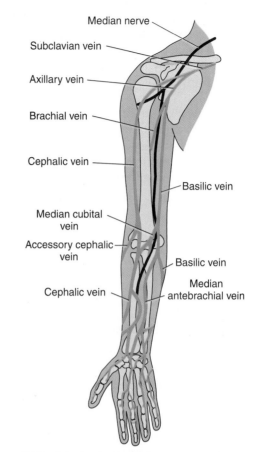

Median nerve
Subclavian vein
Axillary vein
Brachial vein
Cephalic vein
Basilic vein
Median cubital vein
Accessory cephalic vein
Basilic vein
Cephalic vein
Median antebrachial vein

Figure 25-8 Principal veins of the arm including major antecubital veins subject to venipuncture A and B. (Reprinted from McCall R. *Phlebotomy Essentials.* Burlington, MA: Jones & Bartlett Learning, LLC; 2007, with permission.)

5. Ask the patient to make a fist. Do NOT allow the patient to open and close the fist because this will also cause hemoconcentration and lead to inaccurate test results.

Study Skill

It is important that you can tie the tourniquet with the proper amount of tension and without struggling. Practice on yourself. In a sitting position, practice applying the tourniquet to your thigh. Think of your thigh as the patient's arm. You will be able to feel and determine the right amount of tension to apply by feeling it on yourself. When using this practice technique, do not leave the tourniquet too long, <1 minute.

Site Selection

Use the tip of your index finger to palpate, or feel, veins to select a vein for puncture. Palpating helps locate veins and determine their size, depth, and direction. To palpate a vein, extend your index finger and touch the patient's skin with the soft pad at the end of the finger. Then, repeatedly "bounce" this finger on the patient's skin about ⅛ of an inch above the surface in the area you expect to find a vein. Moving in a side-to-side progression, you should go across a patient's arm. When you have crossed the arm, move down the arm about a ¼ inch and go back in the opposite direction. When you feel what you think is a vein, you can attempt to trace the direction of the vein by palpitation. The depth of the vein is determined with practice, experience, and palpitation. A vein may feel like a tight rubber band beneath the surface of the skin.

Select a good vein using the following criteria:

- The direction of the vein should be straight for one or more inches.
- The vein should be sufficiently engorged with blood to make it prominent and firm.
- There is sufficient tissue surrounding the vein to keep it in place.
- The vein is located in an area with no hematoma or bruising.
- The vein selected is beneath skin that is soft and clear of abnormalities.

If you can't find a good vein on one arm, release the tourniquet and repeat the procedure on the other arm. If you can't locate a suitable antecubital vein on either arm, check hand veins and finally, as a last resort, wrist veins. You can try massaging the arm from wrist to elbow to increase blood flow and make veins more palpable. You also can use a warm towel to encourage greater blood flow to the area.

Sites to Avoid

There are specific areas that should be avoided when selecting a location for drawing blood. Those areas include the extremity:

- On the side of the body where a patient had a mastectomy. The specimen from this site might be affected by an increase in lymphatic fluid due to poor lymphatic circulation.
- Where intravenous fluids are being administered. The specimen may be diluted.
- If the tissue appears swollen with edematous tissue, fluid accumulation.
- With evidence of burns or scars.
- With a hematoma, or bruising.

Needle Positioning

If you can't obtain blood once you've punctured a vein, you may have to change the position of the needle. Figure 25-9 shows proper and improper needle positioning.

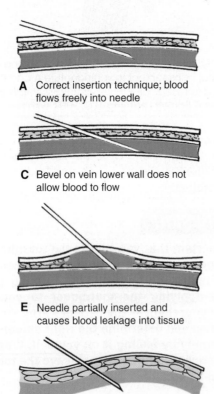

A Correct insertion technique; blood flows freely into needle

C Bevel on vein lower wall does not allow blood to flow

E Needle partially inserted and causes blood leakage into tissue

F When a vein rolls, the needle may slip to the side of the vein without penetrating it

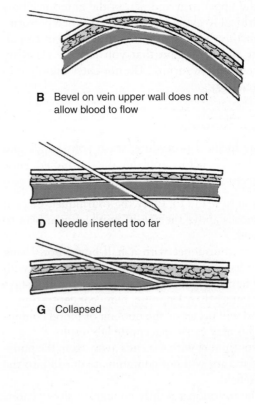

B Bevel on vein upper wall does not allow blood to flow

D Needle inserted too far

G Collapsed

Figure 25-9   Proper and improper needle positioning **A** to **G**. (Reprinted from McCall R. *Phlebotomy Essentials*. Burlington, MA: Jones & Bartlett Learning, LLC; 2007, with permission.)

Here are some of the common problems with needle position:

- The bevel of the needle may be against the wall of the vein. Correct by slightly rotating the needle half a turn.
- The needle may be too shallow and has not penetrated the vein. Correct by slowly advancing the needle farther into the vein.
- The needle may be too deep and has gone too far beyond the vein. Correct by pulling it back a little.
- The tube may not have sufficient vacuum. Correct by changing to another tube before withdrawing the needle.

Never attempt a venipuncture more than twice. If you can't obtain a specimen in two tries, have another person attempt the draw, or perform a skin puncture if possible.

Winged Infusion Set

A winged infusion set should be considered if the veins are small and fragile. Typically, they are used in pediatric and geriatric patients. Figure 25-10 demonstrates the use of a winged infusion set to access a vein in the back of the hand. Notice that the tourniquet is tied above the wrist area.

Order of Draw

The Clinical and Laboratory Standards Institute (**CLSI**) recommends the order in which evacuated tubes should be collected or filled from a syringe. It's important to follow order-of-draw guidelines to avoid any contamination of the specimens. Table 25-1 provides a rationale for the collection order of draw.

After you collect the specimens, label each tube with:

- The patient's first and last name
- An assigned identification number if available
- The date and time
- Your initials to verify that you drew the sample

Complications of Venipuncture

Phlebotomy is a skill that requires specialized knowledge, practice, and attention to detail. Errors can be made during the preparation for the procedure, during

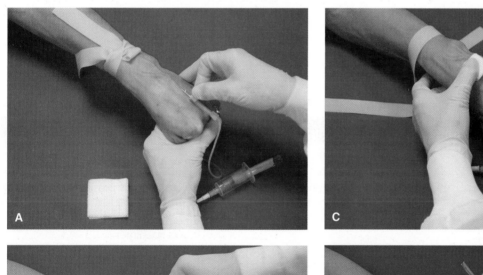
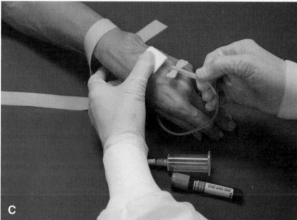
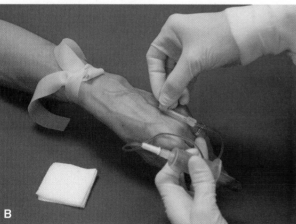
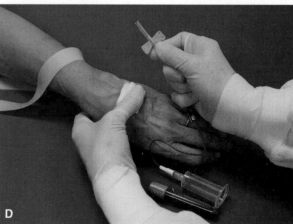

Figure 25-10 Procedure for using butterfly in a hand vein **(A–D)**. (Reprinted from McCall R. *Phlebotomy Essentials.* Burlington, MA: Jones & Bartlett Learning, LLC; 2007, with permission.)

the procedure, or after the procedure is complete. Pay attention to the ways in which errors are made, so you can guard against making them yourself. You must be careful when drawing blood because of the risks involved in venipuncture. These include nerve damage, artery puncture, hematoma formation, and skin infection. Table 25-2 lists some of the errors that may be encountered during venipuncture.

Permanent nerve damage can result from:

- Poor site selection
- Movement of the patient during needle insertion
- Inserting the needle too deeply or quickly
- Excessive blind probing

Another possibly serious complication of venipuncture is the unintentional puncture of an artery. You'll know this has happened by bright red color of the blood and the pulsing of the specimen into the tube. If you accidentally puncture an artery, discontinue the blood draw and apply direct pressure over the site for a full 5 minutes after the needle is removed and apply a pressure bandage. A pressure bandage is made by folding a two-by-two-inch gauze twice to quarter it. It is placed over the venipuncture site and then covered with a bandage.

The most common complication of venipuncture is **hematoma** formation. This happens when blood leaks into the tissues during or after the draw. Hematomas may be painful and may cause unsightly bruising. In rare incidences, they also can cause compression injuries to nerves.

If a hematoma begins to form during the draw, follow these steps:

1. Release the tourniquet immediately.
2. Withdraw the needle.
3. Hold pressure on the site for at least 2 minutes.
4. Apply cold compresses to reduce the pain and swelling.

You can prevent another possible complication, the infection of the site, by following these antiseptic techniques:

- Not touching the site after cleaning
- Removing the needle cap at the last possible moment prior to venipuncture
- Not opening bandages ahead of time

Preventing Hematomas

The following situations can trigger hematoma formation. Being aware of them will help you prevent hematomas from forming in your patients:

- The vein is fragile or too small for the needle.
- The needle is only partly inserted into the vein.
- Excessive or blind probing is used to find the vein.
- The needle is removed while the tourniquet is still tied in place.

Table 25-2	Common Sources of Error in Venipuncture	
Errors in Preparation	**Errors in Procedure**	**Errors After Completion**
Improper patient identification	Failure to dry site completely after cleansing with alcohol	Failure to apply pressure immediately to venipuncture site
Failure to check patient adherence to dietary restrictions	Inserting needle bevel side down	Vigorous shaking of anticoagulated blood specimens
Failure to calm patient prior to blood collection	Use of needle that is too small, causing hemolysis of specimen	Forcing blood through a syringe needle into tube
Use of improper equipment and supplies	Venipuncture in an unacceptable area	Mislabeling of tubes
Inappropriate method of blood collection	Prolonged tourniquet application	Failure to label appropriate specimens with infectious disease precaution
	Wrong order of tube draw	Failure to put date, time, and initials on requisition
	Failure to mix blood collected in additive-containing tubes immediately	Slow transport of specimens to laboratory
	Pulling back on syringe plunger too forcefully	
	Failure to release tourniquet prior to needle withdrawal	

Case Study

Dr. Alhambra's patient, Martha Williams, mentioned that Kim, another medical assistant, caused a huge bruise when she drew blood on her. A bruise is caused from a pool of blood beneath the skin. It is possible that the medical assistant did not apply enough pressure for at least 2 minutes after removing the needle from the puncture site.

Case Question

 What are other reasons that the patient bruised after the blood draw?

Patient Safety During Venipuncture

You're busy drawing blood when the patient says he feels faint. You must respond immediately. Follow these steps to keep the patient safe:

1. Remove the tourniquet and take out the needle as quickly as possible.
2. Talk to the patient to distract him from the procedure and to help keep him alert.
3. Have the patient lower his head and breathe deeply. You should physically support the patient to protect him if he does collapse.
4. Loosen a tight collar or tie if possible.
5. Put a cold compress or washcloth on his forehead and on the back of his neck.
6. Call for the physician if the patient doesn't respond.

Always believe patients who tell you in advance that they faint during venipuncture. For safety, ask these patients to lie down during the procedure. This reduces the chance of **syncope** (fainting). It also ensures that the patient won't fall if he or she does faint. Never draw blood from a patient who is likely to faint unless the physician is in the office.

Complications of Skin Puncture

It can be difficult to obtain a skin puncture specimen without clot formation. This is because the body's clotting system works to stop bleeding as soon as the skin is punctured. Therefore, blood should be drawn in a specific order.

1. First, collect an anticoagulated specimen before blood begins to clot.
2. Next, collect any other additive specimens.
3. Last, collect clotted specimens.

As with venipuncture, there are errors that can occur during collecting blood from a skin puncture. Table 25-3 lists the common sources of errors in skin puncture.

BLOOD EXPOSURE SAFETY

You must be extremely careful when collecting specimens. Blood is classified as a biohazardous material. Use standard precautions at all times when handling blood. Needlestick injuries can cause exposure to blood-borne pathogens, such as hepatitis B, hepatitis C, and human immunodeficiency virus (HIV). Your risk of infection depends on:

Table 25-3	Common Sources of Error in Skin Puncture	
Errors in Preparation	**Errors in Procedure**	**Errors After Completion**
Misidentification of patient	Puncturing wrong area of infant heel	Hemolyzing specimen
	Puncturing bone in infant heel	Failure to seal specimens adequately
	Puncturing fingers of infants	Failure to chill specimens requiring refrigeration
	Puncturing wrong area of adult finger	Erroneous specimen labeling
	Contaminating specimen with alcohol or Betadine	Failure to document skin puncture collection on the requisition or in the computer
	Failure to discard first blood drop	Delaying specimen transport
	Collecting air bubbles in pH or blood gas specimen	
	Excessive massaging of puncture site	
	Bruising site as a result of excessive squeezing	

- The pathogen you were exposed to
- The severity of the needlestick injury
- Whether you have had available, recommended vaccinations prior to the exposure
- Prophylaxis, protective treatment for the prevention of disease once you've been exposed

Cleaning Blood Spills

Accidents do happen. As a medical assistant, you must know how to clean up blood spills and other body fluids. The protocol for cleaning is to:

1. Secure the spill area
2. Locate a spill cleanup kit
3. Wear gloves during cleanup
4. Cover the spill with absorbent material
5. Use a scoop or dustpan to pick up material
6. Wipe up fluids with an absorbent disposable towel
7. Apply a disinfectant to the area
8. Double-bag all cleanup materials in red biohazard bags for disposal

When cleaning up spills of any body fluid, make sure you use disposable gloves that will not tear during cleaning. If your gloves develop holes, tears, or slits, remove them and wash your hands immediately. Then, put on fresh gloves to finish cleaning up the spill. Never wash or reuse disposable gloves.

Spills should be properly cleaned using a hospital-approved chemical disinfectant or a solution of household bleach diluted 1:10 with water. Here are some steps you should take first if there is glass from broken evacuated tubes with the blood:

- Wear double gloves or utility gloves.
- Pick up the glass with forceps, or scoop it up with a broom and dustpan or cardboard. *Never* use your bare hands to pick up the glass.
- Place the broken glass in a sharps container.
- Then, follow the other steps for cleaning up a blood or body fluid spill.

The Biohazard Spill Kit

Your medical office should always have a biohazard spill kit on hand. Everyone in the facility should know where to access the kit. Most clinics store the kit in the immediate area of the blood draw station. There are kits that can be purchased containing all the necessary items to clean a spill or the office may put together a kit with all the recommended items. This kit should contain the following supplies:

- Biohazard spill cleanup instructions
- Nitrile disposable gloves
- Laboratory coat or impervious apron
- Absorbent material, such as absorbent paper towels and granular absorbent material
- All-purpose disinfectant such as household bleach (diluted 1:10) or a hospital disinfectant

- Bucket for diluting disinfectant and can also be used to store kit supplies when not in use
- Dustpan, broom, hand broom (for picking up broken glass and contaminated sharps)
- Sharps waste containers
- Biohazard waste bags

Medical Assistant Safety

To protect yourself and others, immediately dispose of used needles, lancets, and other sharp objects into a sharps container. It is critical that the medical assistant is trained to handle any sharps injury or exposure to bloody fluids. If you encounter a sharps injury or are exposed to a patient's blood or body fluids, you must take immediate action. Follow these steps to protect yourself:

- Wash the needlestick area and cuts with soap and water.
- Flush splashes to the nose, mouth, or skin with water.
- Irrigate eyes with clean water, saline, or sterile irrigant.
- Report the incident to your supervisor.
- Immediately seek medical treatment.

Study Skill

Students usually have more success learning the tube colors in the order of draw by developing a pneumonic that will be helpful in remembering which tube is drawn in order of additive. Use the first letter from each of the tubes and build a sentence that is easy for you to remember. One that many have used is "Sally Brings Really Good Grease and Leaves the Gravy."

S (Sally)—Sterile, yellow culture tube
B (Brings)—Blue, clotting times
R (Really)—Red, no additive
G (Good)—Gold
G (Grease)—Green
L (Leaves)—Lavender
G (Gravy)—Gray

Cultural Connection

In some Asian cultures, specifically the Vietnamese, blood drawing for laboratory tests may be feared or resisted. The traditional Vietnamese people believe that venipuncture results in blood loss that will cause their illness to become worse and that the body cannot replace the blood that was removed. Surgery is also only indicated as a last resort due to the possibility of excessive blood loss that will not be replaced. It is important to reassure patients that only a small quantity of blood is taken during the typical venipuncture and that the body will replace the lost volume. For example, if a 10-ml tube of blood is drawn, that is equal to only two household teaspoons (5 ml/tsp).

Procedure 25-1 — Obtaining a Blood Specimen by Venipuncture

Equipment: The physician's order, the laboratory requisition form and tube labels. Assemble the following equipment: multisample needle, single-use tube holder, or winged infusion set, evacuated tubes, tourniquet, sterile gauze pads, bandages, sharps container, 70% alcohol pad or other antiseptic, permanent marker or pen, and biohazard barriers such as gloves, impervious gown, and face shield. A syringe may also be used with the winged infusion set. Use a syringe that is at least 1 to 1 ½ times larger than the quantity of blood required.

1. Wash your hands and gather your supplies.

2. Complete the requisition form and indicate on the form what lab tests have been ordered. Also note the specimen requirements to determine the appropriate evacuated tubes needed.

3. Check the evacuated tubes to ensure that they are not expired. Using expired tubes may lead to inaccurate test results or inadequate blood collection.

4. Greet and identify the patient. Ask the patient to state and spell their name. Explain the procedure and answer any questions. If the test requires a fasting specimen, ask the patient when they last ate. Most fasting specimens require at least an 8-hour fast.

5. Put on disposable nonsterile latex gloves. Follow standard precautions throughout the entire procedure.

6. Prepare the equipment. Assemble the multisample needle and tube holder. Make sure that the needle is tightly screwed into the adapter. If using a winged infusion set, attach the apparatus to the tube holder or syringe. Extend the tubing of the winged infusion set to straighten it.

7. Ask the patient to sit with a well-supported arm. Veins in the antecubital fossa are easiest to locate when the arm is straight or bent at a 15-degree angle at the elbow.

8. Apply the tourniquet around the patient's arm 3 to 4 inches above the elbow. Check that it is snug but not too tight. Secure by using a half-bow knot. Make sure the tails of the tourniquet go away from the puncture site, toward the shoulder. Ask the patient to make a fist and hold it. Do not allow the patient to pump the fist.

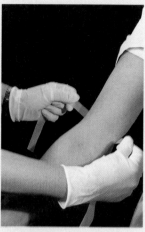

(Reprinted from Kronenberger J, Ledbetter J. *Jones & Bartlett Learning's Comprehensive Medical Assisting.* 5th ed. Burlington, MA: Jones & Bartlett Learning, LLC; 2016.)

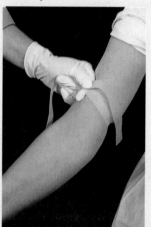

(Reprinted from Kronenberger J, Ledbetter J. *Jones & Bartlett Learning's Comprehensive Medical Assisting.* 5th ed. Burlington, MA: Jones & Bartlett Learning, LLC; 2016.)

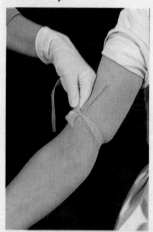

(Reprinted from Kronenberger J, Ledbetter J. *Jones & Bartlett Learning's Comprehensive Medical Assisting.* 5th ed. Burlington, MA: Jones & Bartlett Learning, LLC; 2016.)

Procedure 25-1   Obtaining a Blood Specimen by Venipuncture (*continued*)

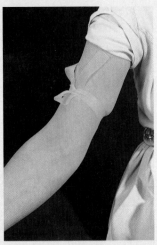

(Reprinted from Kronenberger J, Ledbetter J. *Jones & Bartlett Learning's Comprehensive Medical Assisting.* 5th ed. Burlington, MA: Jones & Bartlett Learning, LLC; 2016.)

9. Using your gloved index finger, palpate to find a vein. Then, trace the vein with your finger to determine the direction and depth of the vein.

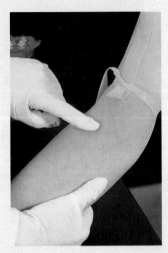

(Reprinted from Kronenberger J, Ledbetter J. *Jones & Bartlett Learning's Comprehensive Medical Assisting.* 5th ed. Burlington, MA: Jones & Bartlett Learning, LLC; 2016.)

10. Release the tourniquet. Remember to never leave a tourniquet in place for more than 1 minute.

11. Cleanse the venipuncture site with an alcohol pad using a circular motion starting from the center and working outward. Allow it to air-dry or dry with sterile gauze. Don't touch or blow on the site after cleansing.

12. Reapply the tourniquet using a half-bow knot. Be sure the tails of the tourniquet extend upward and away from the puncture site.

13. If you're drawing blood for a blood culture, it is critical that the specimen is sterile. This requires additional cleansing of the puncture. Before reapplying the tourniquet, cleanse the area with alcohol and then apply a 2% iodine solution. Cover the clean area with a sterile four-by-four-inch gauze pad for 2 minutes. Cleanse the site with an alcohol pad. Now, reapply the tourniquet.

14. You're ready to penetrate the vein. It's easier to do this if you hold the blood draw equipment with your dominant hand. Grasp the patient's arm with the other hand and use your thumb to draw the skin taut over the site. Never place fingers above the puncture site.

15. With the bevel of the needle facing up, line up the needle with the vein about one-fourth to one-half inch below the site where the vein is to be entered. Insert the needle into the vein at a 15- to 30-degree angle. Remove your nondominant hand, and if using a syringe, slowly pull back the plunger of the syringe allowing blood to flow into the syringe.

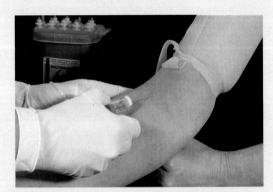

(Reprinted from Kronenberger J, Ledbetter J. *Jones & Bartlett Learning's Comprehensive Medical Assisting.* 5th ed. Burlington, MA: Jones & Bartlett Learning, LLC; 2016.)

16. When using an evacuated tube system, place fingers on the flange of the tube holder, and with the thumb, push the tube onto the needle inside the holder. When blood begins to flow into the tube or syringe, you can release the tourniquet and allow the patient to release the fist.

17. Allow the syringe or tube to fill to capacity. When blood flow stops, remove the tube from the adapter by gripping the tube with your nondominant hand and placing your thumb against the flange during removal. Twist and gently pull out the tube. Hold the needle steady in the vein, without pulling up or pressing down, and insert any other necessary tubes into the adapter and fill each to capacity.

18. Remove the tube from the adapter *before* removing the needle from the arm. This is important because you don't want any blood to drip from the tip of the needle onto the patient. Place a sterile gauze pad over the puncture site as you are withdrawing the needle. Never apply pressure until you are certain that the needle is completely removed from the patient.

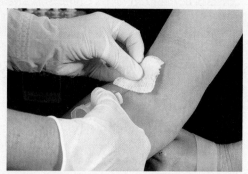

(Reprinted from Kronenberger J, Ledbetter J. *Jones & Bartlett Learning's Comprehensive Medical Assisting.* 5th ed. Burlington, MA: Jones & Bartlett Learning, LLC; 2016.)

19. Engage the safety device on the needle and immediately dispose of the needle and tube holder into the sharps container. The needle is not recapped.

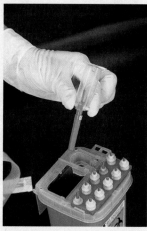

(Reprinted from Kronenberger J, Ledbetter J. *Jones & Bartlett Learning's Comprehensive Medical Assisting.* 5th ed. Burlington, MA: Jones & Bartlett Learning, LLC; 2016.)

20. Apply pressure or have the patient apply direct pressure for 5 minutes. Don't let the patient bend the arm at the elbow.

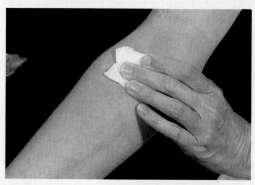

(Reprinted from Kronenberger J, Ledbetter J. *Jones & Bartlett Learning's Comprehensive Medical Assisting.* 5th ed. Burlington, MA: Jones & Bartlett Learning, LLC; 2016.)

21. If a syringe was used, transfer the blood from the syringe into the evacuated tubes using a blood transfer device and following the proper order of draw. If the tubes contain an anticoagulant, you should mix immediately by gently inverting the tube eight to ten times. Do not shake the tube. Label the tubes with the proper information.

22. Check the puncture site to be sure it isn't bleeding. Apply a dressing, a clean two-by-two-inch gauze pad folded in quarters. Secure it with an adhesive bandage or 3-inch strip of tape.

23. Thank your patient when you've finished. Tell your patient to leave the bandage in place for at least 30 minutes.

24. Clean the work area and dispose of other equipment and supplies. Supplies that are visibly soiled with blood are put into a biohazard bag. Remove your gloves and wash your hands.

25. Perform laboratory tests or prepare and store the blood for transport to an outside laboratory. Always follow the protocol of the medical facility for storage and transport of specimens.

26. Document the procedure in the patient's medical record.

Procedure 25-2 — Obtaining a Blood Specimen by Skin Puncture

Equipment: The physician's order, the laboratory requisition form. Assemble the following equipment: single-use skin puncture device, 70% alcohol or other antiseptic, sterile gauze pads, microcollection tubes and sealing clay or microcollection containers, heel-warming device (if necessary), and biohazard barriers such as gloves, impervious gown, and face shield.

1. Wash your hands and gather your supplies.

2. Complete the laboratory requisition slip. Also note the specimen requirements.

3. Greet and identify the patient, or if the patient is a child, confirm the identity with the parent or guardian. Explain the procedure and answer any questions.

4. Put on gloves. Follow standard precautions throughout the procedure.

5. Select the puncture site from one of the following:
   - Just off center of the tip of the middle or ring finger of the nondominant hand; use the fleshy portion of the fingertip; make the puncture perpendicular to the grooves of the fingerprint.
   - The lateral curved surface of the heel.
   - The heel of an infant.

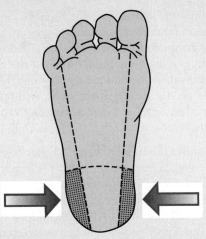

(Reprinted from Kronenberger J, Ledbetter J. *Jones & Bartlett Learning's Comprehensive Medical Assisting.* 5th ed. Burlington, MA: Jones & Bartlett Learning, LLC; 2016.)

6. Make sure the site chosen is warm. Gently massage the finger from the base to the tip to increase the blood flow.

7. Use both hands for this procedure. Grasp the finger or heel firmly with your nondominant hand. Cleanse the area with alcohol and allow to air-dry.

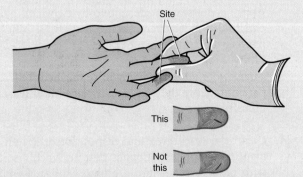

Site

This

Not this

(Reprinted from Kronenberger J, Ledbetter J. *Jones & Bartlett Learning's Comprehensive Medical Assisting.* 5th ed. Burlington, MA: Jones & Bartlett Learning, LLC; 2016.)

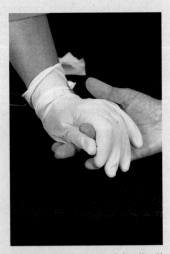

(Reprinted from Kronenberger J, Ledbetter J. *Jones & Bartlett Learning's Comprehensive Medical Assisting.* 5th ed. Burlington, MA: Jones & Bartlett Learning, LLC; 2016.)

| Procedure 25-2 | Obtaining a Blood Specimen by Skin Puncture (*continued*) |

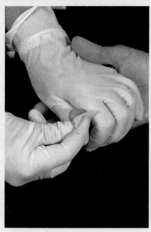

(Reprinted from Kronenberger J, Ledbetter J. *Jones & Bartlett Learning's Comprehensive Medical Assisting.* 5th ed. Burlington, MA: Jones & Bartlett Learning, LLC; 2016.)

8. Place the skin puncture device over the puncture site and activate the lancet.

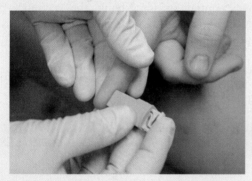

(Reprinted from Kronenberger J, Ledbetter J. *Jones & Bartlett Learning's Comprehensive Medical Assisting.* 5th ed. Burlington, MA: Jones & Bartlett Learning, LLC; 2016.)

9. Wipe away the first drop of blood. It may be contaminated with tissue fluid or residue from the alcohol wipe.

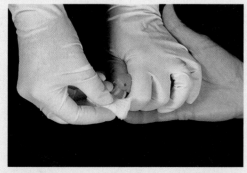

(Reprinted from Kronenberger J, Ledbetter J. *Jones & Bartlett Learning's Comprehensive Medical Assisting.* 5th ed. Burlington, MA: Jones & Bartlett Learning, LLC; 2016.)

10. Collect the specimen touching only the tip of the micro-collection tube or container to the drop of blood. You can encourage blood flow by holding the puncture site downward and applying gentle pressure near the site.

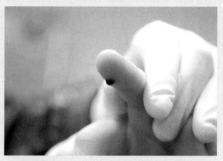

(Reprinted from Kronenberger J, Ledbetter J. *Jones & Bartlett Learning's Comprehensive Medical Assisting.* 5th ed. Burlington, MA: Jones & Bartlett Learning, LLC; 2016.)

11. As each microcollection tubes is filled, place it in sealing clay to cap the end of the tube.

12. Once the blood collection is complete, apply pressure to the site with clean gauze or have the patient apply pressure. Don't release your patient until the bleeding has stopped. Label the containers with the proper information.

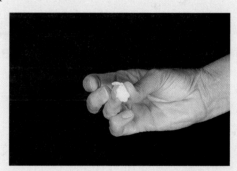

(Reprinted from Kronenberger J, Ledbetter J. *Jones & Bartlett Learning's Comprehensive Medical Assisting.* 5th ed. Burlington, MA: Jones & Bartlett Learning, LLC; 2016.)

13. Thank your patient when you've finished. Tell your patient to leave the bandage in place for at least 30 minutes.

14. Properly dispose of all equipment and supplies. Clean the work area. Remove your gloves and wash your hands.

15. Perform the laboratory tests or prepare the specimen for transfer to an outside laboratory.

16. Document the procedure in the patient's medical record.

Preparing for Externship

Your externship is your opportunity to apply the communication skills you learned and practiced while in the classroom. When working with patients who need to have their blood drawn, there can be many challenges, not just with the actual procedure but also with the interaction that you need to have with the patient before, during, and after the procedure. This also includes the patient's family members who accompany the patient. For example, you may encounter a parent with a young child. Before the procedure, you need to assure the patient of your ability to perform the procedure. Some patients may have questions that you should be prepared to answer. Doing phlebotomy in the classroom with your classmates may be less intimidating than when on your externship performing on actual patients. The externship office should always have an assigned preceptor or supervisor to oversee your phlebotomy procedures until you are confident and they can trust you to perform on your own. If you do not feel comfortable with a specific blood draw, ask for assistance or for someone else to perform that one.

Chapter Recap

- A blood-drawing station has the supplies and equipment needed for phlebotomy procedures.
- The venipuncture procedure utilizes color-coded evacuated tubes, multisample needle, and adapter.
- The winged infusion set is used with the adapter and evacuated tubes or an attached syringe.
- The color-coded tube stoppers are used to identify the additive content of each type of evacuated tube.
- Blood specimens collected by venipuncture must be placed in evacuated tubes using the proper order of draw.

- Single-use lancets are used to pierce the skin to collect drops of blood in a microcollection tube or container.
- It is essential to identify the patient before performing a venipuncture or skin puncture.
- Accurate completion of the laboratory requisition is essential in identifying the patient's personal information and requested lab tests.
- Hematoma is the most common complication of venipuncture.
- Blood spills must be managed appropriately following established safety protocols.

Online Resources for Students

Student Resources available on the text's online site include:
- Audio Glossaries
- Animations
- Competency Evaluation Forms

- Videos
- Anatomy & Physiology Module with Heart and Lung Sounds
- Weblinks
- Worksheets

Exercises and Activities

Certification Preparation Questions

1. Which of these veins is the first choice for drawing blood in the antecubital area?

   a. Median cubital
   b. Cephalic
   c. Basilica
   d. Anterior lateralis
   e. Dorsalis

2. What is the maximum time to keep a tourniquet in place?

   a. 30 seconds
   b. 1 minute
   c. 1 ½ minute
   d. 2 minutes
   e. 3 minutes

3. What is the primary reason not to leave a tourniquet on too long?
   a. It will cause the patient discomfort.
   b. The needle will dislodge.
   c. It could cause an infection at the site of needle insertion.
   d. It will cause a bruise on the patient.
   e. It will cause hemoconcentration of the blood.

4. What is the first action that should take place if the patient feels faint during a phlebotomy procedure?
   a. Complete the blood draw and notify your supervisor.
   b. Remove the tourniquet and discontinue the procedure.
   c. Remove the tourniquet and continue the procedure.
   d. Put a cold compress on the patient forehead.
   e. Loosen the patient's clothing.

5. Which of the following items is not required for a blood draw procedure?
   a. Evacuated tubes
   b. Sterile gloves
   c. Tourniquet
   d. Sharps container
   e. Antiseptic

6. Which gauge needle is used for most normal blood draws from the antecubital area?
   a. 18 to 20
   b. 18 to 23
   c. 21 to 22
   d. 23 to 25

7. The term hemolysis refers to:
   a. a blood clot.
   b. the rupture of blood cells.
   c. a concentration of blood in one area.
   d. a high level of red blood cells.
   e. abnormal clotting.

8. Which of the following tube colors represents the correct order of draw (first, second, and third)?
   a. Gray, green, red
   b. Lavender, red, yellow
   c. Blue, red, yellow
   d. Red, lavender, gray
   e. Red, yellow, lavender

9. Which of the following does not constitute an error after venipuncture?
   a. Immediately shaking the tubes to mix the additives
   b. Applying pressure over the puncture site for 15 seconds
   c. Putting the time and date on the requisition slip, not on the tubes
   d. Labeling the tubes with "See other tubes"
   e. Inverting the tubes to mix the additives

10. Which of the following techniques is least likely to result in permanent nerve damage?
    a. Inserting the needle too deep
    b. Repositioning the needle
    c. Patient movement
    d. Using the cephalic vein
    e. Probing after insertion of the needle

 Internet Activities

Access this Web site for additional information on phlebotomy products and education: Becton, Dickinson and Company; www.bd.com.

26 Immunology and Immunohematology

Chapter Objectives

- Describe the different types of immunity.
- Identify the different types of antibodies.
- List the reasons for immunological testing.
- Describe the antigen–antibody reaction.
- Explain the principles of agglutination testing and ELISA.
- Summarize the proper storage of handling of immunology test kits.
- Describe the ways that quality control is applied to immunology testing.
- List and describe immunology tests most commonly performed in the medical office or physician office lab.
- Perform an HCG pregnancy test.
- Perform a group A rapid strep test.
- Identify the major blood types and explain why differences in blood type exist.
- Describe how blood is typed and explain why this testing is important.

CAAHEP & ABHES Competencies

CAAHEP

- Perform patient screening using established protocols.
- Obtain specimens and perform CLIA-waived immunology test.
- Differentiate between normal and abnormal test results.
- Reassure a patient of the accuracy of the test results.

ABHES

- Practice quality control.
- Perform selected CLIA-waived immunology tests that assist with diagnosis and treatment.
- Perform selected CLIA-waived kit testing including pregnancy and quick strep testing that assist with diagnosis and treatment.
- Collect, label, and process specimens.
- Obtain throat specimens for microbiologic testing.

Chapter Terms

Active induced immunity
Active natural immunity
Agglutination

Antibody
Antigens
Globulins

Immunoglobulin
Immunohematology
Immunology

Passive induced immunity
Passive natural immunity
RhoGAM

Abbreviations

ELISA   HIV   RA   Rh
HCG

Case Study

Brianna Jones has had a sore throat for a week and is concerned that it is not going away. She has a history of postnasal drip due to allergies and thought the sore throat was due to that. She is seeing the doctor today because she needs to feel better so she does not lose any time off work. Carlos, the medical assistant, escorts Brianna to an exam and takes her vitals. Her temperature is slightly elevated at 99.8°F.

Immunology is a branch of medicine that focuses on the study of the immune system. It is the study of how the body distinguishes between self and nonself and how the body works to eliminate infectious agents. As we explore immunology, we better understand how our body remains strong and healthy.

IMMUNOLOGY BASICS

If you're studying immunology in a lab, you'll be looking at or for antigens and antibodies.

Antigens are toxins or other foreign substances that induce an immune response in the body, especially the production of antibodies. They are molecules the body identifies as nonself. They frequently are infecting organisms. However, they also can be part of a normal or cancerous cell in the body itself.

Antibodies are substances the body produces when it detects antigens inside it. They belong to a group of proteins called **globulins**. Since antibodies are involved in the body's immune system, they are referred to as immunoglobulins (Ig).

Types of Immunity

Immunoglobulins are antibodies that appear in your body in four ways. Some are acquired naturally, while others are introduced to your body. The types of immunity include the following:

- Active natural immunity
- Active induced immunity
- Passive natural immunity
- Passive induced immunity

Active Natural Immunity

Active natural immunity occurs when people are exposed to a foreign antigen as a natural process and develop their own antibodies to fight it. For example, when you come in contact with pollen in the air or with an infectious virus or bacteria, your body manufactures antibodies against the foreign antigen, pollen, virus, or bacteria.

Active Induced Immunity

Active induced (acquired) immunity occurs when a person is exposed to a foreign antigen as part of therapy and develops his own antibodies to fight it. An example is injecting a vaccine for the measles, mumps, and rubella (MMR). The body is introduced to the antigen forcing the body to manufacture antibodies. The CDC, Centers for Disease Control and Prevention, maintains a list of current immunization schedules.

Passive Natural Immunity

Passive natural immunity occurs when infants receive already-made antibodies from their mothers. These antibodies cross from mother to fetus through the placenta. These antibodies are also found in the milk of nursing mothers, especially in the first 2 weeks after delivery. This is one of the main benefits of breast-feeding newborns.

Case Question

Brianna asks Carlos why, after a week, her throat is still hurting and seems to be getting worse. How would you respond to Brianna's question?

Passive Induced Immunity

Passive induced (acquired) immunity occurs when a person receives already-made antibodies as part of therapy. An example is injecting an Rh-negative mother with Rh immune globulin (**RhoGAM**), usually in the 28th week of pregnancy, when she is carrying an Rh-positive baby. The RhoGAM counteracts the antibodies the mother's blood will develop.

Study Skill

Study, study, study, now that you are in school, is that all you think about? How do you know when you have studied enough? Researchers found that students retained more information and performed better on exams when they organize their study time into 30 to 50 minute segments taking at least a 10-minute break between the study times. Set a timer just as if you were in a school class or period. Split up information for these study sessions and just focus on that area for the preset time.

Types of Antibodies

There are five general groups of immunoglobulins.

Immunoglobulin M

Immunoglobulin M (IgM) antibodies are the largest in size. They are also the first to appear when the body detects an antigen. IgM antibodies are fairly crude in that they are less specific to particular antigens than the second antibody to appear in an immune response, IgG. IgM antibodies don't cross the placental barrier. Therefore, they neither help nor harm a fetus or newborn child.

Immunoglobulin G

Immunoglobulin G (IgG) antibodies develop after IgM formation. They last longer than IgM and reach higher protective levels. Booster injections increase levels of IgG, and they last longer and longer following each booster. IgG can cross the placental barrier, allowing a mother to pass her immunities to her fetus. This protection remains good for about 6 months after birth, while the child's own immune system is developing.

Immunoglobulin E

Immunoglobulin E (IgE) antibodies function mainly in reaction to intestinal worms (called helminths) and allergic antigens. IgE stimulates the body to release a protein that's toxic for helminths. They also stimulate the release of histamine and other chemicals in allergic reactions. IgE actions are also responsible for a severe allergic reaction called anaphylactic shock.

Immunoglobulin A

Immunoglobulin A (IgA) is found in many secretions, such as mucus, tears, saliva, and breast milk. These antibodies combat microbes in body secretions and give nursing babies some of the mother's immunities through the breast milk.

Cultural Connection

We know it is important to educate new mothers on the benefits of breast-feeding. The mother's milk provides antibodies that support the immune system for the newborn and into the first few months of life. The act of breast-feeding is not accepted globally. It may be difficult to encourage mothers with a diverse cultural background. For example, in Brazil, they say that breast-feeding is an act of love; however, in Indonesia, a new bill was passed in 2009 making it a crime to expose the female breast. Because of this new law, mothers are reluctant to nurse their babies. In Kenya, it is normal and common to see women nursing babies in public; however, in Egypt, it is forbidden in public because of the Egyptian religious beliefs. Fortunately, in 43 states of the United States, laws have been enacted that make it a legal right to breast-feed.

Immunoglobulin D

Immunoglobulin D (IgD) antibodies are found on the surface of some inactive lymphocytes. The small amount present in blood serum is thought to result from the death of the lymphocyte cells. The function of IgD is unknown.

 IMMUNOLOGY TESTING

Immunology testing involves looking for antigens or antibodies in different types of body fluids, such as blood, urine, spinal fluid, and other fluids. Here are some of the conditions immunology tests can identify:

- Bacterial and viral infections, such as hepatitis A and B, strep, human immunodeficiency virus (**HIV**), rubella, and Epstein-Barr virus
- Chlamydia, syphilis, and Rocky Mountain spotted fever
- Pregnancy in women, drugs in urine specimens, and hormones in serum
- Blood types for donors and recipients

Most immunology testing uses blood serum. This is why immunology is also known as serology. When blood is centrifuged, it separates into three parts:

* Serum or plasma, which is the most liquid part of blood. It contains mostly water and the antibodies.
* The buffy coat, which is the middle layer of centrifuged blood. It contains the white blood cells and platelets.
* Red blood cells, which are also called erythrocytes. They are the heaviest part of the blood.

Immunohematology is the testing that blood banks do on red blood cells (RBCs) and serum or plasma. This is done to make sure that blood from a donor (a person who contributes blood) matches the blood of the person who receives it. There are several immunology tests performed in the POL; however, blood typing is performed in a specialized blood bank prior to transfusing a patient.

Antigens and Antibodies

Antigens can enter the body from the outside or they can occur within the body itself. Here are some examples:

* Foreign substances from the environment, such as pollen, bacteria, or viruses
* The hormone the body produces that is detected in a positive pregnancy test
* Proteins in the membranes of the RBCs that cause differences in people's blood (called "blood types")

When the body detects antigens, it produces antibodies. An **antibody** is a blood protein produced in response to and counteracting a specific antigen. The antibodies flow through the bloodstream and bind with antigens they encounter. This binding is the first part of the body's process for destroying the antigens.

Each antibody is designed to recognize and bind with only one kind of antigen. This is called specificity. That antigen may be common to a related group of substances, or it may be unique to a specific substance. The smaller the group of substances in which the antigen can be found, the more specific the antibody is for it.

Antibodies are named after the specific antigen they're attracted to and by adding the prefix anti-. For example, if one type of antigen is called A, the antibodies attracted to it are known as anti-A.

Antibodies have a strong attraction to their antigens. Therefore, only a little of the antigen needs to be in a patient's lab sample for the antibody to find it. This is called sensitivity. Test manufacturers try to increase sensitivity through their tests' content and procedures. For example, temperature and the strength of a solution can affect sensitivity. This is why it is so important to follow test procedures closely. False results may occur if the test is not performed exactly according to manufacturer's instructions.

Immunology Test Methods

Immunology testing is based on this attraction of specific antibodies to specific antigens. Here's how it works.

* To test for the presence of specific antibodies in the patient, a known antigen is mixed with the patient's sample to see if there is a reaction. This method is used to test patients for infectious mononucleosis, rheumatoid arthritis, syphilis, and rubella.
* To test for the presence of a certain antigen in a patient, the antibody, for that antigen, is mixed with the patient's sample to see if there's a reaction. This method is used in some tests for strep infections, such as strep throat.

Most immunology tests are sensitive enough to detect a fairly small amount of antigens or antibodies in a patient's sample that contains millions of other substances. In some cases, the amount of the antigen or antibody present in the patient's sample is measured too.

The reagents used to conduct these tests contain antigens or antibodies that are specific to the kind of test being run. They also contain other substances that allow the test results to be observed. Because the binding of antigens and antibodies usually can't be seen by the naked eye, the reagents also provide ways to make the results more visible. They do this in two main ways.

* Agglutination tests depend on clumping to create visible particles if binding of antigens and antibodies occurs.
* Enzyme-linked immunosorbent assays (**ELISA**) rely on color changes to show positive or negative results.

Agglutination Tests

Agglutination means the clumping together of materials that are suspended in a liquid. Associate the word "glue" to remember agglutination. Agglutination tests are fast and easy to do. They also can be quite inexpensive. To perform agglutination testing, you will need:

* The specimen to be tested
* A reagent containing a known antibody or antigen and a clumping agent such as latex beads

The reagent and the patient's blood, urine, or other specimen are mixed and observed to see if agglutination will take place.

* If agglutination doesn't occur, the solution will appear smooth and milky. In most cases, this is a negative finding, which means the substance being tested for is not present in the specimen.
* If agglutination does occur, antigens and antibodies will bind on the latex beads. The solution will appear rough and grainy, with areas of clumped particles. This result shows that the patient's specimen contains the substance for which it's being tested.

Sometimes, the binding and clumping involve red blood cells (RBCs) instead of latex beads. Because agglutination tests are so sensitive and specific, the results are very accurate and reliable. For these tests, the timing of the procedure must be exact. False positives or false negatives are less likely when using these tests.

- A false positive is a result that says a substance is present in a specimen when it actually is not.
- A false negative is a result that fails to detect the substance being tested for, even though it's present in the specimen.

False results can have many causes. Some are biological conditions in the patient. Others are technical difficulties with samples or with performing the test. For example, here are some problems that can cause false-positive or false-negative results:

- Timing—waiting too long to look for agglutination or looking for it too soon.
- Specimen—samples that are lipemic; they have a high fat level.
- Hemolysis—samples that have damaged RBCs or hemolysis.

Although the patient's biological condition cannot be changed, you can avoid technical problems when collecting the specimen and performing the test.

A false positive on a lab test may show that a patient has a condition he really doesn't have. On the other hand, a false negative might mean that a patient who actually has a problem will not get treatment for it. False results can have serious effects for patients. False positives could lead to treatments a patient doesn't need, which might even harm him. False negatives can harm patients by delaying needed treatments.

When a test's results are positive, a patient's physician may order a second test before beginning treatment. This could be a different type of test or a repeat of the first test. The purpose of doing another test is to recheck the accuracy of the first test's results. If a patient's symptoms do not support the accuracy of a negative result, the physician may order further testing in that case too.

Enzyme-Linked Immunosorbent Assays

ELISA stands for enzyme-linked immunosorbent assays. An assay is a test that analyzes the contents of a substance. ELISA tests have more steps and more reagents than agglutination tests, but they result in an easy-to-read color change.

Most ELISA tests come in kits that contain all the reagents and other materials needed to run them. Some ELISA tests are so simple that all you have to do is put the patient's sample into a cartridge provided in the kit.

The color changes if the sample contains the substance for which you're testing.

Always ensure that the test has been CLIA waived and approved for medical assistants to perform.

HANDLING TEST REAGENTS

Most immunology tests come in kits from a test manufacturer. These kits contain the reagents needed for the test. Many kits also include the pipettes, tubes, cups, and other things needed for the test to be done.

Storing Reagents

Reagent kits must be stored at the temperature the manufacturer states on the kit box or package insert. Some kits can be stored at room temperature (68°F to 72°F or 20°C to 22°C). Others will have to be kept in the lab refrigerator at 40°F to 45°F (4°C to 8°C). Some kits will have to be divided, with some reagents kept at room temperature and others in the refrigerator. Some kits require storing away from direct sunlight. It is best to store the kit contents in the original packaging when possible.

Be sure to read the instructions that come with each kit, so you'll know how to store its contents. If reagents are not stored properly, their quality may be affected. Poor-quality reagents may produce false results if you use them in testing.

Good Practices with Reagents

Each reagent kit is marked with a lot number and expiration date. Kits with the same lot number were manufactured in the same place and at the same time. Only use reagents from kits that have the same lot number. Reagents from kits with different lot numbers shouldn't be used together. Manufacturers won't guarantee a test will work correctly if reagents from different lots are used.

If there's a problem with a test kit, the kit lot number can help you trace the trouble with the manufacturer. Here are some additional tips for using reagents properly:

- Always check the expiration date on the kit box before using any of its reagents. Never use a reagent past its expiration date.
- When you open a new test kit, write the date and your initials on it. Some kits have a new expiration date that starts from the day they are opened.
- Always read the kit's package insert for details about handling its reagents and supplies. The manufacturer may change the kit requirements.

- There may be guidelines with the kit for collecting or handling patient specimens. Be sure to read and follow these instructions.
- Check to make sure the manufacturer or supplier shipped the kits or reagents as recommended. For example, when requesting a delivery, make sure the package doesn't arrive on an afternoon when the office may be closed.

Quality Control

Reagents don't always function correctly, even if not expired. Here are a couple of reasons this might happen:

- The reagent is properly stored in the refrigerator when you take it out to use it. However, a past user left it out too long and it warmed to room temperature before it was put back in the refrigerator.
- A past user accidentally added serum or another solution to the reagent. This changed its composition so that it won't react or respond correctly.

Quality Control for Test Kits

Kits should be tested regularly to make sure their reagents are performing correctly. Here are some basic guidelines for a good quality control (QC) program for test kits.

- A QC test should be done each time a kit's reagents are used.
- Some forms of QC may be needed when a new kit is opened.
- Other forms of QC may be performed daily.
- Record the results of QC on a Quality Control Log.

Your lab also should have its own QC policies and procedures to follow. They will tell you exactly what the standards are for each step of each process. All immunology tests should have written procedures, which should be followed each time you test a sample.

External Controls

An external control is a solution that is used instead of a patient's sample during a QC test. The contents of the control solution are a known value, so if the reagent is okay, the test results should be as expected. Since the contents of the control solution are always the same, the test results should always be the same too. External controls are often part of test kits. In some cases, additional controls can be bought from the test manufacturer.

 POL TESTS

There are many immunology tests, but we will concentrate on the ones most commonly performed in the physician's office laboratory. These include tests for:

- Rheumatoid arthritis
- Infectious mononucleosis
- Pregnancy
- Strep infections

Testing for Rheumatoid Arthritis

Rheumatoid arthritis (**RA**) is an autoimmune disease that affects the joints. An autoimmune disease is a disease caused by a person producing antibodies against their own cells or tissue. It progresses over time and inflames the joints, causing a lot of pain, stiffness, and swelling. RA has been linked to antibodies called rheumatoid factors. Testing a person's blood for these antibodies helps in diagnosing the disease.

The most common tests for rheumatoid factor are based on agglutination of particles. For valid test results, the positive control must agglutinate and the negative control must not agglutinate. If this is what happens, the results can be reported to the patient's physician.

Even when the controls act properly, lab tests are not perfect tools for diagnosing RA. Only about 70% of RA patients test positive for rheumatoid factor. The other 30% have a false-negative result. For this reason, physicians also use physical findings to make clinical decisions about the disease.

Test results also can be positive when the patient doesn't have RA. This is most likely to happen if the patient is elderly or has lupus, syphilis, or certain kinds of hepatitis.

Testing for Infectious Mononucleosis

Infectious mononucleosis is commonly known as "mono" and even the "kissing disease." It's caused by the Epstein-Barr virus. The symptoms are fatigue, swollen lymph glands, sore throat, and sometimes other symptoms. It's fairly infectious and can be transmitted through saliva and other body fluids. Mono is sometimes called the kissing disease because that's one way it can spread from one person to another.

The most common tests for mono include the following:

- Agglutination of RBCs (heterophile antibody test)
- Agglutination of latex particles
- ELISA

Pregnancy Tests

Fertile women are often tested to rule out pregnancy before starting a medical procedure that could harm a fetus. For example, if pregnancy is possible, a test may be performed prior to doing x-ray exams. Pregnancy tests are based on detecting the hormone **HCG** (human chorionic gonadotropin). Some tests are so sensitive that they can determine pregnancy before a woman misses

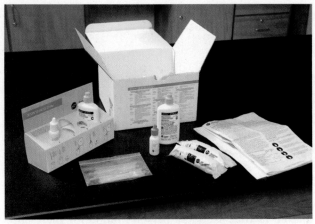

Figure 26-1 Pregnancy test kit. (Reprinted from Kronenberger J, Ledbetter J. *Jones & Bartlett Learning's Comprehensive Medical Assisting*, 5th ed. Burlington, MA: Jones & Bartlett Learning, LLC, 2016.)

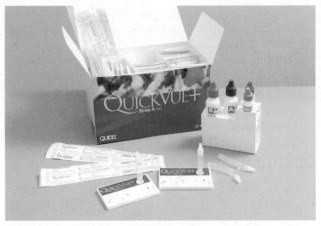

Figure 26-2 Rapid strep test kit. (Reprinted from Kronenberger J, Ledbetter J. *Jones & Bartlett Learning's Comprehensive Medical Assisting*, 5th ed. Burlington, MA: Jones & Bartlett Learning, LLC, 2016.)

her first period. The tests for HCG include agglutination and ELISA. Figure 26-1 is an example of a pregnancy test kit that you typically be used in a physician's office laboratory.

Strep Tests

Group A *Streptococcus* is one of the most common bacterial causes of sore throat and upper respiratory infections. There are two types of tests that can be performed to confirm this infection. One is a serology test and the other is a culture. For both of these, a specimen is obtained by swabbing the patient's throat.

Culturing the specimen to grow bacteria takes 18 to 24 hours. However, a culture is the more sensitive and accurate test. If a rapid strep test is negative, the physician may send another specimen to the lab for a culture. When you're getting a specimen from a patient who might have strep, collect two swabs in case the physician wants to do a culture. Figure 26-3 is an example of a culture tube that would be collected if the physician wants to do a culture and sensitivity of the throat.

Collecting the throat swab specimen requires using proper technique to ensure reliable test results. Other reasons the results may not be reliable are as follows:

- Not obtaining enough specimen
- Swabbing the wrong area
- Letting the test stand too long before reading the results

 BLOOD TYPING

Blood typing is performed in the immunohematology department of the lab, which is also known as the blood bank. Blood to be transfused into a patient must be tested first to make sure it's compatible with the patient's

---

Case Questions

Remember our patient Brianna Jones? After the physician examined her, he ordered a rapid strep test. Carlos, the medical assistant, performed the test and gave the results to the physician. Brianna is started on amoxicillin (antibiotic) and was instructed to stay away from the workplace until she has been on the antibiotic for at least 24 hours.

Why would the physician not want Brianna to go to work until she has been on antibiotics for at least 24 hours? How would you explain this to the patient who is reluctant to follow that direction?

The serology test is a rapid strep test that can detect the bacteria even if they're not alive. One advantage of this test is that it can be done in <15 minutes. This allows the physician to begin treatment immediately if results are positive. Figure 26-2 is an example of a rapid strep test kit used in a physician office laboratory.

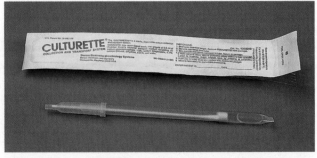

Figure 26-3 Culturette swab used as transport media. (Reprinted from Kronenberger J, Ledbetter J. *Jones & Bartlett Learning's Comprehensive Medical Assisting*. 5th ed. Burlington, MA: Jones & Bartlett Learning, LLC, 2016.)

blood. If it's not, the patient's body will treat it as a foreign substance and begin destroying it. It's critical that a patient who needs a transfusion gets the right type of blood or it could lead to the patient's death.

Blood Group Antigens

Red blood cells (RBCs) contain antigens. The kind of antigens on the surface of the RBCs determines that person's blood type. Every person belongs to one of four blood groups: A, B, O, or AB. Their blood group depends on what antigens are on their red blood cells. In the United States, the population is approximately:

- 40% type A blood
- 11% type B blood
- 45% type O blood
- 4% type AB blood

The ABO Group

Almost everyone has antibodies to the RBC antigens that he or she lacks. These antibodies occur naturally in the body. Here's how it works:

- A person in the A blood group will have the A antigen and antibodies to type B blood.
- A person in the B blood group will have the B antigen and antibodies to type A blood.
- The AB person has both A and B antigens and does not have antibodies to either type A or B.
- A person with O blood has neither the A nor B antigens, but antibodies to both types A and B.

Figure 26-4 shows the four different types of blood and the antigen and antibody specific to each type.

Having antibodies to other types of blood prevents a patient from getting a transfusion using those types of blood. The antibodies in the patient's blood will cause her body to treat the new blood as a foreign substance and reject it. If the patient is transfused with blood to which she has no antibodies, her body will accept it. Table 26-1 shows the blood types and which donors are compatible to receivers.

As you can see from the table, people with AB blood can have blood from any group transfused into them. The reason is that their blood has no A or B antibodies. AB blood type persons are referred to as the universal recipients. However, they can donate blood to only AB recipients.

On the other hand, people with O blood can receive blood only from O donors. That's because their blood contains antibodies to all the other blood groups. However, O blood can be given to patients of all blood types. For this reason, it is known as the universal donor.

Even though O blood has no antigens, some people with other blood types can still react badly to it. To prevent this, plasma is removed from the donor O blood and only the cells are transfused.

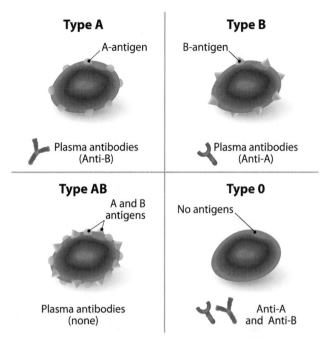

ABO blood group

Type A
A-antigen
Plasma antibodies (Anti-B)

Type B
B-antigen
Plasma antibodies (Anti-A)

Type AB
A and B antigens
Plasma antibodies (none)

Type 0
No antigens
Anti-A and Anti-B

Figure 26-4   ABO blood group. (Image from Shutterstock.)

The Rh Group

A group of antigens called Rh is also important to the blood bank. Within the Rh group are several antigens. Of these antigens, D is the most important. Not all people have this antigen, however. The presence or absence of the D antigen in a person's blood determines what's called the Rh factor. The **Rh** factor got that name when it was discovered doing research using rhesus monkeys.

- Rh positive—when the D antigen (Rhesus factor) is present in the blood
- Rh negative—when the D antigen (Rhesus factor) is not present in the blood

Antibodies to D don't occur naturally. A person without the D antigen must be exposed to blood that has D for anti-D antibodies to develop in his body. This would happen if a patient with Rh-negative blood was transfused with Rh-positive blood. The patient's body would form antibodies against the "foreign" D antigen and try to destroy the RBCs in the new blood.

In addition to the ABO group, the person's Rh factor is another critical consideration when doing blood transfusions. In some cases, mixing blood with different Rh factors can be life threatening, even when the ABO group of the blood is the same.

The best example of this is when a woman who is Rh negative becomes pregnant with an Rh-positive baby. This can happen if the baby's father is Rh positive. She will produce antibodies against the D antigens in the

Table 26-1   Blood Types: Donors and Compatible Receivers

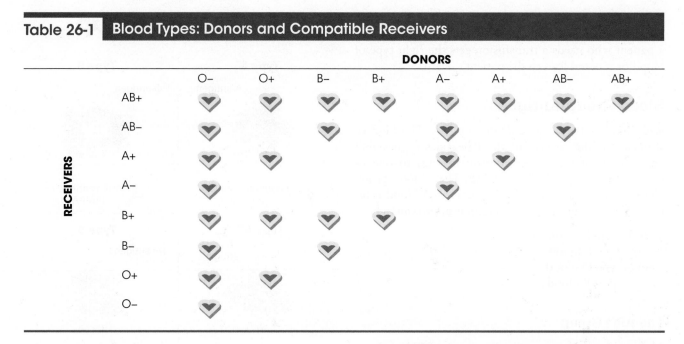

		DONORS							
		O–	O+	B–	B+	A–	A+	AB–	AB+
RECEIVERS	AB+	♥	♥	♥	♥	♥	♥	♥	♥
	AB–	♥		♥		♥		♥	
	A+	♥	♥			♥	♥		
	A–	♥				♥			
	B+	♥	♥	♥	♥				
	B–	♥		♥					
	O+	♥	♥						
	O–	♥							

blood of her fetus. This can endanger the baby but usually not during the first pregnancy; however, it may present a problem for a second pregnancy.

When an Rh-negative mother gives birth to an Rh-positive child, the mother is given a RhoGAM injection. RhoGAM must also be given within 72 hours to any Rh-negative woman whose pregnancy is terminated by miscarriage, stillbirth, or abortion. The RhoGAM injection prevents the mother from producing antibodies that might endanger her next baby by destroying its RBCs.

Patient Education

Expectant Mothers and RhoGAM

If you work with pregnant women who are Rh negative, the physician will explain the RhoGAM injection; however, the medical assistant needs to understand the purpose well enough to restate the information to the patient. Always seek approval from the physician before answering questions. Typically, the offices will have written informational brochures that support the verbal discussion. Here are some suggestions:

- First, explain to the patient's level of understanding what it means to be Rh negative.
- Explain that if the father is Rh positive or has an unknown Rh factor, the baby could have Rh-positive blood. (Also note that if the father has Rh-negative blood, there shouldn't be any need for RhoGAM.)

- Explain that if the baby's blood comes in contact with her blood, her body will make antibodies against the baby's blood. In future pregnancies, these antibodies will work against the fetal blood if it is Rh positive. This can cause severe hemolytic anemia, which can be fatal to the baby.
- Inform the patient that RhoGAM is a treatment to prevent her from producing these antibodies. It's given as early as the 28th week of pregnancy. Tell her that she'll need to sign a consent form to have this treatment.
- Tell the patient that if she miscarries or has an abortion, she will still need RhoGAM.

Be aware that some doctors will automatically give all Rh-negative mothers RhoGAM. This avoids any awkward questions about who is the father of the child. Whenever information is provided to the patient, use simple understandable language that you believe the patient can understand. Many do not want to admit that they don't understand.

THE NATION'S BLOOD SUPPLY

Blood banks often have a difficult time getting enough usable blood and blood products to meet the needs of recipients. This is especially true during holiday times when people increase their travel and there is an increase in the number of auto accidents. There's also a continuing shortage of volunteer donors. The American Red Cross and other agencies use bloodmobiles or worksites to collect blood.

One 450-mL unit of donated whole blood can be divided into three products.

- Packed RBCs can be kept for 42 days if they're stored at a very low temperature. They are used to treat anemia.
- Plasma can be frozen and kept for up to a year. It's used to treat uncontrolled bleeding caused by lack of coagulation factors.
- Platelet concentrates are good for up to 5 days. They are stored at room temperature and are used to treat uncontrolled bleeding caused by damaged platelets or low platelet counts.

Patient Education

Who Can Donate Blood?

The American Red Cross has rules for donating blood. These rules are based on government and other research. Each state also has laws that govern blood donations. You should check the laws in your own state. Potential donors are carefully screened starting with these general conditions:

- Must be at least 17 years old
- Must weigh at least 110 pounds
- Must have a hemoglobin level of at least 12.5 g/dL
- Must have a pulse rate of 50 to 110 beats per minute
- Must have a blood pressure lower than 180 over 100
- Must be willing and able to provide a brief medical history

The actual donation time can take up to 1 hour. Blood can be donated every 2 months, and only one pint may be donated at a time. Donated blood is tested for HIV, hepatitis, syphilis, and at least 20 other conditions.

Procedure 26-1 | Performing an HCG Pregnancy Test

Equipment: Patient specimen, lab requisition, pregnancy test kit, gloves.

Follow these steps to perform an assay on a patient's specimen for pregnancy. Be aware that manufacturers' kits, timing, drops, and control procedures can vary from lab to lab. Follow office policies to ensure accuracy and quality control.

1. Wash your hands and apply gloves.

2. Assemble the test kit's equipment. The kit should be at room temperature.

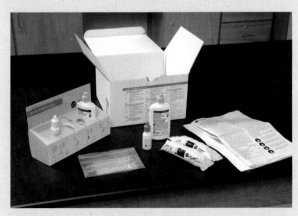

Pregnancy test kit

3. Check that the names on the specimen container and lab form are the same.

4. Use one test pack for the patient and one for each control.

5. Label three test packs as follows: the patient's name, "positive control," and "negative control."

6. In the patient's chart and the control log, record the type of specimen you're obtaining (urine or plasma/serum).

7. Use a transfer pipette to aspirate the specimen. Place four drops in the sample well of the test pack labeled with the patient's name.

8. Carefully aspirate the positive control and place four drops in the sample well of the test pack labeled "positive control."

9. Follow the exact same step for the negative control.

10. Set a timer for the amount of time specified by the manufacturer of the test.

11. Consult the test manufacturer's insert in the kit to interpret test results. The insert will tell you what to look for in reading a positive or negative result.

| Procedure 26-1 | Performing an HCG Pregnancy Test (*continued*) |

12. Report the results when the end-of-assay window is read and after you have checked the controls for accuracy. This will happen at about 7 minutes for serum and about 4 minutes for urine. The end-of-assay window should either change or appear wet. If it doesn't and/or the controls don't work, the test must be redone.

13. Record the controls and patient's information on the worksheet or log form and in the patient's records.

14. Clean up the work area and dispose of all waste properly.

| Procedure 26-2 | Performing a Group A Rapid Strep Test | |

Equipment: Patient specimen, gloves, group A rapid strep test kit.

Follow these steps to perform a group A rapid strep test. Be aware that manufacturers' kits and control procedures can vary from lab to lab. Follow office policies to ensure accuracy and quality control.

1. Wash your hands and apply gloves.

2. Double check that the names on the specimen container and the lab form are the same.

3. Label one extraction tube with the patient's name, one with "positive control," and one with "negative control."

4. Follow the kit directions. Carefully add the correct reagents and drops to each of the extraction tubes.

5. Insert the patient's culture swab (which is one of two swabs collected) into the labeled extraction tube. If only one swab was taken, first swab a beta strep agar plate. Then, use the same swab for the actual test.

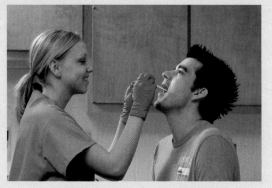

MA collecting throat swab

6. Add the correct controls to each of the two control tubes and place a sterile swab into each control tube.

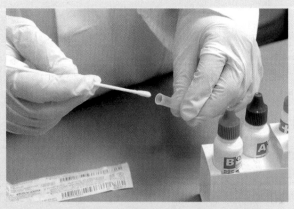

Performing strep test

7. Use the swab to mix each tube's contents by twirling each swab five to six times.

8. Set a timer for the amount of time specified by the manufacturer of the test.

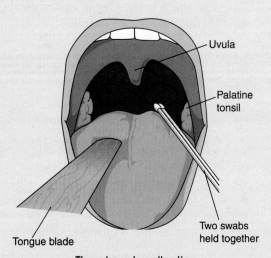

Uvula

Palatine tonsil

Tongue blade

Two swabs held together

Throat swab collection

| **Procedure 26-2** | **Performing a Group A Rapid Strep Test** *(continued)* |

9. Draw the swab up from the bottom of each tube and out of any liquid. Press out all fluid on the swab head by rolling the swab against the inside of the tube before it is withdrawn.

10. Add three drops from the well-mixed extraction tube to the sample window of the strep A test unit labeled with the patient's name. Do the same for each control.

11. Set the timer for the correct amount of time.

12. A positive result will show up as a line in the result window within 5 minutes.

13. A negative result is indicated if no line appears within 5 minutes. However, you must wait exactly 5 minutes to read a negative result, to avoid getting a false negative.

14. Verify the control results before recording any test results. Log the controls and the patient's information into your log or worksheet.

15. You may have to culture all negative rapid strep tests on a blood agar, if your lab requires it. A bacitracin disk may be added to the first quadrant when you set up the blood agar.

16. Clean up the work area and dispose of all waste in the right place.

17. Wash your hands.

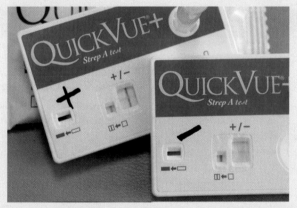

Positive and negative strep results

Preparing for Externship

Your externship is a great opportunity for you to demonstrate the knowledge and skills you learned during the classroom courses; however, it is also a time to leave the company of your classmates and your friends and be on your own. It is tempting to communicate with your classmates and compare the externship experience. Since medical offices are different, you will find that not every office provides an identical opportunity for students. For example, your first few days at the site may have you doing administrative work in the front office, while one of your classmates, at a different location, may be doing back office procedures on day 1. Do not compare this experience because all work in the office is valuable to your development as a medical assistant. Be content with the tasks assigned to you and perform them to the best of your ability. The office may be evaluating how well you handle the front office and work with the staff before they advance you to the back office.

Chapter Recap

- Serological testing includes how antigens and antibodies react.
- Specimens from patients can include many different kinds of body fluids, such as serum, urine, or spinal fluid.
- The most common types of tests are agglutination tests and ELISA.

- There are many types of test kits. You must be familiar with the steps involved in each one used in your lab.
- Each day that tests are performed, quality control (QC) processes must be strictly followed.
- You may have to arrange for your physician's patients to undergo transfusions at places outside the medical office. You must have a good understanding of ABO blood groups and Rh types to correctly answer any questions patients may have.

Online Resources for Students

Student Resources available on the text's online site include:

- Audio Glossaries
- Animations
- Competency Evaluation Forms

- Videos
- Anatomy & Physiology Module with Heart and Lung Sounds
- Weblinks
- Worksheets

Exercises and Activities

Certification Preparation Questions

1. What type of immunity occurs when people are exposed to a foreign antigen as a natural process and develop their own antibodies to fight it?
   a. Active natural immunity
   b. Active induced immunity
   c. Passive natural immunity
   d. Passive natural immunity
   e. Passive acquired immunity

2. Which of these is typically NOT an immunology test that is performed in a physician's office laboratory?
   a. Rheumatoid arthritis
   b. Pregnancy
   c. Human immunodeficiency virus
   d. Infectious mononucleosis
   e. *Streptococcus*

3. Which of these is an accurate statement regarding blood types?
   a. A person with type O blood will have no antigens and no antibodies.

   b. A person with type O blood will have the A and B antigen and antibodies to type A and B blood.
   c. A person with type AB blood has no antigens but does have antibodies to both type A and B blood.
   d. A person with type A blood will have the A antigen and antibodies to type B blood.
   e. A person with type O blood has A antigens and B antibodies.

4. The Rh factor is an important consideration when:
   a. the mother is Rh positive and the fetus is Rh negative.
   b. the mother is Rh negative and the fetus is Rh positive.
   c. the mother is Rh positive, the fetus is Rh positive, and the father is Rh negative.
   d. the mother is Rh negative and the father is Rh negative.
   e. the mother is Rh negative and the fetus is Rh negative.

5. Which of these is the type of immunity that occurs when a person is vaccinated and develops antibodies?

   a. Active natural immunity
   b. Active induced immunity
   c. Passive natural immunity
   d. Passive natural induced immunity
   e. Passive acquired immunity

6. Which of these is a term that means the clumping together of materials that are suspended in a liquid?

   a. Lipemic
   b. Agglutination
   c. Immunology
   d. Antigen reaction
   e. Antibody production
   f. Hemolysis

7. Which type of immunity occurs when a person receives already-made antibodies such as RhoGAM injection?

   a. Active natural immunity
   b. Active induced immunity
   c. Passive natural immunity
   d. Passive natural induced immunity
   e. Passive acquired immunity

8. Which immunoglobulin is the largest and first to detect an antigen in the body?

   a. A
   b. E
   c. D
   d. G
   e. M

9. A false-positive test result:

   a. was performed wrong.
   b. says a substance is present in a specimen when it actually is not.
   c. the patient has the disease tested for.
   d. is reported as a negative result.
   e. happens when the patient's specimen is too old.

10. Infectious mononucleosis is caused by:

   a. *Staphylococcus aureus*.
   b. *Streptococcus*.
   c. Epstein-Barr virus.
   d. human immunodeficiency virus.
   e. rheumatoid factors.

Internet Resource

Visit the CDC, Centers for Disease Control and Prevention, Web site for a list of current immunization schedules available at www.cdc.gov/vaccines/schedules.

27 Urinalysis

Chapter Objectives

- Explain why urinalysis is performed and the role of the medical assistant in this procedure.
- Describe the methods of urine collection.
- Perform a physical analysis of a urine specimen.
- Perform a chemical reagent test strip analysis.
- Explain the purpose of a urine culture.
- Identify the physical properties of urine and cite various conditions that can affect them.
- List the main chemical substances that may be found in urine and their significance.

- Prepare urine specimen for microscopic examination.
- Identify substances that might be present in urine sediment.
- Describe the process of microscopic examination of urine sediment.
- Describe how urine pregnancy tests are conducted.
- Describe how urine drug testing is conducted.

CAAHEP & ABHES Competencies

CAAHEP

- Obtain specimens and perform CLIA-waived urinalysis.
- Identify CLIA-waived tests associated with common diseases.
- Differentiate between normal and abnormal test results.

ABHES

- Perform selected CLIA-waived tests that assist with diagnosis and treatment.

- Perform urinalysis.
- Perform kit testing for pregnancy.
- Collect, label, and process specimens.
- Instruct patients in the collection of clean-catch midstream urine specimen.
- Instruct patient in the collection of a 24-hour urine specimen.
- Practice quality control.

Chapter Terms

Bacteriuria
Casts
Catheter
Culture

Diuretics
Glycosuria
Hematuria
Hyperglycemia

Ketones
Myoglobin
Postprandial
Pyuria

Random urine
Specific gravity
Turbid

Abbreviations

C&S
HCG

pH
POL

PPM

UTI

Case Study

Molly Rayburn, a 29-year-old patient, has a 2:00 PM appointment to see the physician for abdominal pain and a burning sensation each time she urinates. She has had these symptoms for 5 days and now it has become worse. She suspects that she has a urinary tract infection so brought a urine specimen from home that she collected this morning. She put it in a storage container with a lid. The medical assistant, Angela Garcia, asks the patient to collect another urine specimen before escorting her to an examination room.

Urinalysis involves examining and testing urine. Urine tests are often performed in the physician office lab (**POL**), and the CLIA-waived tests can be done by medical assistants. The medical assistant may also prepare urine specimens for other nonwaived tests such as microscopic examination, which will be performed by the physician or other qualified personnel. Knowing the basics of urinalysis will help you carry out these responsibilities.

URINALYSIS

Urinalysis is part of the process the physician uses to assess a patient's health. Like blood testing, urinalysis can reveal things that even the patient may not be aware.

Here are just some of the conditions that might be discovered through urine testing:

- Liver disease
- Kidney disease
- Diabetes
- Malnutrition
- Dehydration
- Infection
- Pregnancy

Urinalysis includes physical (macroscopic and microscopic) and chemical testing of urine. Before a specimen is tested, the appearance and odor are evaluated. Based on the outcome of the basic urinalysis, further testing may be required including performing a culture of the specimen. In order to get reliable results, urine testing must be performed on a quality specimen.

Specimen Collection Methods

The medical assistant is typically responsible for the collection of urine specimens for testing. There are several ways or methods used to collect a urine specimen. The method used depends on what test will be performed. Unless the physician tells you otherwise, a freshly

Case Questions

Why do you think the medical assistant requested another urine specimen? How would you explain this request to the patient?

voided specimen is usually all that is needed. When it is collected at anytime, it is called **random urine**. The patient urinates or voids into a dry, clean specimen container.

The time of collection is sometimes an important factor. The most concentrated urine is voided just after a person wakes up in the morning. Concentrated specimens are useful for many types of tests. For example, pregnancy tests are usually done with "first morning" urine. Other timed tests are **postprandial**, which means after eating a meal. Some postprandial tests measure concentrations of glucose in urine collected 2 hours after the patient has eaten a meal.

Clean Catch

Clean-catch midstream urine is the most commonly ordered random specimen. It is especially useful when an infection is suspected. The reason is that when the specimen is collected correctly, any microorganisms present will be from the urinary tract and not the result of contamination by the patient's skin or other factors.

A clean-catch urine specimen is sent to the laboratory in a clean, dry container with a lid. If the specimen is to be cultured, the container must also be sterile. Figure 27-1 is an example of a sterile specimen cup with a screw-type lid.

A culture can then be performed to detect the microorganism that is causing the disease. A **culture** is a test in which bacteria and other microbes are grown in a lab. Urine cultures are discussed later in this chapter.

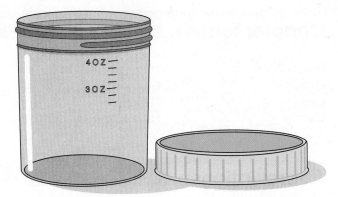

Figure 27-1   Sterile specimen cup with lid. (Reprinted from Kronenberger J, Ledbetter J. *Jones & Bartlett Learning's Comprehensive Medical Assisting.* 5th ed. Burlington, MA: Jones & Bartlett Learning, LLC; 2016.)

Patients generally collect clean-catch specimens themselves. Since the correct collection procedure is so important to accurate test results, instructing patients in the proper methods to use is critical. When instructing a patient, emphasize the proper cleaning of the external urinary meatus and surrounding skin. Figure 27-2 shows the proper technique used to collect a clean-catch midstream specimen for a female patient.

Remember, if a culture is ordered, then a sterile container must be used.

When handling urine specimens, you should wear gloves, and if necessary, other appropriate protective gear such as a face mask and lab coat.

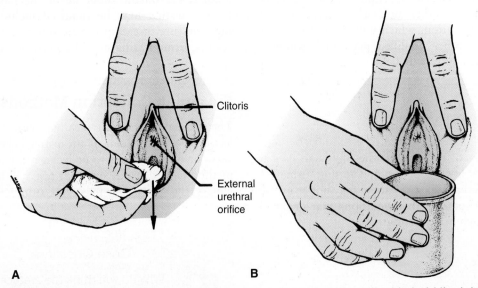

Clitoris

External urethral orifice

A   **B**

Figure 27-2   Obtaining clean-catch midstream urine specimen. **A.** Instruct the patient to hold the labia apart and wash from high up front toward the back with cleansing cloth. **B.** The collection cup is held so that it does not touch the body, and the sample is obtained only while the patient is voiding with the labia held apart. (Reprinted from Kronenberger J, Ledbetter J. *Jones & Bartlett Learning's Comprehensive Medical Assisting.* 5th ed. Burlington, MA: Jones & Bartlett Learning, LLC; 2016.)

When working with patients with various cultural and ethnic backgrounds, it is important to communicate in a way that provides the most effective understanding. Do not assume that all patients understand basic procedures such as collecting a urine specimen. You may have to rely on anatomical drawings to explain the cleansing process prior to a clean-catch midstream collection to both male and female patients. Also when a patient has a UTI, it is not uncommon for the patient to believe that it is due to bad luck, emotional and spiritual distress, lack of balance, and even the "evil eye." It may be difficult to convince the patient that something as basic as drinking more water can help them avoid dehydration that may lead to future infections. Health care providers need to be careful not to insult a person's belief by implying that it is not in any way related to their medical problem.

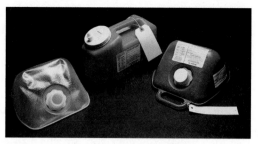

Figure 27-4 24-hour specimen containers. (Reprinted from Kronenberger J, Ledbetter J. *Jones & Bartlett Learning's Comprehensive Medical Assisting.* 5th ed. Burlington, MA: Jones & Bartlett Learning, LLC; 2016.)

Other Collection Methods

The type of urine test and the type of patient can affect how the specimen is collected. Most specimens are collected using the clean-catch midstream method. Other collection methods exist, but they are less common and generally require the direct involvement of a health care professional. Special collection methods include the following:

- Bladder catheterization—a thin sterile, flexible tube called a **catheter** is inserted into the bladder through the urethra; this method is recommended when the patient can't give a urine specimen in a sterile manner using the clean-catch method.
- Suprapubic aspiration—the least common method of urine collection. A needle is inserted directly into the bladder through the abdominal wall above the symphysis pubis, and urine is withdrawn. A physician performs this method using sterile technique. Figure 27-3 demonstrates the technique used to aspirate a urine specimen from the suprapubic region.
- Collection device—is usually used to collect urine from young children. You apply the device around the mons pubis or external genitalia and collect the urine in a bag.

24-Hour Urine Collection

The amount of hormones and some other substances that are excreted in urine can vary during the day. Tests for these substances are more accurate when all urine produced is collected over a 24-hour period. Patients need specific instructions to collect this urine specimen; otherwise, the results will not be reliable and accurate. Figure 27-4 shows some of the collection containers used for the 24-hour urine collection.

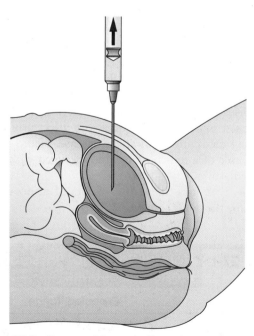

Figure 27-3 Suprapubic aspiration of urine. The full bladder is easily accessible by an abdominal puncture. (Reprinted from Kronenberger J, Ledbetter J. *Jones & Bartlett Learning's Comprehensive Medical Assisting.* 5th ed. Burlington, MA: Jones & Bartlett Learning, LLC; 2016.)

The medical assistant is usually responsible for instructing patients in many procedures. For a 24-hour urine procedure, provide clearly written instructions and review them carefully with the patient to ensure that the patient understands what they are to do. Always document any patient education in the patient's medical record. The general instructions given to the patient for a 24-hour urine collection are as follows:

- Follow these instructions exactly—Your test results are based on the total amount of urine excreted by your body over a 24-hour period.

(continued)

If you don't follow these instructions carefully, the test results may be inaccurate.

- Make sure you drink the amount of fluid you normally would during the 24-hour collection period. (The physician may also request special dietary or medication restrictions, which the medical assistant will instruct the patient.)
- Use the special container you are given to collect the urine. If a preservative (tablet or liquid) is in the container, don't throw it away.
- Preservatives may be caustic or toxic. Be careful not to spill the preservative. If you do spill the preservative, immediately wash your skin with large amounts of water. Then, call the physician or lab to get a new container to collect the specimen.
- Don't urinate directly into the container unless a funnel is provided. Instead, use the collection cups you are given and transfer the urine contents to the large container. Collect your urine often enough that the amount you void each time doesn't exceed the volume of the collection cup.
- Refrigerate the container during collection. The urine must be kept cold.

Instructions for Day 1

- When you wake up in the morning, empty your bladder into the toilet. Record the date and the exact time (to the minute) on your 24-hour urine container.
- Then, collect all specimens during the day, evening, and night for the next entire 24-hour period.
- Add all the specimens to the container. Be careful not to get the cap of the container wet.
- Keep the container refrigerated until you take it to the physician or lab for testing. Some patients use an ice chest with ice cubes to keep the container cold.

Instructions for Day 2

- Exactly 24 hours after you began the collection, completely empty your bladder and add this specimen to the container. This will be your last collection.
- Record the ending date and the exact time (to the minute) on the container.
- Replace the cap and tighten firmly.
- Refrigerate the specimen until you can submit the container. Take the specimen to the physician or lab as soon as possible.
- If you were under any dietary or medication restrictions, you may resume your normal diet after you finish collecting your specimen.

Physical Examination of Urine

The physical properties of a patient's urine can tell a lot about the patient's general health. Physical examination involves looking at the specimen to judge its color and appearance or clarity. Other observations include measuring the specimen's specific gravity and examination of the specimen under a microscope. Table 27-1 lists the normal range for physical properties of urine.

Preserving Specimens for Testing

Urine specimens should be tested within 1 hour after collection because the specimen will begin deteriorating after that time. The microorganisms in the urine will multiply, causing it to change from acidic to alkaline. The microorganisms also may consume glucose in the urine as a nutrient. This will lower the specimen's glucose level. A glucose test in this case would not be measuring the true level of glucose in the patient's urine.

If testing won't be performed within an hour from collection, you should refrigerate the container at 4°C to 8°C (39°F to 46°F). This will slow down changes in the specimen. Urine may be refrigerated for up to 4 hours and still be used for accurate testing.

Urine Color

The normal urine color ranges from pale straw to dark yellow. Pale colored urine usually means that it's diluted. This can happen if the patient has been drinking a lot of fluid. It also can result from diuretic therapy. **Diuretics** are drugs that increase the body's fluid output resulting in more urine production. They're sometimes used to treat hypertension (high blood pressure). They're also prescribed to remove excess fluid from the body's tissues. This build up can result from kidney, lung, liver, or heart disease. The removed fluid dilutes the urine, making it paler in color. Many things can affect urine color including medications, diet, and disease. Figure 27-5 is an example of a red-colored urine specimen with blood in it, hematuria.

Table 27-2 lists the various colors of urine and the causes for the color change.

Table 27-1	Normal Range for Physical Properties of Urine
Property	**Expected Range**
Color	Pale yellow to dark yellow
Odor	Slightly aromatic
Clarity	Clear
Specific gravity	1.003–1.035

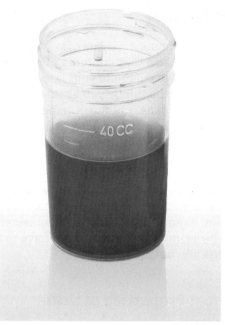

Figure 27-5 Urine specimen for hematuria. (Image from Shutterstock.)

Clarity

Urine is normally clear when it's voided. Urine that's **turbid** (cloudy) probably contains particulate matter, or tiny solid particles. Urine samples that have been sitting a long time can turn cloudy from the precipitation (settling out) of phosphates and urates that are in the solution. Phosphates are compounds made of phosphorous and oxygen. Urates are nitrogen compounds that result when the body burns protein. Urine that's turbid for this reason is considered normal. Other causes of turbidity may be a sign of problems. Here are some substances that can make urine turbid:

- White blood cells (WBCs)
- Red blood cells (RBCs)
- Epithelial cells (skin and organ-lining cells)

- Pus
- Mucus
- Fat droplets
- Blood
- Bacteria

Common terms used to describe the clarity of a urine specimen include clear, hazy, and cloudy. A clear specimen container or a clear centrifuge tube containing the specimen is held up against a white paper with black lines on it. If the black lines can't be seen through the specimen, it's called cloudy. If the specimen is turbid but the lines can still be seen through it, the urine is judged to be hazy.

Specific Gravity

Specific gravity measures the concentration of urine. To find its specific gravity, the weight of urine is compared to the weight of distilled water. Urine is normally slightly heavier than water. That's because it contains substances like sodium, potassium, and chloride, which water does not. This makes urine weigh more than the same amount of water would.

Specific gravity is not an actual weight but a comparison to the weight of water. The specific gravity of water is set at 1.000. The specific gravity of a normal urine specimen will range between 1.003 and 1.035. Urine that's dilute will have a lower specific gravity. This occurs when a person has taken in a lot of fluids and with abnormal conditions that cause dilute urine including diabetes insipidus and kidney infections.

Urine that has a high specific gravity is concentrated. A patient who's dehydrated could easily produce such a specimen because the body tries to conserve water when it becomes dehydrated. Dehydration can result from a number of conditions, including:

- Heavy sweating
- Prolonged vomiting
- Frequent diarrhea

Table 27-2	Common Causes of Color Variations in Urine
Color	**Possible Cause**
Yellow-brown or amber	Bilirubin in the urine as in jaundice; possible liver disease including hepatitis
Dark yellow	Concentrated urine due to low fluid intake, dehydration, inability of the kidney to dilute urine, fluorescein (intravenous dye), multivitamins, excessive carotene
Bright orange-red	Pyridium, an analgesic used to treat urinary tract pain typically due to urinary tract infection
Orange	Ingesting larger quantities of carrots or carrot juice
Red or reddish brown	Hemoglobin pigments, pyrvinium pamoate (Povan) medication for intestinal worms, sulfonamides (sulfa-based antibiotics)
Pink to red	Ingesting larger quantities of beets, rhubarb, and blackberries
Green or blue	Artificial color in food or drugs
Blackish, grayish, or smoky	Hemoglobin or remains of old red blood cells (indicating bleeding in upper urinary tract), chyle, prostatic fluid, yeasts, homogentisic acid

Diabetes mellitus also can cause urine to have a high specific gravity. That's because of the high concentration of glucose the urine contains. IVP dye, the x-ray dye used to visualize the urinary system, can also cause urine to have a high specific gravity. This doesn't reflect the patient's state of hydration, but simply shows the presence of a foreign substance with a high weight. The specimen will frequently look clear and colorless, but have a high specific gravity. Specific gravity is generally determined by one of three ways:

- Reagent strip—the specific gravity pad on a reagent test strip also takes just one drop of urine. The pad's change in color measures the urine's specific gravity. This is the most common method of determining specific gravity.
- Urinometer—this device looks something like an oral thermometer. It floats upright in the specimen and its upper part has a calibrated scale. The specific gravity is measured by how much of the device sinks into the urine.
- Refractometer—this device only requires a drop of urine, compared to about 100 mL that's needed to float a urinometer. It works by measuring how light passing through the urine drop is affected by the particles in it. Figure 27-6 is a refractometer used to measure the specific gravity.

Urine Odors

Urine should have a slightly aromatic odor; however, any unusual odor should be reported since it may indicate certain conditions. For example, a sweet, fruity odor can be a sign that the patient has diabetes. Bacteria in urine can make it smell foul or like ammonia. This is what accounts for the ammonia odor that is detected in a baby's diaper. Urine may smell very strong when it is highly concentrated and when a person has eaten asparagus.

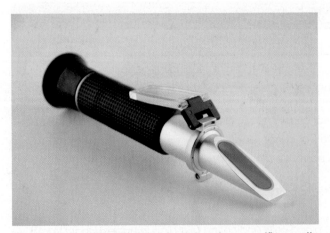

Figure 27-6   Refractometer to determine specific gravity of urine using only one drop of urine.

Chemical Properties of Urine

Urine contains a number of chemicals. Some of these are produced by the body itself. Others are taken in from the environment. The basic urine test for the chemical properties typically uses a strip with ten reagent pads along its surface. The reagent in each pad tests for a specific substance in urine. The pads change color when the strip is dipped in the specimen. The color change indicates if that substance is present in the specimen. Variations in color correspond with the quantity of substance or how much of the substance is in the specimen.

Each pad's color is compared to a color chart provided by the strip's manufacturer. Each row on the chart corresponds to one pad on the strip. Instead of the manual reading of reagent strips, a facility may have an automated strip reader. In that case, follow the manufacturer's directions for machine operation. Figure 27-7 is an example of an automatic dipstick reader.

These tests are basic screening tests only. Table 27-3 lists the expected or "normal" results for these tests.

Determining pH

The **pH** (concentration of hydrogen ions determining the acidity or alkalinity of a substance) of urine is one of the things tested on the reagent strip. It is the measure of a substance to determine if it is acid or alkaline (base). If a pH is >7.0, the liquid is alkaline. Values <7.0 indicate acids. The higher or lower the number, the more alkaline or acidic the liquid is.

Acids are a product of the body's chemical processes. Ammonia is a base that's produced when nitrogen in the body breaks down. The kidneys clean the blood of these and other substances and get rid of them in urine. Urine is usually acidic because the body produces more acids than bases.

The pH of freshly voided urine is slightly acidic at 6.0. But the expected range for a normal pH is from

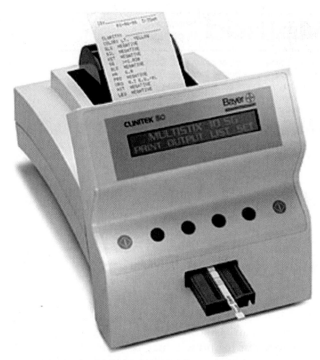

Figure 27-7   Bayer Clinitek Dipstick Reader. (Reprinted from Kronenberger J, Ledbetter J. *Jones & Bartlett Learning's Comprehensive Medical Assisting*. 5th ed. Burlington, MA: Jones & Bartlett Learning, LLC; 2016.)

5.0 (acidic) to 8.0 (slightly alkaline). If the patient has a high-protein diet or uncontrolled diabetes, urine can be more acidic. Alkaline urine can occur after meals and in the following situations:

- The patient follows a vegetarian diet.
- The patient has certain renal (kidney) diseases.
- The patient has a urinary tract infection (**UTI**).

Glucose Testing

Normal urine does not contain glucose. A patient should submit a urine specimen when fasting, nothing to eat or

Table 27-3	Expected Range of Urine's Chemical Properties
Property Tested	**Expected Range or Result**
Glucose	Negative
Bilirubin	Negative
Ketones	Negative
Blood	Negative
pH	5.0–8.0
Protein	Negative to trace
Urobilinogen	0.1–1.0 EU/dL
Nitrite	Negative
Leukocyte esterase	Negative

drink for 8 to 12 hours. **Glycosuria** (glucose in urine) can be a sign of diabetes or some other condition related to **hyperglycemia** (high blood sugar). In the kidney, glucose is filtered from the blood in the nephron. To conserve the glucose for the body, it is reabsorbed into the blood from the tubule portion of the nephron. However, the nephron can only reabsorb glucose up to a blood level of about 180 mg/dL. This is known as the renal blood glucose threshold level. If the blood glucose is higher than 180 mg/dL, the glucose in excess of 180 mg/dL will start to pass out of the nephron in the urine.

Diabetics whose condition is uncontrolled or poorly managed may pass glucose in their urine because of a high level in their blood.

Undetected or uncontrolled diabetes can lead to heart disease, kidney failure, blindness, and even death. Yet a person can be severely diabetic before signs will show up on a urine test. However, since a routine urinalysis is part of nearly every hospital admission and annual physical exam, it remains a primary method of screening for diabetes. The diagnosis is then confirmed by blood glucose tests.

Monitoring the glucose levels of known diabetics was also once done by urine testing. However, since the rise of handheld computerized glucose monitors, urine monitoring has been replaced by testing blood samples taken by finger stick.

Clinitest

The Clinitest was routinely used to confirm urine glucose; however, results can be inaccurate when used simply to confirm a positive strip test result for glucose. That's because other sugars and vitamin C in the specimen will also react with the reagent. However, a negative strip test result combined with a positive Clinitest result strongly suggests that the patient has a carbohydrate metabolism disorder.

This copper reduction test method can detect any reducing sugar in urine. Reducing sugars are sugars that give up electrons easily in chemical reactions. This type of sugars includes the following:

- Glucose
- Galactose
- Lactose
- Fructose

This test is often used to screen young children for galactosuria, or high levels of galactose in urine and blood. This condition results when a newborn lacks an enzyme that metabolizes galactose in the body.

A strong chemical reaction occurs when performing the Clinitest. This reaction gives off a large amount of heat. You should always use glass test tubes, never plastic, when performing this test. The test tubes become very hot so wait 15 seconds after the reaction stops before touching the tubes. This allows them time to cool. Finally, avoid touching the bottoms of the test

5-Drop Method Standard Procedure

DIRECTIONS FOR TESTING:

1. Collect urine in clean container. With dropper in upright position, place **5 drops** of urine in test tube. Rinse dropper with water and add 10 drops of water to test tube.

2. Drop one tablet into test tube. Watch while complete boiling reaction takes place. Do not shake test tube during boiling, or for the following 15 seconds after boiling has stopped.

3. At the end of this 15-second waiting period, shake test tube gently to mix contents. Compare color of liquid to Color Chart below. Ignore sediment that may form in the bottom of the test tube. Ignore changes after the 15-second waiting period.

4. Write down the percent (%) result which appears on the color block that most closely matches the color of the liquid.

NEGATIVE	1/4%	1/2%	3/4%	1%	2% or more

Figure 27-8 Clinitest for reducing sugars. (Reprinted from Kronenberger J, Ledbetter J. *Jones & Bartlett Learning's Comprehensive Medical Assisting.* 5th ed. Burlington, MA: Jones & Bartlett Learning, LLC; 2016.)

tubes. Figure 27-8 is an example of the results from a Clinitest for reducing sugars.

Ketone Testing

Ketones are chemicals the body makes when it metabolizes (breaks down) fat. Most of your energy comes from carbohydrates. When the body doesn't have enough carbohydrates to meet its energy needs, it burns fats. This happens if a person is starving or is eating a low-carbohydrate, high-protein diet. Poorly managed diabetics also get energy from fats and produce ketones.

Normally, there are too few ketones in urine to even measure. When a patient's urine tests positive for ketones, it's a sign the body is burning more fat than normal.

Nitroprusside is used to detect ketones in urine. Nitroprusside is a nitrogen-cyanic compound that reacts with ketones. It's used on reagent strips and in tablet tests. A tablet test called the Acetest is used in many labs to confirm the results of the strip test.

Protein Testing

A small amount of protein is normal in urine. High amounts can be an important sign of renal disease. Other things that can cause protein in urine are as follows:

- Strenuous exercise
- Pregnancy
- Infection
- Hematuria
- **Pyuria** (white blood cells in the urine)
- Multiple myeloma (a cancer of the bone marrow)
- Orthostatic proteinuria

Examining urine under a microscope can help find whether high protein levels are caused by bacteria, casts, or cell-related factors. Urine is screened for proteins on a reagent test strip. When there is a positive result, a confirmatory test for protein may be performed. The most common turbidity or precipitation test mixes sulfosalicylic acid with an equal amount of urine. The urine is centrifuged to remove any particulate matter. Then it's mixed with the acid. If the strip test showed little or no protein, the urine acid mixture in this confirmation test should remain clear. Cloudiness won't appear unless the urine contains at least 20 mg/dL of protein. The more protein in the urine, the cloudier the mixture will be.

Blood in Urine

Small numbers of red blood cells (RBC) sometimes show up in urine. The kidneys have small blood vessels that normally don't allow blood to pass into the urine. However, in the female, blood can be present if the specimen has been contaminated by menstrual blood.

Hematuria, blood in the urine, also can be a sign of bleeding in the urinary tract. Such bleeding could result from the following:

- Renal disorders
- Urinary tract infection (UTI)
- Abnormal tissue growths or tumors
- Trauma to the urinary tract
- Kidney stones (calculi)

The reagent strip tests for blood in urine. The strip reacts to the hemoglobin found in red blood cells. However, the strip also reacts to myoglobin, a protein found in muscles. Myoglobin may be released into the bloodstream because of overexercise, a crushing injury or other trauma, and some kinds of surgery. Then it's excreted in urine. So to avoid a false result, if the strip test is positive for blood, it should be confirmed by looking for RBCs under a microscope. If myoglobin is suspected, a specific test for it can be ordered.

Bilirubin Testing

Bilirubin is made when the body breaks down hemoglobin. It's processed in the liver before it's excreted into the intestines. High levels in urine can be a sign of:

- Liver diseases such as hepatitis
- Bile duct blockage in the liver
- Destruction of red blood cells—for example, in a bad reaction to a blood transfusion

Test for bilirubin as soon as possible because it breaks down when exposed to light. Be sure to shield the specimen until you can do the test. Also remember that if a urine specimen cannot be tested within an hour, refrigerate it.

Bilirubin is another substance tested for on the reagent strip. However, its color can give urine an amber or dark yellow shade. This can make its pad on the test strip hard to read. Therefore, many labs confirm the result by using the diazo tablet method (Ictotest). Figure 27-9 shows the results of the diazo tablet test for bilirubin.

Detecting Urobilinogen

After bilirubin is secreted into the intestines, bacteria that reside in the intestines convert bilirubin into urobilinogen. Some of this chemical is absorbed through the intestines into the bloodstream. When blood is filtered through the kidneys, the urobilinogen is excreted in the urine. The rest passes through the intestines and leaves the body in feces.

Urobilinogen is detected in reagent strip testing. It's measured in Ehrlich units, a special measurement for urobilinogen. An Ehrlich unit is 1 mg/dL of urobilinogen. A value between 0.1 and 1.0 is considered normal. Any test result over 1.0 Ehrlich units/dL can be a warning sign. Here's what high levels of urobilinogen in urine can mean:

- High rate of RBC destruction—this can result from the same things a high bilirubin level indicates.

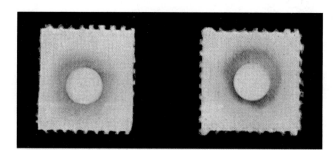

Figure 27-9 Ictotest for testing bilirubin. (Reprinted from Kronenberger J, Ledbetter J. *Jones & Bartlett Learning's Comprehensive Medical Assisting.* 5th ed. Burlington, MA: Jones & Bartlett Learning, LLC; 2016.)

- Bowel obstruction if feces are forced to stay in the intestine—more urobilinogen will be reabsorbed into the blood and excreted by the kidneys in urine.
- Damaged liver—high urobilinogen levels can occur in the early stages of hepatitis or with other liver impairments.

Nitrite Testing

Some bacteria that infect the urinary tract have an enzyme that changes the nitrates in urine to nitrites. In the nitrite test, urine is applied to the reagent pad. If the pad changes color, nitrites are present in the specimen. A positive nitrite test signals that the patient has a urinary tract infection (UTI), or **bacteriuria** (bacteria in urine). However, there is a delay in testing the urine, a small number of bacteria in it can multiply. A false-positive result for nitrites could occur and be falsely interpreted and diagnosed as a urinary tract infection.

Leukocyte Esterase

Leukocytes (WBC) in the urine also mean that a UTI is present. Leukocytes called neutrophils enter the kidneys to fight infection. These neutrophils contain an enzyme called esterase. This is detected on a reagent strip that contains a leukocyte esterase reaction pad. Normal urine may contain a few white cells. Larger numbers must be present to produce a positive leukocyte esterase test. Leukocytes are also confirmed with a microscopic examination of the urine.

Urine Confirmation Tests

Several confirmation tests were discussed for some of the chemical tests when there is a positive result. These tests use a different chemical reaction to look for the substance than was used by the strip test. Confirmation tests are usually performed to make sure the results of the strip test are correct. Some labs automatically do them when strip test results are abnormal. Here is a review of the common confirmation tests for some chemicals found in urine:

- Protein—sulfosalicylic acid test
- Ketones—Acetest
- Bilirubin—Ictotest
- Glucose—Clinitest

 URINE SEDIMENT

Looking at a urine specimen under the microscope can confirm some of the urinalysis results. It may also add more information that will help the physician diagnose the patient. However, microscopic examination of urine is not a CLIA-waived procedure that a medical assistant will perform. CLIA classifies urine sediment exams as moderate-complexity tests. Generally, a lab must have a Certificate of Compliance or Accreditation to perform tests at this level. However, CLIA allows other labs to examine urine sediment if they have a Certificate of Provider Performed Microscopy (**PPM**) Procedures. This certificate allows the following practitioners to perform PPM:

- Physician (MD or DO)
- Midlevel professional under a physician's supervision
- Podiatrist
- Dentist

There are other CLIA requirements for urine sediment testing.

- The lab must have written PPM procedures in place.
- A positive (abnormal results) control must be tested each day urine sediment is examined.
- The centrifuge and microscope must be cleaned and checked for accuracy regularly. And maintenance records must be kept for 2 years.

If your lab is allowed to perform microscopy, you may be asked to prepare specimens for study.

Urine sediment is examined for:

- RBCs
- WBCs
- Casts
- Epithelial cells
- Bacteria
- Crystals

Figure 27-10 shows some of the more common formed elements found in urine sediment.

Blood Cells

When the sediment contains red blood cells or RBCs, the strip test should also be positive for blood. As you've already read, RBCs in urine can mean a number of things including contamination from menstrual blood.

Sometimes, however, a microscopic exam won't find RBCs, even when the reagent strip test is positive. This can happen if the patient is suffering some kinds of hemolysis—for example, a transfusion reaction or a sickle cell crisis.

As stated earlier, a positive strip test result may occur if the patient's urine contains **myoglobin**, a red protein containing heme that carries and stores oxygen in muscle cells. It is structurally similar to a subunit of hemoglobin. No red cells will be found in the urine sediment in this case either.

White blood cells (WBCs), or leukocytes, in the sediment can indicate a urinary tract infection. If there is a large enough number, the leukocyte esterase test on the reagent strip will also be positive. The protein test on the strip may be positive too if some of the WBCs lyse, or break apart. It will also be positive if the infection has reached the tubes of the kidneys.

Casts

Casts are cylinders of proteins and other substances that form and solidify in the nephron tubules in the kidneys. Most casts eventually break free and end up in the urine. Certain casts can indicate disease or infection. For example, in a kidney infection, WBCs become trapped in the protein network and form white cell casts. Figure 27-11 is an example of the various types of casts found in urine sediment, and Figure 27-12 is a WBC cast.

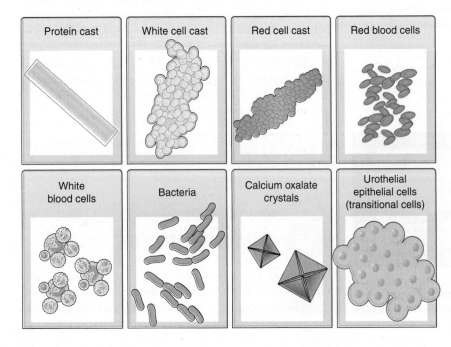

Figure 27-10 Microscopic examination of urine sediment. Common formed elements found in urine. (Reprinted from Kronenberger J, Ledbetter J. *Jones & Bartlett Learning's Comprehensive Medical Assisting.* 5th ed. Burlington, MA: Jones & Bartlett Learning, LLC; 2016.)

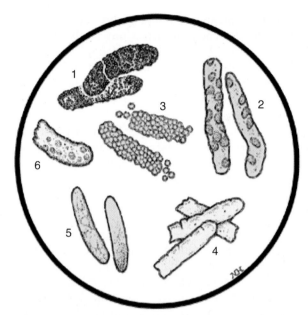

Figure 27-11 Urinary casts. (*1*) Course granular casts. (*2*) Epithelial casts. (*3*) RBC casts. (*4*) Waxy casts. (*5*) Hyaline casts. (*6*) Casts with pyocytes (pus corpuscles). (Reprinted from Hardy NO, Wesport CT. *From Stedman's Medical Dictionary.* 27th ed. Baltimore, MD: Lippincott Williams & Wilkins; 2000.)

Casts are examined using low-power magnification and reduced light. They provide good information about what's going on inside the kidneys' nephron tubules. They are reported as the number of casts counted within the microscope's low-power field. A field indicates a single view of one area of the slide when looking through the eyepieces.

Bacteria and Crystals

Normal urine should not contain bacteria if the clean-catch specimen was properly collected. If it wasn't done properly, bacteria on the skin could have been washed into the specimen. This would contaminate the sample

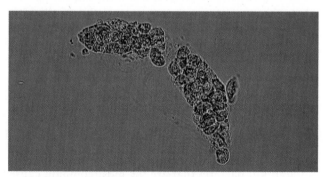

Figure 27-12 WBC cast. Hyaline cast, which has polymorphonuclear neutrophils adhered (bright-field microscopy). (Reprinted from Kronenberger J, Ledbetter J. *Jones & Bartlett Learning's Comprehensive Medical Assisting.* 5th ed. Burlington, MA: Jones & Bartlett Learning, LLC; 2016.)

and could produce a false result on the test strip. On the other hand, large amounts of bacteria in the urine can be a sign of a urinary tract infection.

As you've already read, the test strip relies on the nitrites produced by bacteria for a positive result. However, not all bacteria produce nitrites. Therefore, some kinds of bacteria may be found in urine sediment even when the strip test is negative.

Crystals appear when there is a sufficient quantity of certain chemicals in the urine to form solid structures. These structures are tiny, but they can be seen under the microscope. The following crystals are most commonly found in urine sediment.

- Calcium oxalate crystals can occur in urine that has a pH lower than 7.0.
- Uric acid crystals also may occur in urine with a pH lower than 7.0.
- Triple phosphate crystals can develop in urine with a pH above 7.0.

Crystals by themselves are not necessarily a problem. However, they can contribute to the formation of stones in the urinary tract. Also, uric acid crystals are often found in patients who have fever, leukemia, or gout.

Epithelial Cells

Epithelial cells cover the skin and organs, and line pathways like the digestive tract and urinary tract. Epithelial cells shed and are normally found in urine, but a large number in a specimen can be a sign of inflammation somewhere in the urinary system.

Three types of epithelial cells may be found in urine:

- Squamous epithelial cells cover the body's outer skin surfaces. They are a normal finding in urine because the urine comes in contact with the skin during urination.
- Transitional epithelial cells line the bladder. They are present in conditions including cystitis and other infections of the lower urinary tract.
- Renal epithelial cells line the nephrons of the kidneys. They're seen with infections and inflammations of the upper urinary tract.

There is no chemical test for epithelial cells and are only detected in the microscopic exam of urine. When renal epithelial cells are seen, it is likely that the renal tubules have been damaged. Also, the strip test for protein may be positive if these cells are present.

Other Structures

Other structures may also be found in urine sediment. For example, a patient with a vaginal yeast infection

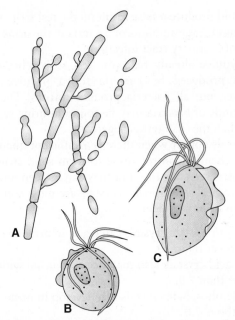

Figure 27-13 Organisms that cause vaginal infections. **A.** *Candida albicans* (yeast). **B, C.** *T. vaginalis* (trichomonas). (Reprinted from Kronenberger J, Ledbetter J. *Jones & Bartlett Learning's Comprehensive Medical Assisting.* 5th ed. Burlington, MA: Jones & Bartlett Learning, LLC; 2016.)

can have a urine specimen contaminated with yeast. Yeast, *Candida albicans*, also can appear in urine if the patient has a UTI. This is especially true of diabetic patients.

The parasite *Trichomonas vaginalis* can contaminate urine from the genital tract of an infected person. Figure 27-13 is an example of these organisms seen under the microscope in the urine sediment.

Mucus can be present in the sediment if the patient's urinary tract is inflamed. Mucus threads are usually reported as few, moderate, or many in number. Sperm may be found in the urine of a male patient who has recently ejaculated.

Upon completion of the physical, chemical, and microscopic examination of the urine, a report is submitted by the laboratory. Figure 27-14 is an example of a urinalysis report.

URINE TESTING FOR PREGNANCY

The blood or urine pregnancy test is used to detect the presence of human chorionic gonadotropin (**HCG**) in the woman's urine or serum. HCG is a hormone that is secreted by the developing placenta shortly after conception takes place.

Most urine pregnancy test kits are easy to use and are sold over the counter for home use. The test simply requires adding urine to the test device and reading

the result. All pregnancy tests measure some part of the HCG molecule. They can detect tiny levels of HCG in urine just 10 to 12 days after conception. This is sometimes even before a woman's first missed period.

When using urine for a pregnancy test, the first morning urine sample is best because it is most concentrated in the morning, which makes the hormone easier to detect. Most labs also do a specific gravity test along with the pregnancy test. A specific gravity below 1.015 indicates very dilute urine and may not be concentrated with enough HCG to yield an accurate test.

Case Question

The patient, Molly Rayburn, completed an antibiotic for the UTI that was diagnosed a week ago. She is back in the medical office to follow up. When the medical assistant is rooming, Ms. Rayburn asks the medical assistant why the antibiotic has not treated the UTI. What would you tell the patient?

Urine Culture and Sensitivity

Chemical testing results and microscopic examination may suggest that a patient's urine contains large amounts of bacteria. This generally means that the patient has a urinary tract infection (UTI). Before the infection can be treated, the organism causing the infection must be identified. To do this, the urine specimen is cultured.

A small amount of the specimen is inoculated onto a culture plate that is filled with media, a substance that contains the nutrients that encourage the growth of bacteria. The culture plate is placed in an incubator, a device that maintains a constant warm environment to make the bacteria grow faster. If bacteria are present in the specimen, colonies of bacteria will form and will be visible to the naked eye in the culture dish. Figure 27-15 is an example of a culture plate with colonies of bacteria that have grown on the surface.

The culture can then be tested to find the right antibiotic to fight the patient's infection. Both the culture and sensitivity (**C&S**) are performed to determine the bacteria causing the infection and then identifying the antibiotic that will affect the growth of the bacteria, killing it.

A physician will usually start a patient on an antibiotic to kill bacteria that are the most common cause of UTIs, even before the culture is completed. Then, when the culture results are known, the doctor may need to change the antibiotic if a type of bacteria is found that isn't killed by the antibiotic the patient has been taking.

CENTRAL MEDICAL CENTER
211 Medical Center Drive • Central City, US 90000-1234 • PHONE: (012) 125-6784 • FAX: (012) 125-9999

11//02/20xx
13:49

```
NAME :  TEST, PATIENT        LOC: TEST        DOB: 2/2/XX       AGE: 38Y
MR#   :  TEST-221                                               SEX: M
ACCT # :  H111111111
```

M63560 COLL: 11/2/20xx 13:24   REC: 11/2/20xx   13:25

```
URINE BASIC
    Color               STRAW
    Appearance          CLEAR
    Specific Gravity    1.010        [1.003 - 1.035]
    pH                  5.5          [5.0 - 9.0]
    Protein             NEG          [0 - 10]          MG/DL
    Glucose             NEG          [NEG]
    Ketones             NEG          [NEG]
    Bilirubin           NEG          [NEG]
    Urine Occult Blood  NEG          [NEG]
    Nitrites            NEG


URINE MICROSCOPIC
    Epithelial Cells    3 to 4                         /HPF
    WBCs                0 to 1                         /HPF
    RBCs                0                              /HPF
    Bacteria            0
    Mucous Threads      0
```

TEST, PATIENT   TEST-221   END OF REPORT   PAGE 1
11/02/20xx   13:49   INTERIM REPORT
INTERIM REPORT COMPLETED

Figure 27-14 Sample urinalysis report. (Reprinted from Kronenberger J, Ledbetter J. *Jones & Bartlett Learning's Comprehensive Medical Assisting.* 5th ed. Burlington, MA: Jones & Bartlett Learning, LLC; 2016.)

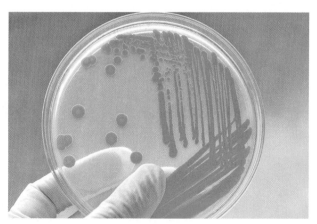

Figure 27-15 Culture plate. (Image from Shutterstock.)

When culturing urine, it's important that the specimen not be contaminated. Contamination can happen when the patient does not follow proper collection procedure. For example, bacteria could get into a clean-catch urine specimen if it came in contact with the patient's skin. Another way the specimen can become contaminated is if it's used for another test. In either case, it would produce false results in a urine culture.

 URINE DRUG TESTING

To test urine for drugs, a lab must use a commercial test approved by the U.S. Food and Drug Administration

(FDA). In addition, the patient must test positive for a drug on two separate tests before a positive result can be reported. When a negative drug test is reported, then either the specimen does not contain the drug tested for or the drug tested for is not concentrated at a level that can be detected by the test. If the first test results in a negative finding, no further testing is done. If that test result is positive, a confirming test is performed. A method called gas chromatography/mass spectrometry (GC/MS) is used in confirmation testing for drugs.

Here are some of the drugs that can be detected in urine:

- Amphetamines
- Barbiturates
- Benzodiazepines
- Cocaine
- Marijuana
- Methadone
- Opioids
- PCP

Urine drug testing may be requested as part of a preemployment physical. The results of the test are released to the employer; however, the patient (employee) may refuse to have the testing performed. Preemployment drug testing may be required for employment so refusing the testing will result in not being hired for that position. Many employers who hire people to drive vehicles and operate equipment require preemployment urine or blood drug testing. When collecting urine specimens for drug testing, the chain of custody must be followed carefully. Procedure 23-1 found in Chapter 23 describes the steps to follow for maintaining the chain of custody for urine collection.

Procedure 27-1   Obtaining a Clean-Catch Midstream Urine Specimen

Equipment: A clean, dry (or sterile) urine container labeled with the patient's name; antiseptic wipes, a bedpan or urinal (if necessary); and gloves if you will be assisting the patient.

Follow these steps to instruct patients how to collect a clean-catch midstream urine specimen:

1. Gather the equipment.

2. Wash your hands. Put on gloves if you will be assisting the patient.

3. Greet and identify the patient. Explain the procedure. Ask for and answer any questions the patient may have.

4. If the patient will perform the procedure, give the patient the proper supplies.

5. Tell patients that they must follow the procedure exactly or the specimen may be contaminated and produce false test results. Also, keep in mind that many patients might not know what the meatus or glans labia are, so be sure to explain in your instructions if necessary.

6. Male patient instructions:
   - Wash your hands upon entering the bathroom. Remove the lid from the container and place the lid flat side down in the designated area. Be careful not to touch the inside of the lid.
   - If uncircumcised, retract the foreskin to expose the glans penis. Clean the meatus with an antiseptic wipe. Use a new wipe for each cleaning sweep.
   - Keep the foreskin retracted and void for a second into the toilet or urinal. It's important to do this first so the specimen will have the least contamination with the skin.
   - While maintaining a stream, bring the sterile container into the urine stream. Collect 30 to 100 mL. Don't touch the inside of the container with the penis.
   - Once a sufficient amount has been collected, finish voiding into the toilet or urinal.
   - Without touching the inside of the lid, replace the lid on the specimen container and wash your hands. Bring the container to the designated area.

7. Female patient instructions:
   - Wash your hands upon entering the bathroom. Remove the lid from the container and place the lid flat side down in the designated area. Be careful not to touch the inside of the lid.

| Procedure 27-1 | Obtaining a Clean-Catch Midstream Urine Specimen (*continued*) |

- Position yourself over a bedpan or toilet. Spread the labia minora to expose the meatus. First, cleanse on each side of the meatus. Wipe from front to back, using a new wipe for each side. Then, using a new wipe, clean the meatus itself. Again, wipe from front to back.
- Keeping the labia separated, initially void for a second into the toilet or bedpan. It's important to do this first so the specimen will have the least contamination with the skin.
- While maintaining a stream, bring the sterile container into the stream and collect 30 to 100 mL.

- Once a sufficient amount has been collected, finish voiding into the toilet or bedpan.
- Without touching the inside of the lid, replace the lid of the specimen container and wash your hands. Bring the container to the designated area.

8. Use gloves when handling the specimen container returned by the patient. Then clean the work area, remove your gloves, and wash your hands.

9. Test, transfer, or store the container according to the office policy and record the procedure.

| Procedure 27-2 | Determining Color and Clarity of Urine |

Equipment: A clear test tube, a sheet of white paper with scored black lines, and a patient report form or data form, gloves, impervious gown, and a face shield.

Follow these steps to determine the color and clarity of a urine specimen. Note that some urine turns cloudy if left standing. Color and clarity must be determined rapidly.

1. Wash your hands and assemble the equipment.

2. Assemble the equipment: a clear test tube, a sheet of white paper with scored black lines, and a patient report form or data form.

3. Put on gloves, and if applicable, an impervious gown, and a face shield.

4. Verify that the patient name on the specimen container and the report form are the same.

5. Pour 10 to 15 mL of urine from the container into the test tube.

6. In a bright light against a white background, examine the color of the urine in the tube.
   - The intensity of yellow color, which is due to urochrome, depends on urine concentration.
   - The most common colors are straw (very pale yellow), yellow, and dark yellow.

7. Determine clarity by holding the tube in front of the white paper scored with black lines.
   - If you can see the lines clearly, record the sample as clear.
   - If the lines are not well defined when viewed through the sample, record it as hazy.
   - If you can't see the lines at all through the sample, record it as cloudy.

8. If further testing is to be done but will be delayed more than an hour, refrigerate the specimen to avoid chemical changes.

9. Properly care for or dispose of equipment and supplies. Clean the work area using a 10% bleach solution. Remove your gown, face shield, and gloves. Wash your hands.

Procedure 27-3 | Performing a Chemical Reagent Strip Analysis

Equipment: Urine specimen, a chemical strip (such as Multistix or Chemstrip), the manufacturer's color comparison chart, a stopwatch or timer, a 15 x 125 mm test tube or Kova system urine tube, patient report form or data form, gloves, impervious gown and a face shield.

Follow these steps to perform a reagent strip test (dipstick test) to screen chemical properties of a urine specimen.

1. Wash your hands and assemble the equipment.

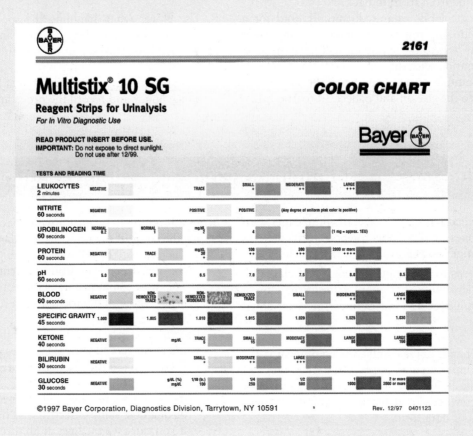

2. Apply PPE including gloves and, if applicable, an impervious gown and a face shield.

3. Verify that the names on the specimen container and the report form are the same.

4. Mix the patient's urine by gently swirling the specimen container. Then pour 12 mL of urine into a Kova system urine tube.

5. Remove a reagent strip from its container and replace the lid to prevent deterioration of the strips by humidity. Don't remove the desiccant package from the container. It keeps moisture levels in the container to a minimum.

6. Immerse the reagent strip in the urine completely, then immediately remove it, sliding the edge of the strip along the lip of the tube to remove excess urine. Turn the strip on its edge and touch the edge to a paper towel or other absorbent paper. Immediate removal and touching its edge to a paper towel prevents colors from leaching due to prolonged exposure to urine.

7. Start your stopwatch or timer immediately after removing the strip from the urine. Reactions must be read at specific times as directed in the package insert and on the color comparison chart.

8. Compare the reagent pads to the color chart. Determine the results at intervals stated by the test strip manufacturer.
    *   Example: Glucose is read at 30 seconds. For that result, examine the glucose pad 30 seconds after dipping and compare it with the color chart for glucose.

Procedure 27-3 — Performing a Chemical Reagent Strip Analysis (*continued*)

9. Read all the reactions at the times indicated and record the results.

10. Discard the used strip in a biohazard container. Discard the urine in accordance with the office policies.

11. Properly care for or dispose of equipment and supplies. Clean the work area using a 10% bleach solution. Remove PPE and wash your hands.

Precautions for chemical strip testing:

- False-positive and false-negative results are possible. Review the manufacturer's package insert to learn about factors that may give false results and how to avoid them.
- If the patient is taking Pyridium, don't use a reagent strip for testing because the medication will interfere with the color.
- Outdated materials give inaccurate results. If the strip's expiration date has passed, discard it.

Procedure 27-4 — Preparing Urine Sediment for Microscopic Examination

Equipment: A centrifuge, urine centrifuge tubes, a transfer pipette, microscope slide and cover slip, and a patient report form or data form, an impervious gown, a face shield, and gloves.

Follow these steps to prepare a urine sediment sample for microscopic examination. Note that if the specimen is to be tested by chemical reagent strip, this can be done before or after centrifuging the urine.

1. Wash your hands and assemble the equipment.

2. Assemble the equipment: a centrifuge, urine centrifuge tubes, a transfer pipette, and a patient report form or data form. Sediment stain may be used to enhance the viewing of the substances in the urine sediment.

3. Put on an impervious gown, a face shield, and gloves.

4. Verify that the names on the specimen container and the report form are the same.

5. Swirl the specimen to mix. Pour 10 or 12 mL of well-mixed urine into a labeled urine centrifuge tube or a tube provided by the test system manufacturer. Cap the tube with a plastic cap.
   - Some test systems use 10 mL and some use 12 mL. The 12 mL volume allows reagent strip testing from the same tube. Check your lab procedures to find out which type of tube to use.

- Some patients cannot produce a large amount of urine. If less than the standard 10 or 12 mL of urine is available, document the actual volume prepared on the report form. This is necessary to ensure proper interpretation of results.
- Preparing a urine sediment sample from <3 mL of specimen is not recommended.

6. Centrifuge the sample at 1,500 rpm for 5 minutes. This ensures that cellular and particulate matter is pulled to the bottom of the tube.

7. When the centrifuge has stopped, remove the tubes. After making sure no tests are to be performed first on the supernatant, pour off all but 0.5 to 1.0 mL of the fluid.

8. Suspend the sediment again in the remaining supernatant by aspirating up into the bulbous portion of a urine transfer pipette.

9. Place a urine slide (Kova slide or other urine system slide) on the counter. Add a drop of the mixed sediment on the slide and place a coverslip over the drop. The concentrated urine is now prepared for microscopic examination.

10. Properly care for or dispose of equipment and supplies. Clean the work area using a 10% bleach solution. Remove your gown, face shield, and gloves. Wash your hands.

Procedure 27-5   Urine Collection from Infants

Urine collection from an infant or young child who isn't toilet trained requires a special collection device and technique.

Equipment:

- Gloves
- Personal antiseptic wipes
- Pediatric urine collection bag
- Completed laboratory request slip
- Biohazard transport container

Follow these steps to correctly apply a urine collection device to an infant.

1. Gather the equipment and supplies and then wash your hands.

2. Explain the procedure to the parents.

3. Place the infant in a lying position on their back. Ask for help from parents as needed.

4. After putting on gloves, clean the genitalia with the antiseptic wipes.
   A. For girls: Cleanse front to back with separate wipes for each downward stroke on the outer labia. The last clean wipe should be used between the inner labia.
   B. For boys: Retract the foreskin if the child isn't circumcised. Cleanse the meatus in an ever-widening circle. Discard the wipe and repeat the procedure. Return the foreskin to its proper position.

5. Holding the collection device, remove the upper portion of the paper backing and press it around the mons pubis. Remove the second section and press it against the perineum. Loosely attach a diaper.

6. Give the infant fluids unless it's otherwise indicated. Check the collection device frequently.

7. When the infant has voided, remove the collection device and diaper. Clean the skin of any adhesive that remains.

8. Prepare the specimen for transport to the laboratory or process it according to the office policy and procedure manual.

9. Remove your gloves and wash your hands.

10. Record the procedure in the patient's chart.

Preparation for Externship

It is easy to become "caught up" in office politics, even a student during externship. Some employees like to play office politics to get ahead in their position or to cause the fall or failure of another employee. You may be tempted to provide your input or opinion to employees about situations in the office. Remember you are a student, not an employee. Your involvement in the "office politics" could be harmful to your overall experience. Some employees play this "game" to get a promotion. They offer false support of individuals in order to get what they want. They will try to lure in and use the new person to build support from anyone who will buy into this scheme. Remember that good relationships are developed from trust and respect, not lies to gain an advantage over others. Avoid the trap of office politics and don't play the game.

Chapter Recap

- Urinalysis helps the physician determine or rule out conditions to make a correct diagnosis.
- The medical assistant's role is to assist in the collection of uncontaminated, quality specimens and to perform reagent strip screening and confirmation tests on patients' urine.
- Clean-catch midstream urine collection is the most common method for collecting a urine specimen.

- Physical examination of urine includes observation of color and clarity and measuring specific gravity.
- Chemical tests include determining the urine's pH and checking for glucose, ketones, proteins, blood, bilirubin, urobilinogen, nitrites, and leukocytes in the specimen.
- Medical assistants also may prepare specimens for urine sediment exams.

- Urine sediment is examined under a microscope by a highly trained professional for things such as blood cells and casts, epithelial cells, bacteria, crystals, and other structures.
- Urine also may be tested to determine pregnancy and the presence of certain drugs in the body.

Online Resources for Students

Student Resources available on the text's online site include:
- Audio Glossaries
- Animations
- Competency Evaluation Forms

- Videos
- Anatomy & Physiology Module with Heart and Lung Sounds
- Weblinks
- Worksheets

Exercises and Activities

Certification Preparation Questions

1. The term postprandial refers to:

   a. the urine test performed after blood glucose testing.
   b. the first morning urine specimen.
   c. a fasting urine specimen.
   d. a urine specimen 2 hours after eating a meal.
   e. a random collected urine specimen.

2. The preferred specimen to perform a C&S is:

   a. a random collection.
   b. 24-hour collection.
   c. a clean-catch midstream collection.
   d. a first morning specimen.
   e. a postprandial specimen.

3. Which of these would be appropriate instructions for a patient who needs to collect a 24-hour urine?

   a. Drink more fluid than you usually would to increase your urine production.
   b. Stop all medications until you have completed the urine collection.
   c. Keep the collection container at room temperature.
   d. On day 1 of the collection, empty your bladder is first thing in the morning but discard the specimen.
   e. Urinate directly into the container.

4. The normal specific gravity range is:

   a. 1.000 to 1.010.
   b. 1.003 to 1.035.
   c. 1.005 to 1.050.
   d. 1.010 to 1.100.
   e. 1.020 to 1.115.

5. Which of these is a normal pH reading of urine?

   a. 3.5
   b. 4.5
   c. 6.0
   d. 8.5
   e. 9.0

6. The term glycosuria is used to describe:

   a. diabetes insipidus.
   b. high blood sugar.
   c. glucose in the urine.
   d. renal threshold.
   e. glucose in the blood and urine.

7. What is the chemical that is formed when fat is metabolized in the body?

   a. Acetone
   b. Albumin
   c. Bilirubin
   d. Ketones
   e. Protein

8. Casts are formed in the:
   a. bladder.
   b. ureters.
   c. nephron.
   d. urethra.
   e. renal pelvis.

9. Uric acid crystals are associated with:
   a. hematuria.
   b. gout.
   c. diabetes.
   d. infection.
   e. liver disease.

10. The ideal specimen for a urine pregnancy is a:
    a. 24-hour specimen.
    b. clean-catch midstream.
    c. first morning.
    d. random.
    e. postprandial.

28 | Clinical Chemistry

Chapter Objectives

- Explain the purpose of performing clinical chemistry tests.
- List the common panels of chemistry tests.
- List the instruments used for chemical testing.
- List tests used to evaluate renal function.
- List the common electrolytes and explain the relationship of electrolytes to body function.
- Describe the nonprotein nitrogenous compounds and name conditions associated with abnormal values.
- Describe the substances commonly tested in liver function assessment.
- Explain thyroid function and identify the hormone that regulates the thyroid gland.
- Describe how laboratory tests help assess for a myocardial infarction.
- Describe how pancreatitis is diagnosed with laboratory tests.
- Explain how the body uses and regulates glucose and summarize the purpose of the major glucose tests.
- Determine a patient's blood glucose level.
- Perform glucose tolerance testing.
- Describe the function of cholesterol and other lipids and their correlation to heart disease.

CAAHEP & ABHES Competencies

CAAHEP

- Perform patient screening using established protocols.
- Obtain specimens and perform CLIA-waived chemistry tests.
- Differentiate between normal and abnormal test results.
- Reassure a patient of the accuracy of the test results.

ABHES

- Practice quality control.
- Perform selected CLIA-waived chemistry tests that assist with diagnosis and treatment.
- Collect, label, and process specimens.

Chapter Terms

Bilirubin
Electrolytes
Hyperkalemia

Hypernatremia
Hyperuricemia
Hypocalcemia

Hypochloremia
Hypoglycemia
Hypokalemia

Hyponatremia
Nitrogenous

Abbreviations

ALT	CK	HbA1C	POL
ALP	CMP	HCO$_3$	PP
AST	FBS	HDL	TSH
BUN	GTT	LDL	

Case Study

Donna Rogers is a 49-year-old patient who was recently diagnosed with prediabetes. She is returning to the clinic today because the physician asked her to schedule to have a complete physical exam.

Anna, the medical assistant, is completing the vital signs for the patient getting her ready to see the physician.

Blood chemistry tests measure important substances in the body. These tests are valuable tools in helping health care providers assess a patient's state of health.

Knowing the amount of various chemical substances in the body helps the provider in two ways:

- It helps assess the function of certain organs. For example, knowing the level of bilirubin in a patient's blood helps show how well the patient's liver is functioning.
- It helps gain a better understanding of the patient's overall health status. For example, knowing a patient's glucose and cholesterol levels can help the physician evaluate the patient's health.

Although most chemistry tests are referred to outside labs for processing, this testing increasingly is being done in physician office labs. Several chemistry tests are CLIA waived and can therefore be performed by medical assistants. No matter where the chemistry tests ordered in your office are performed, you need to have a good general knowledge of these important tests and what their results can mean.

THE SCOPE AND PURPOSE OF CLINICAL CHEMISTRY

Clinical chemistry is laboratory testing for many of the chemical substances found in the body. This is determined by analyzing the following fluids:

- Serum
- Plasma
- Whole blood
- Body fluids that collect in the body's cavities

The chemical substances found in these fluids exist in several different forms. These include the following:

- Electrically charged atoms are called ions; ions are chemical elements that carry an electrical charge, for example, K$^+$, potassium; Na$^+$, sodium; and Cl$^-$, chloride.
- By-products of the body's metabolic processes, for example, urea and creatinine.
- Proteins such as albumin and globulin.
- Hormones including testosterone and thyroid-stimulating hormone (TSH).

Tests and Testing Methods

A large number of chemistry tests can be performed using blood collected either by venipuncture or by skin puncture. Many of these tests are grouped according to body system. These groups of tests are called panels or profiles. An example of a commonly ordered panel is the comprehensive metabolic panel (**CMP**). Panels of chemistry tests can evaluate the following:

- Renal (kidney) function
- Liver function
- Thyroid function

Case Questions

The patient asks Anna why the complete physical exam is necessary because she is really not sick. How should Anna respond to the patient's question? Why is the physician requesting a complete physical on the patient?

- Cardiac function
- Pancreatic function
- Levels of lipids and lipoproteins

Specimen collection, reporting, and follow-up of patient care are critical aspects of your role as a medical assistant. This information directly impacts the patient's treatment and recovery.

Only a few specific tests are performed in the physician office lab (**POL**). However, you must have a basic understanding of all the tests performed at the reference lab so that you can basically understand the lab reports and which results are out of the normal range. You should know what abnormal results may mean for the patient. Plus, you must understand the purpose of those chemistry tests that are conducted in the POL.

Instruments and Methods of Testing

The spectrophotometer is still widely used for measuring various substances in a patient's blood. This is an instrument that measures light in a solution to determine the concentration of substances in it. Color formation or color changes result when certain chemical substances react with other chemicals. By measuring the change in the intensity of the color, the concentration of the substance can be determined.

Reference laboratories use automated systems to perform much of the chemical analysis. These systems mechanically sample, dilute, or add reagents (chemicals) to the patient's blood to measure the chemical substances in it. Automation has many benefits, including:

- Fast test results
- Less operator error
- Controlled testing costs because of less need for human involvement

Remember, the normal ranges for results stated in this chapter may vary from lab to lab because of differences of the various substances on which a chemical acts and temperatures and instruments that may be used in testing.

TESTS FOR RENAL FUNCTION

The kidneys rid the body of waste products. They also help maintain fluid balance and acid–base balance. Acid–base balance is the balance between acid and base (alkaline) in the body.

When the kidneys begin to fail, waste products, such as urea, ammonia, and creatinine, build up in the blood. As a result, the patient may develop edema (swelling due to excess fluid), and the delicate acid–base balance is upset. Abnormal increases or decreases in the substances that affect acid–base balance can harm a patient's health. In some cases, the patient could die.

The physician evaluates renal or kidney function by ordering tests to measure levels of electrolytes, blood urea nitrogen (**BUN**), creatinine, and uric acid. Based on the results of these tests, along with urinalysis, the physician can assess renal function.

Electrolytes

Electrolytes are ions in blood and body fluids. Ions are chemicals that carry an electrical charge. They may have a positive charge or a negative charge. Positively charged ions are called cations, and negatively charged ions are anions. Electrolytes exist in both intracellular (inside cells) and extracellular (outside cells) fluid. The electrolytes found in the blood include the following:

- Sodium
- Potassium
- Chloride
- Calcium
- Magnesium
- Phosphorus
- Bicarbonate (dissolved carbon dioxide)

The renal system helps regulate electrolytes as well as fluid and acid–base balance. If the electrolytes are out of balance, electrical impulses cannot be properly transmitted. The results are fluid and acid–base imbalances and poor functioning of the nervous and muscle tissue.

Sodium

Sodium (Na) is the major cation of the body's extracellular fluid (the fluid outside the cell). Normal serum levels of sodium range from 135 to 145 mEq/L. When sodium levels are below 135 mEq/L, the patient has a condition called **hyponatremia**. This is one of the most common electrolyte imbalances. Hyponatremia can result from many things:

- Gastrointestinal losses (vomiting and diarrhea)
- Severe burns
- Cardiac failure
- Renal failure
- Hypothyroidism (underactive thyroid)

Symptoms of hyponatremia vary depending on how severe the condition is but may include changes in energy levels and seizures. **Hypernatremia** occurs when a patient's sodium levels are above the normal 145 mEq/L level. Drug therapy, Cushing syndrome, and diabetes insipidus are among the causes of hypernatremia.

Potassium

Potassium (K) is the major cation of the body's intracellular fluid, the fluid inside the cell. Because only 2%

of potassium is extracellular, its serum levels are much lower than the sodium serum levels. The normal range for potassium is 3.5 to 5.0 mEq/L. Abnormal levels of potassium in the blood can cause the following:

- Muscle weakness and cramping
- Paralysis
- Cardiac arrhythmias (abnormal heart rhythms)

A serum potassium level below the normal level of 3.5 mEq/L is called **hypokalemia**. This condition can occur because of:

- Insulin therapy
- Gastrointestinal losses
- Renal disease

When a patient's potassium level is above 5.0 mEq/L, the result is known as **hyperkalemia**. Abnormally high potassium levels can be caused by:

- Cell injuries
- Renal failure

A high potassium level may also be due to an artifact caused by outside interference such as a traumatic venipuncture, hemolysis of red blood cells (RBCs), or if the tourniquet is on the patient's arm too long or too tightly applied when blood is being drawn.

Chloride

Chloride (Cl–) is the major anion of the extracellular fluid. The normal range for chloride is 96 to 110 mEq/L. Chloride is necessary to help maintain the body's acid–base balance. In conditions such as diabetic ketoacidosis (high blood glucose caused by a lack of insulin) and metabolic acidosis (increased metabolic acids), a patient's chloride level can become abnormal.

The body normally loses chloride in urine, sweat, and stomach secretions. However, a serum chloride level that drops below 96 mEq/L is known as **hypochloremia**. This condition can occur from heavy sweating, vomiting, and renal failure, as well as several other conditions or diseases. Extremely low chloride levels can be fatal to a patient.

A patient with a serum chloride level above 110 mEq/L has a condition known as hyperchloremia. Dehydration and diarrhea also can cause this condition, as can a number of medications and gastrointestinal and metabolic problems.

Calcium

Calcium (Ca) is another cation. Normal Ca levels in blood range from 8.5 to 10.5 mg/dL.

Serum calcium levels significantly below the normal level of 8.5 mg/dL are known as **hypocalcemia**. This condition can occur as a result of acute or chronic renal

failure or electrolyte imbalance due to hypoparathyroidism, underactive parathyroid glands.

Patients with hypercalcemia have calcium levels that are above 10.5 mg/dL. Hypercalcemia can occur in a patient with hyperparathyroidism. It also can occur if a patient has absorbed excessive amounts of calcium because of a medication he is taking or because of a change in gastrointestinal metabolism.

Magnesium

Magnesium (Mg) is a cation found in intracellular fluid. The normal levels in blood are from 1.3 to 2.1 mEq/L. Hypomagnesemia occurs when a patient's serum magnesium level is below 1.3 mEq/L. This condition may result from shifts in body fluids and other electrolytes.

Hypermagnesemia, or serum magnesium levels above 2.1 mEq/L, also can result from fluid and electrolyte shifts, as well as from impaired excretion of fluids caused by kidney failure. The symptoms of hypermagnesemia and hyperkalemia (high levels of serum potassium) are similar. Cardiac arrhythmia may be a symptom of either hypomagnesemia or hypermagnesemia.

Phosphorus

In the intracellular fluid, phosphorus (P) is a major anion. The normal range for phosphorus levels in blood is from 2.5 to 4.5 mg/dL. Hypophosphatemia, levels below 2.5 mg/dL, can occur in patients for a number of reasons, including:

- Inadequate absorption by the intestines of phosphorus consumed in food
- Gastrointestinal losses, for example, through severe diarrhea
- Electrolyte shifts between the blood and cells
- Endocrine disorders
- The withdrawal process from alcohol abuse

Hyperphosphatemia, serum phosphorus levels above 4.5 mg/dL, can happen when patients experience the following:

- Hypocalcemia
- Hypoparathyroidism
- Renal damage or failure

In patients with renal failure, soft tissue calcification (hardening) is a long-term effect of hyperphosphatemia.

Bicarbonate

In the blood, bicarbonate (HCO_3) occurs when carbon dioxide dissolves in the bloodstream. The bicarbonate forms another negatively charged ion in the extracellular fluid. The normal bicarbonate range is 22 to

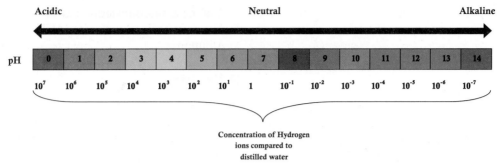

Figure 28-1   pH scale. (Image from Shutterstock.)

29 mmol/L of total CO_2. Bicarbonate plays a major role in the delicate acid–base balance. If bicarbonate levels are increased, the patient develops alkalosis, a condition when the pH is too basic (alkaline). If bicarbonate levels are decreased, the patient develops acidosis, pH is too acidic.

As you've already read, the acid–base balance in the body is very sensitive. The body can't tolerate large changes in pH. Normally, the pH range is 7.35 to 7.45, which is slightly basic. Figure 28-1 is a pH scale that demonstrates the acid and alkaline levels. Notice the 7.0 neutral reading on the scale. The pH of blood is slightly above that level and cannot become too acidic or too alkaline (basic).

Together, the renal and respiratory systems work to regulate the body's acid–base balance. In the renal system, bicarbonate is excreted through the kidneys. In the respiratory system, bicarbonate is exhaled in the form of carbon dioxide. Measuring carbon dioxide is another way to evaluate pH balance. It can also help the physician evaluate overall renal function.

Nonprotein Nitrogenous Compounds

In addition to measuring electrolytes, physicians also may measure three nonprotein nitrogenous compounds to help assess renal function. **Nitrogenous** means relating to, or containing, nitrogen.

When renal function is compromised, urea, creatinine, and uric acid can build up in the blood. However, other conditions also can affect the concentrations of these substances. For this reason, measuring the levels of nonprotein nitrogenous compounds in the blood isn't an absolute indicator of renal function.

Blood Urea Nitrogen

Urea is a waste product that forms in the liver. It's the major end product of protein and amino acid metabolism. The body rids itself of urea by excreting it from the kidneys. Because both the liver and the kidneys process urea, measuring urea levels can tell the physician how the liver and kidneys are functioning.

Urea is usually measured by a chemistry test called BUN, which stands for blood urea nitrogen. The normal range for urea levels in the blood is 10 to 20 mg/dL.

Renal function and liver function aren't the only factors that affect BUN levels. Dietary intake of protein and a patient's level of hydration also affect the BUN level. In acute kidney conditions, the BUN increases before creatinine increases.

Creatinine

Creatinine is the waste product of creatine. Creatine is a chemical compound in the body that's used to store energy. When creatine is used, creatinine forms. While normal values vary somewhat among labs, the generally accepted normal range for creatinine in the blood is 0.8 to 1.4 mg/dL.

Measuring the creatinine present in a patient's blood is actually a better and more specific way to evaluate renal function than the BUN. Here's why. Only trace amounts of creatinine are reabsorbed by the renal system. So the urinary excretion of creatinine is about equal to the amount produced in the body. Urea, on the other hand, is reabsorbed to a certain extent, making it a less reliable indicator of renal function.

Uric Acid

Uric acid, excreted by the kidneys, is a by-product of protein metabolism in the blood. For men, the normal range is 3.5 to 7.2 mg/dL. For women, it's 2.6 to 6.0 mg/dL. Increased amounts of uric acid in the blood are more threatening than decreased amounts.

Hyperuricemia (uric acid levels above the normal range) can occur when a patient experiences renal failure. High uric acid levels are also found in patients undergoing chemotherapy for leukemias and other cancers.

Diets high in proteins (meat, legumes, and yeast) also can cause mild hyperuricemia. Such diets can aggravate a disease called gout, especially if they include food high in a group of amino acids called purines. All meats, fish, and poultry contain purines. But high amounts are found in organ meats like liver, kidney, or brain, as

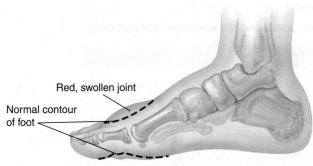

Figure 28-2 Gout of the foot. (Reprinted from Kronenberger J, Ledbetter J. *Jones & Bartlett Learning's Comprehensive Medical Assisting.* 5th ed. Burlington, MA: Jones & Bartlett Learning, LLC; 2016.)

well as in seafood like scallops, shrimp, and anchovies. Figure 28-2 shows the place in the foot where patients may first notice the pain and symptoms of gout.

Cultural Connection

When physicians are treating various conditions that are caused by chemical imbalance within the body, the patient may be prescribed a specific diet, which will add or eliminate certain foods. For example, to treat gout, caused by an increased amount of uric acid crystals, may require a patient to cut back on their intake of alcohol or meat and fish that are high in chemicals called purines. In certain cultures, these foods may be part of the traditional, cultural diet that the patient is unwilling to give up. If the medical assistant is asked to provide the patient with diet education, it is important to first understand the patient's beliefs and culture. It is necessary to provide realistic alternatives to the patient's diet in order to obtain compliance.

TESTS FOR LIVER FUNCTION

The liver is the largest and most complex glands in the body. Some of its major functions include the following:

- The production of bile (the bitter yellow-green secretion of the liver that's stored in the gallbladder)
- The metabolism of many compounds used by the body
- The processing of bilirubin
- Detoxifying substances in the blood

To help evaluate liver function, these tests are commonly performed:

- Bilirubin
- Alkaline phosphatase (**ALP**)
- Alanine aminotransferase (**ALT**)
- Aspartate aminotransferase (**AST**)
- Albumin

Bilirubin

Bilirubin is an amber-colored substance that's produced as a by-product of hemoglobin breakdown. If too much bilirubin settles into the skin and sclera, the patient appears amber, or jaundiced. Bilirubin causes many newborns to appear jaundiced, or yellow, a few days after birth. Often, a newborn's liver isn't developed enough to remove bilirubin from the blood.

Bilirubin is frequently measured, along with liver enzymes present in the blood, to determine the health of the liver. The liver's ability to filter it from the blood is one of the first functions lost in many liver diseases. That's why elevated levels of bilirubin in a patient's blood or urine can be a sign of early liver disease. Bilirubin can be broken down by fluorescent light or sunlight. Any specimen (blood or urine) that will be tested for bilirubin must be protected from exposure to light.

Liver Enzymes

An enzyme is a protein produced by living cells that speeds up chemical reactions. Three of the enzymes present in the liver are alkaline phosphatase (ALP), alanine aminotransferase (ALT), and aspartate aminotransferase (AST). Most of the ALP circulating in the blood is from the liver and bone. High levels are considered normal during periods of bone growth such as childhood growth spurts and during the third trimester of pregnancy. ALT and AST are associated with damage to the heart or liver and can result in increased levels of ALT and AST in the blood.

Albumin

Albumin testing is also part of many liver profiles. Albumin is the smallest and most plentiful of the blood proteins. It binds and transports substances in the blood. Albumin also helps to maintain fluid balance in the body's tissues. Decreased levels of albumin can be due to several factors:

- Malnutrition and muscle-wasting diseases
- Liver disease that makes the liver cells unable to produce albumin
- Excessive loss in urine due to renal disease
- Inflammation of the intestinal tract
- Burns

Testing for Drug-Related Liver Damage

One of the liver's functions is detoxification. With most substances, the liver performs this function with little or no ill effects. Occasionally, drugs or the products of drug breakdown can have harmful effects on the liver.

The physician can detect this damage by measuring enzymes (AST, ALT, and ALP) released into the blood. The greater the damage to the liver, the higher the blood levels of these enzymes will be.

Small elevations in these enzymes may be acceptable if the drug is helping the patient. The dose may be adjusted or the drug stopped while the physician weighs its benefits against the risk of possible harm to the liver. The physician may look for another drug instead, in hopes of reducing or eliminating the harmful effects.

With certain drugs, the patient's enzyme levels must be monitored throughout the course of the treatment. Checking them once is not enough. That's because a drug may be tolerated for a period of time with no increase in enzymes. Then, suddenly, the cumulative effects of taking the drug will result in a sudden increase in enzyme levels.

TESTS FOR THYROID FUNCTION

The thyroid gland regulates the body's metabolism by secreting two hormones—triiodothyronine and thyroxine. The thyroid gland itself is controlled by another hormone, called thyroid-stimulating hormone (**TSH**). This hormone is produced in the anterior pituitary gland, located at the base of the brain.

When no disease is present and additional thyroid hormones are needed, the anterior pituitary gland secretes more TSH to stimulate the thyroid gland. When lesser amounts of the hormones are required, the anterior pituitary gland secretes less TSH. Less TSH causes the thyroid gland to reduce its production of the other hormones.

When the anterior pituitary gland malfunctions, it creates an oversecretion or an undersecretion of TSH. If the thyroid gland isn't working properly, it can't be stimulated no matter how much TSH is secreted. In cases such as these, TSH levels may be very high. In addition to TSH, the tests triiodothyronine (T3) and thyroxine (T4) are commonly ordered in the investigation of thyroid problems. Figure 28-3 demonstrates the production and transport of thyroid-stimulating hormone.

TESTS FOR CARDIAC FUNCTION

When a myocardial infarction occurs, the damaged heart muscle releases large quantities of certain enzymes into the bloodstream. The two enzymes released are creatine kinase-MB and troponin.

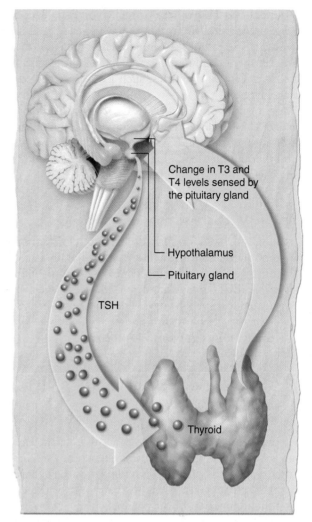

Figure 28-3 Thyroid-stimulating hormone production. (Reprinted from Kronenberger J, Ledbetter J. *Jones & Bartlett Learning's Comprehensive Medical Assisting*. 5th ed. Burlington, MA: Jones & Bartlett Learning, LLC; 2016.)

Creatine Kinase-MB

Creatine kinase (**CK**) is found in three places in the body:

- Skeletal muscle
- Myocardium (the middle layer of the walls of the heart)
- Nervous tissue (in the brain)

CK has three isoenzymes. Isoenzymes are enzymes that are chemically different but functionally the same. That means that although the isoenzymes each have their own chemical properties, they all perform the same job. The three isoenzymes of CK are called:

- MM (muscle enzyme)
- MB (heart enzyme)
- BB (brain enzyme)

When a patient has chest pain, CK-MB levels, along with total CK, are tested to determine whether the patient has had a heart attack. For 2 to 8 hours after a myocardial infarction, CK-MB levels rise and remain high for about 24 hours. They then return to normal if there is no new heart damage. CK levels also increase in crushing injuries, such as those received in car accidents.

Most of the normal levels of CK consist of the MM element. The MB level rises with myocardial infarction. A high total CK can indicate damage either to the heart or to other muscles, but a high CK-MB suggests that the damage was to heart muscle.

Troponin

Troponin, a protein specific to heart muscle, is a valuable tool in diagnosing acute myocardial infarction. Troponin levels in the blood begin to rise within 4 hours after myocardial damage has occurred. These levels may stay elevated for up to 14 days. Troponin levels are used to evaluate the extent of cardiac damage and to help the physician develop a prognosis for the patient.

TESTS FOR PANCREATIC FUNCTION

The pancreas is a gland that functions in both the endocrine system and the exocrine system and produces many secretions. Figure 28-4 is an image of the pancreas showing the pancreatic ducts that are part of the exocrine functioning part of the pancreas.

Amylase and lipase are two exocrine system products of the pancreas. They are released as enzymes into the intestines to help digestion. Insulin and glucagon, two endocrine system products of the pancreas, are

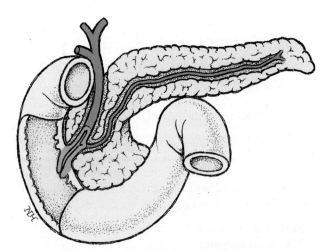

Figure 28-4 Pancreas. (Reprinted from Kronenberger J, Ledbetter J. *Jones & Bartlett Learning's Comprehensive Medical Assisting.* 5th ed. Burlington, MA: Jones & Bartlett Learning, LLC; 2016.)

released into the bloodstream to regulate carbohydrate metabolism.

Amylase and lipase levels are tested to detect pancreatitis, inflammation of the pancreas. When a patient has pancreatitis, the level of amylase in the blood increases quite a bit. The salivary glands also produce amylase, so when a patient has any of the inflammatory diseases of the salivary glands (such as mumps), the level of amylase rises as well.

Pancreatic Hormones and Carbohydrate Metabolism

Sugar has several chemical forms. One of them is glucose, a primary source of energy for the body. When the body metabolizes foods, nutrients including glucose are released into the bloodstream. Blood glucose levels must stay within narrow limits, however, or a person will experience negative physical effects. The pancreatic hormones insulin and glucagon help keep blood glucose levels within the appropriate range.

Insulin

Insulin, an important hormone, transports the glucose into the body's cells. There, it's either used for energy or stored for future use. If enough energy is available for the cells to use, the extra glucose is stored as glycogen in the liver and muscles, or as fat. Glycogen is the stored form of glucose. Cells starve if insulin isn't available or if they can't bring glucose in for energy. Also, by helping with glucose storage, insulin keeps blood glucose levels down. The result is that the body is able to maintain a stable normal range of glucose.

Glucagon

Glucagon is the hormone that stimulates the release of glycogen. Whenever blood glucose levels drop, the glucagon acts on the glycogen. It breaks it apart so that molecules of glucose are available for the cells to use. As a result, blood glucose levels rise again.

Common Glucose Tests

There are several tests a physician can order to determine how well the body's glucose metabolism system is working. These tests include the following:

- Random blood glucose. The specimen can be drawn at any time. The normal result is 60 to 126 mg/dL. Although this test isn't as useful as a fasting blood sugar, it is a good screening tool.
- Fasting blood sugar (**FBS**). A blood glucose level is obtained following an 8- to 12-hour fast in which the patient ingests nothing but water.

- Two-hour postprandial glucose (**PP**). A blood sample is drawn 2 hours after a meal and the glucose level is measured.
- Glucose tolerance test (**GTT**). Blood glucose levels are checked at intervals after the patient takes a large dose of glucose.

Fasting Blood Sugar

The main purpose of determining a fasting glucose level is to detect either diabetes mellitus (usually just called diabetes) or **hypoglycemia** (very low blood sugar). This test can be performed in the medical office or by the patient at home, using a glucose meter. Figure 28-5 shows various blood glucose monitoring systems that are CLIA waived for medical office or home use.

The American Diabetes Association established a cutoff point for normal fasting blood glucose levels at 100 mg/dL. A result of 100 to 125 mg/dL indicates a condition called prediabetes. This means the person has higher-than-normal glucose levels, but not high enough to diagnose diabetes. A diagnosis of diabetes requires the fasting blood glucose of 126 mg/dL or above. Studies show that many people with prediabetes develop diabetes within 10 years.

A 2-hour PP or a GTT is often performed to confirm a high FBS result. A GTT is also used to diagnose hypoglycemia. Hypoglycemia is characterized by FBS levels below 45 mg/dL. A number of symptoms are associated with very low blood glucose levels. These symptoms include the following:

- Sweating
- Weakness
- Dizziness
- Headache
- Trembling
- Lethargy

Two-Hour Postprandial Glucose

The purpose of the 2-hour PP is to screen patients for diabetes and to monitor insulin therapy of diabetic patients. Before the test, the patient must first fast for 12 hours and then eat a high-carbohydrate meal. As a substitute for the meal, patients may drink a glucose solution instead. The standard glucose drink for this test contains 100 g of glucose. The patient can eat exactly 300 g of spaghetti, rice, baked potato, or 150 g of white bread. This is equivalent to about 75 g of sugar. Then, 2 hours later, a blood sample is drawn and the patient's glucose level is measured. Correct timing of the blood collection is extremely important in this test. "Good control" of diabetes is defined by a 2-hour PP value of <140 mg/dL.

Glucose Tolerance Test

The GTT is used to diagnose diabetes and hypoglycemia. The patient ingests a large dose of glucose. Then, blood glucose levels are checked at 30 minutes and 1, 2, and 3 hours after the glucose has been ingested. This checks how the body is metabolizing the glucose. The GTT begins only after a fasting glucose is performed to ensure the initial level is not too high. Figure 28-6 is a chart that demonstrates the pattern of glucose readings based on various blood glucose conditions from normal to severe diabetes.

As in a 2-hour PP, the blood samples must be drawn at the exact times for the diagnosis to be valid. A serum or plasma specimen can be collected, depending on what the lab requires. It's also possible that urine specimens may be collected from the patient during the timed intervals.

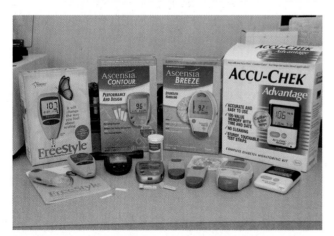

Figure 28-5 Various glucose meters. (Reprinted from Kronenberger J, Ledbetter J. *Jones & Bartlett Learning's Comprehensive Medical Assisting.* 5th ed. Burlington, MA: Jones & Bartlett Learning, LLC; 2016.)

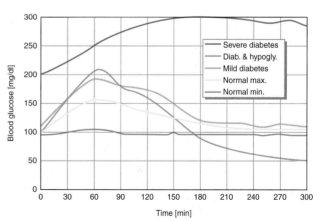

Figure 28-6 Blood glucose chart of GTT testing by disease severity. (Reprinted from Kronenberger J, Ledbetter J. *Jones & Bartlett Learning's Comprehensive Medical Assisting.* 5th ed. Burlington, MA: Jones & Bartlett Learning, LLC; 2016.)

The blood specimens should be centrifuged and separated as soon as possible to prevent the red blood cells from metabolizing the glucose. However, specimens that are collected in gray stopper tubes containing sodium fluoride are stable for up to 3 days even without centrifuging.

Hypoglycemia may also be diagnosed by the GTT, but the test may be extended by additional blood collections at 4, 5, and 6 hours after the glucose was ingested. The patient must be observed carefully for any signs of hypoglycemia.

Unfortunately, a glucose level that's lower than the normal range often does not correspond to the patient's symptoms. The patient's emotional state or level of anxiety, not low glucose levels, may cause the symptoms. Frequently, these same patients improve when their food intake is divided so that they eat many small meals rather than several large ones. This way, smaller glucose loads are introduced to the body.

As a medical assistant, you won't interpret the results of the GTT; however, the National Diabetes Data Group and the World Health Organization proposed criteria that are endorsed by the American Diabetes Association. These criteria recommend a diagnosis of diabetes if the fasting glucose level is >110 mg/dL and the 2-hour measurement is equal to or above 155 mg/dL.

Diabetic Glucose Testing

Blood glucose levels are used to monitor diabetic patients as well as to diagnose diabetes. The preferred test for monitoring patients already known to have diabetes is the hemoglobin A1C test. The normal glycated hemoglobin (**HbA1C**) is <6.5%. The ideal HbA1C for a known diabetic is <7%.

The hemoglobin A1C test measures the average amount of glucose that's been circulating in the patient's blood over a 3-month period.

Obstetric Glucose Testing

Some pregnant patients have increased glucose intolerance in their second and third trimesters. A pregnant patient's glucose level must be monitored because gestational diabetes can endanger the fetus. Gestational diabetes occurs during pregnancy when a woman's body is not metabolizing carbohydrates properly. Usually, this happens because the patient develops an insulin deficiency. This condition usually disappears after delivery.

The most common way to screen a pregnant patient for gestational diabetes is to have her drink a 50 g glucose load and then draw her blood 1 hour later. This test is usually performed during the second trimester. If the test result shows a blood glucose level over 155 mg/dL, a GTT is ordered to confirm a diagnosis of gestational diabetes.

Patient Education

The medical assistant may be required to educate patients on the use of a glucose meter. Diabetic patients often have to monitor their own glucose levels at home. You can help them understand the procedure so they can perform it at home accurately and without difficulty. You should help the patient get familiar with the glucose meter. Instruct the patient to closely follow all the manufacturer's instructions. Most pharmacies and medical supply stores that sell glucose meters also teach patients how to use them. When instructing patients, stress the following points:

- Make sure patients understand the need to test and document their glucose levels regularly. Help them understand why this is so important.
- Following the manufacturer's instructions, instruct patients how to maintain a quality control record for their meters. Demonstrate by using the control materials provided by the manufacturer. Remind patients to pay attention to the expiration date on the control materials.
- Explain the proper technique for getting a blood sample—for example, cleansing the area well before the fingerstick and not milking the finger afterward.
- Caution patients not to self-regulate their glucose levels with insulin. Tell them to call the physician if glucose levels are abnormal.
- Make sure patients know the signs and symptoms of high and low glucose levels and the treatments for each.

Tests for Lipids and Lipoproteins

To assess the risk for heart disease, a physician orders tests to measure the amounts of the following substances present in a patient's blood:

- Cholesterol
- Lipids (free fatty acids)
- Lipoproteins (substances made up of lipids and proteins)

While these compounds have been associated with heart disease for a long time, they're also important building blocks of our bodies. They're part of every cell membrane and of the myelin sheath around the nerves. They also cushion and support organs. The key is that these compounds exist in the body in proper quantities.

Cholesterol

Although we usually associate cholesterol as a bad thing, it actually performs important body functions.

Only when cholesterol exceeds the levels necessary for cell maintenance and other body functions should it be considered a health hazard. Here are just some of the ways that cholesterol is important:

- Cholesterol helps form bile acids that are produced in the liver and stored in the gallbladder. These bile acids are released into the intestine for the digestion of fats.
- Vitamin D is formed from cholesterol at the skin's surface during exposure to sunlight.
- Various hormones, such as cortisol, testosterone, and estrogen, are synthesized from cholesterol.

The American Heart Association recommends that the cholesterol level in the blood be <200 mg/dL. Anyone with a level above 200 mg/dL is considered to be at an increased risk for developing atherosclerosis. Figure 28-7 is a cholesterol meter that is CLIA waived for use in the physician's office.

This condition involves the buildup of fatty plaque on the interior lining of arteries, causing the arteries to narrow and harden.

Low-Density Lipoprotein

Low-density lipoprotein (**LDL**) is a protein found in blood plasma that carries cholesterol from the liver to the walls of large- and medium-sized arteries. LDL is commonly referred to as the "bad cholesterol." Sometimes,

the fatty plaque of atherosclerosis builds up in the arteries. This narrows and thickens the affected vessel and it becomes more rigid. Another result is reduced circulation to the organs and other areas normally supplied by these arteries.

Atherosclerosis is the major cause of coronary heart disease, angina pectoris (chest pain due to a lack of oxygen to the heart), myocardial infarction, and other cardiac illnesses. The risk for heart disease increases when LDL values are above the normal range. Normal levels of LDL are <100 mg/dL. Levels above 129 mg/dL are considered borderline high, and any figure above 159 mg/dL can be dangerously high.

High-Density Lipoprotein

High-density lipoprotein (**HDL**) is the protein molecule that carries cholesterol from the walls of the arteries back to the liver. HDL is commonly referred to as the "good cholesterol." Usually, HDL levels are lower than those for LDL. In men, average HDL levels range from 40 to 50 mg/dL. For women, the average is 50 to 60 mg/dL.

Researchers have been investigating whether there's a way to increase HDL, because higher levels of HDL seem to lower the incidence of heart disease. Unlike LDL, that means the lower a patient's HDL level, the greater the patient's risk for heart disease. Therefore, with HDL, higher levels are better.

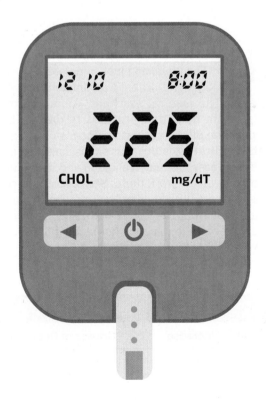
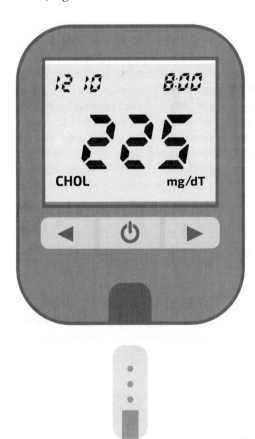

Figure 28-7 Cholesterol meter. (Image from Shutterstock.)

Triglycerides

Triglycerides store energy and are located in adipose (fatty) tissue and muscle. These lipids are released and metabolized between meals according to the body's energy demands.

Normal triglyceride levels vary according to a person's age and gender. However, in general, the level should be <150 mg/dL. Research has identified high triglyceride levels (200 mg/dL or more) as a risk factor in heart disease.

Many people with high triglycerides can bring down their levels through weight loss, regular exercise, and diet. They should limit their intake of carbohydrates to not more than 50% of their total calories. This is because carbohydrates raise triglycerides in some people and lower HDL cholesterol.

Helping Ensure Accurate Lipid Measurements

The medical assistant can help ensure that the most accurate test results are provided for the patient and the physician. Many factors can affect the results of a lipid profile. To a large extent, neither you nor the laboratory can control these factors, but there are some things you can do to help reduce factors that can affect the results:

- Make sure the patient has not performed vigorous physical activity in the 24 hours before testing. Lipids and lipoproteins should be measured only when the patient is in a steady metabolic state.
- Ask the patient to remain seated, resting for at least 5 minutes before the blood is drawn.
- Verify that the patient has maintained his usual diet and weight for at least 2 weeks before the test.
- Fasting or nonfasting specimens can be used for total cholesterol testing but a 12-hour fasting specimen is required for triglycerides and lipoproteins. Make sure you know which type of specimen you need.
- Total cholesterol, triglyceride, and HDL concentrations can be determined in either serum or plasma. Heparin is the preferred anticoagulant if plasma is to be used, avoid EDTA additive tubes.

CHEMISTRY PANEL TESTS

This chapter has presented the basics of clinical chemistry testing. This is a lot of information to remember but the best way to digest it is to recap the key points into a chart. Table 28-1 lists the common chemistry panel tests and the body function it evaluates. The normal values are provided; however, these values may vary from lab to lab depending on the equipment used to perform the test. The table also includes some of the causes when the value is increased or decreased.

Case Question

Remember our patient, Donna Rogers? The physician just completed her physical and ordered a complete metabolic panel. The medical assistant, Anna, returns to the exam room and prepares to draw a blood specimen on the patient for the test. Donna tells the medical assistant that she is confused about the unnecessary medical exam and now she has to have blood work done. She asks the medical assistant how the complete metabolic panel is different from the blood work she had done a few weeks ago to check her blood glucose. How would you answer her question?

Table 28-1	Common Chemistry Panel Tests				
Test	**Body Function**	**Normal Value**	**Causes of Increase**	**Causes of Decrease**
BUN	Metabolic by-product	10–20 mg/dL	Kidney disease, kidney obstruction, dehydration	Liver failure, malnutrition
Calcium	Structural element for bones, teeth, muscles	8.5–10.5 mg/dL	Hyperparathyroidism, hyperthyroidism, Addison disease, bone cancer, multiple myeloma, other malignancies	Hypoparathyroidism, renal failure

Table 28-1	Common Chemistry Panel Tests (*continued*)			
Test	**Body Function**	**Normal Value**	**Causes of Increase**	**Causes of Decrease**
Chloride	Acid–base balance, component of stomach acid	96–110 mEq/L	Dehydration, Cushing syndrome, hyperventilation	Severe vomiting, severe diarrhea, severe burn, pyloric obstruction, heat exhaustion
Cholesterol	Building block for cell membranes, steroid hormones, bile acids	120–200 mg/dL	Atherosclerosis, heart disease, certain liver diseases with obstruction, hypothyroidism	Liver disease, hyperthyroidism, malabsorption syndrome
Creatinine	Metabolic by-product	0.8–1.4 mg/dL	Kidney disease, muscle disease	Muscular dystrophy
Glucose	Energy source	60–100 mg/dL	Diabetes mellitus, Cushing syndrome, liver disease	Excessive insulin, Addison disease, bacterial sepsis, hypothyroidism
Phosphorus	Used in bone, endocrine processes	2.5–4.5 mg/dL	Renal disease, hypoparathyroidism, hypocalcemia, Addison disease	Hyperparathyroidism, bone disease
Potassium	Acid–base balance	3.5–5.0 mEq/L	Kidney disease, cell damage, Addison disease	Diarrhea, starvation, severe vomiting, severe burn, some liver diseases
Sodium	Fluid balance	135–145 mEq/L	Dehydration, Cushing syndrome, diabetes insipidus	Severe burns, diarrhea, vomiting, Addison disease
Triglycerides	Energy source; lipid deposits for stored energy, organ support	Men: 40–160 mg/dL Women: 35–135 mg/dL	Atherosclerosis, liver disease, poorly controlled diabetes, pancreatitis	Malnutrition
Uric acid	Metabolic by-product	Men: 3.5–7.2 mg/dL Women: 2.6–6.0 mg/dL	Renal failure, gout, leukemia, eclampsia	Drug therapy to lower uric acid levels

Procedure 28-1   Determining Blood Glucose

Equipment: A glucose meter, glucose reagent strips, a lancet, an alcohol pad, sterile gauze, a paper towel, an adhesive bandage, and gloves.

The purpose of the blood glucose test is to measure the level of glucose in the blood for diagnosis and treatment of hypoglycemia and hyperglycemia. Follow these steps for using a glucose meter to determine blood glucose correctly:

1. Gather the equipment and supplies.

2. Wash your hands and put on your gloves before you remove the reagent strip from the container.

3. Turn on the glucose meter and make sure that it's calibrated correctly. Otherwise, the test results may be inaccurate.

4. Remove one reagent strip, lay it on the paper towel, and recap the container. The strip is ready for testing and the paper towel serves as a disposable work surface. It will also absorb any excess blood.

5. Greet and identify the patient. Explain the procedure, and ask for and answer any questions the patient might have. Ask the patient when she last ate and document this in her chart.

6. Cleanse the puncture site (finger) with alcohol.

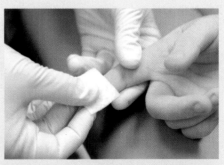

(Reprinted from Kronenberger J, Ledbetter J. *Jones & Bartlett Learning's Comprehensive Medical Assisting.* 5th ed. Burlington, MA: Jones & Bartlett Learning, LLC; 2016.)

Procedure 28-1 Determining Blood Glucose (*continued*)

7. Perform a capillary puncture. Wipe away the first drop of blood.

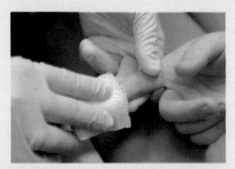

(Reprinted from Kronenberger J, Ledbetter J. *Jones & Bartlett Learning's Comprehensive Medical Assisting*. 5th ed. Burlington, MA: Jones & Bartlett Learning, LLC; 2016.)

8. Turn the patient's hand palm down and gently squeeze the finger so that a large drop of blood forms. You must squeeze gently to avoid diluting the sample with tissue fluid.

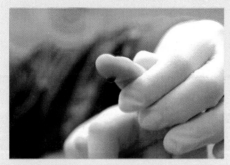

(Reprinted from Kronenberger J, Ledbetter J. *Jones & Bartlett Learning's Comprehensive Medical Assisting*. 5th ed. Burlington, MA: Jones & Bartlett Learning, LLC; 2016.)

Milk the patient's finger to get a hanging drop of blood.

9. Bring the reagent strip up to the finger and touch the strip to the blood. Make sure you don't touch the finger.

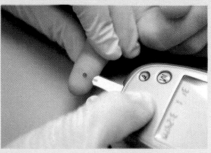

(Reprinted from Kronenberger J, Ledbetter J. *Jones & Bartlett Learning's Comprehensive Medical Assisting*. 5th ed. Burlington, MA: Jones & Bartlett Learning, LLC; 2016.)

Then, insert the reagent strip into the glucose meter. Some devices require the strip to be inserted prior to applying the drop of blood.

10. Apply pressure to the puncture wound with gauze.

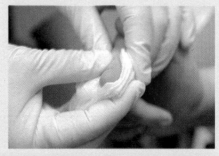

(Reprinted from Kronenberger J, Ledbetter J. *Jones & Bartlett Learning's Comprehensive Medical Assisting*. 5th ed. Burlington, MA: Jones & Bartlett Learning, LLC; 2016.)

While you are doing this, the meter will incubate the strip and measure the reaction.

11. The instrument reads the reaction strip and displays the result on the screen in milligrams per deciliter (mg/dL).

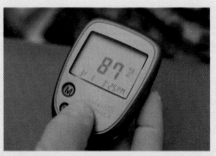

(Reprinted from Kronenberger J, Ledbetter J. *Jones & Bartlett Learning's Comprehensive Medical Assisting*. 5th ed. Burlington, MA: Jones & Bartlett Learning, LLC; 2016.)

Procedure 28-1   Determining Blood Glucose (*continued*)

If the glucose level is higher or lower than expected, review the troubleshooting guide provided by the manufacturer. Controls are available in the low, normal, and high range to ensure that the glucose meter is functioning properly. These controls should be run daily according to the manufacturer's instructions.

12. Apply a small adhesive bandage to the patient's fingertip.

13. Properly dispose the equipment and supplies. Clean your work area. Then, you can remove your gloves and wash your hands.

Note: These are generic instructions for using a glucose meter. Use the package insert to get specific instructions for the meter you are using.

Procedure 28-2   Glucose Tolerance Testing

Equipment: Calibrated amount of glucose solution per physician's order, glucose meter equipment, phlebotomy equipment, glucose test strips, alcohol wipes, a stopwatch (timer), and gloves.

The purpose of the glucose tolerance test (GTT) is to measure the body's ability to metabolize a premeasured quantity of glucose over a specified time. Follow these steps to accurately perform a glucose tolerance test:

1. Gather the following equipment and supplies. The stopwatch (timer) is particularly important because the timing of the blood collections has a direct effect on test results.

2. Greet and identify the patient. Explain the procedure, and ask for and answer any questions the patient might have. Ask the patient when he last ate and document this in his chart.

3. Wash your hands and put on your gloves.

4. Obtain a fasting glucose (FBS) specimen from the patient by venipuncture or capillary puncture. It is recommended that a lab test the fasting blood sample before the patient ingests the glucose drink.

5. If the FBS exceeds 140 mg/dL, do not proceed with the GTT. Instead, inform the physician. Giving more glucose to a patient whose blood glucose level is too high could seriously harm the patient.

6. Give the glucose drink to the patient and ask the patient to drink it all within 5 minutes. The body starts to metabolize the glucose right away, so the patient must drink rapidly.

7. Note the time the patient finishes the drink; this is the official start of the test. Keep the following things in mind during the test:

- The patient should remain mostly inactive during this procedure because exercise alters the glucose levels by increasing the body's demand for energy.
- The patient should not smoke during the test because smoking can artificially increase the glucose level.
- The patient may drink water, but only water.
- If the patient has any severe symptoms (e.g., headache, dizziness, vomiting), obtain a blood specimen at that time. Then, end the test and inform the physician. These symptoms could indicate intolerably high or low glucose levels.

8. Obtain another blood specimen exactly 30 minutes after the patient finishes the glucose drink. Label the specimen with the patient's name and time of collection. Follow the precautions listed in step 7 for the remainder of the test. The physician may want urine glucose tests done with each blood sample taken. Ask the patient to submit a urine sample after you take the blood sample. Never attempt to get the urine sample before the blood sample as it might cause you to miss the time for the blood sample. If the patient doesn't provide a urine sample, don't worry about it. Submit an empty urine cup in place or an actual urine sample and label "patient could not provide urine sample at _____ [time]." Note: It is absolutely vital to the accuracy of the test that you are precise with the timing of the blood collections. Make all proper notations so the results can be accurately interpreted.

9. Exactly 1 hour after the glucose drink, repeat step 8.

10. Exactly 2 hours after the glucose drink, repeat step 8.

Procedure 28-2 | Glucose Tolerance Testing (*continued*)

11. Exactly 3 hours after the glucose drink, repeat step 8. Unless a test longer that 3 hours has been ordered, the test is now complete. Otherwise, continue with the test for the specified period of time. Sometimes, the test can be up to 6 hours to detect hypoglycemia.

12. If the specimens are going to be tested by an outside laboratory, package them carefully and arrange for transportation.

13. Care for and dispose of your equipment and supplies. Clean your work area. Then, you can remove your gloves and wash your hands.

Preparing for Externship

As you approach your externship and completion of your medical assistant program, it is time to think about your employment as a medical assistant. Is your resume ready for your first interview? It is never too soon to start working on a professional resume, which includes your formal medical assistant training and externship experience. As you start developing your resume, think about what separates you or sets you apart from the numerous medical assistant graduates that will be in competition for the same position. What are the special qualities that you can offer the employer? Have you heard of transferrable skills? Transferrable skills transfer from one job to another job. For example, if you worked in a retail or food service environment where you had to apply customer service skills, the knowledge and techniques used for those jobs would easily transfer to working with patients in a health care setting. Providing good customer service is critical, whether in a restaurant or medical office. If you receive poor service in a restaurant, you probably will not return. Patients are no different with their health care provider. If not treated appropriately and in a timely manner, you may not see them again. The patients are the only source of income for a medical practice. A good medical practice thrives on patients. The patients need to trust the physician and staff. The physician and staff need to respect the patients. They are not just another number in the daily schedule but a person with a health problem that needs professional help. Patients are not a bother but the reason you will have and keep a job as a medical assistant.

Chapter Recap

- Blood chemistry tests measure important substances in serum, plasma, whole blood, and other body fluids.
- There are two main purposes for performing chemistry tests: (1) to evaluate organ function and (2) to have a more complete understanding of a patient's overall health. Medical assistants should know what abnormal test results may mean.
- The current trend in clinical chemistry is to refer testing to reference laboratories where large automated analyzers are used. These automated analyzers can conduct tests at a lower cost than smaller labs. But no matter where tests are performed, the results are only as good as the specimen submitted for testing.
- Clinical chemistry tests can help evaluate the following: renal/kidney function, liver function, thyroid function, cardiac function, and pancreatic function. Chemistry tests also measure the levels of lipids and lipoproteins as an indicator of the risks of heart disease.
- To evaluate renal/kidney function, tests measure electrolytes and nonprotein nitrogenous compounds in the blood.
- To assess liver function, these tests are commonly performed: bilirubin, serum albumin, alkaline phosphatase (ALP), alanine aminotransferase (ALT), and aspartate aminotransferase (AST).
- The TSH (thyroid-stimulating hormone) test is the most common test ordered to check thyroid function.
- Myocardial infarction is evaluated by testing the enzymes creatine kinase-MB (CK-MB) and troponin.

- Assessing pancreatic function includes testing for pancreatic enzymes such as amylase and lipase, as well as performing glucose tests of varying types.
- The risk of heart disease can be evaluated using the following tests as risk indicators: cholesterol, low-density lipoprotein (LDL), high-density lipoprotein (HDL), and triglycerides.

- A medical assistant must have a basic understanding of all aspects of the tests performed in the physician office lab, as well as a broad knowledge of tests sent out to larger labs for analysis. This knowledge must include the basic principles of the test, the proper sampling procedures, and the specific handling requirements for the specimen.

Online Resources for Students

Student Resources available on the text's online site include:
- Audio Glossaries
- Animations
- Competency Evaluation Forms

- Videos
- Anatomy & Physiology Module with Heart and Lung Sounds
- Weblinks
- Worksheets

Exercises and Activities

Certification Preparation Questions

1. A BUN test is used to evaluate the function of the:
   a. pancreas.
   b. thyroid.
   c. liver.
   d. kidney.
   e. pituitary gland.

2. Insulin and glucagon are hormones produced by the:
   a. kidneys.
   b. pancreas.
   c. liver.
   d. adrenal glands.
   e. thyroid.

3. The American Diabetes Association established a cutoff point for normal fasting blood glucose levels at:
   a. 45 mg/dL.
   b. 50 mg/dL.
   c. 75 mg/dL.
   d. 100 mg/dL.
   e. 120 mg/dL.

4. Hypokalemia is a term to describe a very low level of:
   a. calcium.
   b. chloride.
   c. potassium.
   d. sodium.
   e. magnesium.

5. One of the most significant symptoms of an increase of bilirubin in the body is:
   a. headache.
   b. jaundice.
   c. nausea.
   d. fever.
   e. dizziness.

6. Which of these is not an electrolyte?
   a. Chloride
   b. Calcium
   c. Sodium
   d. Potassium
   e. Urea

7. ALP, ALT, and AST are associated with testing the function of the:
   a. thyroid.
   b. liver.
   c. kidney.
   d. pancreas.
   e. heart.

8. A1C is associated with:
   a. hypothyroidism.
   b. pancreatitis.
   c. diabetes.
   d. myocardial infarction.
   e. hypernatremia.

9. The American Heart Association recommends that the cholesterol level in the blood be:
   a. more than 250 mg/dL.
   b. less than 200 mg/dL.
   c. between 50 and 75 mg/dL.
   d. less than the HDL.
   e. more than the LDL.

10. An abnormal potassium will commonly cause:
    a. dizziness and headache.
    b. nausea and vomiting.
    c. muscle weakness and cramping.
    d. liver failure.
    e. hypothyroidism.

Internet Resources

For more information regarding diabetes and the management of this disease, visit the Web site for the American Diabetes Association at www.diabetes.org.

For information regarding heart-related topics including recommended cholesterol levels and diet therapy, visit the Web site for the American Heart Association at www.heart.org.

29 | Microbiology

Chapter Objectives

- Describe how cultures are used in medical microbiology.
- Name and describe the different types of bacteria.
- Identify the main types of fungi that may be found in the human body.
- Identify different types of viruses.
- Identify the two main types of Metazoa and give at least one example of each.
- Summarize the medical assistant's responsibilities in microbiological testing.
- List the most common microbiological specimens collected in the physician's office lab.

- Collect a specimen for throat culture.
- Collect a sputum specimen.
- Collect a stool specimen.
- Test a stool specimen for occult blood.
- Explain how to transport a specimen.
- State the difference between primary cultures, secondary cultures, and pure cultures.
- Name at least three kinds of media used in cultures.
- Describe how microscopic examination is used in medical microbiology.
- Prepare a wet mount slide.
- State the purpose of Gram staining.

CAAHEP & ABHES Competencies

CAAHEP

- Obtain specimens and perform CLIA-waived microbiology test.
- Differentiate between normal and abnormal test results.

ABHES

- Practice quality control.
- Perform selected CLIA-waived tests that assist with diagnosis and treatment in microbiology testing.
- Collect, label, and process specimens.

Chapter Terms

Aerobic	Colony count	Mycology	Spores
Anaerobic	Culture	Normal flora	Sputum
Bacteriology	Gram negative	Pathogen	Virology
Colony	Gram positive	Petri dish	Wet mount

Abbreviations

C&S   HAI   KOH   O&P

Case Study

Martin Johnson, a 43-year-old patient, is seeing the physician because he just arrived back in the country from traveling with his job to Europe and Southeast Asia. On his return trip home, he found a worm in the toilet after having a bowel movement. The worm was whitish gray and nearly 3 feet long. Of course, the patient was distressed about this finding. He asked the medical assistant what this could possibly be and how would the physician treat him.

The medical terminology prefix micro- means "very small." So, it won't surprise you to find out that microbiology is the study of very small life. This small life includes bacteria, viruses, fungi, and parasites. For the most part, these microorganisms, or microbes, are so small that you can't see them without a microscope. But even though they're tiny, some microbes can still cause big health problems. Microorganisms that can cause disease are called **pathogens**.

Many microbes, called **normal flora**, live in and on the human body without causing any problems or disease. Some are even helpful to us. Many types of normal flora and pathogens thrive at temperatures between 96°F and 101°F and in a fairly neutral environment. The human body typically offers these conditions.

As a medical assistant, you need to understand microbes and know the conditions in which they could become a problem for patients. Your understanding of microbiology will also help protect patients, your coworkers, and you from health care–acquired infections (**HAI**), formerly known as nosocomial infections. These are infections people can get from being in a medical care setting. There are many biohazard materials in the microbiology lab and work area. Be aware of the biohazard symbol on containers where these items are stored. Figure 29-1 shows the universal symbol used to recognize the presence of biological agents.

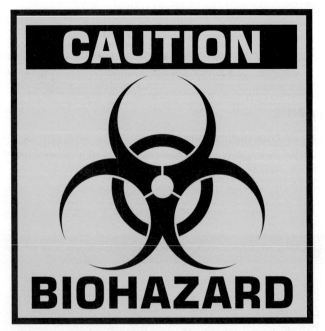

Figure 29-1 Biohazard symbol. (Image from Shutterstock.)

 ## PREVENTING HEALTH CARE–ACQUIRED INFECTIONS

A medical facility is often full of sick people. The lab that tests the office's specimens may be working with many types of pathogens. Health care professionals must take steps to protect themselves and others from infection. There are some common ways infections are spread in a medical setting. These include the following:

- Person to person—includes direct contact with patients who are ill as well as contact among coworkers.
- Contaminated medical equipment—dirty instruments and needles fall into this category, along with other items such as medical devices.

Case Question

 If you were the medical assistant, how would you respond to the patient?

- Bacteria in the environment—includes airborne transmission of microorganisms.
- Failure to follow established procedures—employees who disregard policies and procedures for infection control.

Here are steps you can take to protect yourself, coworkers, and patients from these infections.

- Hand washing—This is the single most important way to prevent the spread of bacteria that cause infections. Some research says that health care workers often think they're washing their hands more than they actually are. It also suggests that many workers aren't washing their hands long enough when they do wash them. Figure 29-2 is a reminder that hand washing may be the most effective means to stop the spread of microorganisms.
- Gloves—These aren't a replacement for hand washing. They provide an extra layer of protection for you and the patient. Make sure you wear gloves whenever you'll be in contact with any body fluids. Also wear gloves when performing any kind of testing. When you remove contaminated gloves, be sure to follow the correct procedure and then wash your hands after your gloves have been removed.

- Decontamination procedures—Follow procedures to properly clean, sanitize, disinfect, and sterilize medical equipment. Plus, as you know, never try to reuse or clean single-use disposable items.
- Single-use disposable equipment—When possible, use single-use disposable equipment and supplies. Make sure you dispose of medical waste properly.
- Personal responsibility—Take personal responsibility for your own safety and protection at work. Recognize that preventing the spread of microbes requires constant thought and attention.

MICROBIOLOGICAL TESTING

Medical microbiology involves testing to find out what kinds of microbes are living in a sample. This is often done by growing cultures from patients' specimens. A **culture** is colonies of bacteria grown under controlled conditions in a container in a lab. A **colony** is a group of identical bacteria that grow in a culture from one "parent" bacteria.

The purpose of growing a culture is to diagnose and treat a disease based on the kinds of bacteria present in the specimen. Cultures are grown in culture media with the help of an incubator. A medium is a special material in a container that helps bacteria present in the specimen to grow. Figure 29-3 shows an example of a transport medium used to collect the specimen to send to the microbiology lab for culturing and identification of the disease organism.

Specimens may be collected from different parts of the body. Here are some of the more common places:

- Wounds
- Throat
- Vagina
- Urethra
- Skin

Specimens also may be drawn from the body, as in drawing blood, or excreted as sputum, stool, or urine.

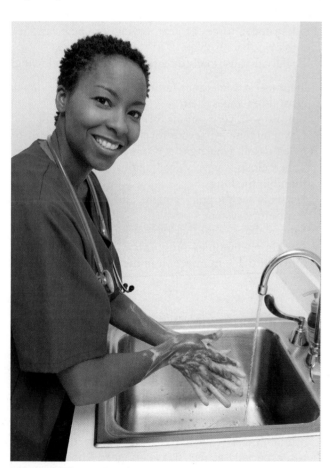

Figure 29-2 Hand washing skills are essential to prohibit the transmission of disease. (Image from Shutterstock.)

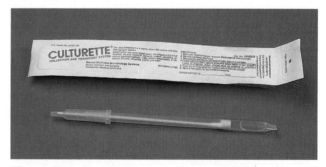

Figure 29-3 Transport media used to deliver culture specimen to the laboratory. (Reprinted from Kronenberger J, Ledbetter J. *Jones & Bartlett Learning's Comprehensive Medical Assisting.* 5th ed. Burlington, MA: Jones & Bartlett Learning, LLC; 2016.)

As a medical assistant, it will often be your job to collect specimens or to assist the physician with specimen collection. You may collect specimens from wounds or from the throat, but the physician will usually collect specimens from the eye, ear, rectum, or reproductive organs. No matter how or where the specimens are collected, you must practice aseptic (sterile) technique so the specimen will provide accurate test results. A test is only as good as the quality of the specimen. You must be very careful to avoid contaminating the specimens you collect.

Bacteria

Bacteria are one-celled simple organisms. Each type has its own characteristics. However, they all need four basic things to survive:

- Nutrients
- Warmth
- Moisture
- Gaseous atmosphere
  - Oxygen—required for growth of **aerobic** bacteria
  - Lack of oxygen—required for growth of **anaerobic** bacteria

The human body provides all four requirements for bacterial growth. Bacteria also can be created in the microbiology lab with the use of culture media and an incubator.

Bacteria can be identified by their own individual shapes and response to chemical tests, how they move, and other ways. There are several groups of bacteria, including the spore-forming bacteria that are very important in medical microbiology. Using culture media and the incubator, bacteria can be grown from patient specimens. Figure 29-4 is an example of Petri plates containing various types of solid media for growing bacteria.

Bacteriology is the science and study of bacteria. Organisms are named with both a genus and species name. The genus is always spelled with a capital letter,

and the species begins with a lowercase letter (e.g., *Staphylococcus aureus*). In print, the bacteria's name is italic or underlined. The name helps describe the characteristics of the bacterium (the singular form of the word bacteria) or the name or place connected with its discovery.

Cocci

The group of spherical bacteria—called cocci—cause many diseases. Figure 29-5 shows the various types of cocci, which include diplococci, streptococci, and staphylococci.

For example, species of streptococci (one genus of bacteria) may cause the following conditions:

- Sore throat
- Scarlet fever
- Rheumatic fever
- Pneumonia
- Skin infections

Bacilli

Rod-shaped bacteria—called bacilli—usually need oxygen to live, which means that they are aerobic. They also may be gram positive or gram negative. Some bacilli form spores. **Spores** are a form of bacteria that can resist the destructive forces of heat, drying, or chemicals. See Figure 29-5, bacilli shape.

Bacilli can cause many diseases, including the following:

- Tetanus—a sometimes fatal infectious disease of the central nervous system
- Botulism—a very serious form of food poisoning
- Gas gangrene—a severe form of gangrene (death of living tissue) where gas is produced in the dead tissue
- Tuberculosis—a very contagious infection usually found in the lungs
- Pertussis—whooping cough, an infection of the respiratory system
- Salmonellosis—another type of food poisoning
- Certain pneumonias—respiratory infections
- Otitis media—an infection in the middle ear

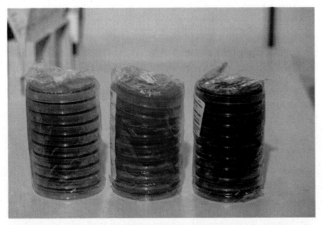

Figure 29-4 Culture plates, also called Petri plates, contain solid media. (Reprinted from Kronenberger J, Ledbetter J. *Jones & Bartlett Learning's Comprehensive Medical Assisting.* 5th ed. Burlington, MA: Jones & Bartlett Learning, LLC; 2016.)

Cultural Connection

Global travel is becoming more and more common for more people either for pleasure or for business. These people are experiencing very diverse cultures, customs, and foods. Unclean food and water can cause travelers' diarrhea and serious illnesses related to diseases only seen in those areas of the world. Those traveling to developing countries are especially at risk. Travelers need to be aware of the risks and should always try to stick to safe food and water habits. Most times, it is safe to eat food that has been cooked and served hot. For example, instead of eating raw or partially cooked eggs, choose hard cooked or boiled eggs. Fruits and vegetables need to be thoroughly washed and peeled if possible. Foods should be avoided if they are prepared by street vendors and open-air merchants since the process for sanitizing and safely storing foods at appropriate temperatures may not be in place. These foods will put the consumer at risk for eating contaminated foods. Raw or undercooked (rare) meat or fish (seafood) should also be avoided. Unclean water can also make a person sick if swallowed or inhaled while bathing, showering, or swimming. In some areas, tap water may not even be safe for brushing your teeth. Bottled water should be used for drinking and personal hygiene.

Spirochetes and Vibrios

The long, spiral, flexible bacteria—called spirochetes—cause disease as well. See Figure 29-5 showing shape of spirochete. Spirochetes cause

- Syphilis, a sexually transmitted disease.
- Lyme disease, an illness caused by a tick bite. Figure 29-6 shows a picture of a deer tick. Based on how small it is, you can imagine why it is very difficult to see on a person.

Some spirochetes have flagella, or whip-like extensions that aid their movement. If the spiral bacteria are rigid (inflexible) rather than flexible, they are called spirilla.

The comma-shaped bacteria—called vibrios—are very motile. Being motile means they move very well on their own too.

SHAPES OF BACTERIA

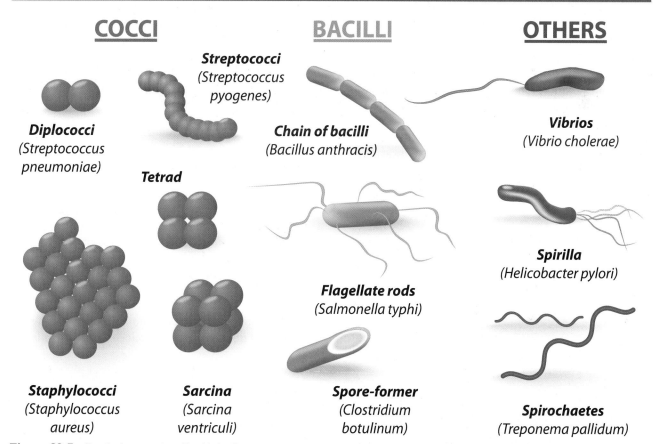

COCCI

Diplococci
(Streptococcus pneumoniae)

Streptococci
(Streptococcus pyogenes)

Tetrad

Staphylococci
(Staphylococcus aureus)

Sarcina
(Sarcina ventriculi)

BACILLI

Chain of bacilli
(Bacillus anthracis)

Flagellate rods
(Salmonella typhi)

Spore-former
(Clostridium botulinum)

OTHERS

Vibrios
(Vibrio cholerae)

Spirilla
(Helicobacter pylori)

Spirochaetes
(Treponema pallidum)

Figure 29-5 Bacteria are classified into five groups according to their basic shapes: cocci, bacilli, spiral (spirilla), vibrios, or corkscrew (spirochetes). (Image from Shutterstock.)

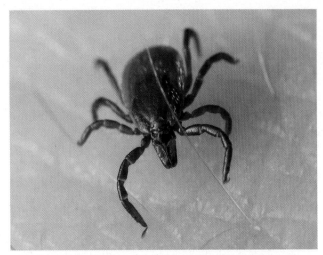

Figure 29-6 Close-up photo of adult female deer tick crawling on white skin. (Image from Shutterstock.)

Rickettsias and Chlamydiae

Certain forms of bacteria fit into their own separate category. These forms are rickettsias and chlamydiae. They both share some common characteristics:

- They are smaller than bacteria but larger than viruses.
- They must have a living host to reproduce and survive. They're known as obligate intracellular parasites because they can't survive unless they're attached to a living host organism.

Rickettsias cause Rocky Mountain spotted fever, typhus, Q fever, trench fever, and others. The rickettsias are carried by a particular kind of tick, louse, or mite. Figure 29-7 shows a tick sucking blood from its host person.

Chlamydiae cause trachoma (an eye disease) and lymphogranuloma venereum (a sexually transmitted disease).

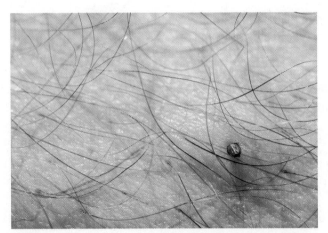

Figure 29-7 Tick parasite sucking blood from human skin. (Image from Shutterstock.)

Informing Patients about Lyme Disease

You may have to instruct patient about the deer tick, which is an arthropod that can transmit *Borrelia burgdorferi*, the spirochete that causes Lyme disease. The bacteria enter the human body when an infected tick bites a person. The bite results in symptoms that include the following:

- A bull's-eye–shaped rash
- Headache, fever, and chills
- Fatigue and general body aches
- If left untreated, severe muscle, joint, heart, and nervous system problems
- Teach patients to protect themselves from Lyme disease by giving them these guidelines.
- Try to avoid places where ticks live (e.g., grassy, wooded, and bushy areas), especially in May to July when they are most active.
- Wear insect repellant, shoes, long socks, long pants, and long sleeves in outdoor areas to keep ticks off your skin. Light-colored clothing will make any ticks on it easier to see.
- Check your clothes each time you come inside after working or playing outdoors. Wash this clothing in hot water with strong soap.
- Perform daily checks for ticks after being outdoors. Include scalp and hair, groin, and armpits as well. Remove any ticks you find using fine-tipped tweezers. If a tick is attached to your skin for <24 hours, your chances of getting Lyme disease are small.

Bacterial Spores

Spores are extremely hardy forms of bacteria that are tough to kill. Some microbes can produce spores to protect themselves from destruction. A spore is a bacterium that forms a capsule around itself. This puts the bacterium into a state of rest keeping it from being destroyed by asepsis. Bacterial spores can be destroyed using an autoclave set at just the right heat, steam, pressure, and time. Once the spore is in the right conditions, the bacterium picks up where it left off and becomes active again.

Examples of bacteria that produce spores include the following:

- *Clostridium botulinum*—a bacteria that causes food poisoning
- *Clostridium tetani*—a bacteria that causes tetanus
- *Clostridium perfringens*—a bacteria that causes gas gangrene
- *Bacillus anthracis*—a bacteria that causes anthrax

Fungi

Like bacteria, fungi are small organisms that can produce disease given the right set of conditions. Also like bacteria, some fungi can be contagious as well as infectious. But fungi are more like plants, while bacteria are more like one-celled animals. Many types of fungi can be seen with the naked eye, but some can only be seen under a microscope. **Mycology** is the science and study of fungi. Diseases caused by fungus are called mycotic infections, or mycoses.

In the human body, fungi can appear in the form of molds or yeasts. Tinea pedis (athlete's foot), tinea corporis (ringworm of the body), tinea capitis (ringworm of the scalp), and tinea unguium (nail fungus) are among the more common conditions caused by molds. Yeasts like candidiasis cause thrush (skin and mouth), vaginitis, and endocarditis. Candidiasis can be spread by contact. Fungi are opportunistic, which means they become able to cause disease when the opportunity presents itself. For example, fungi can cause problems when the host's normal flora can't offset the growth of the fungi. Figure 29-8 is an example of oral candidiasis (yeast infection), also known as thrush.

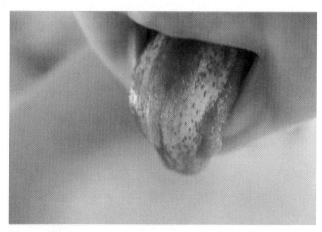

Figure 29-8 Oral candidiasis (thrush) on baby's tongue. (Image from Shutterstock.)

Viruses

Viruses are the smallest microorganisms, but they can be a lot of trouble for a patient. Viruses cause influenza, infectious hepatitis, rabies, polio, and AIDS. **Virology** is the study of viruses. These microbes are so tiny that they can't even be seen with the usual bright-field microscope found in many medical offices. They must be viewed under an electron microscope.

Like rickettsias and chlamydiae, viruses are obligate intracellular parasites. This means that they need a living host to survive and reproduce. However, unlike bacteria, antibiotics can't kill viruses. This makes most viruses difficult to treat. Although there are some antiviral drugs such as the flu vaccine, scientists are developing more antiviral therapies (drugs to slow or stop the growth of viruses) for many of the viruses. Researchers also continue to work on cures for viral diseases such as AIDS and herpes. Figure 29-9 shows an infection of herpes zoster, shingles.

Patient Education

Helping Patients Avoid Athlete's Foot

One common fungal infection is tinea pedis, which is also known as athlete's foot. In spite of this name, patients don't have to be active in sports or even exercise to have this condition. You can help your patients avoid this irritating fungus by giving them the following guidelines:

- After a shower or a swim, dry your feet very thoroughly. Pay particular attention to drying between your toes.
- Wear water shoes or nonskid sandals anytime you're in a public shower or locker room. Don't walk around in your bare feet.
- Don't share shoes, slippers, sandals, or any other kind of footwear with anyone else.
- Use an antifungal powder between your toes. Sprinkle the powder in your shoes, too.
- Make sure your shoes can "breathe." Avoid plastic or vinyl shoes with no air circulation.
- Consider changing your socks once during the day to keep your feet drier. You should also alternate pairs of shoes. Wearing a pair only every other day gives shoes a chance to dry completely.

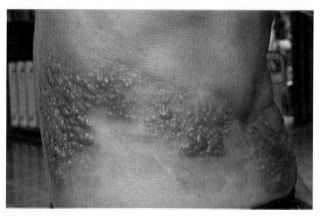

Figure 29-9 Skin infected with herpes zoster virus, shingles. (Image from Shutterstock.)

Protozoa and Metazoa

Protozoa are the single-celled parasitic animals that may be diagnosed in the parasitology laboratory. Parasitology is the study of parasites and parasitism, a relationship in which one organism is dependent on another. Figure 29-10 shows an example of *Trichomonas* that might be found in the vaginal canal.

Here are some common protozoa and the conditions they cause:

- *Entamoeba*—diarrhea, dysentery, and liver and lung disorders
- *Giardia*—giardiasis, diarrhea, and malabsorption of nutrients
- *Trichomonas*—trichomoniasis, vaginitis, and urinary tract infections
- *Plasmodium*—malaria
- *Toxoplasma*—toxoplasmosis and fetal abnormalities

Metazoa are also animal. However, they're multicellular rather than single-celled organisms like protozoa. Metazoa are of two types:

- Helminths (parasitic worms)
- Arthropods (animals with a hard external skeleton, segmented body, and jointed, paired legs)

The family of helminths includes roundworms, tapeworms, and flukes. They can survive almost anywhere in the human body. Some types can move through the body until they find a place to settle. Figure 29-11 shows an example of *Ascaris* worms, giant roundworms that can reach 14 inches in length.

Flatworms

Trematodes and cestodes are both types of flatworms. They can cause these conditions:

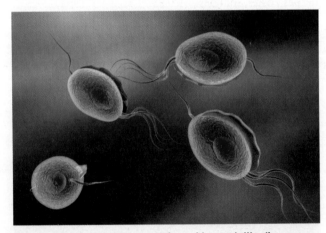

Figure 29-10 Trichomonas found in vaginitis. (Image from Shutterstock.)

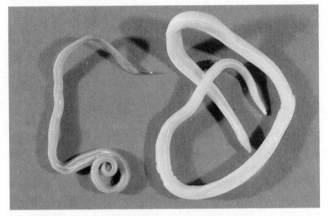

Figure 29-11 Female and male worms of *A. lumbricoides*. (Reprinted from Kronenberger J, Ledbetter J. *Jones & Bartlett Learning's Comprehensive Medical Assisting.* 5th ed. Burlington, MA: Jones & Bartlett Learning, LLC; 2016.)

- Schistosomiasis—Flukes (small, leaf-shaped flatworms) in contaminated water penetrate the skin and get into the bloodstream, bladder, and intestines.
- Liver fluke infestation—Flukes that live on plants or in fish in contaminated water enter the human body through the digestive tract; they migrate through the intestinal wall and settle in the bile ducts of the liver.
- Beef or pork tapeworm infestation—Humans can become infected by tapeworms when eating uncooked infected beef or pork. The parasite is separated from the meat during digestion in the stomach. It then moves into the small intestine where it attaches to the intestine's walls and develops into an adult tapeworm. An adult tapeworm can grow as long as 50 feet.

Roundworms

The roundworms are called nematodes and also can infect humans. Here are some of the conditions they can cause.

- Roundworm infestation (worms hatching and living in the intestines)
- Gastrointestinal blockage
- Bronchial damage
- Pinworm infestation (worms filling the intestines and rectum)
- Trichinosis (disease caused by eating undercooked pork or other wild game)

Figure 29-12 demonstrates how the *Trichinella* invades the body through eating uncooked meat.

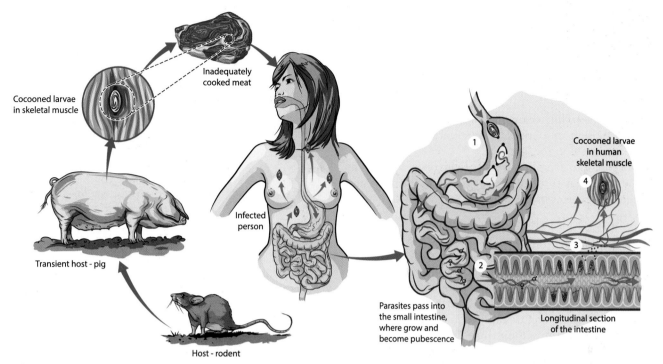

Figure 29-12 *Trichinella* life cycle leading to trichinosis. (Image from Shutterstock.)

Case Question

A F F Remember our patient Mr. Johnson, the world traveler? The physician just talked with the patient to obtain a full history of his travels and foods and drink he had. The physician requested a stool sample to see if there were any segments of worms. He didn't see any on microscopic exam of the specimen. The patient was not exhibiting any symptoms at the time of the visit. The physician referred the patient to an infectious diseases specialist who prescribed an antiprotozoal drug for the patient as a precaution.

After the patient completed the medication, he returned to the original physician's office for follow-up and a final stool specimen evaluation. He asked the medical assistant why a stool specimen is still needed. What would you tell this patient?

Arthropods

Arthropods are the better-known group of Metazoa. They include mites, lice, ticks, fleas, bees, spiders, wasps, mosquitoes, and scorpions. All arthropods can cause injury with their bites or stings. Several also can transmit disease by biting or stinging. Figure 29-13 shows an example of a scorpion that can sting with the tip of the tail. Notice the needle-like stinger at the tip.

Study Skill

It is amazing how many students do not bring their textbook to class each day. Excuses include that it is too heavy to carry around. Do yourself a favor and have your textbook with you during class, and you will quickly see that most of the instructor's presentation is included in the book. Write notes in the margin of any additional information or examples that the instructor discusses that is not included in the textbook. Many students write volumes of notes only to discover that the information is right in the book. Invest in an inexpensive book bag on wheels to help you out. You can also "park" the bag in your study area for easy access to items that you need.

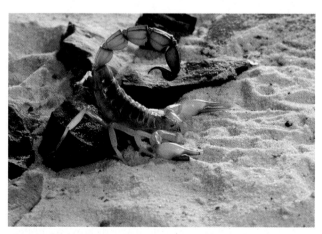

Figure 29-13   Yellow-tailed scorpion. (Image from Shutterstock.)

MICROBIOLOGY AND YOU

Two main procedures are used to identify what possibly harmful bacteria may exist on or in a patient's body. These procedures are

- Culturing—This means growing colonies of the bacteria present in a specimen in a carefully controlled environment in the lab.
- Microscopic examination—This involves looking at the specimen through a microscope to identify any bacteria present in it.

As a medical assistant, you may be involved with both procedures in your medical office or lab. If you are, your responsibilities may be both administrative and clinical. Each medical setting is different. So you may perform tasks that medical assistants in other settings do not. Always remember to work within your scope of training and according to CLIA requirements.

Your administrative duties may include the following:

- Routing specimens
- Handling and filing reports
- Keeping patients safe
- Educating patients
- Billing and insurance filing

Your clinical duties may include the following:

- Collecting and processing specimens
- Assisting the physician and patient, as needed
- Maintaining standard precautions and safety
- Cleaning after testing is complete

Collecting Specimens

In order to determine specific diseases or conditions, the physician may need to obtain specimens from a patient's body. Most lab tests are performed on specimens that are easy to collect. The most commonly tested specimens include

- Blood
- Urine
- Sputum
- Feces
- Wound drainage
- Mucus from the throat and other parts of the body

Testing these substances can reveal much about a patient's condition. Here are just three of many examples.

- A throat culture can detect strep throat.
- A urine culture can show if there's an infection within the urinary system.
- A blood culture can detect infections in the circulatory system.

In previous chapters, you learned how to collect blood and collect urine specimens. This chapter includes information about how to collect other types of specimens, as well as instructions on how to conduct various microbiology tests.

To make sure these tests are accurate, you must collect specimens in the correct manner. You also must handle them according to the accepted medical standards.

Collection Methods

Most specimens for microbiological testing are obtained in one of four ways.

- Swab—A stick topped with cotton or an absorbent manmade fiber. Swabs are used to take samples from the throat, vagina, urethra, skin, and wounds. Figure 29-14 demonstrates collection of a specimen from a wound using a swab.
- Venipuncture—Blood is drawn through a syringe, evacuated tube, or butterfly apparatus and is deposited into culture bottles.
- Centesis (surgical puncture)—This procedure is performed by the physician. Specimens typically collected this way include spinal fluid and pleural fluid (fluid from lung membranes).
- Collection of body excretions—Examples include urine, sputum, and feces or stool. Patients usually collect these specimens, so they need to be educated in the proper collection technique.

Throat Cultures

The physician may order a throat culture to identify the presence of infectious microbes. Throat cultures are useful when a patient has tonsillitis or a sore throat. The results of the throat culture help identify what's causing the problem. A sterile swab gently sweeps the patient's throat to obtain the specimen. You also must use a tongue depressor for this procedure to avoid culturing mouth or cheek microbes that are normal flora. Once the specimen is collected, it can be processed in the office or sent out to a reference lab. If you send the swab to a lab, you must first place it in the correct culture medium.

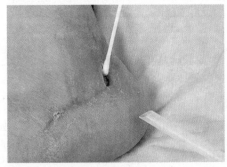

Figure 29-14 Collecting exudate onto culture swab from a heel wound. (Reprinted from Kronenberger J, Ledbetter J. *Jones & Bartlett Learning's Comprehensive Medical Assisting.* 5th ed. Burlington, MA: Jones & Bartlett Learning, LLC; 2016.)

Then label the culture and put it in a biohazard bag. Be sure to include the proper paperwork requesting the test the physician has ordered.

Collecting Sputum

Sputum is mucus from a patient's lungs. It's often tested when diagnosing respiratory diseases such as pneumonia and tuberculosis. The specimen is collected by deep coughing into a sterile container with a lid. It's important that the specimen be a sample of lung secretions and not secretions from the mouth. For this reason, the patient should be instructed to avoid spitting saliva into the sterile container.

It's best to obtain sputum specimens in the morning when the greatest volume is usually present in the lungs. If a patient's mucus is thick and difficult to cough up, a cool-mist humidifier might be ordered for him or her to use at home, to help loosen thick secretions.

You may be responsible for explaining sputum collection procedure to the patient.

Stool Specimens

Many physicians order a stool specimen as part of the routine physical exam of an adult patient. Appointments to collect stool specimens should be scheduled early in the morning. Most people move their bowels soon after getting up. Delaying the appointment may cause the patient discomfort or might result in loss of the specimen. In many cases, the patient may collect the sample at home. No matter where it's collected, it's important that the patient follow the proper procedure. Some stool specimens are collected and transported in special containers. It'll be your responsibility to make sure proper procedures are followed. Patients should be told to bring specimens they collect at home to the office or lab as soon as possible.

Most often, the feces is tested for the presence of occult (or hidden) blood. Blood in a patient's stool can mean there's bleeding in the gastrointestinal (GI) tract. This can be a sign of several conditions, including ulcers or colorectal cancer. Other tests may look for ova (eggs) and parasites (O&P).

The medical assistant will instruct the patient prior to stool collection to ensure a quality specimen. Follow these tips for collecting stool specimens:

- When testing for occult blood, tell the patient to avoid these foods and medications, which can cause false results, for 2 days before collecting the sample:
  ○ Red meat and fruits high in vitamin C
  ○ Cauliflower, broccoli, lettuce, spinach, corn, and other vegetables that contain the enzyme peroxidase
  ○ Aspirin and nonsteroidal anti-inflammatory drugs (NSAIDs)
- When testing for pinworms, collect the sample early in the morning before the patient has a bowel movement or a bath. Pinworms tend to leave the rectum and lay eggs around the anus during the night. Place clear adhesive tape against the anal area. Remove it quickly and place it sticky-side down on a glass slide for the physician or lab to examine. Provide the patient with a slide to take home and use to mount the tape.
- When testing for parasites, tell the patient not to use a laxative or enema before the test. This might destroy the evidence of parasites. If the sample contains blood or mucus, include as much of this as possible in the container.

Transporting Specimens

Most pathogens are not fragile. However, every specimen should be processed or transported for processing as soon as possible after it's collected. Otherwise, some organisms in it could multiply or die off. Either event could cause a false result on the test.

TABLE 29-1	Handling Common Specimens	
Specimen	**Collecting**	**Processing**
Urine	Clean-catch midstream with care to avoid contaminating the inside of the container. Don't let stand more than 1 h after collection.	Refrigerate if test cannot be performed within 1 h.
Blood	Handle carefully. Collect in blood culture bottle. Must remain free of contaminants. Requires special preparation of the venipuncture site.	Deliver to lab immediately.
Feces	Collect in clean container. Leave at room temperature if testing for ova (eggs), parasites, or occult blood.	Deliver to lab at once. If delayed, mix with preservative recommended by lab or use transport medium.
Microbiology specimens	Don't contaminate swab or inside of container by touching either to surface other than site of collection. Protect anaerobic specimens from exposure to air.	Transport as soon as possible.

Specimens that will be processed in an outside lab must first be placed in transport media. A number of companies manufacture this special type of media. It can generally be stored at room temperature until it's needed for use.

Most transport media are self-contained and include a plastic tube with a sterile swab and media appropriate for transporting that type of specimen. You'll usually find all the directions for using the container on the manufacturer's package.

Fill out all paperwork carefully and check the information before releasing specimens for transport. Many specimens that are tested outside the office will be sent to large laboratories. You want to be sure your patient's specimen is identified, processed, and tested properly.

For the most reliable results, lab tests should be performed on specimens within an hour after collection. When that isn't possible, store the specimen properly to preserve all its properties. Never expose a specimen to extreme temperature changes. Table 29-1 provides information on the proper handling of common specimens.

 # CULTURING SPECIMENS

In medical microbiology, much of the testing to diagnose disease is done using cultures. As you've already read in this chapter, the lab can create the warmth, nutrients, and other things microbes need to grow. There are three types of cultures.

- Primary cultures come directly from a patient's specimen. These cultures are used to study any or all of the microorganisms found at the specimen site.
- Secondary cultures, also called subcultures, are taken from the primary culture. Suspicious-looking organisms in the primary culture are removed and encouraged to grow for more study.
- Pure cultures contain only one type of organism. A pure culture may be either a primary or a secondary culture.

Culture Media

You already know that the purpose of media is to encourage the growth of microbes so physicians can identify them easily. When the perfect environment is provided, microorganisms will grow and multiply, making it easier to diagnose and treat a disease.

Whatever the suspected microbe is, all the things it needs to survive must be present for it to grow. The media in the culture container provide nutrients, moisture, and the right pH. The incubator maintains the right temperature and gaseous atmosphere. Depending on the type of suspected microbe, the incubator or the culture containers placed in it provide the correct atmosphere—oxygen for aerobes, no oxygen for anaerobes, or CO_2 (carbon dioxide) for capnophilic organisms, those that require higher concentrations of carbon dioxide to grow.

Types of Media

There are three basic preparations, or forms, in which media come:

- Solid
- Semisolid
- Liquid or broth

Most specimens submitted for lab study are cultured on blood agar. This solid medium is prepared by adding 5% sheep's blood to agar, a firm, transparent, and colorless gelatin-like substance made from seaweed. The agar congeals the blood and forms a firm surface to support the growth of microbes. The firm surface makes it easy to observe the culture growth.

Media Containers

A **Petri dish** is an empty glass or a plastic container that's used to hold a solid culture medium, such as blood agar. Once the container is filled with the medium, it's called a plate. The plate is fitted with a cover to prevent contamination of the specimen. Plates are clear so you can see the culture as it grows.

Agar also may be placed in sterile glass tubes. The tubes are either allowed to harden with a flattop surface (a butt tube) or with a slanted surface (a slant-and-butt combination).

A liquid or broth medium usually comes in a small jar or tube. Many special broth media have swabs to be used for specimen collection and are enclosed in special envelopes for transporting the specimen.

Solid media come on plates wrapped in a plastic sleeve. Plates are always stored medium side up so that condensation does not form on the plates.

Microbiological Inoculation

Microbiological inoculation means introducing a microbe into a culture medium and then putting the medium in an environment likely to make the microbe grow. To make sure a specimen is inoculated in a way that microbes in it will grow best, you'll put it on or in the medium by one of these methods:

- By using a specimen swab
- By removing part of the specimen using a sterile inoculating loop or inoculating needle

The swab and inoculating loop (needle) are used in different situations. Swabs are used when sampling some specimens, such as feces, from specimen containers. Other specimens, such as sputum, are sampled with loops. A swab is usually used when the specimen is being transferred directly from the patient site onto the culture medium. You would then switch to an inoculating loop to prepare the specimen for culture.

A sterile inoculating loop or needle is used when lifting a colony from a culture to inoculate a secondary culture. Specific colonies are lifted from the primary culture plate and streaked onto the second plate. Then those specific colonies will be incubated again for a pure culture and more study.

Plates

To inoculate a solid medium on a plate, you streak the medium using a qualitative or quantitative technique. Qualitative cultures are done to reveal what kinds of bacteria are present. Quantitative cultures tell how many of a certain bacteria are present.

Butt and Slant Tubes

Butt tubes are inoculated by penetrating the center of the media surface with a needle inoculator, stopping about one-fourth inch from the bottom of the tube.

Slant tubes are usually inoculated with a curvy stroke up the surface of the slant. Some slant tubes require that you inoculate by both streaking the slant and penetrating the center of the butt portion.

Sensitivity Testing

When the physician wants a specimen cultured, she will usually order what's called a **C&S**. This stands for "culture and sensitivity." The C&S is a several-step test that involves not only growing any pathogens in a specimen but also finding out which drugs will stop their growth. The physician can then use those drugs to help the patient's body fight off the microbes.

To perform a sensitivity test, a secondary or pure culture of the suspected pathogen is created. A sample from this culture is then inoculated in broth medium and incubated for 18 to 24 hours.

Next, a sterile inoculating loop is used to transfer the growth in this medium into a tube containing another liquid medium. Growth should be added until the second tube is so turbid (cloudy) that print is barely visible through the tube. If not enough growth is available to reach this level of turbidity, the tube can be incubated for 2 to 4 hours, until the correct turbidity is achieved.

The contents of the tube are next used to inoculate a culture plate. After the plate is prepared, it's incubated for 18 to 24 hours. It's then inspected to see if there's a zone around any of the disks where no microbes have grown (called a zone of inhibition). Figure 29-15 shows an example of a Petri dish with sensitivity disks.

- If there's no zone of inhibition around a disk, the pathogen is resistant to that particular drug. Therefore, using the drug wouldn't be effective for treating the patient's infection.
- If there's no microbe growth around a disk, you know that the pathogen is sensitive to that particular drug. It would be effective for treating the patient.
- If there's a small zone around a disk, this would be reported as an intermediate test result. Such a drug would be barely effective against the microbe.

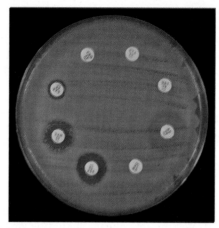

Figure 29-15   Culture plate testing antimicrobial susceptibility (antibiotic sensitivity). (Image from Shutterstock.)

- The best drug to use in treatment will be the one with the largest zone of inhibition. This shows that it is the most effective drug against that microbe.

Urine Colony Counts

Urine cultures often include a colony count in addition to a culture and sensitivity test. A urine **colony count** measures the amount of bacteria growing in one milliliter of urine. The results can tell the physician the severity of the infection if pathogens are present.

To perform this test, urine is generally inoculated onto two or three types of media. For example, a blood agar plate will grow all bacteria present in the specimen. MacConkey media will grow only gram-negative rods, and Columbian CNA media will grow only any gram-positive cocci that may be present.

- 0 to 100 visible colonies on a plate indicate 0 to 10,000 bacteria/mL and means that no infection is present.
- 100 to 1,000 visible colonies on a plate indicate 10,000 to 100,000 bacteria/mL and means that the patient might have a urinary tract infection (UTI).
- More than 1,000 visible colonies on a plate indicate more than 100,000 bacteria/mL and means that an infection is definitely present. The higher the number, the more severe the infection is.

As a medical assistant, you probably won't be making these counts. However, you may be asked to inoculate the plates.

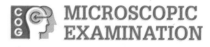 **MICROSCOPIC EXAMINATION**

Bacteria grown on a culture can be spread onto a glass slide so they can be examined under a microscope. Sometimes a swab of the specimen is taken directly from the site and put on the slide. Microscopic examination can help identify the specific pathogen that's causing the patient's problems.

For example:

- Stool specimens are put on slides to look for parasites such as pinworms, tapeworms, and their ova.
- Fungi such as "ringworm" and "yeast" infections are diagnosed by examining skin scrapings and samples from mucous membranes under a microscope.
- The protozoa that cause malaria are found through the microscopic examination of blood.

Wet Mounts and Dry Smears

Some pathogens are easier to identify if they're allowed to move about freely in fluid. This type of slide is called a **wet mount**. Wet mounts always should be viewed right away, or not later than 30 minutes after the slide is prepared. A dry smear is a slide in which the specimen is not suspended in fluid.

Direct smears are slides made from material taken directly from the patient. They may contain epithelial cells (skin cells or cells from organ linings) as well as bacteria or other microbes. Indirect smears are slides made from a culture. They will contain only bacterial cells.

If more than one slide is made from a culture, number the colonies that will be observed on the back of the plate or plates. Then number each slide with the corresponding number using a diamond-tipped pen on the frosted edge of the slide to properly identify its culture site. You may also use a pencil to label the frosted part of the slide.

Gram Staining

Most bacteria are colorless. They're hard to identify or even to see without some kind of special treatment.

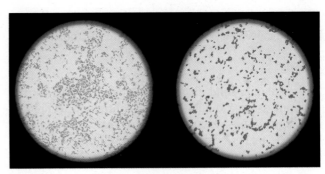

Figure 29-16 Gram-negative **(left)** and gram-positive **(right)** bacteria. (Image from Shutterstock.)

At times, a fixative or a stain is added to the smear. Fixatives are solutions or sprays that "fix" the specimen to the slide. Stains help the physician identify the microbe.

Dutch physician Hans Gram developed the Gram stain process more than 100 years ago. He discovered that after staining with crystal violet and safranin (a red dye). Certain bacteria accept the purple color of the crystal violet dye. These bacteria are known as **gram-positive** bacteria. Other bacteria will stain red with the safranin, which is also called the counterstain. These bacteria are called **gram negative**.

The Gram stain is an important test. Along with factors such as the bacteria's shape and the patient's symptoms, it helps give the physician an idea of the patient's disease. This can allow treatment to begin even before the specimen is cultured. Figure 29-16 is an example of gram-negative and gram-positive bacteria. Typically, gram positive include staphylococci, and gram negative, *E. coli*.

Procedure 29-1 | Collecting a Specimen for Throat Culture

Follow these steps to collect a specimen for throat culture.

1. Gather your equipment and supplies, including a tongue blade, a sterile specimen container and swab, gloves, a commercial throat culture kit (for testing in your office), a laboratory request form, and a biohazard container (for transport to the lab).

2. Wash your hands and put on gloves.

3. Greet and identify the patient. Explain the procedure.

4. Ask the patient to sit so a light source is directed at the throat.

5. Remove the sterile swab from its container.

6. Ask the patient to say "ahhh" as you press on the midpoint of the tongue with the tongue depressor. Saying "ahhh" helps reduce the gag reflex.

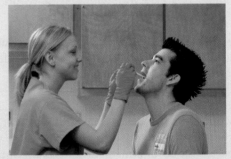

Throat swab patient and medical assistant. (Image from Kronenberger.)

Procedure 29-1 | Collecting a Specimen for Throat Culture (*continued*)

7. Swab the membranes that are suspected to be infected. Normally, you'll touch the side of the throat at the depth of the tissue hanging in the center back of the mouth (uvula). Expose all of the swab's surfaces to the membranes by turning the swab over the membranes. Avoid touching any other structures in the mouth such as the tongue or lips with the swab.

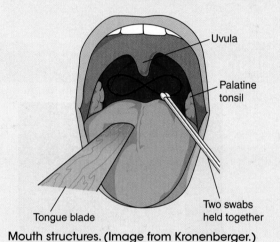

Uvula

Palatine tonsil

Two swabs held together

Tongue blade

Mouth structures. (Image from Kronenberger.)

8. Keep holding the tongue depressor in place while removing the swab from your patient's mouth.

9. Follow the directions on the specimen container for transferring the swab or processing the specimen in the office.

10. Dispose of supplies and equipment in a biohazard waste container. Remove your gloves and wash your hands.

11. If sending to a reference lab, prepare the specimen for transport with the lab requisition form.

12. Document the procedure.

Procedure 29-2 | Collecting a Sputum Specimen

Follow these steps to collect a sputum specimen:

1. Gather your equipment and supplies, including the labeled sterile specimen container, gloves, the laboratory request form, and a biohazard transport container.

2. Wash your hands and put on gloves.

3. Greet and identify the patient. Explain the procedure. Write the patient's name on a label, and put the label on the outside of the container.

4. Ask the patient to cough deeply. Tell the patient to use the abdominal muscles to bring secretions up from the lungs.

5. Ask the patient to expectorate directly into the container. Caution him or her not to touch the inside of the container or the specimen will be contaminated. You'll need 5 to 10 mL for most tests.

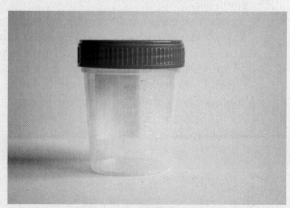

Sputum collection cup. (Image from Shutterstock.)

Procedure 29-2	Collecting a Sputum Specimen (*continued*)

6. Handle the specimen container according to standard precautions. Cap the container right away and put it into a transport container marked biohazard. Fill out the proper laboratory requisition slip.

7. Care for and dispose of your equipment and supplies. Clean your work area. Then you can remove your gloves and wash your hands.

8. Send the specimen to the laboratory immediately.

9. Document the procedure.

Procedure 29-3	Collecting a Stool Specimen

Follow these steps in teaching a patient how to collect a stool specimen:

1. Gather your equipment and supplies, including a stool specimen container (for ova and parasite testing), an occult blood test kit (for occult blood testing), and wooden spatulas or tongue blades. Label the container or test kit with the patient's name.

2. Wash your hands.

3. Greet and identify the patient. Explain the procedure. Also explain any dietary, medication, or other restrictions necessary for the collection. (Don't collect a specimen within 4 days of a barium procedure.)

4. When collecting a specimen for ova and parasites:
   - Tell the patient to collect a small amount of the first and last portion of the stool using the wooden spatula and to place the specimen in the container.
   - Suggest that it's easier if the patient defecates into a disposable plastic container designed to fit on a toilet seat (called a specimen pan, or "top hat") or onto plastic wrap placed over the toilet bowl.
   - Caution the patient not to contaminate the specimen with urine.

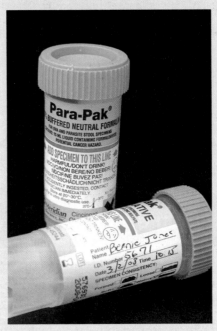

ParaPak. (Image from Kronenberger.)

5. When collecting a specimen for occult blood:
   - Suggest that the patient obtain the sample from the toilet paper he or she uses to wipe after defecating. Tell the patient to use a wooden spatula to collect the sample.
   - Tell the patient to smear a small amount of the sample from the spatula onto the slide windows.

6. After the patient returns the stool sample, store the specimen as directed. If you're instructing the patient to take the specimen directly to a laboratory, give the patient a completed laboratory requisition form.

7. Document the date and time of the procedure as well as the instructions that were given to the patient, including the routing procedure.

Procedure 29-4 Testing a Stool Specimen for Occult Blood

Follow these steps to test a stool specimen for occult blood. This procedure should take 5 minutes:

1. Gather your equipment and supplies including gloves, the patient's labeled specimen pack, and developer (or reagent drops). Make sure you check the expiration date on the developing solution. You could get inaccurate test results from expired solution.

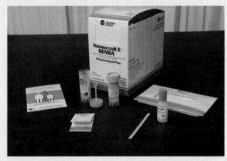

Hemoccult kit. (Image from Kronenberger.)

2. Wash your hands and put on gloves.

3. Open the test window on the back of the pack. Then put a drop of the developer or testing reagent on each window according to the manufacturer's directions.

4. Read the color change within the time specified by the directions. The time is usually 60 seconds.

5. Put a drop of developer (as directed) on the control monitor section or window of the pack. Take note whether the quality control results are positive or negative, as appropriate.

6. Use proper procedures to dispose of the test pack and gloves. Then wash your hands.

7. Record the procedure.

Procedure 29-5 Preparing a Wet Mount Slide

Follow these steps to prepare a wet mount slide:

1. Gather your equipment and supplies, including the specimen, gloves, a slide, sterile saline or 10% potassium hydroxide (**KOH**), a coverslip, petroleum jelly, a microscope, and a pencil or diamond-tipped pen.

2. Wash your hands and put on gloves.

3. Label the frosted edge of the slide with the patient's name and the date using a pencil or diamond-tipped pen.

4. Put a drop of the specimen on a glass slide with sterile saline or ten percent potassium hydroxide (KOH).

5. Use a wooden applicator stick to coat the rim of a coverslip with petroleum jelly.
   - You also can spread a thin layer of petroleum jelly on the heel of your gloved hand and then scrape the edges of the coverslip on it to transfer a thin line to each edge.
   - Change the glove before the next step if you use this method.

6. Put the coverslip over the specimen to keep it from evaporating.

7. Examine the slide with a microscope using the 40-power objective lens with diminished light. The physician will examine and read the slide for findings. Microscopic examination is not CLIA-waived testing for medical assistants.

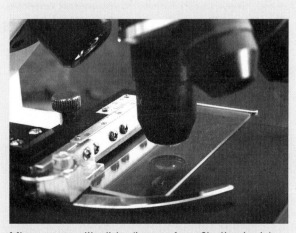

Microscope with slide. (Image from Shutterstock.)

Preparing for Externship

As you complete your externship, remember that there is an evaluation of your skills and knowledge, but who is going to evaluate you and what else will be included in the evaluation report. Your externship supervisor or preceptor typically completes your evaluation. However, others in the office provide input to the final evaluation. Your evaluation may include comments from the physician, other medical assistants, and the administrative staff. It is important to maintain good rapport with all the staff in the office. If your school provides a formal evaluation form, make sure you have reviewed the evaluation areas on the form. It is helpful to do a self-assessment of all these areas throughout the externship. Be very honest with yourself and try to imagine the grade you will receive from the staff for each of these areas. Although some of the areas of the evaluation are objective (measurable), other areas require a subjective opinion from the evaluator. Throughout your externship, ask the staff about your performance. Don't wait for someone to come to you. Be assertive with your approach but not aggressive. Assertiveness shows that you are self-assured and confident with your skills and behavior. Aggressive behavior is usually perceived as negative and bossy. So, get out there and assert yourself and enjoy your externship experience.

Chapter Recap

- Microbiology is an important part of the practice of medicine. Your duties in this area may include collecting, processing, and routing specimens and assisting the physician or patient with specimen collection.
- Commonly collected specimens for microbiological testing include blood, urine, sputum, feces, wound drainage, and mucus. Collection methods include the use of swabs, venipuncture, centesis, and collecting body excretions.
- The major types of microorganisms that you may deal with in your work as a medical assistant include bacteria, viruses, fungi, protozoa (one-celled parasites), and Metazoa (parasitic worms and arthropods).

- Follow procedures carefully to avoid contaminating specimens you collect. Also, know how to maintain the quality of each specimen before it is tested. Follow all handling guidelines in dealing with specimens that will be sent to outside labs for processing.
- Bacterial cultures are one way to identify pathogens that may be causing a patient's health problems. This type of testing involves inoculating various kinds of media with specimen samples and then incubating the culture to encourage the pathogens to grow.
- Microscopic examination is another way of identifying bacteria and some fungi and protozoa that cause disease. Wet mounts, dry smears, and Gram staining are all procedures that aid in this process.

Online Resources for Students

Student Resources available on the text's online site include:
- Audio Glossaries
- Animations
- Competency Evaluation Forms

- Videos
- Anatomy & Physiology Module with Heart and Lung Sounds
- Weblinks
- Worksheets

Exercises and Activities

Certification Preparation Questions

1. A sputum specimen would probably be used to determine the presence of:
   a. malaria.
   b. rabies.
   c. tonsillitis.
   d. trichinosis.
   e. tuberculosis.

2. Tapeworms are classified as:
   a. flukes.
   b. arthropods.
   c. cestodes.
   d. helminths.
   e. trichomonas.

3. Which of these duties would not be in the scope of practice for the medical assistant?
   a. Routing specimens
   b. Educating patients
   c. Reading KOH slide
   d. Billing insurance
   e. Collecting specimens

4. What type of specimen would be used to perform an O&P?
   a. Blood
   b. Urine
   c. Stool
   d. Sputum
   e. Mucus

5. If urine cannot be processed within 1 hour, what should the medical assistant do?
   a. Discard the specimen.
   b. Refrigerate the specimen.
   c. Ask the patient for another specimen.
   d. Reschedule the test date and collect a new specimen.
   e. Freeze the specimen.

6. When a microbe is introduced to a culture medium, it is called:
   a. culturing.
   b. incubating.
   c. swabbing.
   d. inoculating.
   e. transferring.

7. The purpose of sensitivity testing is to:
   a. determine if the patient has an allergy to any drugs.
   b. inoculate the culture medium and grow a bacteria.
   c. determine if the bacteria is gram negative or gram positive.
   d. determine the drug that will kill the bacteria.
   e. grow a pure culture.

8. A colony count measures:
   a. the quantity of specimen submitted by the patient.
   b. the amount of bacteria in one milliliter of urine.
   c. the size of the bacteria.
   d. the quantity of antibiotic needed to treat the patient.
   e. the amount of bacteria in a pure culture.

9. A stool specimen would be examined on a microscope slide to determine the presence of:
   a. pinworms.
   b. ringworm.
   c. malaria.
   d. *Trichomonas*.
   e. gram-negative bacteria.

10. Which of these is not a virus?
    a. Influenza
    b. Rabies
    c. Hepatitis
    d. Trichinosis
    e. Polio

APPENDIX A

Abbreviations

A

AA Alcoholics Anonymous

AAMA American Association of Medical Assistants

AAP American Academy of Pediatrics

ABG arterial blood gas

ABHES Accrediting Bureau of Health Education Schools

ACTH adrenocorticotropic hormone

ADAAA Americans with Disabilities Act Amendments Act (2008)

ADH antidiuretic hormone

ADHD attention deficit hyperactivity disorder

AED automated external defibrillator

ALARA As Low As Reasonably Achievable

ALP alkaline phosphatase, liver function test

ALS amyotrophic lateral sclerosis

ALT alanine aminotransferase, liver function test

AMT American Medical Technologists

ARDS acute respiratory distress syndrome

AST aspartate aminotransferase, liver function test

ATP adenosine triphosphate, necessary for muscle action

AV atrioventricular node

B

BMR basal metabolic rate

BNDD Bureau of Narcotics and Dangerous Drugs

BP blood pressure

BPH benign prostatic hyperplasia

bpm beats per minute

BSA body surface area

BUN blood urea nitrogen

Bx biopsy

C

C&S culture and sensitivity

CAAHEP Commission on Accreditation of Allied Health Education Programs

CAB circulation (chest compression), airway, breathing

CABG coronary artery bypass graft

CBC complete blood count

CC chief complaint

CDC Centers for Disease Control and Prevention

CK creatine kinase, enzyme which is elevated during heart attack

CLIA Clinical Laboratory Improvement Amendments

CLSI Clinical and Laboratory Standards Institute

CMA Certified Medical Assistant

CMP comprehensive metabolic panel

CMS Centers for Medicare and Medicaid Services

CNS central nervous system, brain and spinal cord

CO₂ carbon dioxide

COC chain of custody

COPD chronic obstructive pulmonary disease

CPR cardiopulmonary resuscitation

CPT-4 Current Procedural Terminology—book used to locate insurance codes for procedures

CPX complete physical examination

CSF cerebrospinal fluid

CT computerized tomography

CVA cerebrovascular accident

D

DEA   Drug Enforcement Agency

DIP   distal interphalangeal joint

DJD   degenerative joint disease

DSD   dry sterile dressings

E

E/M   evaluation and management

ECG/EKG   electrocardiograph

EDC   pregnancy due date, the estimated date of confinement

EDTA   ethylenediaminetetraacetic acid, additive in evacuated blood draw tubes

EEG   electroencephalograph

EHR/EMR   electronic health records/electronic medical records

ELISA   enzyme-linked immunosorbent assays

EMS   emergency medical services

EOB   explanation of benefits

EPA   Environmental Protection Agency

ER   emergency room

ESR   erythrocyte sedimentation rate

ESWL   extracorporeal shock wave lithotripsy

F

FBS   fasting blood sugar

FDA   Food and Drug Administration

FH   family history

FMH   family medical history

FSH   follicle-stimulating hormone

G

GERD   gastroesophageal reflux disease

GH   growth hormone

GI   gastrointestinal

GTT   glucose tolerance test

H

HAI   health care–acquired infection

HbA1C   glycated hemoglobin

HBG   hemoglobin

HBV   hepatitis B virus

HCG   human chorionic gonadotropin, hormone secreted by developing placenta

HCl   hydrochloric acid

HCO$_3$ bicarbonate

HCPCS   Healthcare Common Procedure Coding System

HCT   hematocrit

HDL   high-density lipoprotein

Hep B   hepatitis B virus

HHS   Department of Health and Human Services

HIPAA   Health Insurance Portability and Accountability Act

HIV   human immunodeficiency virus

HPI   history of present illness

HPV   human papillomavirus

HRT   hormone replacement therapy

Ht   height

I

I&D   incision and drainage

IBD   inflammatory bowel disease

IBS   irritable bowel syndrome

ICD-10-CM   International Classification of Disease 10 revision clinical modification, book used to locate insurance codes for diseases and conditions

ID   intradermal

IM   intramuscular

IV   intravenous

K

KOH   potassium hydroxide used for wet mount

L

LDL   low-density lipids

LES   lower esophageal sphincter

LH   luteinizing hormone

LMP   last menstrual period

LOC   level of consciousness

M

MCH   mean corpuscular hemoglobin

MCHC   mean corpuscular hemoglobin concentration

MCV   mean cell volume

MI   myocardial infarction

mL   milliliter

MP   metacarpophalangeal joint

MRI   magnetic resonance imaging

MS   multiple sclerosis

MTBI   mild traumatic brain injury

N

NCHS   National Center for Health Statistics

NFPA   National Fire Protection Association

NKA   no known allergies

NPO   nothing by mouth

NPT   new patient

NSR   normal sinus rhythm

O

O&P   ova (eggs) and parasites

O₂   oxygen

OA   osteoarthritis

OCD   obsessive–compulsive disorder

OIG   Office of Inspector General

OPIM   other potentially infectious material

OSHA   Occupational Safety and Health Administration

OTC   over-the-counter (drugs)

OV   office visit

P

P   pulse

PAC   premature atrial contraction

PACS   picture archiving and communication system

PAP   Papanicolaou smear

PASS   pull, aim, squeeze, sweep—directions for using a fire extinguisher

PAT   paroxysmal atrial tachycardia

PDR   Physician's Desk Reference

PERRLA   pupils are equal, round, and reactive to light and accommodation

PET   positron emission tomography

PH   past history

pH   concentration of hydrogen ions determining the acidity or alkalinity of a substance

PHI   protected health information

PI   present illness

PID   pelvic inflammatory disease

PIP   proximal interphalangeal joint

PMH   past medical history

PMS   premenstrual syndrome

PNS   peripheral nervous system

PO   by mouth

POC   point of care

POCT   point of care test

POL   physician office laboratory

POMR   problem-oriented medical record

PP   postprandial, after eating such as glucose testing

PPE   personal protective equipment

PPM   provider-performed microscopy

PRL   prolactin hormone

PSA   prostate-specific antigen

PSDA   Patient Self-Determination Act

PST   plasma separator gel tubes used in blood collection

PT   prothrombin time, physical therapy

PT/INR   prothrombin time/international normalized ratio

PTCA   percutaneous transluminal coronary angioplasty

PTT   partial thromboplastin time

PVC   premature ventricular contraction

Q

QA   quality assurance

QC   quality control

QI   quality improvement

R

R respiration

RA rheumatoid arthritis

RBC red blood cells, erythrocytes

RBRVS Resource-Based Relative Value Scale; guideline used by Medicare to set its physician fee schedule by measuring the relative value of a service in units

Rh Rh factor found in blood cells, blood type, named for experiments using the rhesus monkey

RICE rest, ice, compression, elevation—used to treat sprains, strains, and other injuries

RMA Registered Medical Assistant

ROM range of motion

ROS review of systems

RSV respiratory syncytial virus

RVU relative value unit; assigned by Medicare as a measurement of worth

Rx take, prescribe

S

SA sinoatrial node

SC subcutaneous

SDS safety data sheet

SH social history

SLE systemic lupus erythematosus

SOAP subjective, objective, assessment, plan

SOB shortness of breath

SOMR source-oriented medical record

SPECT single photon emission computed tomography

SQ subcutaneous

SSL secure sockets layer

SST serum separator gel tubes used in blood collection

STAT urgently or immediately

STI sexually transmitted infection

T

T temperature

T1DM type 1 diabetes mellitus

T2DM type 2 diabetes mellitus

TAH total abdominal hysterectomy

TB tuberculosis

TSH thyroid-stimulating hormone

U

UCR usual, customary, and reasonable

URI upper respiratory infection

USDA U.S. Department of Agriculture

USP United States Pharmacopeia

UTI urinary tract infection

W

WBC white blood cells, leukocytes

WHO World Health Organization

Wt weight

Key English-to-Spanish Health Care Phrases

Although English is the primary language spoken in North America, a variety of languages are heard. Prominent among them is Spanish. According to the U.S. Census Bureau, Hispanics are the second largest minority group in the United States. Their number is projected to more than double in the next 50 years.

The client and family can be at ease and feel more relaxed if someone on the staff speaks their language. Some health care facilities, especially in areas with a large population of Spanish-speaking people, provide interpreters. In smaller communities, this may not be possible. For this reason, the following table of English-to-Spanish phrases has been prepared. Keep in mind that this is not a complete list. Rather, it contains key words and simple phrases that the medical assistant can use to communicate with a Spanish-speaking individual.

Here's how to use this table: Look for the word or phrase in English in the first column. Then, look across to the second column for the word or phrase in Spanish. Use the third column, which contains the phonetic pronunciation, as a guide to speaking the word or phrase. The syllable in each word to be accented is printed in italic type.

Even if proficiency in English to Spanish is lacking, Spanish-speaking clients will appreciate the attempt to converse in their language. Begin with "Buenos días. ¿Cómo se siente?" And remember "por favor[a]."

Introductory Phrases

English	Spanish	Pronunciation
Please[a]	Por favor	Por fah-*vor*
Yes/no	Si/no	See/no
Thank you	Gracias	*Grah*-see-ahs
Good morning	Buenos dias	*Bway*-nos *dee*-ahs
Good afternoon	Buenas tardes	*Bway*-nas *tar*-days
Good evening	Buenas noches	*Bway*-nas *noh*-chays
My name is	Mi nombre es	Me *nohm*-bray ays
I am a student nurse.	Soy estudiante enfermera.	Soy ays-stoo-dee-*ayn*-tay *ayn*-fay-*may*-rah
What is your name?	¿Cómo se llama?	Koh-moh say *yah*-mah
How old are you?	¿Cuántos años tiene?	*Kwan*-tohs ahn-yos tee-*ayn*-ays
Do you understand me?	¿Me entiende?	Me ayn-tee-*ayn*-day
Speak slower.	Hable más despacio.	*Ah*-blah mahs days*pah*-see-oh
How do you feel?	¿Cómo se siente?	*Koh*-moh say see-*ayn*-tay

[a]Begin or end any request with the word PLEASE (POR FAVOR).

Numbers

Zero	Cero	*Se*-roh
One	Uno	*Oo*-noh
Two	Dos	Dohs
Three	Tres	Trays
Four	Cuatro	*Kwah*-troh
Five	Cinco	*Sin*-koh
Six	Seis	Says
Seven	Siete	See-*ay*-tay
Eight	Ocho	Oh-choh
Nine	Nueve	New-*ay*-vay
Ten	Diez	*Dee*-ays

Days of the Week

Sunday	Domingo	Doh-*ming*-goh
Monday	Lunes	*Loo*-nays
Tuesday	Martes	*Mar*-tays
Wednesday	Miércoles	Mee-*er*-cohl-ays
Thursday	Jueves	*Hway*-vays
Friday	Viernes	Vee-*ayr*-nays
Saturday	Sábado	*Sah*-bah-doh

General Terms

Good	Bien	Bee-ayn
Bad	Mal	Mahl
Physician	Médico	*May*-dee-koh
Hospital	Hospital	*Ooh*-spee-tall
Midwife	Comadre	Koh-*mah*-dray
Native healer	Curandero	Ku-ren-*day*-roh
Right	Derecha	Day-*ray*-chah

Left	Izquierda	Ees-kee-*ayr*-dah
Week	Semana	Say-*mah*-nah
Month	Mes	Mace
A prescription	Una receta	Oo-na ray-*say*-tah
Pulse	Tomar su pulso	*Pool*-soh
Temperature	Temperatura	Taym-pay-rah-*too*-rah
Blood pressure	Presión	Pray-see-*ohn*
IV line	Intravenosa	Een-trah-vayn-*oh*-sah
Pain medicine	Medicación para dolor	May-dee-kah-see-*ohn* pah-rah doh-*lohr*
Enema	Lavado	Lah-*vah*-doh
Unusual vaginal bleeding?	¿Hemorragia vaginal fuera de los periodos?	Ay-moh-*rah*-hee-ah *vah*-hee-nahl foo-*ay*-rah day lohs pay-ree-*oh*-dohs
Hoarseness?	¿Ronquera?	Rohn-*kay*-rah
A sore throat?	¿Le duele la garganta?	Lay doo-*ay*-lay lah gahr-gahn-tah
Does it hurt to swallow?	¿Le duele al tragar?	Lay doo-ay-lay ahl trah-gar
Difficulty in breathing?	¿Dificultad al respirar?	Dee-fee-kool-*tahd* ahl rays-*pee*-rahr
Is your memory good?	¿Es buena su memoria?	Ays *bway*-nah soo may-moh-*ree*-ah
Have you any pain in the head?	¿Le duele la cabeza?	Lay doo-*ay*-lay lah kah-*bay*-sah
Do you feel dizzy?	¿Tiene usted véigo?	Tee-*ay*-nay ood-*stayd vehr*-tee-goh
Are you tired?	¿Está usted cansado?	Ay-*stah* ood-*stayd* kahn-*sah*-doh
Can you eat?	¿Puede comer?	*Pway*-day koh-*mer*
Are you constipated?	¿Está estreñido?	Ay-*stah* ays-trayn-*yee*-do
Do you have diarrhea?	¿Tiene diarrea?	Tee-*ay*-nay dee-ah-*ray*-ah
Have you any difficulty passing water?	¿Tiene dificultad en orinar?	Tee-*ay*-nay dee-fee-kool-*tahd* ayn oh-ree-*nahr*
Do you hear voices?	¿Oye los voces?	Oy-eh los *vo*-ses

Bedside Care

Warm	Calor	Kahl-*or*
Cold	Frío	Fr*ee*-oh
Milk	Leche	*Leh*-chay
Tea	Té	Tay
Coffee	Café	Kah-*fay*

Times of the Day

Early in the morning	Temprano por la mañana	Tehm-*prah*-noh por lah mah-*nyah*-na
In the daytime	En el día	Ayn el *dee*-ah
At noon	A mediodía	Ah meh-dee-oh-*dee*-ah
At bedtime	Al acostarse	Al ah-kos-*tar*-say
At night	Por la noche	Por la *noh*-chay
Today	Hoy	Oy
Tomorrow	Mañana	Mah-*nyah*-nah
Yesterday	Ayer	Ai-*yer*
Before meals	Antes de las comidas	*Ahn*-tays day lahs koh-*mee*-dahs
After meals	Después de las	*Days*-poo-ehs day lahs koh-mee-dahs
Every day	Todos los días comidas	*Toh*-dohs lohs *dee*-ah
Every hour	Cada hora	*Kah*-dah *oh*-rah

Questions to Begin Phrases

Do you have …?	¿Tiene …?	Tee-*ay*-nay
Are you …?	¿Tiene …?	Tee-*ay*-nay
How long …?	¿Hace cúanto?	*Ah*-say *kwahn*-toh
How much …?	¿Cuánto …?	*Kwahn*-toh
How …?	¿Cómo …?	*Ko*-mo

Signs and Symptoms

English	Spanish	Pronunciation
Pain?	¿Dolor?	Doh-*lorh*
Stomach cramps?	¿Calambres en el estómago?	Kah-*lahm*-brays ayn el ays-*toh*-mah-goh
Chills?	¿Escalofrios?	Ays-kah-loh-*free*-ohs
Hemorrhage?	¿Hemorragia?	Ay-moh-*rah*-hee-ah
Nosebleeds?	¿Hemorragia por la nariz?	Ay-moh-*rah*-hee-ah por-lah nah-*rees*
Where is the pain?	¿Donde está el dolor?	*Dohn*-day ay-*stah* ayl doh-*lorh*
Do you want medication for your pain?	¿Quire medicación para su dolor?	Key-*ay*-ray may-dee-kah-see-*ohn* *pa*-rah soo doh-*lorh*
Are you comfortable?	¿Está comfortable?	Ay-*stah* kohm-for-*tah*-blay
Are you hungry?	¿Tiene hambre?	Tee-*ay*-nay *ahm*-bray
Are you thirsty?	¿Tiene sed?	Tee-*ay*-nay sayd
You may not eat/drink.	No coma/beba.	Noh *koh*-mah/bay-*bah*
You can drink only water.	Sólo puede tomar agua.	Soh-loh *pway*-day toh-mar *ah*-gwah
You can take only ice chips.	Solo puéde tomár pedacitos de hiélo.	Soh-loh *pway*-day toh-*marh* pay-da-*zee*-tohs day eee-*ay*-loh
Keep very quiet.	Estése muy quieto.	Ays-*tay*-say moo-ay key-*ay*-toh

(Reprinted from Rosdahl CB, Kowalski MT. *Textbook of Basic Nursing.* 10th ed. Philadelphia, PA: Wolters Kluwer Health; 2012.)

APPENDIX C

Valuable Internet Resources

Frequently, students are assigned classroom activities that require further research of specific topics. Although the textbook and classroom discussions provide a wealth of information, listed here are many Web sites containing additional information on these topics. Lifelong learning is encouraged in post secondary education programs. Medical assistant instructors encourage students to seek out answers to questions and teach them the techniques of researching information.

Agency for Healthcare Research and Quality (AHRQ) **www.ahrq.gov**

American Association of Medical Assistants (AAMA) **www.aama-ntl.org**

American Medical Technologists (AMT) **www.americanmedtech.org**

Centers for Disease Control and Prevention (CDC) **www.cdc.gov**

Clinical and Laboratory Standards Institute (CLSI) **www.clsi.org**

Centers for Medicare and Medicaid Services (CMS) **www.cms.org**

Department of Health and Human Services (HHS) **www.hhs.gov**

Department of Labor (DOL) **www.dol.gov**

Equal Employment Opportunities Commission (EEOC) **www.eeoc.gov**

Federal Emergency Management Agency (FEMA) **www.fema.gov**

Food and Drug Administration (FDA) **www.fda.gov**

Immunization Action Coalition (IAC) **www.immunize.org**

Mayo Clinic **www.mayoclinic.org**

National Health Information Center (NHIC) **www.health.gov**

National Institutes of Health (NIH) **www.nih.gov**

National Institute of Mental Health (NIMH) **www.nimh.nih.gov**

Occupational Safety and Health Administration (OSHA) **www.osha.gov**

Postal Service (USPS) **www.usps.com**

World Health Organization (WHO) **www.who.int**

Glossary

A

abandonment occurs when the physician ends the relationship without proper notice while the patient still needs treatment

abduction moving away from the midline of the body

abortion general term that means the loss of the embryo or fetus prior to week 20 of the pregnancy

abrasion a scratch or scrape on the skin's surface

accommodation refers to the ability of the pupils to adjust when focusing on objects at different distances

accounting an organized system for keeping track of a business's finances

accounts payable money the office owes for operating expenses

accounts receivable money owed to the office from patient accounts

acromegaly growth condition in adults causing the bones of the face, hands, and feet to enlarge

active induced immunity occurs when a person is exposed to a foreign antigen as part of therapy and develops his own antibodies to fight it

active natural immunity occurs when people are exposed to a foreign antigen as a natural process and develop their own antibodies to fight it

acute used to describe a condition with a sudden onset of symptom(s)

adduction moving toward the midline of the body

adipose fatty tissue

adjustments deducting or subtracting from the amount owed with no monetary exchange

aerobic requiring oxygen for growth; aerobic bacteria

aerosol particles suspended in gas or air

afebrile without fever

agglutination the clumping together of materials that are suspended in a liquid

aging schedule amount of time an account balance has been outstanding

albinism lack of pigment in the skin, hair, and eyes

allergen a substance that causes a person to have an allergic reaction

allergy hypersensitivity to a substance, excessive reaction

alphanumeric a code composed of letters and numbers

ampule small glass containers that must be broken at the neck to withdraw the fluid in the ampule

amputation loss of all or part of an extremity

anabolism the building up of tissues through growth and repair

anaerobe microbes that do not need oxygen to survive

anaerobic does not require oxygen for growth, anaerobic bacteria

anaphylactic shock a type of shock due to a severe allergic reaction requiring immediate medical intervention

anaphylaxis severe, potentially life-threatening, allergic reaction

anatomy refers to the structure of the body

anemia condition resulting from reduced numbers of RBCs in the blood or decreased hemoglobin

aneurysm   bulging or ballooning sac of a vessel due to weakness in the wall of the vessel

anisocytosis   variations in the size of a blood cell

anorexia   chronic loss of appetite

antagonism   opposes or resists the action of another, effect in which one drug makes the other less effective

antecubital space   the inside area of the elbow, location of veins preferred for use in blood collection

anthropometric   physical measurements of the patient's body

antibody   a blood protein produced in response to and counteracting a specific antigen

anticoagulant   substance or medicine used to prevent blood clotting in conditions caused by clot formation and blocked blood vessels

antigens   toxins or other foreign substances that induce an immune response in the body

antiseptics   agent that blocks the growth of bacteria, example is 70% isopropyl alcohol used to cleanse the skin

apex   rounded lower end of the heart

appendicitis   inflammation of the appendix due to infection or obstruction

appendicular   the bones of the extremities

approximation   bringing the edges of the wound as close together as possible to their original position

arbitration   an alternative method to settle a dispute without going to court

arrhythmia   an abnormal heart rhythm

arteriosclerosis   hardening of the arteries caused by loss of elasticity of the arterial wall

arthrocentesis   draining accumulated fluid from a joint cavity

arthroplasty   surgical joint replacement

arthroscopy   a procedure using an arthroscope (endoscope), a lighted instrument, to examine the inside of a joint

articular cartilage   cartilage located at and covering the ends of the bones

asepsis   a condition in which there are no living pathogens, a state of sterility

assault   threatening a person or acting in a way that causes the person to fear harm

assessment   the process of gathering information in order to determine the patient's problem

asymmetry   inequality of size and shape

atherosclerosis   condition caused by a buildup of plaque (fatty deposits)

atrioventricular   pertaining to the atria and ventricles of the heart

atrophy   decrease in size or lack of development

auscultation   listening to body sounds

autoclave   a device that uses steam heat under high pressure to sterilize objects

avulsion   a wound with a flap of skin torn loose; the flap may remain hanging or tear off altogether

axial   the bones of the head and torso

axons   neuron fibers that conduct impulses away from the cell body

B

bacteria   tiny one-celled creatures found in soil or water, or on other organisms

bacteriology   the science and study of bacteria

bacteriuria   bacteria in urine

battery   unlawful touching, whether or not the touching causes bodily harm

beneficence   doing good, especially doing things that will benefit other people

bevel   the slant end of the needle where the opening is located

bilirubin   amber-colored substance produced as a by-product of hemoglobin breakdown

biopsy removal of a tissue sample for diagnostic examination

bioterrorism terrorist attack involving the deliberate release of biological agents used to cause illness or death

blood-borne pathogens dangerous organisms that can exist in the blood, body fluids, and secretions of an infected person

bookkeeping maintaining office financial accounts; basic bookkeeping formula is Previous Balance + Charges – Payments – Debits = Current Balance

bradycardia slow heart rate of <60 bpm

breach failure to do what is required or what you have been expected to do under contract

bronchodilators medication used to open up or dilate the bronchioles of the lungs

bronchoscope flexible fiberoptic instrument used for visual examination of the inside of the lungs

bundled procedure codes that are combined together under one code; example laboratory panels such as a thyroid panel

C

cancellous spongy bone

capillaries small blood vessels in the skin

carbaminohemoglobin carbon dioxide combined with hemoglobin

cardiogenic shock a type of shock which is an extreme form of heart failure occurring when the heart's left ventricle is so impaired; blood is not adequately pumped to body tissues

cardiologist heart specialist

casts cylinders of proteins and other substances that form and solidify in the nephron tubules in the kidneys

catabolism the breakdown of complex substances into simpler compounds

cataract cloudiness of the lens of the eye causing gradual loss of vision

catheter a thin sterile, flexible tube inserted into the bladder through the urethra to drain the bladder of urine

catheterization an invasive procedure used to diagnose or treat conditions affecting circulation in the coronary arteries

caustic corrosive or abrasive

centrifuge a machine that separates liquids into their different parts, uses centrifugal force or spinning that exerts force outward

cerebrum largest part of the brain divided into a right and left hemisphere

cerumen earwax

ceruminosis impacted earwax

cesarean section involves a surgical incision made in the abdominal wall and uterus to remove the baby

charges/debits fees owed by the patient or responsible party for services performed

chemical burns burns due to corrosive substances contacting the skin or mucous membranes

cholecystectomy surgical removal of the gallbladder

cholelithiasis development of stones that may become large enough to block the bile ducts of the gallbladder

chronic symptoms or condition that persist for a long time or is constantly reoccurring

chyme a semiliquid substance found in the stomach due to breakdown of food

cicatrix a scar

circumduction moving in a circular pattern as when moving the outstretched arm in a circle

cirrhosis chronic disease of the liver

clustering appointment scheduling method when patients with similar needs are seen in the same time period—bunched together in a "cluster"

coinsurance contracted percentage owed by the insured/patient per service

collagen a protein substance, required to strengthen structures in the body including bones

collections process of collecting payments due on all accounts

colony a group of identical bacteria that grow in a culture from one "parent" bacteria

colony count measures the amount of bacteria growing in 1 mL of urine or quantity of specimen

comorbidity more than one disease or condition occurring at the same time

conjunctivitis inflammation of the conjunctiva

constellation of symptoms a group of symptoms that happen together signaling a specific problem

consultation another physician reviews a patient's case and examines the patient to render an opinion and offer recommendations

contagious a disease that can spread easily from one person to another

contaminated has been touched by a source of pathogens, unsterile

contract a voluntary agreement between two parties from which each party benefits

contusion a collection of blood under the skin or in damaged tissue, a bruise

cookies tiny files that many internet Web sites will leave in the hard drive

co-payment amount owed by the insured/patient at time of service; usually a set dollar amount

coronary from the word crown, which is how the vessels encircle the heart

coronary angiography injection of contrast dye into the coronary arteries to highlight any vessel damage or blockage

cryptorchidism undescended testicle

culture colonies of bacteria grown under controlled conditions in a container in a lab

cyanosis bluish discoloration of the skin when there is not enough oxygen in the blood

cycle billing billing system in which accounts are divided alphabetically and billed separate intervals during the month

cystitis inflammation of the bladder

cytology the study of cells

D

deductible annual amount owed by the insured prior to insurance payment

defecation the process of eliminating waste from the body

defendant person accused of breaking the law

defibrillation the process of using electric shock to restore normal heart rhythm

dehiscence the separation of wound edges

dehydration an excessive loss of fluid from the body

dendrites neuron fibers that conduct impulses *to* the cell body

denial when a person rejects a fact that's painful or difficult to accept

deoxygenated blood with less oxygen

dermatosis general term used for any skin disease

diabetes mellitus condition of the body not producing enough insulin or utilizing the insulin properly

diagnosis the process of identifying a disease or illness

diagnostic codes insurance codes used to identify the reason the patient is seeking care

dialysis hemodialysis, uses a dialysis machine to filter the blood

diaphoresis profuse sweating

diaphysis the narrow shaft of long bones

diastole resting, relaxing phase of the heart

dilemma a problem caused by a conflict between choices

diluent diluting agent, usually sterile water or saline

disinfection destruction of pathogens by direct exposure to chemical or physical agents

dislocation structures of the joint become deranged

dissect cut apart

diuretics drugs that increase the body's fluid output resulting in more urine production

diverticulosis development of large numbers of diverticula, small pouches in the wall of the intestine

dorsiflexion moving the foot upward toward the body decreasing the angle between the foot and the lower leg

double-booking two patients are given the same appointment slot

downcoding coding for less than the actual service provided

dunning computer option in billing that allows you to set messages to be added onto statements within specific parameters, usually determined by age of account

dysmenorrhea painful or difficult menstruation

dysrhythmia an abnormal heart rhythm

E

ecchymosis a bruise; resulting from blood pooling under the skin following trauma

edema swelling; collection of fluid in an area due to injury or inflammation

effusion accumulation of fluid

electrolytes ions in blood and body fluids; chemicals that carry an electrical charge

embezzlement wrongful taking of money or property

encryption translates data into special codes limiting access to the information

endocarditis inflammation of the lining of the heart

endocardium innermost lining of the heart

endometriosis condition when the endometrial tissue grows outside the uterus

endometrium inner lining of the uterus

endoscopy use of a lighted scope to visualize the gastrointestinal tract

endosteum lines the bone marrow cavity

enuresis form of involuntary urination usually occurring at night; bed wetting

epicardium outermost covering of the heart

epidermis the top layer of the skin and contains no blood vessels

epinephrine hormone produced in the adrenal medulla

epiphyseal plates where continued growth of the bone takes place

episiotomy small incision between the vagina and the anus to increase the size of the delivery area

epistaxis nosebleed

erythema redness of the skin

erythropoietin hormone that is released from the kidneys and influences the production of RBCs

ethics guidelines for determining proper behavior

etiology cause of disease or condition

etiquette rules for polite behavior

eversion turning the sole of the foot outward so the bottom of the foot faces away from the body

excise cut out tissue

excretory urinary system

extension increases the angle of the joint

extension of credit allowing payments to set fixed payments, with or without interest

extracellular fluid fluid outside the cell; includes blood plasma and lymphatic fluid

F

familial disorder a problem that is unusually common within a family

febrile has a fever

fee schedule a list of charges for specific medical procedures

felony serious crimes punishable by long prison sentences or even by death

fenestrated drape   a surgical drape with an opening to expose the operative site while covering other areas

fidelity   faithfulness and loyalty to others

firewalls   computer programs or devices that prevent unauthorized users from accessing private information on a computer network through the internet

fixed scheduling   form of scheduling in which patients are assigned to a specific appointment time slot

flexion   decreases the angle of the joint

fontanelles   membrane areas found in the infant skull, called "soft spots"

forceps   instrument used for grasping and holding things

fraud   any deceitful act with the intention of concealing the truth

fungi   a type of plant

G

gait   refers to the style or way in which a person walks

gastritis   any inflammation of the stomach lining

gauge   the size of an opening or lumen; the larger the gauge number, the smaller the opening of the needle

generic   the name assigned to the drug during research and development; the chemical ingredients that make up the drug

gigantism   causing the child to grow abnormally tall

glaucoma   excessive pressure of the aqueous humor of the eye

global surgical follow-up   an inclusive package of all the procedures and visits surrounding a surgical procedure

glomerulonephritis   malfunctioning glomeruli causing increased protein and red blood cells in the urine

glycosuria   sugar or glucose in the urine usually indicates diabetes mellitus

gram negative   a type of bacteria that stain red with safranin dye

gram positive   a type of bacteria that stain purple with crystal violet dye

H

hematocrit   percentage of RBCs in whole blood

hematology   the study of blood, blood-forming tissues, and blood diseases

hematoma   blood leaks into body tissues due to trauma or injury; may occur during or after blood draw

hematopoiesis   the process of blood cell production

hematuria   blood in the urine usually indicates injury or disease in the urinary system

hemoconcentration   pooling; increased collection of blood components; occurs from application of tourniquet for long time

hemoglobin   the part of the red blood cell that binds oxygen and carbon dioxide

hemolysis   the rupture of the blood cells

hemorrhage   excessive bleeding caused by damage to a blood vessel

hemorrhagic shock   type of shock produced from excessive blood loss

hemostasis   to control bleeding or stop flow of blood from the body

hemostat   instrument used to grasp and clamp blood vessels to establish hemostasis; the stopping of blood flow or bleeding

hepatitis   inflammation of the liver

hereditary disorder   passed from parents to their off-spring

histology   the study of tissue

homeopathic   the use of substances that would produce the symptoms of the disease being treated

homeostasis   state of internal balance in the normal body

hydronephrosis   accumulation of fluid in the kidney

hyperextension extending a body part beyond the anatomical position

hyperglycemia high blood sugar

hyperkalemia potassium level is above 5.0 mEq/L

hypernatremia sodium levels above the normal 145 mEq/L level

hyperpyrexia extremely high temperature, 105°F to 106°F

hypertension high blood pressure

hyperthermia a general condition of excessive body heat

hypertrophy increase the size or bulk of a body part, for example, a muscle

hyperuricemia uric acid levels above the normal range

hyperventilation abnormally rapid breathing; respirations that are too fast

hypocalcemia calcium levels below the normal level of 8.5 mg/dL

hypochloremia serum chloride level that drops below 96 mEq/L

hypoglycemia low blood sugar

hypokalemia serum potassium level below the normal level of 3.5 mEq/L

hyponatremia sodium levels below 135 mEq/L

hypotension low blood pressure

hypothermia an abnormally low body temperature

hypovolemic shock type of shock occurring from excessive loss of fluids

I

immobilized to secure in a manner that prevents normal movement

immunity refers to the body's ability to fight specific pathogens

immunoglobulin protein-based antibodies in the body

immunohematology testing that blood banks do on red blood cells (RBCs) and serum or plasma to make sure that blood from a donor matches the blood of the person who receives it

immunology a branch of medicine that focuses on the study of the immune system

impetigo type of infection caused from a staphylococcal bacteria

implementation the process used to perform patient education; the actual teaching

incident reports written accounts of negative events experienced by patients, visitors, or staff; should be completed for even minor negative events

incision cutting into tissue

incontinence involuntary loss of urine

incus tiny bone of the ear shaped like an anvil

infarction obstruction of blood flow to an area

informed consent a legal document that explains the course of treatment, including the risks and benefits to the patient

ingestion process of taking food into the mouth

inhalation administered through the lungs

initial encounter first time seeing the patient by a health care practitioner

inscription on a prescription, the name of the medication, the desired form, and the strength

insertion the moveable end of a muscle attached to the bone that is moved

inspection looking at areas of the body to observe physical features

instillation administration into the eyes, ears, and nose

integrity the quality of strongly sticking to your principles

interaction the effect or action that occurs between drugs and the human body

intracellular fluid fluid inside the cells; maintains the homeostatic internal environment of the cell

intranet an internal business system that provides quick access to company information

inventory detailed listing of supplies and equipment with accurate accounting of quantity

inversion turning the sole of the foot inward so the bottom of the foot faces the other foot

ischemia lack of blood supply resulting in a decrease in oxygen supply to a body part

isometric muscle tension increases, but the size remains the same; the word means equal or same measure

isotonic muscle tension remains the same, but it changes in length; the word literally means equal or same tension

itinerary a detailed plan of a trip including transportation and hotel (housing)

J

jaundice yellowish skin discoloration which may be caused by excessive amounts of bile pigments

K

keratin hardened protein found in finger and toenails

ketones chemicals the body makes when it metabolizes (breaks down) fat

key components used for insurance coding to determine E/M codes; include history, physical examination, and medical decision making

L

late effects conditions that result from a past injury or illness

learning goal what a patient should achieve at the end of patient education

learning objectives tasks to help reach patient education goals; objectives are performed at different points in the program

leukemia disease in which unusually high numbers of abnormal WBCs are produced

leukocytosis too many WBCs in the body

leukopenia too few WBCs in the body

libel damaging a person's reputation in writing

ligaments connect bone to bone around synovial joints

lithotripsy procedure used to crush kidney stones into small pieces that are able to be passed through the urinary tract

luxation the end of a bone is displaced from its normal position in a joint, also referred to as dislocation

M

malfeasance the performance of a wrong and unlawful act

malleus tiny ear bone shaped like a hammer

malpractice professional person is negligent in his or her duties

mammogram an x-ray study of the breast to detect even small growths

manipulation moving a body part or joint

mastication the process of chewing food

matrix model used to set physician's schedule for appointments

meaningful use use of certified electronic health records to improve quality of care and reduce medical errors

mediastinum central area of the chest cavity, slightly to the left of the midline of the body

medical asepsis practices used to stop microbes from spreading from one patient to another

medical necessity the procedure or service being billed was reasonable for the patient's medical condition

medullary cavity the center of the diaphysis where the bone marrow is located

melanin a dark pigment that colors the skin and protects it from the harmful rays of the sun

melanoma a malignant tumor of melanocytes

melena blood in the stool

meninges three membranes covering the spinal cord and brain

mensuration the process of measuring

metabolism the sum of all chemical and physical changes that occur in the body's tissues

microorganisms living organisms that are only visible with a microscope

micturition urination

misdemeanor less serious crimes punishable by fines or short jail sentences

misfeasance the performance of a lawful act in an improper manner

modified wave scheduling blocks of patients are scheduled into a set time frame with specific parameters, for example, each half hour would have one major appointment with three to four minor appointments mixed in

modifiers used to alter or modify insurance codes by providing additional information

murmur abnormal sounds of the heart caused by a faulty heart valve that fails to close tightly and blood leaks back

mycology the science and study of fungi

myelin whitish, fatty substance that covers some of the axons

myocarditis inflammation of the heart muscle

myocardium muscular layer of the heart

myoglobin a red protein containing heme that carries and stores oxygen in muscle cells

myopia nearsightedness

N

nausea feeling of queasiness that usually precedes vomiting

necrosis death of tissue

negative feedback a method that reverses any shift from normal range by upward or downward changes

negligence results from failing to act with reasonable care

nerve a bundle of neuron fibers

neurogenic shock type of shock caused by a dysfunction of the nervous system following an injury to the spinal cord

neurons highly specialized cells of the nervous system

neuropathy any disease of the nervous system

neutropenia a low number of neutrophils

neutrophilia an increase in the percentage of neutrophils

nitrogenous relating to, or containing, nitrogen

noncompliance the patient's inability or refusal to follow a prescribed order

nonfeasance the failure to perform a necessary act

nonsufficient funds check check (NSF) returned by the bank due to lack of funds in the account; it was written form

normal flora microbes that live in and on the human body without causing any problems or disease; nonpathogenic

normal values refers to the acceptable ranges for laboratory test results

O

ophthalmoscope a medical tool used to inspect the interior structures of the eyes

oral thrush a fungal infection that affects the mouth usually due to yeast

origin the less moveable, fixed end of a muscle

osseous tissue the living tissue that composes bone tissue

ossicles three tiny bones in each middle ear (incus, malleus, stapes)

ossification the process of converting cartilage to bone

osteoblast the cells responsible for building bone tissue

osteoclast the cells responsible for resorption, the breakdown of bone tissue

osteocyte mature bone cell

otitis media infection and inflammation of the middle ear

otorhinolaryngologist a physician who specializes in treating disorders and diseases of the ears, nose, and throat

otoscope allows the examiner to see inside the ear canal and inspect the tympanic membrane

ovulation process of releasing an egg from the ovary follicle

oxygenated blood that is rich in oxygen

oxyhemoglobin binding of oxygen with hemoglobin

P

palpation touching or moving body areas with the fingers or hands

paraphrasing rephrasing what the patient said in your own words

paraplegia paralysis of both lower limbs

parenteral administration routes other than the digestive tract, injection, and intravenous

parotitis inflammation of the parotid salivary glands

participating provider a provider that is in a plan's network

passive induced immunity occurs when a person receives already-made antibodies as part of therapy

passive natural immunity occurs when infants receive already-made antibodies from their mothers

pathogen disease-causing microorganisms

payments/credits funds received to cover charges on an account

percussion tapping or striking parts of the body with the hand or an instrument to produce sounds

pericarditis inflammation of the sac around the heart

pericardium fibrous sac enclosing the heart

periosteum the membrane covering bones

peristalsis the rhythmic action of moving this material through the large intestine

Petri dish an empty glass or plastic container used to hold a solid culture medium, such as blood agar

pharmacokinetic pertaining to how drugs move through the body after swallowed or injected

phlebotomist person trained to obtain blood specimens from patients

phlebotomy process of collecting blood from a vein

physical status modifier describes the patient's condition, at the time of anesthesia administration

physiology refers to the function of body parts

plaintiff person or party that charges the wrongdoing

plantar flexion bending the foot downward as in standing on the tiptoes; increases the angle between the foot and lower leg

plaque fatty deposits

plasma the liquid part of the blood with the clotting agents

pnea refers to breathing

poikilocytosis condition of irregular shape of RBCs

poliomyelitis viral disease of the nervous system

posting recording of charges, payments, and adjustments to an account

postprandial after eating a meal

potentiation occurs when one drug extends or multiplies the effect of another drug

precedents previous cases tried under the same law to determine how the law was applied

precertification obtaining authorization from the insurance company prior to performing certain procedures or hospitalization; payment is not guaranteed

pressure points specific places where you can press an artery against a bone; arteries located close to the surface of the skin

primary diagnosis patient's chief complaint or the reason medical attention was sought that day

privileged information information regarding patients that cannot be released without proper authorization

procedure codes insurance codes used to explain services provided

pronation facing down and turning the palm of the hand down; backward when in anatomical position

protozoa tiny parasites—animals that live in or on another organism

psoriasis an overgrowth of keratinocytes in the epidermis

purulent drainage with a color other than pink, usually yellow

pyelonephritis inflammation of the renal pelvis, the lower portion of the kidney

pyrexia fever of 102°F or higher (rectally) or 101°F or higher (orally)

pyuria pus in the urine indicating possible infection in the bladder or kidneys

Q

quadriplegia paralysis of all four limbs

quality assurance written policies and procedures to make sure lab employees meet the standards required by CLIA

quality control processes used to ensure accuracy in testing by monitoring

R

radiation burns result from overexposure to ultraviolet light or from any extreme exposure to radiation

random urine urine specimen collected at any time

rationalization the process of finding excuses for thoughts or feelings that would otherwise be hard to accept

reagent substance used to produce a test reaction

referral a physician transfers the care of a patient to another provider for a specific issue

reflecting repeating back what the patient said, using open-ended statements

reflex an involuntary response to a stimulus

repression the process the mind uses to block uncomfortable or distressing ideas from conscious awareness

res ipsa loquitur Latin term that means "the thing speaks for itself"

rescue breathing used in emergency situations when the patient has a pulse, however, is not breathing adequately

resident flora bacteria that normally live in your body and do not cause disease

resistance refers to how well the human body fights disease

respondeat superior Latin term that means "let the master answer"

restrictive endorsement endorsement or signature on the back of a check to be deposited that limits the use of the check

retractor instrument used to separate the edges of a wound and to hold open layers of tissue

RhoGAM Rh immunoglobulin injected when there is Rh incompatibility during pregnancy

risk management the process of identifying problems before they cause injury to patients or staff

rotation the action of turning a bone on its own axis

rule of nines method used to calculate the percentage of total surface area affected by a burn

S

safety data sheets provides the manufacturer's instructions for how to store, handle, and dispose of the chemical or substance

sanitization cleaning items using soap or detergent

sanitizing   reducing the microorganisms on a surface by using low-level disinfection practices

scalpel   surgical knife with a handle and a straight or curved cutting blade

sciatica   compression of the sciatic nerve of the lower back causing pain, numbness, and tingling from the lower back continuing down the leg

sebum   oil which lubricates the skin and hair preventing dryness

seizure   abnormal electrical activity in the brain which might be due to infection, trauma, or high fever; causes uncontrollable muscle contractions

semilunar   resembling a half moon shape such as semilunar valves of the heart

septic shock   shock caused by a general infection of the bloodstream

sequela   follow-up encounters

serum   the liquid part of the blood with the clotting agents removed

service contract   an arrangement with a company to care for office equipment

sesamoid   small bone found around joints such as the patella, kneecap

shock   life-threatening condition in which the body system begins to shut down

signs   objective information, observed or seen by someone other than the patient

sinus rhythm   normal heart rhythm

skin puncture   piercing the skin with a sharp object for the purpose of obtaining a small blood sample

slander   speaking lies about another person that harms the person's reputation or employment

spasm   a sudden and involuntary contraction of a muscle

specific gravity   comparing the consistency of a substance compared to the weight of water

speculum   a medical tool that enlarges and separates the opening of a body cavity so the examiner can see the interior structures and mucosa

sphygmomanometer   blood pressure cuff

spirometer   machine used to measure and record the volume of air moved with each inhalation and expiration

spores   a form of bacteria that can resist the destructive forces of heat, drying, or chemicals

sprain   an injury to a joint capsule and supporting ligaments

sputum   mucus from a patient's lungs, used to prepare a culture

stapes   tiny ear bone shaped like a stirrup

stare decisis   Latin term that means "let the decision stand"

statutes   laws passed by Congress or by state legislatures

stenosis   narrowing of a structure such as a heart valve opening

sterile field   a specific area that is considered free of microbes

sterilization   the complete elimination or destruction of all microbes, including spores

stethoscope   an instrument used for listening to body sounds

strain   an injury to a muscle and supporting tendons

streaming   assigning the number of time slots required for a patient's visit; patient's reason for the visit is required for this type of scheduling to be effective

sublingual   administration under the tongue

subluxation   a bone pulled from its socket, but all structures in the joint, such as ligaments and tendons, keep their proper relationships, also known as a partial dislocation

subpoena   order issued by the court to obtain evidence

subscription   the section of a prescription that indicates how much of the drug to dispense

subsequent encounter   follow-up visit(s)

supination turn face up as turning the palm of the hand up; forward when in anatomical position

surgical asepsis set of practices that stop microbes from getting into the patient's body during an invasive procedure

symmetry equality of size and shape

symptoms subjective information; reflect changes in the body sensed by the patient

synapse transmission of a nerve impulse from the axon of one neuron to the dendrite of another neuron

syncope fainting; temporary loss of consciousness

synergism to work together; medications that work together

systole active, contracting phase of the heart

T

tachycardia rapid heart rate of more than 100 bpm

tendons dense connective tissues that attach the muscles to bones

third party someone other than the patient or responsible party is held accountable for the charges from service

third-party payers liability cases, in which another individual's liability insurance covers expenses, or legal cases where payments are received directly from the attorney

thrombocytopenia too few platelets

thrombocytosis too many platelets

thrombosis blood clot formation

tort wrongs committed against a person or property

tortfeasor person who commits a tort

tourniquet a soft, flexible rubber strip wrapped around the arm to block the flow of blood in the veins, used during venipuncture to enlarge the veins, making them easier to find and puncture with a needle

transdermal administration through the skin

turbid used to describe cloudy urine, probably contains particulate matter or tiny solid particles

U

ulcerative colitis inflammation and ulceration of the colon and rectum

unbundled submitting a code for each piece of a service package, instead of the single code for the entire package

unsecure information information provided on an Internet Web site that might be seen by unauthorized people

upcoding submitting a code for a service the physician did not perform

uremia excess of nitrogen waste substances in the blood due to kidneys inability to properly filter the blood

ureterocele herniation of the ureter as it enters the bladder

urethritis inflammation of the urethra

urticaria hives causing intense itching usually due to allergic reaction

V

vacuum a space from which the air has been removed, or evacuated; evacuated tubes are used to collect blood during phlebotomy

vasodilation dilation of blood vessels increasing blood flow to an area

vector an object that contains pathogens

venipuncture use a hollow needle to puncture a vein to obtain a blood specimen

veracity being truthful and honest

verdict the decision or outcome of a criminal case

viable alive—capable of living

vial a glass or plastic container sealed at the top by a stopper

villi finger-like projections found on the wall of the intestines

virology the study of viruses

virus tiny bits of protein-coated nucleic acid that invade and take over cells in other living organisms

viruses plural form of virus; also a computer related action that invades a computer and destroys files and software, a major security problem

vitiligo blanching of the skin to near whiteness, due to the defective action of the melanocytes

W

wave scheduling appointment scheduling of several patients, or group of a patients, into one time frame allowing patients to arrive at any time within that block of time

wet mount microscopic exam of bacteria freely moving in fluid

Index

Note: Page numbers in *italics* denote figures; page numbers followed by b indicate boxes; those followed by t indicate tables.